Rehabilitation After Traumatic Brain Injury

Rehabilitation After Traumatic Brain Injury

BLESSEN C. EAPEN, MD
Section Chief, Polytrauma Rehabilitation Center
Director, Polytrauma/TBI Rehabilitation
Fellowship Program Site Director
Defense and Veterans Brain Injury Center (DVBIC)
South Texas Veterans Health Care System
San Antonio, TX, United States

Associate Professor
Department of Rehabilitation Medicine
UT Health-San Antonio
San Antonio, TX, United States

DAVID X. CIFU, MD
Herman J. Flax, MD Professor and Chairman
Department of Physical Medicine and Rehabilitation
Virginia Commonwealth University School of Medicine
Richmond, VA, United States

Senior TBI Specialist
U.S. Department of Veteran Affairs

Director, Sports Science
NHL Florida Panthers

Principal Investigator
VA-DoD Chronic Effects of NeuroTrauma Consortium

ELSEVIER

ELSEVIER

3251 Riverport Lane
St. Louis, Missouri 63043

Content Strategist: Kayla Wolfe
Content Development Manager: Taylor Ball
Content Development Specialist: Meredith Madeira
Publishing Services Manager: Deepthi Unni
Project Manager: Janish Ashwin Paul
Designer: Gopalakrishnan Venkatraman

Printed in United States of America

Last digit is the print number: 9 8 7 6 5 4 3 2 1

Working together
to grow libraries in
developing countries

www.elsevier.com • www.bookaid.org

List of Contributors

Elizabeth V. Adamova, DO
Department of Physical Medicine and Rehabilitation
Harvard Medical School
Boston, MA, United States, Spaulding Rehabilitation
    Hospital
Boston, MA, United States

Ruth Alejandro, MD, FAAPMR
Assistant Clinical Professor
Columbia University Dept. of Rehabilitation and
    Regenerative Medicine
New York, NY, United States, Attending Physiatrist
TBI Inpatient Unit & Day Hospital at Blythedale
    Children's Hospital
New York, NY, United States

Michael Armstrong, MD
Department of Physical Medicine and Rehabilitation
Minneapolis Veterans Affairs Health Care System
Minneapolis, MN, United States

Sheital Bavishi, DO
Dodd Hall
Columbus, OH, United States

Heather G. Belanger, PhD
James A. Haley Veterans Hospital
Tampa, FL, United States, Department of Psychiatry
    and Behavioral Neurosciences
University of South Florida Medical School
Tampa, FL, United States, Defense and Veterans Brain
    Injury Center (DVBIC)
Silver Spring, MD, United States

Kathleen R. Bell, MD
Professor and Chair
Physical Medicine and Rehabilitation
University of Texas Southwestern
Dallas, TX, United States

Erin D. Bigler, PhD, ABPP
Departments of Psychology and Neuroscience
Brigham Young University
Provo, UT, United States

Marcia Bockbrader, MD, PhD
Dodd Hall
Columbus, OH, United States

Lisa A. Brenner, PhD, ABPP
Rocky Mountain Mental Illness Research Education
    and Clinical Center (MIRECC)
Denver, CO, United States, Departments of Physical
    Medicine and Rehabilitation, Psychiatry and
    Neurology
University of Colorado Anschutz Medical Campus
    and Marcus Institute for Brain Health
University of Colorado Anschutz Medical Campus
Aurora, CO, United States

David Cancel, MD, JD
Director
Pediatric Rehabilitation Medicine Fellowship
Albert Einstein College of Medicine/Montefiore
    Medical Center
Bronx, NY, United States

Kerri Chung, DO
Department of Physical Medicine and Rehabilitation
Minneapolis Veterans Affairs Health Care System
Minneapolis, MN, United States

David X. Cifu, MD
Associate Dean of Innovation and System
    Integration
Virginia Commonwealth University School of
    Medicine
Richmond, VA, United States

Edan A. Critchfield, PsyD, ABPP-CN
Staff Neuropsychologist
South Texas Veterans Healthcare System
San Antonio, TX, United States

Barbara J. Darkangelo, PT, DPT, NCS
James A. Haley Veterans Hospital
Tampa, FL, United States

Nyaz Didehbani, PhD
Assistant Professor
Department of Psychiatry
University of Texas – Southwestern Medical Center
Dallas, TX, United States

Nathalie Dieujuste, BA
Rocky Mountain Mental Illness Research Education
    and Clinical Center (MIRECC)
Denver, CO, United States

Sangeeta Driver, MD, MPH
Attending Physician
Shirley Ryan Ability Lab
Assistant Professor
Department of Physical Medicine and Rehabilitation
Northwestern University Feinberg School of Medicine
Chicago, IL, United States

Blessen C. Eapen, MD
Section Chief
Polytrauma Rehabilitation Center
Polytrauma/TBI Fellowship Program Director
Site Director
Defense and Veterans Brain Injury Center
South Texas Veterans Health Care System
San Antonio, TX, United States, Associate Professor
Department of Rehabilitation Medicine
UT Health-San Antonio
San Antonio, TX, United States

Andrew J. Gardner, PhD
Hunter New England Local Health District Sports
    Concussion Program
John Hunter Hospital
Callaghan, NSW, Australia, Centre for Stroke and
    Brain Injury
School of Medicine and Public Health
University of Newcastle
Callaghan, NSW, Australia

Bryan Garrison, RKT, CDRS
James A. Haley Veterans Hospital
Tampa, FL, United States

Ekua Gilbert-Baffoe, MD
Clinical Fellow, Department of Physical Medicine
    and Rehabilitation
Baylor College of Medicine
Houston, TX, United States

David H. Glazer, MD
Polytrauma Rehabilitation Center
Hunter Holmes McGuire VA Medical Center
Richmond, VA, United States

Shankar P. Gopinath, MD
Chief of Neurosurgical Service
Ben Taub General Hospital
Houston, TX, United States, Associate Professor
Department of Neurosurgery
Baylor College of Medicine
Houston, TX, United States

Geoffrey Grammer, MD
Defense and Veterans Brain Injury Center
Silver Spring, MD, United States

Brian D. Greenwald, MD
JFK Johnson Rehabilitation Institute
Edison, NJ, United States

Stephen Hampton, MD
Department of Physical Medicine and Rehabilitation
University of Pennsylvania
Philadelphia, PA, United States

Mary Himmler, MD
Department of Physical Medicine and Rehabilitation
Minneapolis Veterans Affairs Health Care System
Minneapolis, MN, United States

Sandra Hong, DO
Clinical Fellow
Polytrauma/Traumatic Brain Injury
South Texas Veterans Health Care System
San Antonio, TX, United States

Faiza Humayun, MD
James A. Haley Veterans Hospital
Department of Physical Medicine and Rehabilitation
Medical Director
Brain Injury Program
Tampa, FL, United States
University of South Florida School of Medicine
Department of Neurology
Tampa, FL, United States

Carlos A. Jaramillo, MD, PhD
Staff Physician/Clinical Investigator
Polytrauma Rehabilitation Center
South Texas Veterans Health Care System
San Antonio, TX, United States
Assistant Professor
Department of Rehabilitation Medicine
UT Health- San Antonio
San Antonio, TX, United States

Neil Jasey, MD
Kessler Institute for Rehabilitation
West Orange, NJ, United States

James M. Kaplan, MEd, CTRS, ATP, CBIS
James A. Haley Veterans Hospital
Tampa, FL, United States

Kathryn Kieffer, MS, CCC-SLP
Speech-Language Pathologist
Polytrauma Rehabilitation Center
James A. Haley Veterans' Hospital
Tampa, FL, United States

Sunil Kothari, MD
Department of Physical Medicine & Rehabilitation
Baylor College of Medicine
Disorders of Consciousness Program
TIRR-Memorial Hermann Hospital
Houston, TX, United States

Tracy Kretzmer, PhD
James A. Haley Veterans Hospital
Tampa, FL, United States

Mithra Maneyapanda, MD
Brain Injury Program
Bryn Mawr Rehab Hospital
Malvern, PA, United States

Michael H. Marino, MD
MossRehab at Elkins Park/Einstein Healthcare
   Network
Elkins Park, PA, United States

Suzanne McGarity, PhD
Rocky Mountain Mental Illness Research Education
   and Clinical Center (MIRECC)
Denver, CO, United States

Diane Mortimer, MD, MSN
Clinical Fellow, Department of Physical Medicine and
   Rehabilitation
Minneapolis Veterans Affairs Health Care System
Minneapolis, MN, United States

Katherine A. O'Brien, PhD
Department of Physical Medicine & Rehabilitation
Baylor College of Medicine
Disorders of Consciousness Program
TIRR-Memorial Hermann Hospital
Houston, TX, United States

Justin J.F. O'Rourke, PhD, ABPP-CN
Staff Neuropsychologist
South Texas Veterans Healthcare System
San Antonio, TX, United States

Linda M. Picon, MCD, CCC-SLP
Department of Veteran Affairs
Veterans Health Administration
Rehabilitation and Prosthetic Services
Washington, DC, United States

Robert Rinaldi, MD
Associate Professor
Dept of Physical Medicine and Rehabilitation
UT Southwestern Medical Center
Dallas, TX, United States

David L. Ripley, MD, MS
Section Chief
Brain Injury Medicine
Shirley Ryan Ability Lab
Associate Professor
Department of Physical Medicine and Rehabilitation
Northwestern University Feinberg School of Medicine
Chicago, IL, United States

William Robbins, MD
Assistant Professor
Department of Physical Medicine and Rehabilitation
Virginia Commonwealth University
Richmond VA, United States
Director
Polytrauma Transitional Rehabilitation Program
Director
Service Member Transitional Advanced Rehabilitation
Richmond VAMC
Richmond, VA, United States

Claudia S. Robertson, MD
Professor
Department of Neurosurgery
Baylor College of Medicine
Houston, TX, United States

Joseph Rosenthal, MD, MPH
Dodd Hall
Columbus, OH, United States

Octavio A. Santos, PhD
Neuropsychology Postdoctoral Fellow
Mayo Clinic
Jacksonville, FL, United States

Joel Scholten, MD
Department of Veteran Affairs
Veterans Health Administration
Rehabilitation and Prosthetic Services
Washington, DC, United States

Billie A. Schultz, MD
Department of Physical Medicine and Rehabilitation
Mayo Clinic
Rochester, MN, United States

Jason R. Soble, PhD, ABPP-CN
Staff Neuropsychologist
South Texas Veterans Healthcare System
San Antonio, TX, United States

Ryan Stork, MD
Medical Director
Brain Injury Rehabilitation Program
Clinical Instructor
Department of PM&R
University of Michigan
Ann Arbor, MI, United States

Bruno Subbarao, DO
Medical Director
Polytrauma & Transitional Care Management Program
Phoenix VA Health Care System
Phoenix, AZ, United States

David F. Tate, PhD
Associate Professor
Research Senior Scientific Director
Missouri Institute of Mental Health
University of Missouri, St. Louis
Berkeley, MO, United States

Brionn Tonkin, MD
Department of Physical Medicine and Rehabilitation
Minneapolis Veterans Affairs Health Care System
Minneapolis, MN, United States

Aditya Vedantam, MD
Neurosurgery Resident
Department of Neurosurgery
Baylor College of Medicine
Houston, TX, United States

Thomas K. Watanabe, MD
MossRehab at Elkins Park/Einstein Healthcare
    Network
Elkins Park, PA, United States

Elisabeth A. Wilde, PhD
Departments of Physical Medicine and Rehabilitation,
    Neurology, and Radiology
Baylor College of Medicine
Houston, TX, United States, Michael E. DeBakey VA
    Medical Center
Houston, TX, United States

Hal S. Wortzel, MD
Rocky Mountain Mental Illness Research Education
    and Clinical Center (MIRECC)
Denver, CO, United States, Departments of Physical
    Medicine and Rehabilitation, Psychiatry and
    Neurology
University of Colorado Anschutz Medical Campus
Aurora, CO, United States

Gerry E. York, MD
Alaska Radiology Associates
TBI Imaging and Research
Anchorage, AK, United States

Ross D. Zafonte, DO
Department of Physical Medicine and Rehabilitation
Harvard Medical School
Spaulding Rehabilitation Hospital
MassGeneral Hospital for Children Sport
    Concussion Program
Red Sox Foundation and Massachusetts General
    Hospital Home Base Program
Brigham and Women's Hospital
Boston, MA, United States

Preface

Traumatic brain injury (TBI) remains the most common cause of significant disability in young adults, a major factor in youth and professional sports, and an area of intense scrutiny and research across the Departments of Defense and Veterans Affairs. As such, TBI continues to garner significant media attention, given the short- and long-term effects of TBI in these sports, military, and veteran populations. As TBI is a major cause of morbidity worldwide and a serious public health concern, better understanding of and caring for TBI must be a priority for the healthcare systems. This first edition of *Rehabilitation after Traumatic Brain Injury* highlights the current state of rehabilitation medicine for the evaluation and treatment of individuals with brain injury.

The illustrious and diverse authors of this book review the acute management of TBI, levels of rehabilitation care, epidemiology, and management of common medical and neurologic complications after brain injury. In addition, the text reviews unique populations of brain-injured patients, including pediatrics, sports, geriatrics, military, and veterans, individuals who have suffered an anoxic injury and the cohort with a disorder of consciousness. There are also chapters on the pharmacologic management of brain injury, posttraumatic pain conditions, and management of neuropsychiatric sequelae after brain injury. Finally, we discuss the use of advanced neuroimaging techniques, neuroprosthetics, cognitive rehabilitation, and community reintegration in this unique population.

As with any work that relies on decades of clinical experience as the framework of knowledge, supplemented by intensive, confirmatory research, we are indebted to the thousands of individuals with brain injury and their family and caregivers, without whom we would know nothing; this edition is dedicated to your sacrifices and to your indomitable spirit of hope. We would also like to thank our colleagues who contributed their time and efforts in making this first edition a huge success. Meredith Madeira and the editorial team at Elsevier have been tireless in their efforts to bring this book to production, and we are so grateful. We hope this book will provide a framework for the students, residents, fellows, and clinical providers to help brain injury survivors on their pathway toward recovery.

Contents

CHAPTER 1

Acute Management of Traumatic Brain Injury

ADITYA VEDANTAM, MD • SHANKAR P. GOPINATH, MD •
CLAUDIA S. ROBERTSON, MD

INTRODUCTION

Traumatic brain injury (TBI) is an important cause of morbidity and mortality, accounting for more than 1.4 million annual cases in the United States and an estimated 10 million cases globally.[1] The adherence to well-researched trauma guidelines as well as an efficient trauma system has contributed to improved outcomes after TBI.[2] Our understanding of the pathophysiology of TBI has also improved over the years, and this has helped refine the acute clinical management of patients with TBI. Advances in critical care have also played a major role in improved outcomes for patients with TBI.

In this chapter, we describe current management protocols for acute TBI, particularly moderate and severe TBI. Although the Brain Trauma Foundation (BTF) has provided updated evidence-based guidelines for the management of TBI, the lack of high-quality evidence for many of the interventions has limited the strength of recommendations. The American College of Surgeons Trauma Quality Improvement Program (ACS TQIP) has published a best practices document for the management of TBI that provides practice recommendations for clinicians taking care of patients with TBI. We have incorporated recommendations from both the BTF and ACS TQIP in this chapter and discuss prehospital care, evaluation, and acute critical care management of patients with TBI.

PREHOSPITAL CARE

Prehospital care in the United States is often initiated by emergency medical service providers, who are trained to provide basic emergency care in the field. The evaluation and treatment of the patient with acute TBI begins with a rapid assessment and interventions for airway, breathing, and circulation. Maintaining an airway in the unconscious patient may require interventions ranging from a laryngeal mask airway to intubation. Supplemental oxygen to avoid hypoxemia (cyanosis, <90% oxygen saturation) is recommended.[3] The avoidance of hypotension (systolic blood pressure <90 mm Hg) is also important,[4] and a peripheral intravenous line or intraosseus line may be required to administer isotonic fluids en route to the trauma center. Recording a Glasgow Coma Scale (GCS) score (Table 1.1) in the field provides an important baseline assessment for these patients and should be repeated at frequent intervals to identify an improvement or deterioration in the neurologic status. Based on the GCS, TBI has been classified as mild (13–15), moderate (9–12), and severe (<9) TBI. It is important to recognize that the initial GCS can change as a result of secondary insults. Patients with an initial moderate TBI can potentially deteriorate rapidly to GCS consistent with a severe TBI. Therefore treatment protocols should not be established based solely on the initial GCS. In addition to the GCS, the size and reaction of pupils to light should be recorded after resuscitation. All patients should be rapidly evaluated for active blood loss from open injuries and signs of polytrauma. The patient should be rapidly transferred to a trauma center with available computed tomography (CT) imaging and neurosurgical care. Cervical immobilization should be performed with a hard cervical collar during transport. Continuous monitoring of blood pressure and pulse oximetry should be instituted during transport with additional intravenous fluid resuscitation using bolus doses of isotonic fluids if necessary. An organized trauma care system and the development of protocols for prehospital providers can streamline and reduce delays in prehospital care. The importance of avoiding early hypoxemia and hypotension in the prehospital setting for patients with acute TBI cannot be overemphasized.

TABLE 1.1
Glasgow Coma Scale—Calculated by Adding up the Scores for Eye Opening, Verbal Response, and Motor Response

Components	Score
EYE OPENING (E)	
Spontaneous	4
To voice	3
To pain	2
No eye opening	1
VERBAL RESPONSE (V)	
Oriented	5
Confused	4
Inappropriate words	3
Incomprehensible sounds	2
No verbal response	1
MOTOR RESPONSE (M)	
Obeys commands	6
Localizes stimulus	5
Withdraws from stimulus	4
Abnormal flexion	3
Abnormal extension	2
No motor response	1

The minimum score is 3, and the maximum score is 15.

EVALUATION OF THE PATIENT WITH ACUTE TRAUMATIC BRAIN INJURY

Once the patient is brought to the emergency room at the trauma center, a rapid clinical evaluation by the trauma team is essential. Clinical history on the mechanism of injury, GCS, and pupil examination in the field, as well as interventions performed by the emergency service providers, should be clearly stated on arrival for all trauma team members. Securing the airway is an important first step, and this may involve endotracheal intubation (if GCS <9) or conversion of a laryngeal mask airway to endotracheal tube. A formal primary and secondary survey by the trauma team should be performed, and the patient should be log-rolled to perform a thorough examination. If the patient is intubated, the position of the endotracheal tube should be confirmed with a chest X-ray, and any resuscitation for hypotension should be initiated with a blood transfusion empirically. If there is evidence of hemorrhagic shock due to an open

injury, attempts to temporarily control the bleeding should be initiated in coordination with a massive transfusion protocol. The hemodynamically stable patient should be soon transferred to the CT scanner, and a noncontrast CT imaging of the head and neck should be performed. Additional CT imaging of the chest, abdomen, and pelvis should be performed in patients with polytrauma and patients with unexplained hypotension. It is important to note that blood loss from a closed head injury cannot produce hemorrhagic shock, and investigations should be directed at other sources of traumatic bleeding (abdomen, pelvis, chest injuries, or long bone fractures) to explain the hypotension.

If the initial CT imaging shows a mass lesion with impending or gross cerebral herniation (Fig. 1.1), emergent decompressive surgery is required, and the patient needs to be transferred to the operating room immediately. If no emergent neurosurgical intervention is anticipated, the patient is transported to the critical care unit.

EMERGENT SURGERY IN TRAUMATIC BRAIN INJURY

In patients with a large unilateral mass lesion (subdural/epidural hematoma or contusion [Figs. 1.1 and 1.2]) with midline shift, effacement of basal cisterns, and impending or obvious transtentorial herniation, emergent surgical intervention is recommended. It is important to ensure that patients undergoing emergent surgical intervention are hemodynamically stable or being actively resuscitated before entering the operating room. Guidelines for surgical neurotrauma care recommend evacuation of a subdural hematoma >10 mm in size or with mildline shift >5 mm,[5] or an epidural hematoma >30 cc.[6] However, surgical decisions are made based on the clinical status of the individual patient, and relying solely on imaging findings is not advised. For unilateral subdural or epidural hematomas, decompressive surgery involves a craniotomy with evacuation of the hematoma. For patients with subdural hematomas and significant cerebral edema, a lax duraplasty is required to avoid the constricting effect of the dura on underlying brain. If the brain is too edematous at surgery, a decision is made in the operating room to not replace the bone flap. The bone flap is placed in a freezer, with the plan for a cranioplasty at a later time point. Other indications for early surgery in TBI include an open depressed skull fracture and a large contusion with associated clinical deterioration.

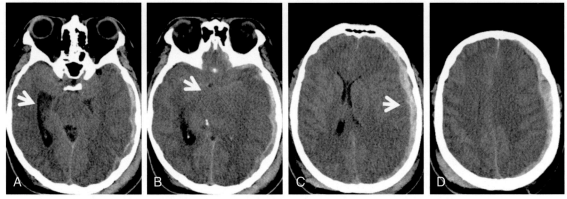

FIG. 1.1 Select axial CT head images from the base of skull to vertex showing a traumatic acute left hemispheric subdural hematoma. **(A)** Effacement of ipsilateral temporal horn and dilated contralateral temporal horn (*arrow*); **(B)** effacement of basal cisterns (*arrow*) due to midline shift and cerebral edema; **(C)** midline shift toward the right created by a left hemispheric acute subdural hematoma (*arrow*); **(D)** cerebral edema and effacement of cerebral sulci at the vertex. *CT*, computed tomography.

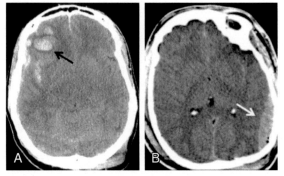

FIG. 1.2 **(A)** Axial head CT showing traumatic right frontal contusion (*arrow*); **(B)** axial head CT showing left parietal epidural hematoma (*arrow*). *CT*, computed tomography.

CRITICAL CARE MANAGEMENT
Blood Pressure Management
Critical care management is important for the maintenance of circulation, ventilation, and homeostasis in the patient with TBI, as well as for frequent monitoring of the neurologic examination. In all patients with TBI, avoiding hypotension is important to avoid secondary brain injury due to associated cerebral hypoperfusion. The current BTF guidelines recommend maintaining a systolic blood pressure ≥100 mm Hg for patients 50–69 years old. For patients 15–49 years old and those older than 70 years, the threshold is ≥110 mm Hg.[7] Isotonic fluids, as well as blood transfusions and vasopressors, if required, are necessary to maintain blood pressure thresholds. The maintenance of appropriate blood pressure is also determined by the target cerebral perfusion pressure

(CPP), which is dealt in the following sections. In patients with intracranial pressure (ICP) monitoring, an arterial catheter (preferably radial artery) is recommended to provide accurate mean arterial pressure (MAP) measurements. In addition, bedside assessment of inferior vena cava (IVC) diameter and collapsibility using ultrasound provides a measure of volume status and can guide fluid resuscitation in critically ill patients with TBI.[8]

Intubation and Ventilation
Intubation and mechanical ventilation in severe TBI is necessary for airway protection, to maintain adequate tissue oxygenation and avoid hypercarbia. In mechanically ventilated patients, a normal partial pressure of carbon dioxide ($PaCO_2$) of 35–45 mm Hg should be targeted by titrating tidal volume and respiratory rate. Prolonged hyperventilation to a $PaCO_2$ of 25 mm Hg or more is not recommended because this can exacerbate cerebral ischemia by reducing cerebral blood flow.[9] Transient hyperventilation is recommended only as a temporizing measure to reduce ICP in patients with impending cerebral herniation who are being transported to the operating room. In some patients, mild hyperventilation to $PaCO_2$ 30–35 mm Hg may be maintained as a second-tier treatment for ICP management; however, the effect is often transient and there is a risk of rebound intracranial hypertension if the hyperventilation is withdrawn rapidly.

Sedation and Analgesia
Critical care management of patients with TBI requires a careful approach to sedation and analgesia. In an

TABLE 1.2
Goals of Treatment for Patients with TBI

Pulse oximetry ≥ 95%	ICP 20–25 mm Hg	Serum sodium 135–145 Meq/L
PaO_2 ≥ 100 mm Hg	$PbtO_2$ ≥ 15 mm Hg	INR ≤ 1.4
$PaCO_2$ 35–45 mm Hg	CPP ≥ 60 mm Hg	Platelets ≥ 75,000/mm³
SBP ≥ 100 mm Hg	Temperature 36.0–38°C	Hemoglobin ≥ 7 g/dL
pH 7.35–7.45	Glucose 80–180 mg/dL	

CPP, cerebral perfusion pressure; ICP, intracranial pressure; INR, international normalized ratio; $PaCO_2$, partial pressure of carbon dioxide; PaO_2, partial pressure of oxygen; $PbtO_2$, local brain tissue oxygen; SBP, systolic blood pressure; TBI, traumatic brain injury.
From ACS TQIP. *Best Practices in the Management of Traumatic Brain Injury*; 2015. https://www.facs.org/~/media/files/quality programs/trauma/tqip/traumatic brain injury guidelines.ashx; with permission.

unintubated patient with mild to moderate TBI, the use of narcotics and sedatives is avoided owing to the risk of obscuring the neurologic examination. Intubated patients require adequate sedation and analgesia to treat patient agitation, pain, and increases in ICP. Low-dose opioid infusions using morphine or fentanyl can be used initially for analgesia. Short-acting sedative infusions, such as propofol or midazolam, are options in intubated patients. The need for sedative infusions should be reevaluated often and the levels, ideally, titrated to maintain an RASS (Richmond Agitation Sedations Scale) score of −2. Sedatives and analgesics should be withheld at least once a day to perform a reliable neurologic examination. In patients with persistent elevated ICP, neuromuscular blockade, using cisatracurium, may be considered, and this should always be given in combination with a sedative infusion.

Intracranial Pressure Monitoring

Monitoring ICP in patients with severe TBI is vital to detect intracranial hypertension crises, which contribute to poorer outcomes. ICP monitoring guides clinicians in the intensive care unit (ICU) and offers the opportunity for timely interventions to alleviate ICP crises and reduce secondary injury. The consensus remains that ICP monitoring is a valuable tool despite data from the BEST TRIP (Benchmark Evidence from South American Trials: Treatment of Intracranial Pressure) trial showing that patients with severe TBI can be managed without ICP monitoring in a resource-constrained setting, using only clinicoradiologic evaluations.[10] ICP monitoring is indicated for patients with severe TBI and abnormal CT imaging of the head on admission. In patients with severe TBI with a normal CT imaging of the head on admission, ICP monitoring is indicated if two or more of the following factors are present: age >40 years,

unilateral or bilateral motor posturing, and one or more episodes of systolic blood pressure <90 mm Hg.[11] ICP monitoring should also be considered in obtunded patients with moderate TBI, in whom serial neurologic examinations cannot be obtained owing to nonneurosurgical procedures or injuries.

ICP monitoring is commonly performed using an external ventricular drain, intraparenchymal ICP catheter, or a combination catheter. These devices are connected to a pressure transducer, zeroed at the level of the tragus, and provide real-time monitoring of ICP. External ventricular drains are preferred, as they offer the opportunity to drain cerebrospinal fluid (CSF) to reduce ICP, as well as provide a more global estimate of the ICP as compared with intraparenchymal devices. The normal ICP is 10–15 mm Hg, and treatment is often initiated for sustained increases in the ICP >20 mm Hg. The ACS TQIP provides practical parameters and thresholds for the acute management of TBI (Table 1.2). Our protocol involves intermittent CSF drainage for sustained ICP more than 20 mmHg and is guided by the clinical examination as well as CPP/brain oxygenation data. Current BTF guidelines recommend continuous CSF drainage over intermittent use and an ICP threshold of 22 mm Hg based on a recent retrospective study[12]; however, these data need to be validated in prospective studies. If continuous CSF drainage is used, an additional intraparenchymal monitor will be required to continuously monitor ICP while CSF is being drained.

Cerebral Perfusion Pressure Monitoring

CPP is calculated as MAP − ICP and represents the principle determinant of cerebral blood flow. In the uninjured brain, cerebral autoregulation maintains an adequate and steady CPP over a range of MAPs;

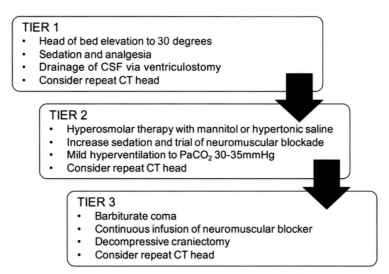

TIER 1
- Head of bed elevation to 30 degrees
- Sedation and analgesia
- Drainage of CSF via ventriculostomy
- Consider repeat CT head

TIER 2
- Hyperosmolar therapy with mannitol or hypertonic saline
- Increase sedation and trial of neuromuscular blockade
- Mild hyperventilation to $PaCO_2$ 30-35mmHg
- Consider repeat CT head

TIER 3
- Barbiturate coma
- Continuous infusion of neuromuscular blocker
- Decompressive craniectomy
- Consider repeat CT head

FIG. 1.3 Three-tiered management of intracranial hypertension after TBI. *CSF*, cerebrospinal fluid; *CT*, computed tomography; *TBI*, traumatic brain injury.

however, this process is often impaired in patients with TBI. In patients with impaired autoregulation, close monitoring of CPP is essential to avoid dramatic changes in the CPP due to changes in systemic blood pressure. The recommended goal of CPP per the BTF guidelines is 50–70 mm Hg. Targeting high CPP ≥70 mm Hg has not been shown to be beneficial in patients with TBI and is associated with an increased risk of acute respiratory distress syndrome (ARDS).[13] The maintenance of a stable blood pressure is critical to CPP management, and central venous pressure monitoring with a subclavian central venous catheter can guide fluid management. Fluid resuscitation and use of vasopressors (norepinephrine, phenylephrine, or dopamine), if necessary, may be required to maintain an adequate CPP.

Brain Oxygenation Monitoring

Monitoring brain oxygenation allows clinicians to detect ongoing cerebral ischemia and institute appropriate interventions to ameliorate this. Global cerebral oxygenation can be measured using jugular venous saturation oxygen ($SJVO_2$), which is measured by a monitor in the internal jugular vein. Local brain tissue oxygen ($PbtO_2$) is measured using a small intraparenchymal monitor that is often inserted adjacent to the entry site for a ventriculostomy. The $PbtO_2$ is a measure of the oxygenation in the brain tissue adjacent to the tip of the monitor. Both devices provide continuous measurement of oxygenation, and the indications are the same as that for ICP monitoring.

The recommended treatment goals are $SJVO_2$ ≥50% and $PbtO_2$ ≥15 mm Hg. Reduced cerebral oxygenation is often related to increases in ICP and reductions in CPP and resolves with optimization of one or both of these parameters. If no specific cause is found, increasing the FiO_2 may be required to produce hyperoxia and improve oxygenation.

Intracranial Pressure Management

Multiple local and systemic factors affect the ICP, and a systematic approach to the evaluation and treatment of increased ICP is needed in patients with TBI with ICP monitoring. The ICP may be elevated as a result of increased cerebral edema, expanding contusion, altered CSF dynamics, cerebral venous obstruction, patient agitation, fever, and increased $PaCO_2$. The ACS TQIP Best Practices[14] proposes a three-tier approach to ICP management, which is a useful guide in the ICU (Fig. 1.3). In clinical practice, these tiers may overlap and ICP management is often individualized based on the patient's clinical examination, imaging findings, and trend in cerebral hemodynamics.

Tier 1

The first step in the evaluation of a patient with persistent elevated ICP >20 mm Hg requires confirmation that the pressure transducer is zeroed at the level of the tragus and a good ICP waveform is observed on the monitor. A head of bed elevation at 30 degrees is recommended to improve cerebral venous outflow.[15] Constricting cervical collars or tight neck ties to secure the endotracheal tube should be loosened, if needed, to avoid compression of neck veins. If the patient is agitated, a bolus of sedative or analgesia may be necessary. Ventricular drainage of CSF can be performed by opening the ventriculostomy to drain 2–3 cc till the ICP falls below 20 mm Hg. A clinical neurologic examination for GCS and pupil reactivity to light should always be performed to confirm no change from baseline. If there is a concern for an expanding contusion or hematoma based on prior imaging, repeat CT head imaging may be needed to evaluate a sudden persistent elevation in ICP. If the ICP remains >20 mm Hg despite these interventions, tier 2 treatment options can be instituted.

Tier 2

Hyperosmolar therapy should be considered as a second-tier approach to increased ICP. Mannitol should be administered as intermittent boluses (0.25–1 mg/kg) intravenously. Patients who receive mannitol should have frequent monitoring (every 6 h) of serum sodium and osmolality, and additional doses should be avoided if osmolality is >320 mOsm/L or the patient is hypovolemic. Alternatively, intermittent boluses of hypertonic saline (3% or 23.4%) can be given to reduce the ICP, with monitoring of serum sodium and avoiding sodium >160 mEq/L. An increase of sedation in agitated patients and use of neuromuscular blockade can also be tried. In some patients, a continuous infusion of cisatracurium may be required, which is often considered a tier 3 treatment. Mild hyperventilation to PaCO2 of 30–35 mm Hg can also be tried if patients do not show low brain tissue oxygenation. Once again, repeat CT head imaging should be considered at this stage. Tier 3 treatments may be required if the ICP remains >20 mm Hg after these interventions.

Tier 3

Therapeutic interventions at this stage require a nuanced approach, taking into account the clinical examination, imaging findings, associated injuries, and overall clinical status of the patient. The major options include decompressive craniectomy or barbiturate coma.

Decompressive craniectomy for the management of refractory intracranial hypertension has been shown to reliably reduce ICP. The Decompressive Craniectomy in Diffuse Traumatic Brain Injury (DECRA) trial showed that early decompressive craniectomy for patients with TBI did reduce ICP but did not contribute to improved clinical outcomes.[16] The RescueICP trial found that patients undergoing decompressive craniectomy as part of a tier 3 approach failed to show a significantly greater probability of a favorable outcome.[17] Outcomes after decompressive craniectomy are possibly related to timing of surgery and patient selection. Decompressive craniectomy is performed as a unilateral frontotemporoparietal craniectomy with expansile duraplasty in patients with a large unilateral lesion (contusion or hematoma) and midline shift to the contralateral side. An ideal bone flap for a unilateral craniectomy is at least 12 cm in the longest diameter with adequate subtemporal decompression. In patients without a large unilateral lesion, a bifrontal decompressive craniectomy can be performed. Continued multimodal monitoring after decompressive craniectomy using a ventriculostomy and PbtO$_2$ is recommended to detect the expansion of ipsilateral or contralateral lesions after surgery.

Barbiturate coma, using pentobarbital or thiopentone, is an alternative to decompressive craniectomy. Propofol may also be used to induce a coma to control intractable intracranial hypertension. Barbiturates reduce cerebral metabolism and can acutely reduce ICP in select patients.[18] Both propofol and barbiturates produce hypotension, and so they are relatively contraindicated in hypotensive patients. Patients should be euvolemic before the barbiturate infusion is started and may require vasopressors during treatment. Continuous electroencephalography (EEG), although not required, is useful to document burst suppression. Barbiturate therapy is associated with an increased risk of ARDS, infections, and coagulopathy. Daily serum levels of pentobarbital, if used, should be obtained. ICP control with barbiturate therapy is the single most important predictor of survival in patients undergoing barbiturate therapy for intractable intracranial hypertension. Therefore, for patients who do not respond to barbiturate therapy, decompressive craniectomy should be considered early.

Seizures/EEG

Posttraumatic seizures can be early (within 7 days of injury) or late (after 7 days). Patients with recurrent seizures more than 7 days following the injury are deemed to have posttraumatic epilepsy. Early clinical seizures may be seen in 2.1%–16.9% of patients with TBI[19]; however, not all seizures are clinically evident. Subclinical seizures may be noted in more than 30% of patients with TBI and are detected only on continuous EEG monitoring.[20] Randomized clinical trials have shown that prophylactic anticonvulsants are useful in preventing early posttraumatic seizures but not late posttraumatic seizures.[21] For patients with abnormal CT imaging after trauma, a loading dose of anticonvulsants (phenytoin or levetiracetam) is administered, followed by a 7-day course of anticonvulsants. If patients have early posttraumatic seizures while on anticonvulsants, these may be continued beyond 7 days and stopped after discharge based on the physician's discretion. Continuous EEG monitoring for 48–72 h is recommended in patients with neurologic deterioration not explained by CT imaging or other systemic cause.

Nutrition

Enteral nutrition should be started as early as possible after TBI, preferably within 24 h of the injury. If there are no contraindications to enteral feeding due to abdominal injuries, patients should have a nasogastric or orogastric feeding tube placed and receive feeds that provide energy for 140% of the resting metabolism. Early enteral nutrition has been shown to improve survival in patients with severe TBI.[22] Total parenteral nutrition should be considered for those patients who cannot receive enteral feeds. All patients should be started on a proton-pump inhibitor on admission to the ICU. Intravenous fluids mixed in 0.9% saline should be given in the ICU. Dextrose-containing fluids are often avoided in the acute treatment of patients with moderate and severe TBI owing to the risk of exacerbating cerebral edema. Hyponatremia (serum sodium <135 mEq/L) should be avoided, and if hyponatremia develops, 3% saline may be considered early.

Both hyperglycemia and hypoglycemia can impair neurologic recovery after TBI. High blood glucose levels can contribute to lactic acidosis in the injured brain and worsen cerebral hemodynamics. An insulin sliding scale should be instituted to maintain blood glucose between 80 and 180 mg/dL. It is preferred to avoid episodes of hypoglycemia, which can exacerbate secondary brain injury, and therefore very tight glucose control should not be attempted.[23]

Transfusions

Blood loss anemia and coagulopathy may be seen in patients with polytrauma with TBI. Decisions on transfusion of packed red cells should be made based on hemodynamic stability and brain oxygenation. Recent data have shown that maintaining a hemoglobin of at least 7 g/dL is adequate and targeting a higher hemoglobin value may lead to progressive hemorrhagic injury in the brain,[24] as well as a higher incidence of systemic complications. For coagulopathic patients, the target international normalized ratio is 1.4 and

platelet count is 75,000/μL. Serial blood counts and coagulopathic studies should be performed to guide treatment.

Deep Vein Thrombosis

Deep vein thrombosis (DVT) is an important issue in TBI. Many patients with TBI have hemorrhagic lesions (hematomas or contusions) in the brain, and so early pharmacologic prophylaxis carries the risk of progressive hemorrhagic injury. Up to 20%–25% of patients with TBI may develop DVT without any prophylaxis,[25,26] whereas up to 7% of patients with TBI who receive pharmacologic prophylaxis may develop DVT.[27] Subcutaneous low-molecular-weight heparin is recommended for pharmacologic prophylaxis. The use of intermittent pneumatic compression devices and/or graduated compression stockings should be started in all patients with TBI. The timing of pharmacologic DVT prophylaxis needs to be determined on an individual patient basis. The Berne-Norwood risk stratification (Table 1.3) provides guidance on the risk of progressive hemorrhagic injury and appropriate prophylaxis. If pharmacologic DVT prophylaxis is not possible for at least 72 h, a retrievable IVC filter should be considered. One study evaluated the use of a combined IVC-femoral central venous catheter that can be placed at the bedside for patients with TBI.[28] The use of similar retrievable dual-purpose venous catheters that can be placed at the bedside is ideal for patients with TBI. Once patients are safe to begin pharmacologic prophylaxis, the IVC filter may be removed. DVTs should be suspected clinically in febrile patients or in those with lower or upper extremity swelling. The diagnosis is made with Doppler ultrasound studies of the extremities. Patients who develop an upper or lower limb DVT need a maximum tolerated level of anticoagulation, which in some cases may be less than full anticoagulation because of intracranial hemorrhage. Patients with a diagnosis of DVT should also undergo placement of a long-term IVC or superior vena cava filter.

Temperature Management

Maintaining normal body temperature is an important component of the critical care management of patients with TBI. Hyperthermia worsens brain injury and can directly contribute to secondary brain injury as well as increased ICP. Fever after TBI should be aggressively investigated and treated. Infections are common after moderate to severe TBI, particularly, respiratory tract infections. Many patients do not have a strong gag reflex after the injury and may have aspirated stomach

TABLE 1.3		
Modified Berne-Norwood Criteria		
Low Risk	**Moderate Risk**	**High Risk**
• No moderate- or high-risk criteria for DVT	• Small subdural or epidural hematoma • Small contusion or intraventricular hemorrhage • Multiple contusions per lobe • Subarachnoid hemorrhage with abnormal CT angiogram • Evidence of progression at 24 h after injury	• ICP monitor placement • Craniotomy • Evidence of progression of hemorrhage on CT head at 72 h after injury
Initiate pharmacologic prophylaxis if CT is stable at 24 h after injury	Initiate pharmacologic prophylaxis if CT is stable at 72 h after injury	Consider placement of retrievable IVC filter

CT, computed tomography; *DVT*, Deep vein thrombosis; *ICP*, intracranial pressure; *IVC*, inferior vena cava.
From the ACS TQIP. *Best Practices in the Management of Traumatic Brain Injury*; 2015. https://www.facs.org/~/media/files/quality programs/trauma/tqip/traumatic brain injury guidelines.ashx; with permission.

contents at the time of injury. Microaspirations in the ICU are also common because of gastroparesis, emesis, gastroesophageal reflux, and frequent turning. Febrile patients with TBI should have blood, urine, and sputum cultures as early as possible and be started on empiric intravenous antibiotics till the antibiotic sensitivity results are available. Maintaining a body temperature of 36–38°C is ideal, and acetaminophen should be used as the first line of treatment. Persistent hyperthermia may require cooling blankets and, if necessary, intravascular cooling catheters. The use of induced hypothermia as a neuroprotective strategy in TBI has been evaluated in large clinical trials and has not shown statistically significant benefit.[29,30] In addition, systemic side effects of hypothermia, such as coagulopathy, infection, and cardiac arrhythmias, can complicate the management of these patients. Induced hypothermia, therefore, is not recommended for patients with TBI.

Tracheostomy
Patients with severe TBI, who cannot be extubated early, should be considered for tracheostomy. The timing of tracheostomy is often determined on the clinical status of the individual patient, based on the likelihood that a patient will need long-term airway protection. Prior studies have shown that early tracheostomy does not improve outcome but can reduce the time spent on the ventilator.[31] Day 10–14 after the injury is a practical time point to perform a tracheostomy in most patients. At this time point, patients are seldom being actively treated for intracranial hypertension and an accurate assessment of the need for long-term airway protection is possible. In some patients with severe TBI

(initial GCS 3–5), who have poor recovery in the first few days after the injury, an early tracheostomy may be considered.

OTHER NEUROSURGICAL PROCEDURES
In addition to primary and secondary decompressive surgery for patients with TBI, other surgical procedures may be required based on the type of injury. Patients with craniofacial trauma may have active CSF rhinorrhea or otorrhea after the injury. The use of prophylactic antibiotics for these conditions has not been shown to reduce the risk of meningitis.[32] Up to 85% of cases with posttraumatic CSF rhinorrhea resolve spontaneously by day 7,[33] and early surgical repair may be considered for patients with persistent CSF leaks after 7 days. In some cases of persistent, profuse CSF otorrhea, a lumbar subarachnoid drain may be required for a few days (3–5 days) till CSF otorrhea resolves. CSF otorrhea, however, has a greater likelihood of spontaneous resolution than CSF rhinorrhea.

Up to a third of patients[34,35] undergoing decompressive craniectomy may show imaging features of hydrocephalus at 3–4 weeks after surgery.[36] Hydrocephalus may be due to arachnoid adhesions, impaired venous drainage via the cortical veins, and loss of pulsatile intracranial dynamics due to the direct effect of atmospheric pressure on the brain.[37,38] After decompressive craniectomy, patients with worsened neurologic examination, increasing size of the pseudomeningocele, or dramatic plateauing in their clinical improvement should undergo CT imaging to evaluate for

---

BOX 1.1
Measures to Prevent Common ICU Complications in Patients With Traumatic Brain Injury

- Aspiration
  - Head of bed elevation
  - Chlorhexidine mouth wash
  - Avoid high residuals in patients receiving nasogastric feeds
  - Swallow evaluation before starting oral diet
- Pneumonia
  - Reduce duration of ventilation
  - Chest physiotherapy
  - Early tracheostomy
- Hypermetabolism
  - Early nutrition within 24 h of injury
- Glycemic control
  - Avoid hypoglycemia and hyperglycemia, appropriate insulin sliding scale
- Hyperthermia
  - Antipyretics, cooling blankets, intravenous cooling catheters

- Deep vein thrombosis
  - Retrievable IVC filter if not a candidate for pharmacologic prophylaxis
  - Sequential compression devices, stockings
  - Passive limb exercises
- Pressure ulcers
  - Scheduled turning/change in position in bed
  - Padding of pressure zones
- Constipation
  - Bowel regimen—suppositories, oral laxatives
- Stress-induced gastric ulcers
  - Proton pump inhibitors
- Others
  - Central line and arterial line care
  - Wound care for lacerations, abrasions
  - Eye care—lubricating ointment, artificial tears

ICU, intensive care unit; *IVC*, inferior vena cava.

---

hydrocephalus. The presence of subdural CSF hygromas on CT imaging is often predictive of hydrocephalus[39] as well as the need for shunting in patients with posttraumatic hydrocephalus.[40]

PROGNOSIS

Multiple prior studies have incorporated admission clinical and imaging data to establish prognostic models in acute TBI.[41] These prognostic models have important applications in helping physicians explain prognosis to patient families as well as for research applications. These prognostic models are useful to guide therapy and goals of care, although the statistical accuracy of prognosis for the individual patient is limited. Therefore there is considerable scope for clinician judgment and experience in determining the best treatment plan for each patient with TBI.

CONCLUSION

The acute management of TBI requires a interdisciplinary team capable of taking care of the cranial injury, as well as concomitant injuries and comorbidities (Box 1.1). Early recovery from TBI is a multifactorial process affected by both local and systemic processes. Guidelines written by the BTF and ACS

help provide a framework for acute TBI management; however, clinical judgment is necessary to further shape the care for the individual patient with TBI.

REFERENCES

1. Hyder AA, Wunderlich CA, Puvanachandra P, Gururaj G, Kobusingye OC. The impact of traumatic brain injuries: a global perspective. *NeuroRehabilitation.* 2007;22(5):341–353.
2. Gerber LM, Chiu YL, Carney N, Hartl R, Ghajar J. Marked reduction in mortality in patients with severe traumatic brain injury. *J Neurosurg.* 2013;119(6):1583–1590.
3. Badjatia N, Carney N, Crocco TJ, et al. Guidelines for prehospital management of traumatic brain injury 2nd edition. *Prehosp Emerg Care.* 2008;12(suppl 1):S1–S52.
4. Chesnut RM, Marshall LF, Klauber MR, et al. The role of secondary brain injury in determining outcome from severe head injury. *J Trauma.* 1993;34(2):216–222.
5. Bullock MR, Chesnut R, Ghajar J, et al. Surgical management of acute subdural hematomas. *Neurosurgery.* 2006;58(3 suppl):S16–S24. Discussion Si–Siv.
6. Bullock MR, Chesnut R, Ghajar J, et al. Surgical management of acute epidural hematomas. *Neurosurgery.* 2006;58(3 suppl):S7–S15. Discussion Si–Siv.
7. Carney N, Totten AM, O'Reilly C, et al. Guidelines for the management of severe traumatic brain injury, fourth edition. *Neurosurgery.* 2017;80(1):6–15.

8. Seif D, Perera P, Mailhot T, Riley D, Mandavia D. Bedside ultrasound in resuscitation and the rapid ultrasound in shock protocol. *Crit Care Res Pract.* 2012;2012:503254.

9. Yundt KD, Diringer MN. The use of hyperventilation and its impact on cerebral ischemia in the treatment of traumatic brain injury. *Crit Care Clin.* 1997;13(1):163–184.

10. Chesnut RM, Temkin N, Carney N, et al. A trial of intracranial-pressure monitoring in traumatic brain injury. *N Engl J Med.* 2012;367(26):2471–2481.

11. Narayan RK, Kishore PR, Becker DP, et al. Intracranial pressure: to monitor or not to monitor? A review of our experience with severe head injury. *J Neurosurg.* 1982;56(5):650–659.

12. Nwachuku EL, Puccio AM, Fetzick A, et al. Intermittent versus continuous cerebrospinal fluid drainage management in adult severe traumatic brain injury: assessment of intracranial pressure burden. *Neurocrit Care.* 2014;20(1):49–53.

13. Contant CF, Valadka AB, Gopinath SP, Hannay HJ, Robertson CS. Adult respiratory distress syndrome: a complication of induced hypertension after severe head injury. *J Neurosurg.* 2001;95(4):560–568.

14. ACS TQIP. *Best Practices in the Management of Traumatic Brain Injury*; 2015. https://www.facs.org/~/media/files/quality programs/trauma/tqip/traumatic brain injury guidelines.ashx.

15. Feldman Z, Kanter MJ, Robertson CS, et al. Effect of head elevation on intracranial pressure, cerebral perfusion pressure, and cerebral blood flow in head-injured patients. *J Neurosurg.* 1992;76(2):207–211.

16. Cooper DJ, Rosenfeld JV, Murray L, et al. Decompressive craniectomy in diffuse traumatic brain injury. *N Engl J Med.* 2011;364(16):1493–1502.

17. Hutchinson PJ, Kolias AG, Timofeev IS, et al. Trial of decompressive craniectomy for traumatic intracranial hypertension. *N Engl J Med.* 2016;375(12):1119–1130.

18. Cormio M, Gopinath SP, Valadka A, Robertson CS. Cerebral hemodynamic effects of pentobarbital coma in head-injured patients. *J Neurotrauma.* 1999;16(10):927–936.

19. Frey LC. Epidemiology of posttraumatic epilepsy: a critical review. *Epilepsia.* 2003;44(suppl 10):11–17.

20. Ronne-Engstrom E, Winkler T. Continuous EEG monitoring in patients with traumatic brain injury reveals a high incidence of epileptiform activity. *Acta Neurol Scand.* 2006;114(1):47–53.

21. Temkin NR, Dikmen SS, Wilensky AJ, Keihm J, Chabal S, Winn HR. A randomized, double-blind study of phenytoin for the prevention of post-traumatic seizures. *N Engl J Med.* 1990;323(8):497–502.

22. Chiang YH, Chao DP, Chu SF, et al. Early enteral nutrition and clinical outcomes of severe traumatic brain injury patients in acute stage: a multi-center cohort study. *J Neurotrauma.* 2012;29(1):75–80.

23. Oddo M, Schmidt JM, Mayer SA, Chiolero RL. Glucose control after severe brain injury. *Curr Opin Clin Nutr Metab Care.* 2008;11(2):134–139.

24. Vedantam A, Yamal JM, Rubin ML, Robertson CS, Gopinath SP. Progressive hemorrhagic injury after severe traumatic brain injury: effect of hemoglobin transfusion thresholds. *J Neurosurg.* 2016;125(5):1229–1234.

25. Kaufman HH, Satterwhite T, McConnell BJ, et al. Deep vein thrombosis and pulmonary embolism in head injured patients. *Angiology.* 1983;34(10):627–638.

26. Denson K, Morgan D, Cunningham R, et al. Incidence of venous thromboembolism in patients with traumatic brain injury. *Am J Surg.* 2007;193(3):380–383. Discussion 383–384.

27. Dudley RR, Aziz I, Bonnici A, et al. Early venous thromboembolic event prophylaxis in traumatic brain injury with low-molecular-weight heparin: risks and benefits. *J Neurotrauma.* 2010;27(12):2165–2172.

28. Tapson VF, Hazelton JP, Myers J, et al. A clinical trial of a device combining an inferior vena cava filter and a central venous catheter for preventing pulmonary embolism among critically ill trauma patients. *J Vasc Interv Radiol.* 2017;28(9):1248–1254.

29. Clifton GL, Miller ER, Choi SC, et al. Lack of effect of induction of hypothermia after acute brain injury. *N Engl J Med.* 2001;344(8):556–563.

30. Andrews PJ, Sinclair HL, Rodriguez A, et al. Hypothermia for intracranial hypertension after traumatic brain injury. *N Engl J Med.* 2015;373(25):2403–2412.

31. Bouderka MA, Fakhir B, Bouaggad A, Hmamouchi B, Hamoudi D, Harti A. Early tracheostomy versus prolonged endotracheal intubation in severe head injury. *J Trauma.* 2004;57(2):251–254.

32. Ratilal BO, Costa J, Pappamikail L, Sampaio C. Antibiotic prophylaxis for preventing meningitis in patients with basilar skull fractures. *Cochrane Database Syst Rev.* 2015;(4):CD004884.

33. Bell RB, Dierks EJ, Homer L, Potter BE. Management of cerebrospinal fluid leak associated with craniomaxillofacial trauma. *J Oral Maxillofac Surg.* 2004;62(6):676–684.

34. Choi I, Park HK, Chang JC, Cho SJ, Choi SK, Byun BJ. Clinical factors for the development of posttraumatic hydrocephalus after decompressive craniectomy. *J Korean Neurosurg Soc.* 2008;43(5):227–231.

35. Honeybul S, Ho KM. Incidence and risk factors for post-traumatic hydrocephalus following decompressive craniectomy for intractable intracranial hypertension and evacuation of mass lesions. *J Neurotrauma.* 2012;29(10):1872–1878.

36. Stiver SI. Complications of decompressive craniectomy for traumatic brain injury. *Neurosurg Focus.* 2009;26(6):E7.

37. Waziri A, Fusco D, Mayer SA, McKhann 2nd GM, Connolly Jr ES. Postoperative hydrocephalus in patients undergoing decompressive hemicraniectomy for ischemic or hemorrhagic stroke. *Neurosurgery.* 2007;61(3):489–493. Discussion 493–484.

38. De Bonis P, Pompucci A, Mangiola A, Rigante L, Anile C. Post-traumatic hydrocephalus after decompressive craniectomy: an underestimated risk factor. *J Neurotrauma.* 2010;27(11):1965–1970.

39. Kaen A, Jimenez-Roldan L, Alday R, et al. Interhemispheric hygroma after decompressive craniectomy: does it predict posttraumatic hydrocephalus? *J Neurosurg.* 2010;113 (6):1287–1293.

40. Vedantam A, Yamal JM, Hwang H, Robertson CS, Gopinath SP. Factors associated with shunt-dependent hydrocephalus after decompressive craniectomy for traumatic brain injury. *J Neurosurg.* 2017:1–6. Epub ahead of print.

41. Perel P, Edwards P, Wentz R, Roberts I. Systematic review of prognostic models in traumatic brain injury. *BMC Med Inform Decis Mak.* 2006;6:38.

CHAPTER 2

TBI Classifications and Rehabilitation Intensities

MICHAEL ARMSTRONG, MD • KERRI CHUNG, DO • MARY HIMMLER, MD • DIANE MORTIMER, MD, MSN • BRIONN TONKIN, MD

DEFINITION

One of the earliest attempts to clinically define traumatic brain injury (TBI) was made by the Congress of Neurological Surgeons in 1966.[1] Although subsequent definitions issued by numerous organizations, including the American Congress of Rehabilitation Medicine,[2] Centers for Disease Control via the National Center for Injury Prevention and Control (CDC/NCIPC),[3] the World Health Organization,[4] and the Concussion in Sport Group,[5] have further evolved the definition, all the definitions have shared the common theme of an alteration of consciousness (AOC) or other transient neurologic abnormality resulting from biomechanical forces. The additions of other qualifiers for TBI only serve to compound the difficulty of a common definition. Regardless of the addition of qualifiers, a TBI of any type or severity manifests itself, either transiently or permanently, as a deficit of neurologic function following a precipitating biomechanical event. This deficit in neurologic function may include AOC, memory, or any of the other myriad roles the brain plays that can be subjectively reported or objectively measured. These deficits can include but are not limited to subjective reports of symptoms affecting cognitive, emotional, or physical domains; sleep disturbance; and objective measurements such as by Glasgow Coma Scale (GCS), neuroimaging, neurocognitive testing, or other means.

TRAUMATIC BRAIN INJURY SEVERITY

TBIs are heterogeneous by nature. Individual injuries vary markedly in mechanism and effect. Even injuries with seemingly identical-appearing imaging can lead to widely variable clinical phenotypes. This heterogeneity complicates attempts to classify injuries. Standard classification systems are thus admittedly imperfect.

However, the use of common terminology allows clinicians and researchers to more effectively discuss and study TBI cases.[6]

CLASSIFICATION OF TRAUMATIC BRAIN INJURY SEVERITY

Table 2.1 includes accepted criteria for determining TBI severity. GCS (Table 2.2), length of loss and alteration of consciousness, length of posttraumatic amnesia (PTA), and presence or absence of imaging findings are important components of this schema.[7]

The GCS quantifies the level of consciousness on the basis of eye opening, verbal response, and motor response.[8] GCS scores have been shown to be affected by factors separate from the TBI and can affect the validity of the scale. Patients with associated polytraumatic injuries, such as jaw or facial fractures, or concurrent substance use or individuals who are sedated, intubated, or require critical interventions may be unable to participate fully in an assessment of GCS thus limiting its interpretation. When using GCS to assess severity, clinicians should use the highest GCS score in the first 24 h. In addition, clinicians should consider the context of assessment. GCS alone should not be the sole determinant of injury severity.[7]

Loss of consciousness (LOC) and AOC are also important in the assessment of severity after TBI. During LOC, an individual is unresponsive and unaware of oneself or the surroundings. AOC involves wakefulness impaired by factors such as confusion, disorientation, and slowed thinking. Any LOC or AOC reflects neurologic deficit. Longer periods are correlated with the presence of more intense or widespread damage to the brain. The duration of LOC is more reliably reported by witness if available. In general, the length of AOC may be determined by witness report and/or patient

TABLE 2.1
Classification of TBI Severity

	Glasgow Coma Scale (Best Available in the First 24h)	Loss of Consciousness	Alteration of Consciousness/ Mental State	Imaging	Posttraumatic Amnesia
Mild	13–15	0–30 min	Up to 24h	Normal	0–1 day
Moderate	9–12	>30 min and <24h	>24h	Normal or abnormal	>1 day and <7 days
Severe	3–8	>24h	>24h	Normal or abnormal	>7 days

TBI, traumatic brain injury.
Adapted from Veterans Affairs/Department of Defense. *VA/DoD Clinical Practice Guideline for the Management of Concussion-Mild Traumatic Brain Injury*. Washington, DC: Veterans Health Administration; 2016, with permission.

TABLE 2.2
Glasgow Coma Scale

Eye opening	1-none 2-to pain 3-to speech 4-spontaneous
Best verbal response	1-none 2-incomprehensible speech 3-inappropriate speech 4-confused conversation 5-oriented
Best motor response	1-none 2-extension (decerebrate posturing) to painful stimuli 3-abnormal flexion (decorticate posturing) to painful stimuli 4-flexion/withdrawal to painful stimuli 5-localizing response 6-follows directions

Adapted from Teasdale G, Jennett B. Assessment of coma and consciousness: a practical scale. *Lancet*. 1974;2:81–84, with permission.

memory. Substances, both recreational and those provided by emergency personnel, may affect the assessment of consciousness.[7]

PTA includes any loss of memory for events that occurred at the time of injury. Retrograde amnesia involves memory loss for events occurring before the injury, whereas anterograde amnesia describes the inability to remember events occurring after the injury. Longer PTA is associated with more severe injuries and poorer outcomes. As with the assessment of GCS and LOC/AOC, accurate discernment of the length of

PTA, especially in mild injuries, may be affected by substances.[7]

Imaging findings are also considered in the evaluation of severity. Any injury with positive imaging findings should be classified as at least moderate in severity.[7] Alternatively, some other authors advocate separating mild injuries into uncomplicated mild (normal imaging) and complicated mild (imaging findings for TBI that would otherwise be classified as mild).[9] This distinction may evolve further as more sensitive imaging techniques are developed.

Additional severity-based classification of TBI uses other less commonly accepted scales. The Abbreviated Injury Scale (AIS) provides information about the threat to life from traumatic injury. The AIS was first published in 1969 and remains one of the most commonly used anatomic-based trauma severity scales. TBI is included as a component of this assessment.[10] The Revised Trauma Score (RTS) provides a physiologic-based assessment, which also describes injury severity. The RTS comprises the GCS, blood pressure, and respiratory rate early in the acute period and can be useful for predicting mortality in patients with trauma. These assessments can help characterize the severity of the overall trauma, with TBI playing a prominent role.[11]

Incidence and Epidemiology

An estimated 2.15 to more than 2.8 million TBIs occur in the United States each year. However, the surveillance data used to derive this estimate are exclusive to emergency rooms and hospitals and the use of accurate International Classification of Diseases (ICD) coding. The estimate excludes those with TBI who were not accurately classified using ICD coding, those who experienced a TBI but did not present for medical care, those who presented to outpatient clinics, and those who received care through the Department of Defense or Veterans Affairs. As a result of these exclusions, this overall incidence estimate is an underrepresentation of the true incidence of TBI in the United States.[12-14]

The vast majority of TBIs evaluated in US emergency departments are mild in nature, and the patients are treated and released. Although the incidence of hospitalization or death from TBI is far less than the number of mild TBIs by comparison, more than 283,000 hospitalizations and more than 52,000 deaths result from TBI each year.[12] Approximately 70% of all TBIs occur concomitantly with other traumatic injuries.[15] Between 2007 and 2013, rates of emergency department presentation for TBI have increased from 534 per 100,000 in 2007 to 787.1 per 100,000 in 2013. Over the same period of time, TBI hospitalization rates have remained relatively stable (87.6 in 2007 compared with 85.4 in 2013), whereas TBI-related deaths decreased slightly (17.9 in 2007 compared with 17.0 in 2013),[14] suggesting that greater recognition of mild TBI may contribute to the increasing rates of emergency visits.

Falls and motor vehicle crashes (MVCs) are the leading causes of TBI in the United States. Falls represent the overall leading cause of all TBI, are highest in children aged 0–4 years and adults 75 years and older, and represent the greatest number of emergency department visits and hospitalizations. MVCs are the leading cause of TBI in young adults aged 15–24 years and represent the leading cause of TBI-related death over the past decade.[12-14,16]

The impact of TBI in sports has garnered special attention in recent years. TBI accounts for approximately 10%–15% of all sports-related injuries. An estimated 300,000 adolescent athletes sustain a TBI playing organized sports each year in the United States. In general, collision sports have the highest incidence of TBI. American football and women's soccer rank number one and two, respectively, for the highest incidence of sports-related TBI. Of special note, female athletes sustain TBIs at two times the rate as their male counterparts in matched sports.[17,18]

TBI has been called a "signature injury" of military personnel serving in the Operation Enduring Freedom and Operation Iraqi Freedom (OEF/OIF). Between 2000 and 2016, the Department of Defense has identified more than 360,000 TBIs across all severities in deployed service members. The primary mechanism of injury is undoubtedly blast related. An estimated 86%–98% of all military TBIs in OEF/OIF were secondary to blast exposure. Between 2005 and 2009, blast rates ranged from 1.7 to 4.5 blast injuries per 1000 deployed military service members.[19,20]

Pathophysiology

The understanding of TBI pathophysiology and its complexities continues to evolve. Although variation across the heterogenous injury mechanisms and subtypes exists, there are principles of pathophysiology common to all TBIs. Common factors include derangements in large cerebral structures, connections between brain regions, cellular functions, and neuronal microstructures resulting from primary injury, secondary injury, or both. Primary injuries result from the direct effects of the mechanical forces and may include damage to both small and large brain structures. Secondary injuries, ranging from focal to diffuse in nature, involve spreading tissue damage in response to the primary injury's structural or metabolic sequelae.

Mechanism

Closed or blunt force injuries may involve direct impacts to the head, as well as acceleration-deceleration and rotational force mechanisms. These injuries may result from falls, assaults, sports collisions, MVCs, blast exposures, and other forces sufficient enough to be transmitted to the brain. A common cause of TBI results from rotational movement of the brain in the anteroposterior plane while the brainstem is fixed in place. The subsequent effects, which can be focal or diffuse, are related to the location and extent of injury.[21]

MILD TRAUMATIC BRAIN INJURY

Mild TBI, or concussion, results when the head encounters a mechanical force significant enough for transmission to the brain. The resulting motion of the brain within the skull may result in stretching of and damage to axonal membranes and associated cascade of detrimental effects. Damage to axonal membranes lead to an abnormal efflux of intracellular potassium through voltage-gated channels. As more channels open and more potassium exits the cell, the membranes depolarize further, resulting in excessive amounts of excitatory amino acids and neurotransmitters being released from presynaptic terminals. These chemicals, including glutamate, in turn stimulate receptors and ligand-gated potassium channels, leading to even greater potassium efflux from the cell. Glutamate also binds to N-methyl-D-aspartate–binding receptor protein, causing opening of potassium-calcium channels and allowing for free flow of calcium and potassium in and out of the cell. Intracellular calcium deposits lead to further damage by activating proteases and reactive oxygen species and by preventing mitochondrial function.[22]

As this cascade progresses and gives way to a period of depressed neuronal function in affected areas, cells develop hypoxia. The damaged and overmatched mitochondria are unable to meet cells' metabolic demands, resulting in a significant delay in restoring normal ionic balance. Neurons enter into short periods of glycolysis, which leads to a buildup of lactic acid. The resulting acidosis causes breakdown of the blood brain barrier (BBB), more oxidative stress, persisting mitochondrial dysfunction, and cell swelling and death.[22]

Local metabolic perturbations lead to the recruitment and activation of local inflammatory responses within 4–6h following injury. The microglia mediate the work of cytokine mediators, proteases, and reactive free radicals. These inflammatory cells scavenge cellular debris and wall off damaged axons in what is likely an initial phase in recovery.[22]

FOCAL INJURIES AND CONTUSIONS

Focal contusions result from direct or indirect impact, as well as from contact of the brain with the internal skull components. The latter may result in contusions when the brain is forcibly jostled within the cranium and makes contact along interior and protuberant structures, such as the greater wing of sphenoid, petrous temporal bone, crista galli, sella turcica, tentorium cerebelli, and falx cerebri.[23]

Contusions are often divided into categories based on the relationship of the damage to the location of head impact. Coup injury occurs at or near the site of impact resulting from direct force on the brain. In contrast, contrecoup injury results from the brain forcefully moving within the skull, generally on the opposite side of the brain from the coup injury. For example, a blunt trauma resulting in a frontal coup injury may cause an associated occipital contrecoup injury because of subsequent motion of the brain.[23]

Focal injuries are also classified by their relationship to the brain's protective dura. Epidural hematoma involves blood collecting outside of the dura, which does not cross suture lines owing to dural adhesion at these sites. Epidural hematomas typically result from damage to an artery, such as the middle meningeal artery. Subdural hematomas are caused by damage to cortical bridging veins. In subdural hematoma, blood collects in the subdural space and can extend past suture lines to affect the entire hemisphere. Traumatic subarachnoid hemorrhage involves blood collecting in the subarachnoid space. Intraventricular hemorrhage involves bleeding in the ventricular system and may lead to hydrocephalus. Skull fractures, which may or may not involve damage to underlying dura and brain, result from blunt trauma and penetrating injury.[23]

DIFFUSE AXONAL INJURY

Unlike focal injuries, diffuse axonal injury (DAI) occurs when transmitted forces result in damage to axons spread over wide regions of the brain, contributing significantly to morbidity and mortality. Axonal damage in DAI may be caused by the cascade of calcium-mediated events following stretching and pulling forces on the axonal membrane. These events result in obstruction of axonal transport and focal axonal swelling. Traumatic disconnection of axons in DAI also leads to deafferentation of axonal projections, synaptic loss, and Wallerian degeneration.

DAI is classified on the basis of the extent of damage. Grade I DAI affects gray-white matter interfaces, generally in the parasagittal regions of frontal lobes, periventricular temporal lobes, and, to a lesser extent, parietal and occipital lobes, internal and external capsules, and the cerebellum. Grade II DAI affects the aforementioned structures as well as the corpus callosum. The damage to the corpus callosum is most commonly located in the areas of the posterior body and splenium. Grade III DAI includes damage to the brainstem, most commonly in the areas of the rostral midbrain, superior cerebellar peduncles, medial lemnisci, and corticospinal tracts. Although he presence of severe DAI is predictive of a worse prognosis, the clinical implications of more localized injury are less clear.[21]

PENETRATING INJURIES

When brain tissue is directly penetrated with armaments, including bullets, knives, shrapnel, and other objects, affected regions suffer mechanical damage. Infection and seizures are common sequelae. Penetrating injuries can also lead to diffuse problems if excitotoxicity, metabolic issues, vascular injury, and inflammatory changes lead to widespread edema and cell death.[21]

BLAST INJURY

Blast injuries result from exposure to explosion-related pressure waves. Even without direct contact between the head and an object, blast-related forces are sufficient to cause injury to the brain. As is the case with other TBIs, blasts damage neuronal, axonal, and glial structure and function. Blasts can have particularly harmful effects on white matter, the BBB, and gray-white matter junctions, in both focal and diffuse patterns. Cellular sequelae include apoptotic and necrotic pathways and subsequent neuronal death. Axonal injury leads to problems with axonal transport and accumulation of phosphorylated neurofilament proteins in neuronal cell bodies. Oxidative damage, dysfunction of the BBB, and inflammatory mishaps lead to further problems.[24]

Blasts exposures result in injuries across the severity spectrum. More mild injuries, such as those from other mechanisms, involve focal disruption in cellular membranes, ion changes, axonal injury, and inflammatory abnormalities. More severe injuries, which affect broader areas of the brain, occur when there is a higher degree of blast exposure. This may result from a larger blast, closer proximity to it, or some other physical factors that allow the blast wave to affect the brain with more force or longer force duration.[24]

SECONDARY INJURY

Primary injuries often give way to diffuse secondary damage. In severe injuries, cascades of abnormal neuronal cell depolarization occur in a more widespread and therefore more damaging manner than in mild injuries. As the injured brain's metabolic demand uncouples from perfusion, it leads to even greater perfusion abnormalities and subsequent hypoxia and cell death.[25] Altered transport and release of neurotransmitters also occurs. Glutamate, an excitatory amino acid, is secreted in abnormally high quantities. Axonal damage, from mechanical forces and from metabolic sequelae, can have precarious consequences.[26] Ionic changes, including transient depolarization, occur immediately after the axon is injured. Influxes of sodium and calcium are accompanied by activation of calcium-dependent proteins proteins, which disrupt the cell's structural elements. The calcium influx occurs between 1.5 and 6 h post injury. During this time, fast axonal transport is lost and the microtubules become incapacitated. This leads to neurofilament changes and dysfunction of cell transport, resulting in further abnormalities in cellular metabolism. Within approximately 4 h, axonal interconnection disrupts.[26]

Cerebral edema, either vasogenic or cellular/cytotoxic, is another deleterious sequela of diffuse brain injury. Vasogenic cerebral edema results from disruption of the BBB and is characterized by the inflow of the blood's protein-rich fluid into the brain's interstitial fluid. This inflow leads to an increase in oncotic pressure in the extracellular fluid, increase in total brain volume, additional neuronal swelling, and microglial activation. Vasogenic edema occurs within the first few hours of injury and then again about 3–5 days later. Cellular, or cytotoxic, edema results from an abnormal buildup of neurochemicals within the neuron in the setting of dysfunctional ion pumps at the cell membrane. Cells become hyperosmotic compared with their environment, resulting in fluid inflow and further swelling. The resultant effects on cell function and interconnectivity lead to further cell damage.[27]

Inflammatory events in the brain also contribute to secondary injury. The inflammatory response within the brain is mediated by astrocytes and microglia. Astrocytes, including oligodendrocytes and ependymal cells, maintain BBB integrity and cellular homeostasis in the healthy brain. After TBI, these cells change shape and are unable to maintain the BBB. They are also unable to maintain homeostatic concentrations of intercellular and extracellular neurochemicals/transmitters, such as glutamate. Microglia mount the brain's immune response after TBI through the release of multiple cytokines, chemokines, and growth factors. Although they mediate the repair and recovery of the damaged brain, it is likely these chemicals lead to at least some increase in edema and metabolic derangement during the acute phase of TBI.[28]

The net effect of the combination of primary injury, cerebral edema, axonal injury, metabolic mismatches, and inflammatory abnormalities is neuronal failure. Within approximately 24 h after injury, some of these neurons undergo apoptosis and die, whereas others begin to recover. Neuronal function returns to its normal state after the normal physiologic homeostasis is achieved. However, emerging injury models demonstrate that the disrupted connections between neurons, inevitably affected by neuronal damage and death, are critical factors in late impairments.[21]

Although irreparable damage may occur as a result of TBI, degrees of recovery do occur. Neuroplasticity is a nonspecific but widely used term that describes the adaptability and flexibility of neurons. As a result of this adaptability and flexibility, neurons have the ability to reorganize, develop new linkages, and assume new activities that lead to remapping and recovery of brain functions. It is believed that neuroplasticity plays an instrumental role in recovery after brain injury.[21]

PROGNOSIS

Owing to the heterogeneous nature of TBI and subsequently its outcomes, accurate prognosis following TBI is difficult to determine and challenging to discuss with patients or their family. Despite the predictive challenges presented by its heterogeneity, numerous studies have identified factors valuable in predicting outcomes after TBI using broader outcome classification categories such as those used in the Glasgow Outcome Scale (GOS). These predictive factors include, but are not limited to, age, etiology of injury, clinical severity, structural abnormalities on neuroimaging, secondary insults (e.g., hypoxia, hypotension), duration of coma, duration of PTA, and numerous other premorbid factors. In general, older age, greater clinical severity, and longer duration of coma and PTA predict worse functional and occupational outcomes, whereas younger age, lesser clinical severity, and shorter duration of

coma and PTA predict better outcomes. Although the use of broad outcome measures, such as the GOS, is limited in predicting outcomes beyond the most generalist domains, they are nevertheless useful in medical, rehabilitation, and disposition decision making, as well as in assisting patients and families with establishing realistic expectations of outcomes after TBI.[29]

LEVELS OF REHABILITATION CARE

Individuals affected by TBI benefit from an interdisciplinary approach to rehabilitation. The appropriate setting for rehabilitation is determined by the type and intensity of an individual's needs. These needs reflect functional status, amount of assistance needed, and the therapies required to meet rehabilitation goals.[30,31]

Inpatient Settings

Inpatient postacute settings of care include long-term acute care hospitals (LTACHs), inpatient rehabilitation facilities (IRFs), and skilled nursing facilities (SNFs) for short or long-term stays (Table 2.3). At the more intense end of the spectrum, LTACHs and IRFs include

TABLE 2.3
Inpatient Settings of Care

	Long-Term Acute Care Hospital (LTACH)	Inpatient Rehabilitation Facility (IRF)	Skilled Nursing Facility (SNF)	Long-Term/Custodial Care
Functional status	• Medically complex needs that cannot be met at a lower level of care • Failure of two or more major organ systems • Ventilator weaning failure after more than 3 weeks at a prior hospitalization • Complex wounds	• Some degree of ADL and mobility impairment • Cognitively able to participate in therapy • Significant practical functional improvement is expected	• Some degree of ADL and mobility impairment or other skilled need • Some functional improvement is expected	• Some degree of mobility or ADL impairment • Needs cannot be managed at a lower level of care • May or may not have cognitive deficits • Has not reached independent level to be managed at home setting • No longer making progress where they can benefit from skilled intervention
Nursing and medical services required	• Requires ongoing acute medical management • Requires 24 h licensed nursing care	• Requires ongoing acute medical management • Requires 24 h rehabilitation nursing care • Need for IDT	• Skilled nursing staff is required to meet individual's medical needs, promote recovery, and ensure medical safety	• Daily skilled nursing or intervention not required

TABLE 2.3
Inpatient Settings of Care—cont'd

	Long-Term Acute Care Hospital (LTACH)	Inpatient Rehabilitation Facility (IRF)	Skilled Nursing Facility (SNF)	Long-Term/Custodial Care
Therapies required	• Therapy as an adjunct to medical treatment	• Requires two or more therapies, one of which must be PT or OT	• Requires one or more therapies **OR** • Patient has daily skilled nursing need	• May require therapy, but the total must be less than five times per week
Number of therapy hours required	• No minimum number of hours required	• Tolerates at least 3 h per day of therapy for 5 days per week	• No minimum number of tolerated hours required • Skilled need is sufficient	• No minimum number of hours required
Discharge plan and social support		• Probable discharge to community • Adequate community support resources are available to meet needs based on functional prognosis	• Completed psychosocial needs assessment • Possible discharge to community	• SNF transfer must include long-term plan of care • Completed psychosocial needs assessment and discussion with family regarding financial requirements

ADLs, activities of daily living; *IDT,* interdisciplinary team; *OT,* occupational therapy; *PT,* physical therapy; *SNF,* skilled nursing facility.[32]
From Association of Rehabilitation Nurses. *The Essential Role of the Rehabilitation Nurse in Facilitating Care Transitions*; 2013. [Online]. http://www.rehabnurse.org/uploads/files/healthpolicy/ARN_Care_Transitions_White_Paper_Journal_Copy_FINAL.pdf, with permission.

daily visits with medical providers. In IRFs, patients participate in at least two therapy disciplines for at least 3 hours per day, at least 5 days per week. IRFs are accredited by the Joint Commission and may also be accredited by the Commission on Accreditation of Rehabilitation Facilities. Interdisciplinary teams typically include the patient and family, rehabilitation physician(s), other nonrehabilitation medical providers, rehabilitation nurses, occupational therapists, physical therapists, speech language pathologists, recreational therapy specialists, psychologists, pharmacists, dietitians, social workers, and assistive technology specialists. These teams help plan and coordinate rehabilitation care.[31]

SNFs provide both short- and long-term care. Over the short term, patients can participate in a subacute or less intense level of rehabilitation consisting of therapy for at least an hour per day, 5 days per week. Patients are seen by a provider at least weekly, and care is planned and coordinated by the interdisciplinary team. Skilled nursing needs are also addressed. SNFs may also provide more traditional long-term nursing care when needed.[31]

Outpatient Settings

For patients who do not require inpatient medical rehabilitation or once postacute inpatient rehabilitation has been completed and patients are ready for discharge to the community, rehabilitation services may be continued in a variety of outpatient settings. Table 2.4 lists the various settings and levels of outpatient rehabilitation care. Individuals can move through this continuum as their rehabilitation needs dictate.[30,31]

REHABILITATION OUTCOMES

Numerous measurement scales have been developed to assess recovery, functional status, and global outcomes after TBI. A comprehensive list of these measures and scales is available through The Center for Outcome Measurement in Brain Injury website maintained by

TABLE 2.4
Outpatient Settings of Care

	Integrated Outpatient Therapy/Day Treatment/ Residential Rehabilitation	Home Health	Standard Outpatient Therapy
Functional status	• Able to be cared for at home • Skilled IDT or MDT intervention required • Potential to make significant functional improvement in ADLs, mobility, or cognition/ language • Able to do a home exercise/activity program	• Homebound owing to some degree of ADL and mobility impairment • Completed cognitive evaluation	• Impairments that requires only supervision or minimal assistance with mobility or ADLs • Cognitively able to participate in therapy
Nursing and medical services required	• Outpatient rehabilitation RN, PM&R, case manager, and medical social worker are part of the IDT or MDT	• May require home health nursing	• Referred to outpatient rehabilitation RN, case manager, and medical social worker if needed
Therapies required	• Requires at least two therapies	• Requires one or more therapies with a nurse or social worker	• Requires one or more therapies
Number of therapy hours required and tolerated	• Tolerates at least 1 h per day **OR** • Has a skilled need and a functional goal with good rehabilitation prognosis	• Tolerates at least 0.5 h per day **OR** • Has a skilled need and a functional goal with good rehabilitation prognosis	• Tolerates at least 0.5 h per day either in the clinic or doing at-home exercises **OR** • Has a skilled need and a functional goal with good rehabilitation prognosis
Discharge plan and social support	• Must have transportation to therapy location • Has accessible environment at home and appropriate durable medical equipment to meet needs • Has support to continue exercise and activity program at home	• Must be able to get to/from therapy visits • Has accessible environment at home and appropriate durable medical equipment • Has social support to continue exercise and activity program at home	• Confined to home • Has accessible environment at home and appropriate durable medical equipment

ADL, activities of daily living; *IDT*, interdisciplinary team; *MDT*, multidisciplinary team; *PM&R*, physical medicine and rehabilitation; *RN*, registered nurse.[32]
From Association of Rehabilitation Nurses. *The Essential Role of the Rehabilitation Nurse in Facilitating Care Transitions*; 2013. [Online]. http://www.rehabnurse.org/uploads/files/healthpolicy/ARN_Care_Transitions_White_Paper_Journal_Copy_FINAL.pdf, with permission.

the Rehabilitation Research Center at Santa Clara Valley Medical Center.[33]

The most commonly used outcome scale in the acute inpatient rehabilitation setting is the Functional Independence Measure (FIM). The FIM is an 18-item scale for the measurement of function across multiple activities of daily living and scaled to allow rating of progress toward functional independence. Although the FIM is consistently used for the measurement of progress during inpatient TBI rehabilitation, it is not specific to brain injury rehabilitation and is used across the spectrum of conditions appropriate for inpatient rehabilitation. The Functional Assessment Measure is a 12-item measure that, when used in conjunction with the FIM, allows for greater measurement of function across cognitive, behavioral, and communication domains. The inclusion of these additional TBI-related domains allows for greater measurement of TBI-specific inpatient rehabilitation interventions. The Disability Rating Scale (DRS) is an eight-item scale validated across moderate to severe TBI population receiving inpatient rehabilitation. Although this scale is not as universally used as the FIM and is more generalized in nature, the scale's specificity for TBI populations and community applicable measures warrant consideration for use in the inpatient TBI rehabilitation setting. The aforementioned GOS has little utility in the measurement of TBI rehabilitation; however, it was frequently used as a broad measure of outcome in TBI prognosis and outcome-based research. The scale is made up of five categories, including dead, vegetative state, severely disabled, moderately disabled, and good recovery. For the assessment of functional status years after TBI, the Revised Craig Handicap Assessment and Reporting Technique, Neurobehavioral Functioning Inventory, Patient Competency Rating Scale, and the DRS employability scale show a more comprehensive picture of the patient's overall functioning in the community.[33,34]

DEVELOPMENT OF CARE SYSTEMS

Rehabilitation clinicians who provide services along the continuum are all too aware of the limitations in access and difficulties with transitions between care settings that patients and families confront. In addition to contending with physical, emotional, and financial effects of the TBI, individuals often also struggle to receive appropriate rehabilitation services to address their needs. In one example of clinicians and policy makers trying to address this significant problem, the Department of Veterans Affairs developed the Polytrauma System of Care. Veterans and service members with TBI and polytrauma move through the continuum of rehabilitation services with the assistance and coordination of case managers and dedicated rehabilitation teams. Specialized services, including planning for long-term follow-up and the implementation of telehealth technology, have also been developed to provide the extensive ongoing care required in the lifelong management of TBI. The overriding goal of systems such as this is to facilitate optimal provision of high-quality rehabilitation services to individuals with conditions such as TBI across the spectrum of severity.[35,36]

SUMMARY

TBI may be defined as AOC or other transient neurologic abnormality resulting from biomechanical forces and manifesting itself, either transiently or permanently, as a deficit of neurologic function. TBI represents a significant public health concern with more than 2.5 million injuries and more than 50,000 TBI-related deaths occurring in the United States each year. Each TBI varies by mechanism, pathophysiology, severity, and sequelae. The variability of these factors combined with the complexity of the brain and its functions results in a heterogeneous mix of health effects and outcomes across the spectrum of TBI. Because of this heterogeneity, a multifaceted continuum of care capable of addressing the broad and variable needs of TBI survivors is required to optimize outcomes and reduce disability.

REFERENCES

1. Gurdjian ES, Volis HC. Congress of Neurological Surgeons Committee on head injury nomenclature: glossary of head injury. *Clin Neurosurg.* 1966;12:386–394.
2. Kay T, Harrington D, Adams R, et al. Definition of mild traumatic brain injury. *J Head Trauma Rehabil.* 1993;8(3):86–87.
3. National Center for Injury Prevention and Control. *Report to Congress on Mild Traumatic Brain Injury in the United States: Steps to Prevent a Serious Public Health Problem.* Atlanta, GA: Centers for Disease Control and Prevention; 2003.
4. Carroll LJ, Cassidy JD, Holm L, et al. Methodological issues and research recommendations for mild traumatic brain injury: the WHO Collaborating Center Task Force on mild traumatic brain injury. *J Rehabil Med.* 2004;43:113–125.
5. McCrory P, Meeuwisse W, Dvorak J, et al. Consensus statement on concussion in sport - the 5th international conference on concussion in sport held in Berlin, October 2016. *Br J Sports Med.* 2017;51(11):838–847.
6. Saatman KE, Duhaime AC, Bullock R, et al. Classification of traumatic brain injury for targeted therapies. *J Neurotrauma.* 2008;25:719–738.
7. Veterans Affairs/Department of Defense. *VA/DoD Clinical Practice Guideline for the Management of Concussion-Mild Traumatic Brain Injury.* Washington, DC: Veterans Health Administration; 2016.
8. Teasdale G, Jennett B. Assessment of coma and consciousness: a practical scale. *Lancet.* 1974;2:81–84.
9. Kay T, Adams R, Anderson T, et al. Definition of mild traumatic brain injury. *J Head Trauma Rehabil.* 1993;8:86–87.
10. Gennarelli TA, Wodzin E. *The Abbreviated Injury Scale.* Des Plaines, IL: American Association for Automotive Medicine; 2008.
11. Champion HR, Sacco WJ, Copes WS, et al. A revision of the trauma score. *J Trauma.* 1989;5:623–629.

12. Centers for Disease Control and Prevention. *Report to Congress on Traumatic Brain Injury in the United States: Epidemiology and Rehabilitation.* Atlanta, GA: National Center for Injury Prevention and Control; Division of Unintentional Injury Prevention; 2015.

13. Albrect JS, Hirshon JM, et al. Increased rates of mild traumatic brain injury among older adults in US emergency departments, 2009-2010. *J Head Trauma Rehabil.* 2016;5:E1–E7.

14. Taylor CA, Bell JM, Breiding MJ, Xu L. Traumatic brain injury–related emergency department visits, hospitalizations, and deaths — United States, 2007 and 2013. *MMWR Surveill Summ.* 2017;66(No. SS-9):1–16.

15. Cancelliere C, Coranado VG, Taylor CA. Epidemiology of isolated versus nonisolated mild traumatic brain injury treated in emergency departments in the United States, 2006-2012: sociodemographic characteristics. *J Head Trauma Rehabil.* 2017;32:E37–E46.

16. Allen CJ, Hannay WM, et al. Causes of death differ between elderly and adult falls. *J Trauma Acute Care Surg.* 2015;79:617–621.

17. Schallmo MS, Weiner JA, Hsu WK. Sports and sex-specific reporting trends in the epidemiology of concussions sustained by high school athletes. *J Bone Joint Surg Am.* 2017;99:1314–1320.

18. Register-Mihalik JK, Kay MC. The current state of sports concussion. *Neurol Clin.* 2017;35(3):387–402.

19. Greer N, Sayer N, et al. *Prevalence and Epidemiology of Combat Blast Injuries from the Military Cohort 2001-2014. VA Evidence-Based Synthesis Program Reports (Internet).* Department of Veterans Affairs; 2016.

20. Defense and Veterans Brain Injury Center. *DoD Worldwide Numbers for TBI.* http://dvbic.dcoe.mil/dod-worldwide-numbers-tbi.

21. McGinn MJ, Povlishock JT. Pathophysiology of traumatic brain injury. *Neurosurg Clin N Am.* 2016;27:397–407.

22. Choe MC. The pathophysiology of concussion. *Curr Pain Headache Rep.* 2016;20:42–52.

23. Yokobori S, Bullock MR. Pathobiology of primary traumatic brain injury. In: Archineagas DB, Bullock MB, Kreutzer JS, eds. *Brain Injury Medicine: Principles and Practice.* 2nd ed. New York: Demos; 2013.

24. Hicks RR, Fertig SJ, Desrocher RE. Neurological effects of blast injury. *J Trauma.* 2010;68:1257–1263.

25. Salehi A, Zhang JH, Obenaus A. Response of the cerebral vasculature following traumatic brain injury. *J Cereb Blood Flow Metab.* 2017;37:2320–2339.

26. Blanco MMB, Prashant GN, Vespa PM. Cerebral metabolism and the role of glucose control in acute traumatic brain injury. *Neurosurg Clin N Am.* 2016;27:453–463.

27. Winkler AW, Minter D, Yue JK, et al. Cerebral edema in traumatic brain injury: pathophysiology and prospective therapeutic targets. *Neurosurg Clin N Am.* 2016;27:473–488.

28. Karve IP, Taylow JM, Crack PJ. The contribution of astrocytes and microglia to traumatic brain injury. *Br J Pharmacol.* 2015;173:692–702.

29. Lingsma HF, Roozenbeek B, et al. Early prognosis in traumatic brain injury: from prophecies to predictions. *Lancet Neurol.* 2010;9(5):543–554.

30. Brusco NK, Taylor NF, Watts JJ, et al. Economic evaluation of adult rehabilitation: a systematic review and meta-analysis of randomized controlled trials in a variety of settings. *Arch Phys Med Rehabil.* 2014;95:94–116.

31. Veterans Health Administration. *VHA Handbook 1170.04: Rehabilitation Continuum of Care.* Washington, DC: Veterans Health Administration; 2014.

32. Association of Rehabilitation Nurses. *The Essential Role of the Rehabilitation Nurse in Facilitating Care Transitions;* 2013. [Online] http://www.rehabnurse.org/uploads/files/healthpolicy/ARN_Care_Transitions_White_Paper_Journal_Copy_FINAL.pdf.

33. *The Center for Outcome Measurement in Brain Injury.* www.tbims.org/list.html.

34. Hall K, Bushnik T, et al. Assessing traumatic brain injury outcome measures for long-term follow-up of community based individuals. *Arch Phys Med Rehabil.* 2001;82:367–374.

35. Darkins A, Cruise C, Armstrong M, et al. Enhancing access of combat-wounded veterans to specialist rehabilitation services: the VA Polytrauma System of Care. *Arch Phys Med Rehabil.* 2008;89:182–187.

36. Sigford BJ. "To care for him who shall have born the battle and for his widow and his orphan" (Abraham Lincoln): the Department of Veterans Affairs Polytrauma System of Care. *Arch Phys Med Rehabil.* 2008;89:160–162.

CHAPTER 3

Medical Complications After Moderate to Severe Traumatic Brain Injury

BLESSEN C. EAPEN, MD • SANDRA HONG, DO • BRUNO SUBBARAO, DO • CARLOS A. JARAMILLO, MD, PHD

INTRODUCTION

A 2017 multicenter cohort study of 12,887 patients admitted for traumatic brain injury (TBI) care found that 22.6% of those patients also suffered nonneurologic complications and 3.6% had neurologic complications. These complications resulted in significant increases in mortality (85% for neurologic complications) and length of stay (twofold increase for nonneurologic complications).[1] Optimal care for this specialized and complex patient population includes prevention and/or treatment of these secondary complications, which is most appropriately done with an interdisciplinary rehabilitation team approach.

SPASTICITY

Spasticity, a known complication of moderate and severe TBI, is defined as a velocity-dependent and involuntary resistance to passive range of motion. It occurs when there is a central injury above the level of the α motor neuron leading to a loss of descending inhibitory signals that ends in altered activity of the stretch reflex. This leads to an increase in muscle tone, which is the continuous contraction of a muscle in a resting state. If left untreated, spasticity may ultimately result in contractures, which are stiffened or hardened myotendinous tissue with a velocity-independent resistance or rigidity that significantly limits range of motion.[1,2]

To measure spasticity, the two most widely used clinical scales are the Modified Ashworth Scale (MAS) and the Tardieu Scale. The Ashworth Scale was developed in 1964 and was then modified by Bohannon and Smith in 1987 to become the MAS. In 2006 the MAS was again modified by Ansari et al. to become the Modified MAS. Both scales are compared in Table 3.1. Of note, the MAS is still widely used and recognized both clinically and in the recent literature. The MAS has been shown to have moderate to good test-retest reliability and interrater reliability when used for spasticity assessment by trained professionals, but it has been found to have limitations when used to measure changes in tone, such as with spasticity treatments.[2,3]

The Tardieu Scale was originally developed in 1954 and was later modified in 1969 and again in 1999 to become the Modified Tardieu Scale (MTS). This scale is thought to have some strength over the MAS because it assesses spasticity at both slow and fast velocities. Unfortunately, there is an insufficient literature validating the MTS, and because most of the existing studies have been on children, validation across age groups is missing. When using the MTS, passive range of motion (R2) is measured during slow, passive stretch (V1), and the angle of muscle reaction (R1) is obtained during fast, passive stretch (V3).[3,4] The MTS grades muscle resistance during fast passive stretch from 0 to 4 as follows[3]:

Modified Tardieu Scale

0: No resistance throughout the course of passive movement

1: Slight resistance throughout the course of passive movement with no clear catch at precise angle

2: Clear catch at precise angle, interrupting the passive movement, followed by release

3: Fatigable clonus (<10 s when maintaining pressure) occurring at precise angle

4: Infatigable clonus (>10 s when maintaining pressure) occurring at precise angle

Patients with spasticity often experience discomfort or pain, decreased mobility, postural issues, and difficulty with hygiene and self-care activities. These individuals are also at risk for developing contractures and pressure ulcers if untreated. In severe cases, it is indicated to treat spasticity to improve quality of life.

TABLE 3.1
Modified Ashworth Scale (MAS) and Modified Modified Ashworth Scale (MMAS)

Grade	MAS	MMAS
0	No increase in muscle tone	No increase in muscle tone
1	Slight increase in muscle tone with or without a catch followed by relaxation/minimal resistance at end of range of motion (ROM)	Slight increase in muscle tone with a catch and then a release/minimal resistance at the end of ROM
1+	Slight increase in muscle resistance throughout ROM Catch followed by minimal resistance throughout less than half of ROM	
2	Moderate increase in muscle tone throughout ROM Affected part easily moved	Marked increase in muscle tone with a catch midrange and resistance throughout the remainder of ROM, affected part easily moved
3	Marked increase in muscle tone throughout ROM Difficult passive movement of affected part	Considerable increase in muscle tone Difficult passive movement of affected part
4	Marked increase in muscle tone Affected part rigid	Affected part rigid

Adapted from Abolhasani H, Ansari NN, Naghdi S, Mansouri K, Ghotbi N, Hasson S. Comparing the validity of the modified modified Ashworth scale (MMAS) and the modified Tardieu scale (MTS) in the assessment of wrist flexor spasticity in patients with stroke: protocol for a neurophysiological study. *BMJ Open*. 2012;2(6); Li F, Wu Y, Li X. Test-retest reliability and inter-rater reliability of the modified Tardieu scale and the modified Ashworth scale in hemiplegic patients with stroke. *Eur J Phys Rehabil Med*. 2014;50(1):9–15, with permission.

Management begins with a thorough physical examination to look for and treat deep venous thrombosis (DVT), wounds, infection, and possible musculoskeletal or visceral pathologies as potential contributors to worsening spasticity.[5] Once complete, nonpharmacologic modalities, such as stretching, splinting, serial casting, and electrical stimulation, can be considered, although efficacy of these modalities requires further research.[2,6]

When initiating pharmacotherapy for spasticity, special consideration must be made for the TBI population. Many of the commonly used medications for spasticity (see Table 3.2) act centrally and could impede neurorecovery.[5] With botulinum toxin and phenol injections, physicians can specifically target spastic muscles to avoid a generalized weakness.[6] However, injection therapy can be time consuming and technically challenging. Injectable intramuscular chemodenervation is often used in the subacute and/or chronic phase of TBI to allow for potential natural recovery. The effect of botulinum toxin usually appears about 3–5 days after injection and can last for approximately 3–6 months. Repeat injections can be performed but no earlier than 3 months. In contrast, the effect of phenol and alcohol blocks can be appreciated within hours of injection and persists for 6 months to 1 year. However, phenol and alcohol injections require more expertise to administer and

can be more uncomfortable for the patient than botulinum toxin therapy.[6,7]

If patients have had no improvement in spasticity with two or more oral or injectable therapies, or have failed oral baclofen owing to side effects, they may be candidates for intrathecal baclofen (ITB). Unlike oral baclofen, ITB can deliver a higher dose directly to the CNS with fewer side effects. In addition, ITB is known to have a greater effect on lower-limb than upper-limb tone. As with all therapies, ITB should treat spasticity without loss of the functional advantages of tone. Increased tone can be functionally more beneficial than flaccidity by providing assistance with head control, upright sitting, transfers, ambulation, and even utensil use.[2,6,9] Therefore, before pump implantation, it is necessary for patients, physicians, and the interdisciplinary team to set functional goals of ITB therapy, such as improved mobility, increased ability to perform activities of daily living, and improved positioning. Once these goals are set, patients undergo a screening test that involves the administration of an initial test dose of 50 μg through a temporary catheter or lumbar puncture. They are then monitored for efficacy and side effects. If little or no effect is observed with the initial dose, a subsequent test bolus of 75 μg and then 100 μg may be given. Each bolus should be given 24 h after the previous administration. If desired results are achieved,

TABLE 3.2
Commonly Used Medications for Spasticity Management

Medication	Mechanism of Action	Side Effects and Special Considerations
Baclofen (oral)	Centrally acting GABA analog that binds to $GABA_B$ receptor to inhibit muscle stretch reflex and decrease motor neuron activity at the spinal cord level	Somnolence, fatigue, muscle weakness, xerostomia, urinary retention, constipation, elevated LFTs Abrupt cessation associated with withdrawal seizures, altered mental status, hallucinations, and increased muscle tone and spasm
Baclofen (intrathecal)	Same as oral baclofen	Reduced systemic side effects compared with oral administration because intrathecal delivery allows for higher concentration at lower dose Withdrawal symptoms secondary to catheter or pump malfunction Effect greater in lower extremities than in upper extremities
Tizanidine	a2-Agonist that inhibits the release of excitatory neurotransmitters (glutamate, aspartate) from spinal interneurons	Somnolence, dizziness, hypotension, xerostomia, elevated LFTs
Dantrolene	Inhibits the release of calcium from the sarcoplasmic reticulum of muscle, interfering with skeletal muscle contraction	Muscle weakness, drowsiness, diarrhea, hepatotoxicity Often preferred for TBI-induced spasticity because it acts peripherally
Gabapentin	GABA analog, but MOA is not fully understood	Drowsiness, dizziness, edema
Diazepam	Binds to $GABA_A$ receptor, facilitating chloride influx and inducing neuronal inhibition	Sedation, cognitive impairments Abrupt cessation may lead to withdrawal symptoms
Clonidine	Centrally acting a2-agonist that decreases sympathetic outflow	Hypotension, rebound hypertension, bradycardia, xerostomia, drowsiness, constipation, depression
Botulinum toxin	Inhibits presynaptic acetylcholine release by cleaving the SNAP-25 protein in the SNARE complex	Weakness, fatigue, flulike symptoms, dysphagia, complications associated with procedure, such as infection, bleeding, and pain Short-term effect (3–6 months) Possible antibody formation
Phenol	Neurotoxin that denatures proteins in the area surrounding the injection site	Dysesthesias, hypotension, prolonged pain, complications associated with procedure, such as infection, bleeding, and pain Longer lasting than botulinum toxin (6 months–1 year)

GABA, γ-aminobutyric acid; *LFT*, liver function tests; *MOA*, mechanism of action; *TBI*, traumatic brain injury.
Data from Iaccarino MA, Bhatnagar S, Zafonte R. Rehabilitation after traumatic brain injury. *HandbClin Neurol.* 2015;127:411–422. https://doi.org/10.1016/B978-0-444-52892-6.00026-X; Bhatnagar S, Iaccarino MA, Zafonte R. Pharmacotherapy in rehabilitation of post-acute traumatic brain injury. *Brain Res.* 2016;1640(Pt A):164–179. https://doi.org/10.1016/j.brainres.2016.01.021; Karri J, Mas MF, Francisco GE, Li S. Practice patterns for spasticity management with phenol neurolysis. *J Rehabil Med.* 2017;49(6):482–488. https://doi.org/10.2340/16501977-2239; Eapen BC, Allred DB, O'Rourke J, Cifu DX. Rehabilitation of moderate-to-severe traumatic brain injury. *Semin Neurol.* 2015;35(1):e1–e3. https://doi.org/10.1055/s-0035-1549094.

planning begins for ITB pump implantation. Patients must be educated on the potential complications of the ITB pump and the importance of regular long-term monitoring, as a mechanical failure of the pump or battery, a catheter block, or a lack of consistent follow-up can cause an abrupt cessation of ITB, which leads to life-threatening withdrawal symptoms such as fever, hallucinations, and seizures.[2,6,10]

Because of its invasive and irreversible nature, surgical interventions should be considered only after other treatment options have been exhausted. Orthopedic surgeries, such as tenotomy, myotomy, tendon transfer, and tendon lengthening procedures, can be considered to address deformities and contractures that may cause pain or increase the risk for complications such as wounds. Selective dorsal rhizotomy is a surgical intervention that has been performed to reduce spasticity, most commonly in children with spastic cerebral palsy. It has been indicated in spastic diplegia or quadriplegia but not spastic hemiplegia. During this procedure, selected dorsal roots are resected to decrease sensory input to the spinal reflex arc. Although selective dorsal rhizotomy has been used in TBI, there is limited information available in the current TBI literature.[2,11]

DEEP VENOUS THROMBOSIS

Although true incidence in the TBI population remains uncertain, there is undoubtedly substantial risk for development of venous thromboembolism (VTE), such as DVT and pulmonary embolism, in those hospitalized after moderate to severe TBIs. One 2011 multicenter trial investigating prophylaxis for VTE in the critically ill estimated that patients with TBI were four times more likely to develop VTE than patients in the medical and surgical intensive care unit (ICU).[12] Unfortunately, owing to the dearth of literature in the TBI population, controversy arises as to if and when to initiate pharmacologic prophylaxis when there is an underlying risk of progression of intracranial bleeds.[13]

A post hoc analysis of the erythropoietin in traumatic brain injury trial demonstrated that independent risk factors for VTE in the TBI population include severity of injury, older age, and increased weight. However, it was also noted that VTE was not independently associated with increased mortality.[13] Although findings were uncertain as to the effects of delayed chemoprophylaxis in that particular trial, a study by Tracy et al. that retrospectively reviewed 1425 patients sustaining either a TBI or spinal injuries found that pharmaceutical prophylaxis for VTE in patients with TBI was delayed twice as long and was associated with twice as many VTE events than that of patients with traumatic spinal injury.[14]

The American College of Chest Physicians reviewed this topic in their ninth iteration of the Antithrombotic Therapy and Prevention of Thrombosis consensus guidelines. They provide grade 2C evidence (a weak recommendation based on lower-quality evidence) to suggest use of chemoprophylaxis or mechanical prophylaxis over no prophylaxis for VTE in patients with TBI. They additionally suggest mechanical prophylaxis, specifically intermittent pneumatic compression stockings, when chemoprophylaxis is contraindicated owing to risk of bleeding. However, pharmacologic prophylaxis, either low-dose unfractionated heparin or low-molecular-weight heparin, should be added when that risk diminishes. Lastly, an IVC filter should not be a primary means of VTE prevention in this population, and periodic surveillance with ultrasound is not recommended.[15]

A 2015 literature review by Abdel-Aziz et al. offered more specific guidelines to aid in the administration of chemoprophylaxis after TBI. They recommend that chemoprophylaxis should be given when low-risk patients have not had enlargement of any intracerebral bleed within 48 h post injury, or on day 3 if they had developed hemorrhagic enlargement. In addition, chemoprophylaxis can be started in patients with diffuse axonal injury without intracranial bleed within 72 h. However, patients with moderate to severe TBI should not be given chemoprophylaxis within 3 days of injury. The authors also cautioned that the incidence of DVT increased when administration of chemoprophylaxis was delayed more than 1 week.[16]

PAROXYSMAL SYMPATHETIC HYPERACTIVITY

Paroxysmal sympathetic hyperactivity (PSH) has been defined in a 2014 consensus statement by Baguley et al. as "…a syndrome, recognized in a subgroup of survivors of severe acquired brain injury, of simultaneous, paroxysmal transient increases in sympathetic (elevated heart rate, blood pressure, respiratory rate, temperature, sweating) and motor (posturing) activity."[17] Previously, the syndrome has been known by several other names, including but not limited to sympathetic storming, dysautonomia, and paroxysmal autonomic instability with dystonia (Table 3.3).[18]

The pathophysiology of PSH has been hypothesized to be a disconnect between higher-order inhibitory centers of the brain and afferent stimuli from the spine, such that even innocuous stimuli can become overamplified and oversensitized, leading to hypersympathetic discharge.[19] This is evident with occurrence of symptomatology after mere touching, passive movement, and endotracheal tube suctioning, for example. Of course, more obvious conditions including constipation, catheter irritation, urinary retention, pressure

TABLE 3.3
Signs and Symptoms of PSH, With Graded Severity

Symptoms	Severity	Normal	Mild	Moderate	Severe
Heart rate		<100	100–119	120–139	≥140
Respiratory rate		<18	18–23	24–29	≥30
Systolic blood pressure		<140	140–159	160–179	≥180
Temperature		<37.0	37.0–37.9	38.0–38.9	≥39.0
Sweating		None	Mild	Moderate	Severe
Posturing		None	Mild	Moderate	Severe

PSH, paroxysmal sympathetic hyperactivity.
Adapted from Baguley IJ, Perkes IE, Fernandez-Ortega J-F, et al. Paroxysmal sympathetic hyperactivity after acquired brain injury: consensus on conceptual definition, nomenclature, and diagnostic criteria. *J Neurotrauma*. 2014;31(17):1515–1520, with permission.

wounds, and other painful or uncomfortable circumstances are culprits as well.

It is important to remember that PSH remains a diagnosis of exclusion,[20] and that the differential should remain wide to include seizures, intracranial hypertension, hydrocephalus, alcohol or sedative withdrawal, infection, and VTE, among other entities. Diagnostic likelihood may increase if symptoms occur simultaneously, are paroxysmal, occur with benign stimuli, persist longer than three consecutive days, persist greater than 2 weeks post injury, persist after treatment of potential alternative diagnoses, occur at greater than or equal to two episodes per day, appear without parasympathetic features, and/or lack other potential etiologies.[17] Studies show that the presence of PSH is associated with poor outcomes, including longer ICU stays, higher healthcare costs, decreased likelihood of emergence from vegetative state, and worse functional outcomes.[21,22]

In considering treatment options, an overall strategy to subdue sensory afferents to prevent allodynia, inhibit sympathetic outflow, and/or block the end organ response to that sympathetic outflow is suggested, but only after identifying and treating any possible triggers.[21] There is no consensus on treatment protocol, although a variety of medication options exist for potential management, including opioids, benzodiazepines, muscle relaxants, α-agonists, β-blockers, antiepileptics, and dopamine agonists. Morphine is a frequently used medication to subdue most symptoms of PSH, including hypertension and tachycardia, as allodynia can be an inciting factor overall in PSH. Caution must be taken, as side effects include constipation, sedation, tolerance, and respiratory depression.[23] Propranolol can also be used to help manage

tachycardia, hypertension, diaphoresis, and potentially dystonia, as it readily crosses the blood-brain barrier, reduces the metabolic rate, and has been shown to be independently associated with lower mortality as compared with other β-blockers. However, side effects include bradycardia and hypotension.[24,25] In certain cases, PSH may warrant the use of multiple medications to effectively control symptoms.[25] Regardless of choice, more research into effective treatment strategies is necessary.

NEUROENDOCRINE DYSFUNCTION

Neuroendocrine dysfunction, once considered a rare complication in the TBI population, has a prevalence that is estimated to be between 15% and 68%[26] according to a 2007 review by Schneider et al. This wide range is most likely because of the variation in the studies in patient selection, comorbidities, severity of TBI, and timing of evaluation[27]; therefore the prevalence and the incidence of neuroendocrine disturbances remain unclear.

There are several possible explanations for the pathophysiology of TBI-induced hypopituitarism, but it is most likely multifactorial. Because of the pituitary gland's anatomic location and blood supply, it is vulnerable to various insults such as direct trauma, compression secondary to edema, and vascular injury.[28] The gland sits within the bony sella turcica, with the diaphragm sellae located superiorly. Most of the blood supply to the anterior pituitary lobe comes from the long hypophyseal vessels, which are susceptible to injury or occlusion as they cross the diaphragm sellae, especially in the setting of skull base fractures or shearing injuries.[29]

In addition, there is a physiologic stress response that occurs in the acute phase of TBI. Thus consideration must be taken when evaluating for and replacing hormone deficiencies in the acute stage, because many of the stress-related deficiencies are transient.[27] Preliminary studies have shown a possible role of autoimmunity in TBI-induced hypopituitarism, but further studies are required to elucidate the presence of these antipituitary antibodies in patients with TBI.[30-32]

In the acute phase, or the first 10–14 days after TBI, evaluation of the hypothalamic-pituitary-adrenal axis and posterior pituitary function is recommended for patients with moderate to severe TBI and symptomatic patients with mild TBI.[33] Patients with TBI without pituitary gland injury have a physiologic increase in plasma cortisol concentration that normalizes after several days. In contrast, patients with a compromised pituitary gland may have inappropriately low cortisol levels requiring intravenous hydrocortisone. Because low levels of cortisol secondary to adrenocorticotropic hormone (ACTH) deficiency have been linked with hyponatremia, hypotension, and increased mortality, possible glucocorticoid deficiencies need to be identified and treated with glucocorticoid replacement.[27,34] An ACTH insufficiency should be considered when the plasma cortisol concentration is <300 nmol/L or when a patient has vague symptoms of fatigue, nausea, anorexia, or orthostasis with a plasma cortisol of 300–500 nmol/L.[8,29,33] Empiric glucocorticoid replacement should be initiated until dynamic testing is able to be performed. Symptomatic patients should be treated with parenteral glucocorticoids (hydrocortisone 200 mg daily), whereas asymptomatic patients may be administered oral hydrocortisone 20 mg three times daily.[29]

Posttraumatic central diabetes should be considered if a patient is found to have polyuria or hypernatremia. Diabetes insipidus (DI) can be diagnosed if plasma sodium is >145 nmol/L, urine osmolality is <300 mosmol/kg, and urine output is >3 L/day or >300 mL/h for two consecutive hours. Usually DI occurs within 2 days of pituitary injury and resolves by the third postoperative day. If it has not improved after 48 h, one dose of subcutaneous or intramuscular desmopressin should be given. It has been reported that failed recovery of vasopressin secretion is associated with increased mortality. Also, persistent DI may indicate increasing intracranial pressure or poor outcome.[29]

If hyponatremia is present, syndrome of inappropriate antidiuretic hormone (SIADH) or cerebral salt wasting should be considered. However, before treating hyponatremia, plasma cortisol concentrations should be checked. Several patients with hyponatremia have also been observed to be glucocorticoid deficient. When treated with hydrocortisone instead of fluid restriction, these patients were found to be responsive, suggesting that SIADH may be related to hypocortisolemia in the TBI population. After considering a glucocorticoid deficiency, the volume status of a patient should be assessed. SIADH is a euvolemic hyponatremia defined by a plasma osmolality <275 mosmol/kg, a urine osmolality >100 mosmol/kg, and a urinary sodium >40 mmol/L. The treatment for SIADH is fluid restriction. Cerebral salt wasting, although documented, is rarely seen in patients with TBI. Like SIADH, it is characterized by a plasma osmolality <275 mosmol/kg, a urine osmolality >100 mosmol/kg, and a urinary sodium >40 mmol/L, but it is a hypovolemic hyponatremia, not euvolemic. The treatment for cerebral salt wasting is intravenous saline fluid replacement.[29]

Aside from investigating for ACTH deficiency or DI, pituitary function should be assessed at a follow-up evaluation 3–6 months after TBI.[27,33] The current literature states pituitary dysfunctions observed are often transient and recover in the first few months. Furthermore, new deficiencies that were not present during the acute phase may appear months after injury, but they rarely develop after 6 months. Also, this chronic stage is more likely to be conducive for dynamic testing required for a neuroendocrine evaluation.[29] Baseline thyroid function tests should be obtained, because hypothyroidism has been linked with cognitive deficits in executive functioning, information processing, and memory.[30] Patients with hypothyroidism may complain of cold intolerance, fatigue, hair loss, and weight gain. In addition, testosterone, luteinizing hormone, and follicle-stimulating hormone levels should also be obtained. Symptoms of hypogonadism include sexual dysfunction, menstrual irregularities, secondary hair loss, and decreased bone mass.[33] In the rehabilitation setting, lower testosterone levels in men have been found to correlate with lower functional independence measure (FIM) scores on admission and at discharge.[34a] Once treated with hormone replacement therapy, all deficiencies should be reassessed at a 1-year follow-up visit. During this evaluation, growth hormone deficiency should be ruled out because of its association with poor stamina, dyslipidemia, insulin resistance, and decreased bone mass, as well as impaired cognitive performance, depression, and higher disability scores.[30,33,35] Because growth hormone may recover up to 5 years after TBI, it should not be checked and replaced until at least 12 months post injury.[30]

HETEROTOPIC OSSIFICATION

The abnormal formation of ectopic lamellar bone in soft tissue is known as heterotopic ossification (HO), which can be seen in 4%–23%[36] of patients with TBI. HO tends to deposit around larger joints, such as the hips, knees, and shoulders.[37] The resulting effects can include loss of range of motion, limitations on mobility and function, chronic pain, and decreased quality of life.

Diagnosis is first established through physical examination, whereby HO can initially present with pain, swelling, erythema, and motion limitation across a joint. With such nonspecific symptoms, it is important to keep a broad differential in mind, including VTE, cellulitis, occult fracture, and septic joint.[38]

If and when HO is suspected, a choice of imaging modalities can be considered, but it is important to remember that HO may be radiographically undetectable until at least 3 weeks post injury. In addition, specificity is low for bone scans and MRI. Blood markers are also nonspecific and include erythrocyte sedimentation rate, C-reactive peptide, and serum alkaline phosphatase.[38,39] Ultrasound imaging has recently gained traction as a potential aid in early diagnosis owing to ease and cost-effectiveness but requires a significant level of competency.[40] A combination of these diagnostic modalities may be the best option, especially when diagnosis remains equivocal.

Prophylactic treatment options should be considered early as to limit functional disability and pain. Nonsteroidal antiinflammatory drugs (NSAIDs), such as indomethacin, help in the prevention of HO through cytotoxic inhibition of osteoblast cells.[41] Unfortunately, NSAIDs carry with them a side-effect profile that includes a risk of long bone nonunion, which is an important consideration in patients with comorbid orthopedic injuries.[42] Concern for gastrointestinal ulcers with NSAID use also exists and may warrant consideration of cyclooxygenase-2 inhibitors as an alternative, as they have been shown to have comparable efficacy.[43] Bisphosphonates are a third option, but controversy exists as to their overall efficacy, and they carry a side-effect profile that includes gastrointestinal distress and jaw osteonecrosis.[44] Finally, radiation has been proved to be effective for preventative treatment of HO at the hip joint, but further studies are required to determine efficacy at other joints, and it carries the risk of delayed wound healing, soft tissue contractures, nonunion, and, theoretically, cancer.[45]

Debate exists as to whether a contributing factor to the development of HO is excessive movement versus limited movement, thus creating uncertainty of physical therapy as a direct treatment option. However, it can be a valued modality to maintain strength, improve mechanics, and assess the need for durable medical equipment.[46]

Surgical excision is currently the mainstay treatment when HO begins to elicit intractable pain, create functional limitations, or cause other severe medical consequences. However, questions remain in regards to timing of excision. A systematic review by Almangour et al. reports that timing, severity of sequelae, or size of the HO may not be associated with the risk of recurrence after excision. Thus surgical excision is recommended as soon as HO is fully formed.[36]

NUTRITION

Secondary to the endocrine disturbances and inflammatory cascade that occur after brain injury, patients with TBI experience metabolic changes that lead to increased energy expenditure.[47] According to Foley et al., the mean energy expenditure during the first 30 days post injury ranged from 75% to 200%, with the lowest values representing patients with brain death who have decreased oxygen consumption. The review also showed that sedatives, paralyzing agents, and barbiturates reduce metabolic rates, whereas steroids do not.[48]

Hypermetabolism, which is proportional to the severity of TBI, can result in malnutrition, hyperglycemia, poor wound healing, and hypercatabolism of proteins, resulting in muscle wasting and increased urinary nitrogen excretion.[49] To achieve nitrogen equilibrium, the general recommended protein dose is at least 2.0–2.5 g/kg/day.[49,50] According to the Brain Trauma Foundation guidelines, basal caloric replacement should be achieved in 5–7 days post injury to decrease mortality.[51,52] In a small prospective study of 59 patients, Chourdakis et al. suggest that early enteral feeding, defined as within 24–48 h of admission, may improve TBI-induced neuroendocrine disturbances.[53]

Often, oral intake for patients with TBI is not possible because of to facial trauma, swallowing dysfunction, or altered consciousness. In these cases, the placement of a nasogastric tube (NGT) or a percutaneous endoscopic gastrostomy (PEG) is necessary to ensure that appropriate nutrition is provided. Although an NGT may be adequate initially, a PEG is eventually required because of the prolonged recovery of TBI.[54] The route of feeding has been found to have no statistically significant impact on the mortality or length of stay in the intensive care unit.[47,55] However, there seems to be a general consensus that enteral nutrition is the recommended method, whereas parenteral supplementation is to be utilized when enteral nutrition is not obtainable or insufficient because of factors such as dysphagia and gastroparesis.[47,49,56] No significant difference in the rate of pneumonia has been established between parenteral and enteral nutrition,[47,52] but there may be a decreased rate of ventilator-associated pneumonia in patients with transpyloric feedings compared with those who received gastric feedings.[57]

Although most nutritional studies refer to patients with severe TBI in the acute setting, Horn et al. addressed enteral nutrition in the inpatient rehabilitation setting. The study showed that patients who received enteral nutrition for 25% or more of the rehabilitation stay had better discharge FIM motor and cognitive scores than those who did not receive enteral nutrition, but no statistical significance was found for length of stay. Unfortunately, this study was limited, because the patients' acute hospitalization course, which includes previous nutritional supplementation, was not available.[57]

BLADDER/BOWEL DYSFUNCTION

Bowel and bladder dysfunction in TBI is frequently encountered and often complicated by cognitive deficits, inability to communicate needs, and behavioral conditions.[58] The incidence of urinary incontinence within 6 weeks of acute TBI is 62%.[58] In TBI, urinary incontinence is often due to detrusor overactivity.[59,60] It has been found to significantly correlate with diffuse and bilateral injury, the presence of aphasia, and diabetes. In addition, it has been associated with a longer acute length of stay before rehabilitation. Once admitted to the rehabilitation unit, patients with urinary incontinence tend to have a longer length of stay, poorer functional status on admission, and lower functional level at discharge. Similarly, urinary retention, with only an 8% incidence, has been strongly associated with poorer functional status, fecal impaction, diabetes, and aphasia.[58] Bladder dysfunction overall in this population has been linked to an increased risk of urinary tract infections and decubitus ulcer.[61]

Before initiating treatment, common causes of urinary disturbances such as urinary tract infection and benign prostatic hyperplasia should be ruled out. All medications should be reviewed for possible urinary side effects. Treatments for bladder dysfunction include bladder/pelvic floor training and timed voiding. Medications such as oxybutynin have been prescribed to treat bladder overactivity, but caution is warranted, as anticholinergics are generally discouraged in TBI because of their undesired effects on cognition.[60] Except in hypotensive patients, urinary retention can be treated with α-blockers, such as tamsulosin. Intermittent catheterization and indwelling catheterization are treatment options for urinary retention, especially when patients present with pressures sores or require strict input and output monitoring. Indwelling catheters can also be considered for patients with poor functional hand use or cognitive impairment. Unfortunately, there are many potential complications of catheterization, which include urinary tract infection, bladder distention, urethral trauma, bladder stones, epididymitis, and bladder cancer. It is for these reasons that catheterization should be utilized after all other interventions.[62]

Neurogenic bowel can present as incontinence, constipation, or both. Insults to the voluntary defecation center in the frontal lobe may lead to incontinence because of a loss of external sphincter control. On admission to inpatient rehabilitation, the incidence of bowel incontinence has been found to be 68%. This high incidence has been attributed to the motor and cognitive deficits in patients with moderate to severe TBI. The incidence of fecal incontinence at discharge and at 1-year follow-up is reported to be 12.4% and 5.2%, respectively.[63] Treatment of fecal incontinence includes increased fiber and fluid intake, bulking medications, and scheduled assistance to the toilet.[64] Without treatment, patients with incontinence are at risk for skin infections and pressure ulcers.[63]

Constipation in TBI occurs because of an upper motor neuron injury leading to hyperreflexive bowel, increased rectal compliance, and increased anal sphincter tone resulting in stool retention. The initial management of constipation should include adequate hydration and increased fiber intake. Medications often used for constipation are stool softeners, prokinetic agents, and suppositories.[64]

Although bowel and bladder dysfunctions are well-known complications of TBI, the current literature is sparse in regards to this specific population. More research is needed in this area to allow for improved, evidence-based, standardized care.

SLEEP DISTURBANCES

Sleep disturbances are complications affecting 30%–70% of individuals following a TBI.[65] These disturbances include insomnia, pleiosomnia (hypersomnia), excessive daytime sleepiness, and circadian sleep-wake disorders.[66] The pathophysiology of posttraumatic sleep disorder is proposed to be dependent on the location of injury within regions of the brain that regulate sleep, providing a possible explanation for the various symptoms encountered in the TBI population. Damage to the basal forebrain, an area involved in sleep initiation, may result in insomnia, whereas injury to the regions responsible for wakefulness, specifically the brainstem reticular formation and posterior hypothalamus, could lead to hypersomnia.[65] Compromise of the hypothalamic suprachiasmatic nuclei, known as the control center of circadian rhythms, is implicated in the dysregulation of circadian sleep-wakefulness secondary to changes in melatonin levels.[65,67]

Diagnosis of posttraumatic sleep disturbances should begin with a patient history that provides a timeline of the sleep disorder in relation to the brain injury, ruling out a preexisting sleep condition.[65] The nature and severity of symptoms can be revealed with a sleep diary and self-reported questionnaires, whereas polysomnography, actinography, and multiple sleep latency testing can be useful to objectively support a diagnosis of posttraumatic sleep disorder.[65,68]

When choosing a treatment course, sleep hygiene education is an appropriate first step. Patients should be counseled on regular sleep-wake times, daytime exercise, decreased evening caffeine consumption, decreased use of alcohol or illicit substances, and avoidance of television in bed.[6,69] Meditation, acupuncture, and cognitive-behavioral therapy show promise as additional nonpharmacologic treatment options, but further research is required with large clinical trials.[65,66,68] Medical and psychiatric comorbidities, such as obstructive sleep apnea, pain, depression, and posttraumatic stress disorder, should be considered and addressed before initiating medication for sleep.[65]

Although there are several medications that can be used to treat sleep disorders (see Table 3.4), there is insufficient evidence showing the use of these pharmacologic treatments in TBI. Most of the current literature does not include the TBI population, provides conflicting reports, or is limited by sample size. Therefore, until more research becomes available, information must be inferred from research with patients of other neurologic conditions.[6,70]

SEXUALITY/INTIMACY

TBI has been well-documented to have a negative impact on social relationships and intimacy. More than 50% of individuals with TBI experience changes in sexuality up to 5 years after injury.[73] These changes include hypersexuality, decreased sexual drive, decreased arousal, inability to achieve orgasm, ejaculatory dysfunction, or dissatisfaction with sex.[74]

Anatomically, the frontal lobes and limbic and paralimbic regions of the brain have been linked to libido, sexual assertiveness and initiation, and sexual preferences. The pituitary gland and hypothalamus are major components of the neuroendocrine system, regulating levels of testosterone, progesterone, and estrogen levels.[75] Physiologically, dopamine has been shown to have an excitatory effect on sexual desire, whereas serotonin has been found to possess an inhibitory effect. TBI has the potential to damage these anatomic structures and physiologic pathways to ultimately lead to alterations in sexual function.[76]

Hypersexuality is an increase in sexual drive that can potentially lead to inappropriate sexual behaviors. With a prevalence rate of 8.9%, behaviors such as inappropriate sexual talk (most common), nongenital touching, self-exposure, and genital touching are believed to be due to a lack of inhibition and are often associated with frontal lobe dysfunction and right hemisphere lesions.[77] According to the current literature, a higher TBI severity, younger age, a lower level of social participation, and greater neuropsychiatric problems increase the risk for inappropriate sexual behaviors. Preinjury psychosocial conditions, such as unemployment, substance abuse, psychiatric history, and intelligence quotient, have been found to have no relevance.[78,79]

Individuals with TBI have reported decreased sexuality more frequently than hypersexuality. In these cases, it is important to realize that sexual function is complex and requires consideration of multiple factors. Owing to their injury, patients can have diminished sexual responses, which include erection and ejaculation for men and lubrication for women. They can have physical limitations secondary to headaches, fatigue, auditory and visual impairments, decreased functional mobility, and spasticity. Oral-motor dysfunction can hinder kissing and romantic vocalizations, whereas urinary and fecal incontinence can cause undesired anxiety or embarrassment. Also, patients with TBI are often prescribed medications that have side effects that interfere with sexual functioning. Antihypertensives, antidepressants, stimulants, anticonvulsants, and antipsychotics can be culprits for decreased sexuality.[75] Furthermore, the TBI population struggles with social integration because of cognitive changes as well as impairments in communication and emotional functioning that eventually lead to loss of friendships

TABLE 3.4
Medications Used for the Treatment of Sleep Disturbances

Medication	Mechanism of Action	Side Effects and Special Considerations
Benzodiazepine	Bind to $GABA_A$ receptor nonselectively to increase GABA inhibitory activity	Drowsiness, dizziness, weakness, fatigue, respiratory depression, hypotension Should be avoided in TBI owing to cognitive side effects May alter sleep architecture: increase non-REM N2 sleep and decrease REM and non-REM N3 (slow-wave) sleep Not appropriate for long-term use Abuse potential
Nonbenzodiazepine GABA receptor agonist (zolpidem)	Selectively binds to $GABA_A$ receptor 1 subtype	Drowsiness, dizziness, headache Shorter half-life than benzodiazepines Possible unknown cognitive side effects similar to benzodiazepines
Trazodone	Serotonin receptor antagonist	Drowsiness, dry mouth, dizziness, headache, priapism Risk for QT prolongation when used with SSRIs
Methylphenidate	Unknown, but thought to block dopamine reuptake	Tachycardia, hypertension, palpitations, weight loss, hyperactivity, insomnia Tolerance may develop
Modafinil	Unknown, but may act to increase levels of dopamine	Headache, nausea, anxiety, insomnia
Prazosin	α1 adrenergic antagonist	Drowsiness, dizziness, headache, weakness, nausea, palpitations
Melatonin	Endogenous hormone that acts on MT_1 and MT_2 receptors in the suprachiasmatic nucleus to regulate sleep-wake cycle	Drowsiness, dizziness, fatigue, headache, abdominal cramping May decrease sleep latency
Ramelteon	Melatonin receptor agonist that targets the MT_1 and MT_2 receptors in the suprachiasmatic nucleus	Somnolence, dizziness, headache, fatigue, nausea May increase total sleep time

GABA, γ-aminobutyric acid; REM, rapid eye movement; SSRI, selective serotonin reuptake inhibitor; TBI, traumatic brain injury.
Data from Bhatnagar S, Iaccarino MA, Zafonte R. Pharmacotherapy in rehabilitation of post-acute traumatic brain injury. Brain Res. 2016;1640(Pt A):164–179. https://doi.org/10.1016/j.brainres.2016.01.021; Larson EB, Zollman FS. The effect of sleep medications on cognitive recovery from traumatic brain injury. J Head Trauma Rehabil. 2010;25(1):61–67. https://doi.org/10.1097/HTR.0b013e3181c1d1e1; Kallweit U, Bassetti CL. Pharmacological management of narcolepsy with and without cataplexy. Expert OpinPharmacother. 2017;18(8):809–817. https://doi.org/10.1080/14656566.2017.1323877; Lequerica A, Jasey N, Portelli Tremont JN, Chiaravalloti ND. Pilot study on the effect of Ramelteon on sleep disturbance after traumatic brain injury: preliminary evidence from a clinical trial. Arch Phys Med Rehabil. 2015;96(10):1802–1809. https://doi.org/10.1016/j.apmr.2015.05.011.

and difficulty forming new relationships.[80] An attention deficit may appear as disinterest to a sexual partner, especially when it affects arousal. The role change of the spouse to a caregiver position can shift the wife-husband partnership to a parent-child relationship, discouraging an intimate and sexual relationship.[75,80] The psychological symptoms of TBI, such as adjustment troubles, perception of unattractiveness, anxiety, and depression, can further affect sexual well-being

and, unfortunately, initiate an emotional distance between partners. The separation or divorce rate in TBI has been reported to be 15%–54%.[80]

To manage and treat disorders of sexuality, a comprehensive and holistic approach should be utilized. Physicians should begin with a thorough medication review and a complete workup that screens for neuroendocrine dysfunctions and medical comorbidities that may affect sexual function. A gynecologic or urologic examination may also be necessary. Medications to address issues such as erectile dysfunction, pain, or spasticity can be considered.

An interdisciplinary approach may be beneficial. Physicians can refer to physical therapy for education on optimizing positioning or occupational therapy for adaptive aids and equipment. A speech therapist can assist with cognitive barriers to sexuality, and a family therapist can counsel on emotional and social issues. Lastly, a sexual health educator or sex therapist may help provide education on safe sex practices and sex strategies.[75,79]

TRAUMATIC BRAIN INJURY AND SPINAL CORD INJURY

Incidence of TBI in spinal cord–injured patients has been estimated to approach 60%,[81] but TBI often remains undiagnosed. In fact, a 2014 Canadian study of 92 spinal cord–injured patients found that TBI went undiagnosed in 58.5% of their sample.[82] This may be due to the overshadowing of the spinal cord injury (SCI) itself, lack of standardization of diagnostic criteria for TBI, the inability to assess for TBI because of sedation or intubation, or the resolution of mild TBI symptomatology before evaluation.[82,83]

Regardless, the potential for TBI to interfere in the rehabilitation of spinal cord–injured patients is significant, and, without proper identification and management, it could lead to an increased length of stay or, worse, a serious adverse event. Difficulty with memory, attention, and executive functioning due to TBI may limit the typical course of recovery in spinal cord–injured patients. Agitation and irritability may appear as voluntary noncompliance.[84] Furthermore, medications to address either clinical entity may negatively affect the other.

Of note, the presence of a dual diagnosis does not necessarily portend poor outcome. A prospective study by Macciocchi et al. of 189 spinal cord–injured patients found that in the tetraplegic population, co-occurring TBI was not related to FIM motor outcomes, and, in the paraplegic population, only severe TBI, but not mild or moderate TBI, worsened FIM motor outcomes.[81] A more recent case-matched cohort study by Nott et al. had similar positive findings, demonstrating that patients with dual diagnosis achieved comparable or better functional outcomes and employment and community participation than the SCI or TBI alone group, although longer lengths of rehabilitation may have played a role.[85]

As we await standardized clinical practice guidelines for this subset of patients, it remains essential to maintain a high level of suspicion for a diagnosis of TBI in spinal cord–injured patients. A prompt diagnosis will better equip the team to make appropriate accommodations and interventions for successful rehabilitation programs.

SUMMARY

Complications are many when caring for patients with TBI, and the evidence base for management strategies is not as robust as some areas of medical practice. However, it is of utmost importance to remain vigilant and with a mindset on prevention to provide the best possible outcomes in this specialized population.

REFERENCES

1. Omar M, Moore L, Lauzier F, et al. Complications following hospital admission for traumatic brain injury: a multicenter cohort study. *J Crit Care*. 2017;41:1–8. https://doi.org/10.1016/j.jcrc.2017.04.031.

2. Kheder A, Nair KPS. Spasticity: pathophysiology, evaluation and management. *Pract Neurol*. 2012;12(5):289–298. https://doi.org/10.1136/practneurol-2011-000155.

3. Abolhasani H, Ansari NN, Naghdi S, Mansouri K, Ghotbi N, Hasson S. Comparing the validity of the modified modified Ashworth scale (MMAS) and the modified Tardieu scale (MTS) in the assessment of wrist flexor spasticity in patients with stroke: protocol for a neurophysiological study. *BMJ Open*. 2012;2(6). https://doi.org/10.1136/bmjopen-2012-001394.

4. Li F, Wu Y; Li X. Test-retest reliability and inter-rater reliability of the modified Tardieu scale and the modified Ashworth scale in hemiplegic patients with stroke. *Eur J Phys Rehabil Med*. 2014;50(1):9–15.

5. Iaccarino MA, Bhatnagar S, Zafonte R. Rehabilitation after traumatic brain injury. *Handb Clin Neurol*. 2015;127:411–422. https://doi.org/10.1016/B978-0-444-52892-6.00026-X.

6. Bhatnagar S, Iaccarino MA, Zafonte R. Pharmacotherapy in rehabilitation of post-acute traumatic brain injury. *Brain Res*. 2016;1640(Pt A):164–179. https://doi.org/10.1016/j.brainres.2016.01.021.

7. Karri J, Mas MF, Francisco GE, Li S. Practice patterns for spasticity management with phenol neurolysis. *J Rehabil Med*. 2017;49(6):482–488. https://doi.org/10.2340/16501977-2239.

8. Eapen BC, Allred DB, O'Rourke J, Cifu DX. Rehabilitation of moderate-to-severe traumatic brain injury. *Semin Neurol*. 2015;35(1):e1–e3. https://doi.org/10.1055/s-0035-1549094.

9. Pérez-Arredondo A, Cázares-Ramírez E, Carrillo-Mora P, et al. Baclofen in the therapeutic of sequele of traumatic brain injury: spasticity. *Clin Neuropharmacol*. 2016;39(6):311–319.https://doi.org/10.1097/WNF.0000000000000179.

10. Boster AL, Bennett SE, Bilsky GS, et al. Best practices for intrathecal baclofen therapy: screening test. *Neuromodulation*. 2016;19(6):616–622. https://doi.org/10.1111/ner.12437.

11. Gump WC, Mutchnick IS, Moriarty TM. Selective dorsal rhizotomy for spasticity not associated with cerebral palsy: reconsideration of surgical inclusion criteria. *Neurosurg Focus*. 2013;35(5):E6. https://doi.org/10.3171/2013.8.FOCUS13294.

12. PROTECT Investigators for the Canadian Critical Care Trials Group, Australian and New Zealand Intensive Care Society Clinical Trials Group, Cook D, et al. Dalteparin versus unfractionated heparin in critically ill patients. *N Engl J Med*. 2011;364(14):1305–1314. https://doi.org/10.1056/NEJMoa1014475.

13. Skrifvars MB, Bailey M, Presneill J, et al. Venous thromboembolic events in critically ill traumatic brain injury patients. *Intensive Care Med*. 2017;43(3):419–428. https://doi.org/10.1007/s00134-016-4655-2.

14. Tracy BM, Dunne JR, O'Neal CM, Clayton E. Venous thromboembolism prophylaxis in neurosurgical trauma patients. *J Surg Res*. 2016;205(1):221–227. https://doi.org/10.1016/j.jss.2016.06.049.

15. Guyatt GH, Akl EA, Crowther M, Gutterman DD, Schuünemann HJ, American College of Chest Physicians Antithrombotic Therapy and Prevention of Thrombosis Panel. Executive summary: antithrombotic therapy and prevention of thrombosis, 9th ed: American College of Chest Physicians evidence-based clinical practice guidelines. *Chest*. 2012;141(suppl 2):S7–S47. https://doi.org/10.1378/chest.1412S3.

16. Abdel-Aziz H, Dunham CM, Malik RJ, Hileman BM. Timing for deep vein thrombosis chemoprophylaxis in traumatic brain injury: an evidence-based review. *Crit Care Lond Engl*. 2015;19:96. https://doi.org/10.1186/s13054-015-0814-z.

17. Baguley IJ, Perkes IE, Fernandez-Ortega J-F, et al. Paroxysmal sympathetic hyperactivity after acquired brain injury: consensus on conceptual definition, nomenclature, and diagnostic criteria. *J Neurotrauma*. 2014;31(17):1515–1520. https://doi.org/10.1089/neu.2013.3301.

18. Perkes IE, Menon DK, Nott MT, Baguley IJ. Paroxysmal sympathetic hyperactivity after acquired brain injury: a review of diagnostic criteria. *Brain Inj*. 2011;25(10):925–932. https://doi.org/10.3109/02699052.2011.589797.

19. Baguley IJ, Nott MT, Slewa-Younan S, Heriseanu RE, Perkes IE. Diagnosing dysautonomia after acute traumatic brain injury: evidence for overresponsiveness to afferent stimuli. *Arch Phys Med Rehabil*. 2009;90(4):580–586. https://doi.org/10.1016/j.apmr.2008.10.020.

20. Rabinstein AA, Benarroch EE. Treatment of paroxysmal sympathetic hyperactivity. *Curr Treat Options Neurol*. 2008;10(2):151–157.

21. Lump D, Moyer M. Paroxysmal sympathetic hyperactivity after severe brain injury. *Curr Neurol Neurosci Rep*. 2014;14(11):494. https://doi.org/10.1007/s11910-014-0494-0.

22. Baguley IJ. Autonomic complications following central nervous system injury. *Semin Neurol*. 2008;28(5):716–725. https://doi.org/10.1055/s-0028-1105971.

23. Baguley IJ, Cameron ID, Green AM, Slewa-Younan S, Marosszeky JE, Gurka JA. Pharmacological management of dysautonomia following traumatic brain injury. *Brain Inj*. 2004;18(5):409–417. https://doi.org/10.1080/02699050310001645775.

24. Schroeppel TJ, Sharpe JP, Magnotti LJ, et al. Traumatic brain injury and β-blockers: not all drugs are created equal. *J Trauma Acute Care Surg*. 2014;76(2):504–509. Discussion 509, https://doi.org/10.1097/TA.0000000000000104.

25. Meyfroidt G, Baguley IJ, Menon DK. Paroxysmal sympathetic hyperactivity: the storm after acute brain injury. *Lancet Neurol*. 2017;16(9):721–729. https://doi.org/10.1016/S1474-4422(17)30259-4.

26. Schneider HJ, Kreitschmann-Andermahr I, Ghigo E, Stalla GK, Agha A. Hypothalamopituitary dysfunction following traumatic brain injury and aneurysmal subarachnoid hemorrhage: a systematic review. *JAMA*. 2007;298(12):1429–1438. https://doi.org/10.1001/jama.298.12.1429.

27. Glynn N, Agha A. Which patient requires neuroendocrine assessment following traumatic brain injury, when and how? *Clin Endocrinol (Oxf)*. 2013;78(1):17–20. https://doi.org/10.1111/cen.12010.

28. Renner CIE. Interrelation between neuroendocrine disturbances and medical complications encountered during rehabilitation after TBI. *J Clin Med*. 2015;4(9):1815–1840. https://doi.org/10.3390/jcm4091815.

29. Palta JR, Ayyangar KM, Suntharalingam N, Tupchong L. Asymmetric field arc rotations. *Br J Radiol*. 1989;62(742):927–931. https://doi.org/10.1259/0007-1285-62-742-927.

30. Tanriverdi F, Schneider HJ, Aimaretti G, Masel BE, Casanueva FF, Kelestimur F. Pituitary dysfunction after traumatic brain injury: a clinical and pathophysiological approach. *Endocr Rev*. 2015;36(3):305–342. https://doi.org/10.1210/er.2014-1065.

31. Tanriverdi F, De Bellis A, Bizzarro A, et al. Antipituitary antibodies after traumatic brain injury: is head trauma-induced pituitary dysfunction associated with autoimmunity? *Eur J Endocrinol*. 2008;159(1):7–13. https://doi.org/10.1530/EJE-08-0050.

32. Tanriverdi F, De Bellis A, Ulutabanca H, et al. A five year prospective investigation of anterior pituitary function after traumatic brain injury: is hypopituitarism long-term after head trauma associated with autoimmunity? *J Neurotrauma*. 2013;30(16):1426–1433. https://doi.org/10.1089/neu.2012.2752.

33. Tritos NA, Yuen KCJ, Kelly DF, AACE Neuroendocrine and Pituitary Scientific Committee. American Association of Clinical Endocrinologists and American College of Endocrinology disease state clinical review: a neuroendocrine approach to patients with traumatic brain injury. *Endocr Pract*. 2015;21(7):823–831. https://doi.org/10.4158/EP14567.DSCR.

34. Hannon MJ, Crowley RK, Behan LA, et al. Acute glucocorticoid deficiency and diabetes insipidus are common after acute traumatic brain injury and predict mortality. *J Clin Endocrinol Metab*. 2013;98(8):3229–3237. https://doi.org/10.1210/jc.2013-1555.

34a. Carlson NE, et al. Hypogonadism on Admission to Acute Rehabilitation Is Correlated with Lower Functional Status at Admission and Discharge *Brain Injury*. 2009;23(4):336–344. https://doi.org/10.1080/02699050902788535.

35. Kreber LA, Griesbach GS, Ashley MJ. Detection of growth hormone deficiency inadults with chronic traumatic brain injury. *J Neurotrauma*. 2016;33(17):1607–1613. https://doi.org/10.1089/neu.2015.4127.

36. Almangour W, Schnitzler A, Salga M, Debaud C, Denormandie P, Genêt F. Recurrence of heterotopic ossification after removal in patients with traumatic brain injury: a systematic review. *Ann Phys Rehabil Med*. 2016;59(4):263–269. https://doi.org/10.1016/j.rehab.2016.03.009.

37. Brady RD, Shultz SR, McDonald SJ, O'Brien TJ. Neurological heterotopic ossification: current understanding and future directions. *Bone*. 2017. https://doi.org/10.1016/j.bone.2017.05.015.

38. Gil JA, Waryasz GR, Klyce W, Daniels AH. Heterotopic ossification in neurorehabilitation. *R I Med J 2013*. 2015;98(12):32–34.

39. Sung Hsieh HH, Chung MT, Allen RM, et al. Evaluation of salivary cytokines for diagnosis of both trauma-induced and genetic heterotopic ossification. *Front Endocrinol*. 2017;8:74. https://doi.org/10.3389/fendo.2017.00074.

40. Stefanidis K, Brindley P, Ramnarine R, et al. Bedside ultrasound to facilitate early diagnosis and ease of follow-up in neurogenic heterotopic ossification: a pilot study from the intensive care unit. *J Head Trauma Rehabil*. 2017. https://doi.org/10.1097/HTR.0000000000000293.

41. Chang J-K, Li C-J, Liao H-J, Wang C-K, Wang G-J, Ho M-L. Anti-inflammatory drugs suppress proliferation and induce apoptosis through altering expressions of cell cycle regulators and pro-apoptotic factors in cultured human osteoblasts. *Toxicology*. 2009;258(2–3):148–156. https://doi.org/10.1016/j.tox.2009.01.016.

42. Sagi HC, Jordan CJ, Barei DP, Serrano-Riera R, Steverson B. Indomethacin prophylaxis for heterotopic ossification after acetabular fracture surgery increases the risk for nonunion of the posterior wall. *J Orthop Trauma*. 2014;28(7):377–383. https://doi.org/10.1097/BOT.0000000000000049.

43. Vasileiadis GI, Sioutis IC, Mavrogenis AF, Vlasis K, Babis GC, Papagelopoulos PJ. COX-2 inhibitors for the prevention of heterotopic ossification after THA. *Orthopedics*. 2011;34(6):467. https://doi.org/10.3928/01477447-20110427-23.

44. Ranganathan K, Loder S, Agarwal S, et al. Heterotopic ossification: basic-science principles and clinical correlates. *J Bone Joint Surg Am*. 2015;97(13):1101–1111. https://doi.org/10.2106/JBJS.N.01056.

45. Hamid N, Ashraf N, Bosse MJ, et al. Radiation therapy for heterotopic ossification prophylaxis acutely after elbow trauma: a prospective randomized study. *J Bone Joint Surg Am*. 2010;92(11):2032–2038. https://doi.org/10.2106/JBJS.I.01435.

46. Sullivan MP, Torres SJ, Mehta S, Ahn J. Heterotopic ossification after central nervous system trauma: a current review. *Bone Jt Res*. 2013;2(3):51–57. https://doi.org/10.1302/2046-3758.23.2000152.

47. Costello L-AS, Lithander FE, Gruen RL, Williams LT. Nutrition therapy in the optimisation of health outcomes in adult patients with moderate to severe traumatic brain injury: findings from a scoping review. *Injury*. 2014;45(12):1834–1841. https://doi.org/10.1016/j.injury.2014.06.004.

48. Foley N, Marshall S, Pikul J, Salter K, Teasell R. Hypermetabolism following moderate to severe traumatic acute brain injury: a systematic review. *J Neurotrauma*. 2008;25(12):1415–1431. https://doi.org/10.1089/neu.2008.0628.

49. Vizzini A, Aranda-Michel J. Nutritional support in head injury. *Nutr Burbank Los Angel Cty Calif*. 2011;27(2):129–132. https://doi.org/10.1016/j.nut.2010.05.004.

50. Dickerson RN, Pitts SL, Maish GO, et al. A reappraisal of nitrogen requirements for patients with critical illness and trauma. *J Trauma Acute Care Surg*. 2012;73(3):549–557. https://doi.org/10.1097/TA.0b013e318256de1b.

51. Brain Trauma Foundation, American Association of Neurological Surgeons, Congress of Neurological Surgeons, et al. Guidelines for the management of severe traumatic brain injury. XII. Nutrition. *J Neurotrauma*. 2007;24(suppl 1):S77–S82. https://doi.org/10.1089/neu.2006.9984.

52. Carney N, Totten AM, O'Reilly C, et al. Guidelines for the management of severe traumatic brain injury, fourth edition. *Neurosurgery*. 2017;80(1):6–15. https://doi.org/10.1227/NEU.0000000000001432.

53. Chourdakis M, Kraus MM, Tzellos T, et al. Effect of early compared with delayed enteral nutrition on endocrine function in patients with traumatic brain injury: an open-labeled randomized trial. *J Parenter Enteral Nutr*. 2012;36(1):108–116. https://doi.org/10.1177/0148607110397878.

54. Chaudhry R, Kukreja N, Tse A, et al. Trends and outcomes of early versus late percutaneous endoscopic gastrostomy placement in patients with traumatic brain injury: nationwide population-based study. *J Neurosurg Anesthesiol*. 2017. https://doi.org/10.1097/ANA.0000000000000434.

55. Wang X, Dong Y, Han X, Qi X-Q, Huang C-G, Hou L-J. Nutritional support for patients sustaining traumatic brain injury: a systematic review and meta-analysis of prospective studies. *PLoS One*. 2013;8(3):e58838. https://doi.org/10.1371/journal.pone.0058838.

56. Horn SD, Kinikini M, Moore LW, et al. Enteral nutrition for patients with traumatic brain injury in the rehabilitation setting: associations with patient preinjury and injury characteristics and outcomes. *Arch Phys Med Rehabil*. 2015;96(8 suppl):S245–S255. https://doi.org/10.1016/j.apmr.2014.06.024.

57. Acosta-Escribano J, Fernández-Vivas M, Grau Carmona T, et al. Gastric versus transpyloric feeding in severe traumatic brain injury: a prospective, randomized trial. *Intensive Care Med*. 2010;36(9):1532–1539. https://doi.org/10.1007/s00134-010-1908-3.

58. Chua K, Chuo A, Kong KH. Urinary incontinence after traumatic brain injury: incidence, outcomes and correlates. *Brain Inj*. 2003;17(6):469–478. https://doi.org/10.1080/0269905021054268.

59. Giannantoni A, Silvestro D, Siracusano S, et al. Urologic dysfunction and neurologic outcome in coma survivors after severe traumatic brain injury in the postacute and chronic phase. *Arch Phys Med Rehabil.* 2011;92(7):1134–1138. https://doi.org/10.1016/j.apmr.2011.02.013.

60. Sakakibara R. Lower urinary tract dysfunction in patients with brain lesions. *Handb Clin Neurol.* 2015;130:269–287. https://doi.org/10.1016/B978-0-444-63247-0.00015-8.

61. Masel BE, DeWitt DS. Traumatic brain injury: a disease process, not an event. *J Neurotrauma.* 2010;27(8):1529–1540. https://doi.org/10.1089/neu.2010.1358.

62. Nseyo U, Santiago-Lastra Y. Long-term complications of the neurogenic bladder. *Urol Clin N Am.* 2017;44(3):355–366. https://doi.org/10.1016/j.ucl.2017.04.003.

63. Foxx-Orenstein A, Kolakowsky-Hayner S, Marwitz JH, et al. Incidence, risk factors, and outcomes of fecal incontinence after acute brain injury: findings from the traumatic brain injury model systems national database. *Arch Phys Med Rehabil.* 2003;84(2):231–237. https://doi.org/10.1053/apmr.2003.50095.

64. Martinez L, Neshatian L, Khavari R. Neurogenic bowel dysfunction in patients with neurogenic bladder. *Curr Bladder Dysfunct Rep.* 2016;11(4):334–340. https://doi.org/10.1007/s11884-016-0390-3.

65. Viola-Saltzman M, Musleh C. Traumatic brain injury-induced sleep disorders. *Neuropsychiatr Dis Treat.* 2016;12:339–348. https://doi.org/10.2147/NDT.S69105.

66. Baumann CR. Sleep and traumatic brain injury. *Sleep Med Clin.* 2016;11(1):19–23. https://doi.org/10.1016/j.jsmc.2015.10.004.

67. Shekleton JA, Parcell DL, Redman JR, Phipps-Nelson J, Ponsford JL, Rajaratnam SMW. Sleep disturbance and melatonin levels following traumatic brain injury. *Neurology.* 2010;74(21):1732–1738. https://doi.org/10.1212/WNL.0b013e3181e0438b.

68. Ouellet M-C, Beaulieu-Bonneau S, Morin CM. Sleep-wake disturbances after traumatic brain injury. *Lancet Neurol.* 2015;14(7):746–757. https://doi.org/10.1016/S1474-4422(15)00068-X.

69. Tapia RN, Eapen BC. Rehabilitation of persistent symptoms after concussion. *Phys Med Rehabil Clin N Am.* 2017;28(2):287–299. https://doi.org/10.1016/j.pmr.2016.12.006.

70. Larson EB, Zollman FS. The effect of sleep medications on cognitive recovery from traumatic brain injury. *J Head Trauma Rehabil.* 2010;25(1):61–67. https://doi.org/10.1097/HTR.0b013e3181c1d1e1.

71. Kallweit U, Bassetti CL. Pharmacological management of narcolepsy with and without cataplexy. *Expert Opin Pharmacother.* 2017;18(8):809–817. https://doi.org/10.1080/14656566.2017.1323877.

72. Lequerica A, Jasey N, Portelli Tremont JN, Chiaravalloti ND. Pilot study on the effect of Ramelteon on sleep disturbance after traumatic brain injury: preliminary evidence from a clinical trial. *Arch Phys Med Rehabil.* 2015;96(10):1802–1809. https://doi.org/10.1016/j.apmr.2015.05.011.

73. Ponsford J. Sexual changes associated with traumatic brain injury. *Neuropsychol Rehabil.* 2003;13(1–2):275–289. https://doi.org/10.1080/09602010244000363.

74. Downing MG, Stolwyk R, Ponsford JL. Sexual changes in individuals with traumatic brain injury: a control comparison. *J Head Trauma Rehabil.* 2013;28(3):171–178. https://doi.org/10.1097/HTR.0b013e31828b4f63.

75. Moreno JA, Arango Lasprilla JC, Gan C, McKerral M. Sexuality after traumatic brain injury: a critical review. *NeuroRehabilitation.* 2013;32(1):69–85. https://doi.org/10.3233/NRE-130824.

76. Ponsford JL, Downing MG, Stolwyk R. Factors associated with sexuality following traumatic brain injury. *J Head Trauma Rehabil.* 2013;28(3):195–201. https://doi.org/10.1097/HTR.0b013e31828b4f7b.

77. Sander AM, Maestas KL, Nick TG, et al. Predictors of sexual functioning and satisfaction 1 year following traumatic brain injury: a TBI model systems multicenter study. *J Head Trauma Rehabil.* 2013;28(3):186–194. https://doi.org/10.1097/HTR.0b013e31828b4f91.

78. Simpson GK, Sabaz M, Daher M. Prevalence, clinical features, and correlates of inappropriate sexual behavior after traumatic brain injury: a multicenter study. *J Head Trauma Rehabil.* 2013;28(3):202–210. https://doi.org/10.1097/HTR.0b013e31828dc5ae.

79. Turner D, Schöttle D, Krueger R, Briken P. Sexual behavior and its correlates after traumatic brain injury. *Curr Opin Psychiatry.* 2015;28(2):180–187. https://doi.org/10.1097/YCO.0000000000000144.

80. Gill CJ, Sander AM, Robins N, Mazzei DK, Struchen MA. Exploring experiences of intimacy from the viewpoint of individuals with traumatic brain injury and their partners. *J Head Trauma Rehabil.* 2011;26(1):56–68. https://doi.org/10.1097/HTR.0b013e3182048ee9.

81. Macciocchi S, Seel RT, Thompson N, Byams R, Bowman B. Spinal cord injury and co-occurring traumatic brain injury: assessment and incidence. *Arch Phys Med Rehabil.* 2008;89(7):1350–1357. https://doi.org/10.1016/j.apmr.2007.11.055.

82. Sharma B, Bradbury C, Mikulis D, Green R. Missed diagnosis of traumatic brain injury in patients with traumatic spinal cord injury. *J Rehabil Med.* 2014;46(4):370–373. https://doi.org/10.2340/16501977-1261.

83. Kushner DS, Alvarez G. Dual diagnosis: traumatic brain injury with spinal cord injury. *Phys Med Rehabil Clin N Am.* 2014;25(3):681–696, ix–x. https://doi.org/10.1016/j.pmr.2014.04.005.

84. Sommer JL, Witkiewicz PM. The therapeutic challenges of dual diagnosis: TBI/SCI. *Brain Inj.* 2004;18(12):1297–1308.

85. Nott MT, Baguley IJ, Heriseanu R, et al. Effects of concomitant spinal cord injury and brain injury on medical and functional outcomes and community participation. *Top Spinal Cord Inj Rehabil.* 2014;20(3):225–235. https://doi.org/10.1310/sci2003-225.

CHAPTER 4

Neurologic Complications After Traumatic Brain Injury

BRIAN D. GREENWALD, MD • STEPHEN HAMPTON, MD •
NEIL JASEY, MD • DAVID H. GLAZER, MD

INTRODUCTION

There is a continuing demand for patients who suffer moderate to severe traumatic brain injury (TBI) to leave the acute care setting for the next step in the continuum of care as early after injury as possible. Many of the multisystem problems that start in the acute care remain active when these patients get to the rehabilitation setting. Previous studies have shown that these medical complications may flare up in the acute rehabilitation setting and new problems may arise.[1] Many of these patients require years, if not a lifetime, of follow-up with a specialist with experience in treating these long-term complications that if not unique to this population are more common after TBI. This chapter focuses on posttraumatic seizures (PTSs), hydrocephalus, cranial nerve disorders, visual dysfunction, movement disorders, neurosensory deficits, sleep/wake disorders, and fatigue. These complications and disorders range from surgical and medical complications seen early on to those that medical professionals need to be aware of to maximize function in the postacute stages after TBI.

POSTTRAUMATIC SEIZURES

The classification of PTSs is based on the time of seizure post injury: immediate (<24h), early (24h–7 days), or late (>7 days). Late PTS is often used interchangeably with posttraumatic epilepsy (PTE). The clinical definition of epilepsy, revised in 2014 by the International League Against Epilepsy, includes the condition of two unprovoked seizures more than 24h apart (the old definition) or one unprovoked seizure when the risk for another is known to be high (>60%). The recurrent seizure risk following a single, unprovoked seizure >7 days post-TBI is high enough to consider late PTS as an epileptic condition.[2,3]

Reported rates of PTS after moderate to severe TBI vary widely pending on study design and population characteristics.[4] The study by Ritter et al. using the civilian TBI Model Systems National Database found that PTS incidence during acute hospitalization was highest immediately (<24h) after TBI (8.9%). New-onset PTS incidence was greatest between discharge from inpatient rehabilitation and year 1 (9.2%). Late PTS cumulative incidence from injury to year 1 was 11.9% and reached 20.5% by year 5.

Risk factors for the development of PTS include biparietal contusions, dural penetration with bone and metal fragments, multiple intracranial operations, multiple subcortical contusions, subdural hematoma with evacuation, midline shift greater than 5 mm, and multiple/bilateral cortical contusions. The more severe the initial TBI, based on the initial Glasgow Coma Scale (GCS) score, the higher the risk for PTS.[5] Mazzini et al. found that PTS correlated with significantly poorer outcome, as measured by the Glasgow Outcome Scale, Disability Rating Scale, Functional Independence Measure (FIM), and subscales of the Neurobehavioral Rating Scale, at 1 year after severe TBI.[6] Harrison-Felix et al., using the TBI Model Systems National Database, found seizures to be an important contributor to premature death among individuals who were hospitalized and received inpatient rehabilitation for TBI.[7]

Phenytoin had long been the preferred antiepileptic drug of choice for seizure prophylaxis and symptomatic treatment primarily because of its availability in oral and intravenous forms that can be administered easily in the acute care setting. The most recent edition of the Brain Trauma Foundation Guideline for the Management of Severe Traumatic Brain Injury continues to recommend phenytoin to decrease the incidence of early PTS.[8] Prophylaxis is not recommended to prevent late PTS. The guidelines note that levetiracetam is commonly used for seizure prophylaxis. The guidelines note that there is a lack of evidence to support levetiracetam over phenytoin regarding efficacy in preventing early PTSs and toxicity. Psychiatric and behavioral side effects should be considered when using levetiracetam at any time after TBI.[9]

It is beyond the practical scope of this chapter to critically examine the pertinent literature regarding the treatment of PTE. Diagnosis of a seizure in patients who have sustained TBI is complicated by the variety of clinical presentations as well as significant cognitive and behavioral dysfunction in this patient population. Movement disorders and syncopal episodes should be considered in the differential diagnoses. Electroencephalogram (EEG) should be obtained in patients with suspected PTSs. The limitations of sensitivity of EEGs should be considered when reviewing the results.[10] The choice of drug to treat PTS should include a risk-benefit analysis regarding the effects the drug has on the common cognitive and psychiatric profile seen after TBI. After initiating pharmacotherapy, ongoing monitoring is necessary to evaluate for dose-related and idiosyncratic adverse effects.

SLEEP/WAKE/FATIGUE

A person's day truly begins at night. With a proper night's sleep, a person has the energy and capabilities to proceed through the day with vigor. Sleep is meant to be restorative. It takes a tired person through a 6- to 8-h process that replenishes and rejuvenates a person back to a fully functional level both physically and cognitively. When a person progresses through sleep stages, the brain is actively working. The reticular activating system, suprachiasmatic nucleus, hypothalamus, reticular nucleus of the thalamus, and area surrounding the third ventricle function at high capacity to properly regulate sleep. When one experiences a brain injury of any severity level, these structural areas of the brain can be affected. In addition, biochemical interactions are also disrupted. With both structural and chemical pathways altered, sleep dysfunction will likely occur.[11,12]

When assessing for sleep dysfunction in a patient, it is important to recognize that, in addition to intrinsic physiology and anatomic insults, other causes, such as environmental, medicinal, and nutritional variables, can affect sleep. Pain levels, daytime napping, caffeine intake, bedtime routine, medical history, and prior sleep disorders can all disrupt sleep in the brain-injured patient. It would seem that fatigue in the brain-injured patient would be solely due to poor sleep, but this is not necessarily true. Fatigue can occur in 21%–80% of all brain-injured patients.[13] Peripheral fatigue is one that is usually associated with musculoskeletal symptoms, which can limit mobility or cardiac status. A brain-injured patient's fatigue is considered central, which makes cognitive activity more challenging in addition to voluntary physical activities. Its impact limits a brain-injured patient's abilities to achieve tasks during the day both in rehabilitation settings and community. The basal ganglia is often determined to be the culprit in fatigue because of disruption of the dopamine levels that help to control motor tasks. The brain is then placed under greater stress, which leads to fatigue. When assessing central fatigue, one must identify fatigue during cognitive tasks rather than during physical tasks, such as walking. Furthermore, a thorough medication review is required in addition to investigating the patient's metabolic, infectious, and endocrine status and any other concomitant medical diagnoses.[14]

Treatment of sleep dysfunction starts with improving "sleep hygiene." This includes first changing the environment so that a person is in a cool and calm room, with pain controlled. Elimination of caffeine products should be the goal, especially if these products are ingested in the evening hours. Screen time on a phone, computer, and television should be minimized as the sleeping hours approach. Cognitive therapy has been found to be helpful. Over-the-counter medication, such as melatonin, can be considered in addition to chamomile tea. Prescription medications, such as trazodone, benzodiazepines, and z-drugs such as zolpidem, can be used. These medications come with cognitive effects such as delaying neurorecovery and decreased coordination, sedation, and confusion.[15]

As with sleep dysfunction, treatment of fatigue often requires environmental adjustments. A patient's medications should be evaluated for potential side effects that cause/exacerbate fatigue. Medications such as modafinil, methylphenidate, amantadine, and selective serotonin reuptake inhibitors can help to treat fatigue. Nutrition should be maximized. Complementary and alternative interventions, such as exercise, cognitive-based activities, biofeedback, and light therapy, have been investigated. As of the time of this writing, evidence is inconclusive in regards to the effectiveness of these complementary and alternative interventions.[16]

Cranial Nerves

The 12 cranial nerves, which arise from the brainstem, are frequently injured in all severities of brain injury. As more people survive their brain injury, an increasing number of cranial nerve injuries are diagnosed.[17] Each cranial nerve has its individualized anatomic location and function. Direct trauma, edema, fracture, and penetration can injure the nerves. This then leads to further functional challenges.

Olfactory nerve (CN I)

This provides the sensation of smell. As a result of smell distortion, the perception of taste is often flawed. It passes through the cribriform plate where shearing injuries often occur. Because olfaction is often not assessed in the acute care setting the dysfunction may not be recognized for weeks or longer after injury. Cerebrospinal fluid (CSF) rhinorrhea is often a sign of possible CN I disturbance. If recovery is seen, it is usually within the first 6 months and complete by 12 months after the injury. Injury to this nerve occurs at an incidence rate of 19.4% after moderate TBI and 24.5% after severe TBI.[18]

Optic nerve (CN II)

The optic nerve provides the sense of sight through transmission of light sensation from rods and cones. It is often injured by shearing forces. Blindness and partial vision field loss are common. Injury to this nerve occurs at an incidence rate of 2.78%–5%.[18,19]

Oculomotor nerve (CN III)

The oculomotor nerve provides the functions of eye movement, pupil reaction, and lid retraction. One study found injury to this nerve in 17% of brain-injured patients.[20] Because there is outward movement of the eye when this nerve is injured, double vision can occur. Eyelid ptosis can occur. In the unconscious patient, pupillary light reflex and doll's eye maneuver can help diagnose this palsy. In the conscious patient, one can have the patient actively move the eyes in various directions to diagnose.[18]

Trochlear nerve (CN IV)

This nerve innervates the superior oblique muscle. Injury to this nerve causes the eye to not be able to have intorsion and downward movements. Injury to this nerve occurs at a rate of 0.2%–1.4%.[21]

Trigeminal nerve (CN V)

The trigeminal nerve provides facial sensation, chewing movements, and corneal sensation. It has three major branches: ophthalmic, maxillary, and mandibular. Orbital fractures often cause injury to the nerve. Trigeminal neuralgia can result and is often treated with anticonvulsants, such as gabapentin or carbamazepine.[22] Injury to this nerve occurs at a rate of 1.4%–2%.[23]

Abducens nerve (CN VI)

The abducens nerve innervates the lateral rectus muscle of the eye. It is responsible for lateral eye movements. Injury to this nerve prevents such movement. Injury to this nerve can cause double vision. Owing to its lengthy nature, multiple areas of the nerve have the potential to be damaged, whether at its nucleus or along cranial bone areas. It is difficult to locate the area of damage. But if this nerve is damaged, other cranial nerves are frequently also injured.[18] Injury to this nerve occurs at a rate of 0.4%–4.1%.[21]

Facial nerve (CN VII)

The facial nerve provides movement of the face, eyelid closure, and taste to the anterior two-thirds of the tongue. It is often damaged with temporal bone fractures. It is important to prevent an exposure keratitis due to the lack of eyelid closure with an eye patch and lubricant. The surgical procedure, tarsorrhaphy, can be performed to aid in closing the eyelid. Injury to this nerve occurs at a rate of 4.53%.[19]

Vestibulocochlear nerve (CN VIII)

The vestibulocochlear nerve provides for hearing and balance. Patients with this nerve injury oftentimes have vertigo, tinnitus, and hearing impairment. Hearing loss due to TBIs is more frequently a sensory loss than a conductive loss. Patients may often complain of the sensation of the room spinning around them. Nystagmus can also be seen. The Dix-Hallpike test should be performed to help in differentiating between peripheral and central vertigo. Injury to this nerve occurs at a rate of 1.51%.[19] Vestibular therapy can help a patient recover from this nerve palsy.

Glossopharyngeal nerve (CN IX)

The glossopharyngeal nerve provides for swallowing functions and taste of the posterior one-third of the tongue. Injury to this nerve often results in dysphagia. As brain-injured patients are in a hypermetabolic state early after injury, increased nutritional supports are required. Dysphagia can oftentimes lead to aspiration and makes the provision of nutrition more challenging. Gag reflex testing can help diagnose injury to this nerve.

Vagus nerve (CN X)

The vagus nerve provides innervation of laryngeal striated muscles in addition to parasympathetic innervation of the heart and smooth muscles of the trachea, bronchi, esophagus, and gastrointestinal tract. Injury to this nerve occurs at a rate of 0.05%–0.16%.[23]

Spinal accessory nerve (CN XI)

This spinal accessory nerve provides for shoulder shrug and side movements of the neck. Injury to this nerve prevents this movement.

Hypoglossal nerve (CN XII)

The hypoglossal nerve provides for motor action of the tongue. Injury to this nerve can cause dysphagia and dysarthria.

Most patients with low cranial nerve (IX–XII) injury require supplemental nutrition oftentimes through a percutaneous endoscopic gastrostomy tube or nasogastric tube. At this time, it is thought that decompression of the nerve combined with the latest microsurgical techniques can help save complete destruction of these nerves in the brain-injured patient.[17]

VISUAL DYSFUNCTION

Dysfunction of the visual system is a serious problem that has adverse effects on rehabilitation of mobility and activities of daily living (ADL) after TBI. Blurred vision, reading problems such as slower reading speed and loss of place when reading, diplopia or eyestrain, vestibular symptoms in visually crowded environments, peripheral vision restrictions, increased sensitivity to light, and color vision deficits are common symptoms following the spectrum of severity of TBI. These vision anomalies may occur because of traumatic lesions to the primary and secondary visual pathways, as well as possibly the primary and associated visual cortices.[24]

Anomalies along the oculomotor nerve–mediated accommodative pathway may occur following TBI, resulting in constant or intermittent blur, difficulty reading because of impaired ability to maintain clear vision of near objects for sustained time periods without fatigue, headache, eyestrain, decrease visual efficiency, and difficulty looking from far to near and far again.[25] The ciliary muscles of the eye are responsible for this function and are innervated by the oculomotor nerve and autonomic nervous system. The most common accommodative dysfunction in those with mild TBI and moderate TBI is accommodative insufficiency, which is diagnosed by the examination finding of reduced accommodation amplitude.[25]

Versional ocular motility refers to conjugate eye movements with regard to objects in the field of view. This includes oculomotor functions such as smooth pursuit, saccades, and fixation, all of which can be evaluated during the extraocular motility assessment. Smooth pursuit refers to the ability to track objects smoothly or to move one's eyes smoothly. Conversely, saccades refer to one's ability to track objects visually as they move rapidly from one position to another or to move one's eyes rapidly from one target to another, as with reading-related eye movements. Fixation refers to the ability to maintain one's eyes on a target. Versional ocular motor deficits may present as difficulty reading because of slow reading speed, loss of place when reading, misreading/rereading words or paragraphs, text appearing to float or shimmer, and dizziness or visual motion sensitivity.[26]

Vergence ocular motility refers to disjunctive changes in eye position as one regards objects at varying distances in the visual field. Vergence deficits may be nonstrabismic or strabismic (such as due to damage to cranial nerves III, IV, or VI) in nature. Symptoms related to vergence deficits occur under binocular viewing conditions and may include diplopia, eyestrain, vision-related headaches, dizziness, and fatigue. Diplopia and eyestrain evident under binocular viewing conditions are common in those with TBI, which may affect rehabilitation of ADLs and mobility adversely. Diplopia and eyestrain under binocular viewing conditions may occur when both eyes are unable to align correctly toward the object of regard. The most common type of vergence dysfunction among those with TBI is convergence insufficiency, which may result from trauma along the oculomotor nerve and/or to the medial recti muscles, thereby impairing convergence.[25]

Gaze stabilization refers to the control of the vestibuloocular reflex (VOR). The VOR's primary responsibility is to stabilize images on the retina while the head is in motion by producing eye movements in the direction opposite to that of head movements. VOR depends indirectly on the visual input, but it is directed by signals from the vestibular apparatus of the inner ear. Head rotation is detected by the semicircular canals, and translation is detected by the otoliths.[27] The pathway for horizontal VOR commences with the semicircular canals being stimulated by head rotation. This initial stimulation is followed by a consequent interaction among the oculomotor (CN III), abducens (CN VI), and acoustic (CN VIII) nerves via the medial longitudinal fasciculus to move the eyes in a direction opposite to the head movement to stabilize gaze.[27]

Those with TBI may have visual-vestibular disturbances, which may be due to abnormalities of the VOR system. This results in symptoms of dizziness, disequilibrium, vertigo, nausea, oscillopsia, photosensitivity to fluorescent lighting, and increased sensitivity to visual motion in visually stimulating environments (i.e., malls, supermarkets, crowds). Reading may be difficult because words may seem to float or shimmer, and computer tasks may be troublesome because of difficulty with scrolling or flickering of the screen.[25,28]

Visual field defects (VFDs) in those with TBI may be restricted overall, present with scattered defects throughout the visual field, or manifest as a lateralized visual defect evident with or without visual inattention. VFDs may be due to trauma along the visual pathway anywhere from the optic chiasm through the optic radiations of the visual cortex. Lateralized VFDs, such as homonymous hemianopsia, may cause a patient to ignore half of the objects in space because they are located on the affected side. Symptoms associated with lateralized VFDs include difficulty reading, with a slower speed of reading, bumping into objects on one side, forgetting food on one side of the plate, difficulty dressing one side of the body, or difficulty navigating streets. Homonymous hemianopsia may pose a safety hazard because affected patients are not always aware of their VFD, which is referred to as visual inattention or, in more severe cases, visual anosognosia.[27]

Photosensitivity is ocular discomfort in the presence of light without ocular inflammation or pain. Photosensitivity may be evident with all lighting or selectively fluorescent lighting. Although the exact underlying neurology for photosensitivity remains unclear, some hypothesize that it may be related to anomalous light and dark adaptation regarding general photosensitivity. Regarding selective light sensitivity to fluorescent lighting, anomalous critical flicker fusion frequency threshold may be a contributing component.[28]

POSTTRAUMATIC HYDROCEPHALUS

Hydrocephalus following TBI, or posttraumatic hydrocephalus (PTH), is an important consideration for the rehabilitation provider. In patients with severe TBI, the presence and severity of PTH has been strongly correlated with functional outcomes 1 year after injury.[28] Ventricular enlargement, from all etiologies, has been detected in as much as 70% of patients at 2 months following moderate to severe TBI.[29] On exclusion of other causes of ventriculomegaly, such as atrophy, incidence rates of PTH diagnosis range from 3.7% to 45%.[28,30,31] Differences in diagnostic criteria likely contribute to this variation. For example, the study showing 3.7% incidence used placement of a shunt as the

only indicator of PTH, whereas the other reported 45% of subjects with evidence of hydrocephalus on magnetic resonance imaging (MRI) but only 11% with PTH severe enough to require intervention.[28,30] In addition, studies focused on the acute stage following TBI likely underestimate PTH rates. In a retrospective cohort of patients admitted to an acute rehabilitation unit following TBI, patients were diagnosed with PTH at a median of 69 days following injury, with one patient diagnosed at day 309.[32]

Risk factors for the development of PTH include older age, more severe TBI on initial GCS, longer coma duration, craniectomy, and intracranial bleeding, primarily due to subarachnoid or intraventricular hemorrhage.[28,31,33] PTH occurs in 12%–43% of patients following craniectomy after TBI.[34] Craniectomies performed bilaterally or within 25 mm from the midline are particularly associated with hydrocephalus development.[31,35] Of note, presence of anoxic injury and severity of diffuse axonal injury do not seem to be associated with PTH, although they have been correlated with ventriculomegaly due to atrophy.[28]

There are several proposed mechanisms for the development of PTH, including outflow obstruction (e.g., due to clot formation, mass effect) and impaired CSF resorption.[33,36] Animal studies have further explored the association of intraventricular hemorrhage with hydrocephalus, even without trauma. In one study, injections were performed into the lateral ventricles and resultant hydrocephalus evaluated with MRI, immunohistochemistry, and Western blot protein analysis.[37] Hydrocephalus was produced when autologous blood or isolated thrombin was injected. Furthermore, electron microscopy following thrombin injection found damage to ependymal cells with loss of cilia. Ependymal cilia dysfunction results in impaired CSF flow and subsequent hydrocephalus.[38] Even without overt bleeding, TBI seems to result in ependymal cilia loss and altered CSF motion in animal models.[39] In addition to thrombin, other blood products have been implicated in the formation of hydrocephalus, including iron and platelets.[40]

In the rehabilitation setting, PTH should be suspected with a plateau or decline in functional status. Although the classic signs of normal-pressure hydrocephalus (NPH) (i.e., urinary incontinence, cognitive dysfunction, and gait impairment) may be present, their absence does not exclude PTH, especially for individuals with disorders of consciousness following TBI.[41] Other clinical signs associated with PTH include headache, nausea, emesis, papilledema, lateral rectus palsy, motor impairment, or other new focal neurologic deficit.[33,42,43] Given the overlap of these clinical signs with direct sequelae of TBI, thorough, serial examinations, preferably in a structured format, is important for detection.[44]

Following clinical suspicion of PTH development, radiographic imaging should be obtained. Both computed tomography (CT) and MRI are useful in evaluation. Quantification of the ventricle size aids in serial comparisons. Two common methods are the ventricle-brain percent ratio (VBR) and Evan's ratio.[30] The VBR is the percentage of the maximum outer width of the ventricles relative to the inner table of the skull. For the Evan's ratio, or frontal horn index, the greatest outer width of the frontal horns of the lateral ventricles is divided by the greatest outer width of the brain on a single axial image. An Evan's ratio of 0.3 or greater indicates ventriculomegaly. These measurement methods should be used with caution when brain anatomy is altered by mass lesions.[28]

Once ventriculomegaly is detected, hydrocephalus must be distinguished from atrophy, or ex vacuo ventricular dilation. Brain sulci appear more prominent with atrophy and may be reduced or absent in the setting of hydrocephalus.[28] Movement of fluid across the ependymal layer surrounding the ventricles is correlated with PTH.[45] This transependymal flow appears as decreased density on CT or increased T2 intensity on MRI. Reduced T2 signal in the cerebral aqueduct connecting the third and fourth ventricles may be an additional indicator of PTH.[45]

Additional techniques include elevated opening pressure on lumbar puncture, although opening pressure in the normal range does not exclude clinically significant hydrocephalus.[46,47] A so-called tap test can be performed in which 20–50 mL of CSF is removed during a lumbar puncture.[32,48,49] Improvements in neurologic or functional status indicate a positive test with likely benefit from ventriculoperitoneal shunt (VPS) placement. However, more prolonged removal of fluid may be necessary to remove stress from periventricular structures; thus use of a lumbar drain with removal of >300 mL over several days can be useful.[49,50] Various methods to evaluate CSF dynamics, such as measuring resistance to flow, have demonstrated utility in predicting response to VPS placement.[49,51] Single-photon emission computed tomography (SPECT) provides information about brain pathways. Decreased brain perfusion appears diffusely in the setting of atrophy on SPECT but may be more concentrated in the temporal lobes with PTH.[28]

Shunt placement, typically between one of the lateral ventricles and peritoneal space, is the most common definitive treatment for PTH. PTH is included in the category of secondary normal-pressure hydrocephalus (sNPH) along with NPH owing to subarachnoid hemorrhage, malignancy, infection, and cerebrovascular disease. A review of the sNPH literature from 1965 to 2015 found that sNPH has a higher rate of response to shunting than idiopathic NPH and that clinical improvement after shunting was noted in 83% of patients with NPH following head trauma.[52] A retrospective cohort of patients admitted to an acute inpatient rehabilitation unit following TBI found that, among those diagnosed with PTH, TBI severity predicted score on the FIM at admission but later VPS placement was correlated with lower FIM at discharge as well as longer duration of posttraumatic amnesia.[32]

Complication rates following VPS placement for PTH range from 18% to 42%, and complications include problems with the shunt device (e.g., obstruction, tubing migration), infection, bleeding, and CSF leakage.[53,54] Most infections occur in the perioperative period after shunt placement, typically from contamination by skin flora.[55] Shunt malfunction may present with similar symptoms and functional decline as initial PTH; however, the onset of symptoms may be more rapid. Brain imaging and an x-ray shunt series provide information about system integrity, position, and ventricle size relative to preoperative imaging.

INTRACRANIAL PRESSURE MANAGEMENT: CRANIECTOMY AND CRANIOPLASTY

Decompressive craniectomy is a routine practice for addressing elevated intracranial pressure (ICP) following TBI, particularly when nonoperative measures are unsuccessful. The rehabilitation provider is typically not involved in acute ICP management; therefore factors in the decision making regarding craniectomy are outside the scope of this chapter. A randomized trial comparing decompressive craniectomy with nonoperative medical treatment demonstrated improved survival at 6 months for the craniectomy group.[56] However, the craniectomy group also had higher rates of severe disability and vegetative state at the same time point.

Craniectomy is associated with various complications such as PTH as described earlier. Given the lack of protective bone, patients are encouraged to wear helmets to prevent further injury. Cranioplasty involves either replacing removed bone or placement of other autologous bone or synthetic material to cover the craniectomy defect. Once felt to be cosmetic, cranioplasty has been shown to improve cerebral blood flow as well as neurologic status.[57] Cranioplasty has historically been delayed at least 3 months following craniectomy, although recent studies have suggested that performance as early as 2 weeks after craniectomy may not result in increased complication rates.[58]

Over the course of weeks the craniectomy site typically develops a more concave shape. In some cases when cranioplasty is delayed, there is functional and neurologic decline that is independent of original injury. This decline has variably been called the syndrome of the trephined (SoT) and sinking skin flap syndrome (SSFS).[57] A systematic review of SoT noted onset of symptoms at an average of 5 months following craniectomy, although the range of reported timings was wide.[59] Symptoms of SoT and SSFS resolve in 25%–34% of patients following cranioplasty.[57,59]

MOVEMENT DISORDERS

The presentation of movement disorders after TBI is generally considered an infrequent occurrence.[60] However, much depends on the definitions used for the disorders in question. For this review, movement disorders are broadly characterized as hypokinetic or hyperkinetic disorders and include tremors, dystonia, athetosis, ballism, chorea, myoclonus, parkinsonism, and tics. Motor disorders, defined as plegia, ataxia, and spasticity, are excluded.[60]

Historically, the terms "movement disorder" or dyskinesia, meaning "abnormal movement" as well as "extrapyramidal," have classically referred to dysfunction of the basal ganglia. Broadly, movement disorders can be categorized by speed (hypokinesia vs. hyperkinesia) and whether they occur at rest or are accentuated by motion.[43] A tremor can be slow or fast and is defined by a rhythmic or oscillatory movement and is further characterized by the position, activity, or posture required to trigger its emergence. Dystonia is defined as involuntary, sustained, patterned muscle contractions of opposing muscles and can be focal (e.g., writer's cramp), segmental, or generalized. It may be present at rest or be triggered by activity. Athetosis is a term applied to dystonic movements that are more phasic and writhing, whereas in chorea, movements are rapid and unpredictable, spreading from one muscle group to another. Along the same spectrum of disorders, ballism has been defined as continuous, nonpatterned, purposeless movements involving primarily the proximal portions of limbs.[61] In addition, patients with a frontal lobe disorder may have a type of rigidity termed paratonia or gegenhalten, whereby the resistance to passive movement is more active, inconsistent, or seemingly voluntary. Myoclonus is felt to be the fastest of the movement disorders and is defined as a rapid muscular jerk that can be focal, unilateral, or bilateral.[43]

After a TBI, movement disorders can emerge individually or be part of a broader clinical syndrome. In addition, they may be transient in nature, present during the more chronic course of treatment, or be the result of medications used to address agitation or deficits in arousal and cognition. Because of these variations, precise quantification and description of these disorders may be difficult in this population. In addition, as movement disorders can present later in life, it is often difficult to establish a connection between a remote brain injury and the emergence of hypokinesia or hyperkinesia. This point is made by O'Suilleabhain and Dewey[62] who report that in a movement disorder clinic, of the 3500 cases identified over the course of 5 years, only 30 could be traced back to a brain injury. Also, time from injury to emergence of the disorder, such as dystonia, has been reported between 14 days and 9 years, with more severe injuries potentially presenting later than mild to moderate injuries, whereas the presentation of parkinsonism related to repeated trauma may occur decades after the injury.[61,63]

O'Suilleabhain and Dewey have reported that the most common movement disorders after TBI are tremors, followed by dystonia, parkinsonism, myoclonus, ballism, chorea, and tics.[62] Movement disorders occur most frequently in patients with severe injury, with rates of 20% and 22% noted in a retrospective German university hospital study in patients with GCS <9.[62] However, in 2002 Krauss and Jankovic reported a more variable incidence with 13%–66% of patients with severe injury developing a movement disorder.[61] In addition, in this population, dystonia can present as part of a more general syndrome characterized by sympathetic outflow termed paroxysmal autonomic instability with dystonia (PAID) as described by Blackman et al.[64] In this 2004 article, the authors describe PAID as "a syndrome of intermittent agitation, diaphoresis, hyperthermia, hypertension, tachycardia, tachypnea, and extensor posturing." Unfortunately, likely owing to lack of recognition or reporting, a prevalence is not available.

After mild to moderate TBI, the incidence of movement disorders seems to be less frequent and is often transient in nature. In a 1997 article, Krauss et al. reported 16 of 156 (10.1%) cases of movement disorder in patients with mild to moderate injury.[65] Of the 16 cases, 12 were transient in nature and only 4 had persistent symptoms. The primary disorder in these patients was a postural/intentional tremor that was not disabling.[65] This estimation of occurrence is consistent with O'Suilleabhain and Dewey as well, who propose that movement disorders occur at about half the rate in mild to moderate injuries as they do in severe injuries, roughly 10%.[62]

Anatomically, the areas of the brain that seem to be most closely linked to movement disorders are the basal ganglia, thalamus, subthalamus, cerebellum, and white matter tracts.[43,61,62] However, myoclonus may have a variety of possible locations beyond the basal ganglia, including the cerebral cortex, brain stem, or spinal cord. It may also be seen after anoxic brain injury, encephalitis, or encephalopathy.[43] In a study by Lee et al. in 1994, 29 cases of dystonia after brain injury were reported and investigated with CT or MRI. The types of dystonia varied, including focal, hemifocal, multifocal, and generalized, with some progression noted from the more focal to more generalized presentations. On imaging, the most common lesion site was in the contralateral basal ganglia or thalamus, although two had normal findings.[63] In a case report of a person with a mild traumatic injury and resting tremor, MRI with diffuse tractography demonstrated damage to the dentorubrothalamic tract.[66] In addition, parkinsonism may present as a result of chronic subdural hematoma or hydrocephalus.[62] Subdural hematoma has been reported to cause dystonia as well.[61]

Further complicating the diagnosis and subsequent treatment are potential causes of movement disorders beyond the injury itself. The primary areas of concern are pharmacologic side effects or peripheral nerve injury. Pharmacologically, substances that are noradrenergic can potentially cause a tremor.[67] This is particularly pertinent in patients with severe brain injury, as these agents are often used to promote arousal and improve concentration and attention. Other general classes of medication known to potentially cause movement disorders include those that block dopamine, including antiemetic or antipsychotic medications. Here, the movement disorder may be delayed or "tardive," thus leading to the term tardive dyskinesia.[43] In regards to peripheral nerve injury, in a 2010 review van Rooijen et al. identified 133 publications discussing patients with "peripherally induced movement disorders."[68] Of the patients identified, most presented with a "fixed" dystonia, 26% had a peripheral nerve injury, 15% were diagnosed with "psychogenic" movement disorder, and more than one-third had complex regional pain syndrome.[68]

Treatment for each type of movement disorder is dependent on the type of disorder, where it may fall on the spectrum (fast to slow), and the level of disability associated with it. The first step is to eliminate other potential causes, such as medications or neurosurgical issues like hydrocephalus or subdural hematoma, that may be reversible. Once these possibilities are eliminated, the clinician may consider pharmacologic or surgical intervention. For tremors, weighting the walker or utensils may be beneficial.[62] A variety of medications have also been reported as possible treatments, including propranolol, primidone, carbamazepine, benzodiazepines, levetiracetam, gabapentin, glutethimide, isoniazid, and L-tryptophan.[43,61,62] If medications are not effective, then botulinum toxin injection or surgical options may be considered, including deep brain stimulation (DBS) stereotactic surgery with targets in the ventrolateral thalamus and the subthalamic region.[61,62] Stereotactic surgery and DBS may also be considered for patients with disabling and generalized dystonia, whereas pharmacologic intervention may include oral antiepileptic or anticholinergic medications or intrathecal infusion of baclofen.[61,62] For more focal dystonia, botulinum toxin injections may be considered as well.[62,69] With myoclonus, valproic acid and clonazepam are the first-line options, whereas tryptophan, phenytoin, and levetiracetam have also been used.[62]

SPATIAL NEGLECT

Spatial neglect involves an impairment of attention toward the side contralateral to the primary neurologic injury.[70] It can involve perception (i.e., visual, auditory, tactile, and proprioceptive), movement, and memory in the affected region. Most current knowledge about spatial neglect comes from studies of patients after stroke, where it has been more predictive of functional impairment and caregiver burden than stroke severity.[70] Information regarding the impact of neglect on individuals after TBI has primarily been limited to case reports. Studies conducted in inpatient and outpatient rehabilitation have detected spatial neglect in 30%–45% of patients after TBI.[71,72] A retrospective study of patients admitted to acute inpatient rehabilitation after TBI found those diagnosed with spatial neglect had increased length of stay, decreased functional independence measure (FIM) score at discharge, and a trend toward decreased rate of home discharge.[72] A variety of rehabilitative treatment approaches for spatial neglect have been proposed following different theoretical frameworks such as using "top-down" cues from a therapist to attend to an affected side or "bottom-up" manipulation of sensory input, for example, with prism goggles.[73] More study is needed to establish evidence-based approaches for treatment of neglect, especially resulting from TBI. Systematic identification of patients with neglect following TBI is important in developing individualized treatment approaches based on specific deficits. This screening may be aided by structured tools that extend beyond visual deficits.[74]

DIZZINESS/BALANCE DISORDERS

Reports of impaired balance or dizziness are common across the spectrum of TBI. Dizziness may be considered a vaguer term that includes symptoms of disorientation, lightheadedness, vertigo, and imbalance.[75] Balance disorders have been reported to occur in 30%–65% of people during their recovery, whereas dizziness after TBI has been reported in as high as 80% of patients.[75,76] These entities are often subdivided into different categories according to possible etiology and when attributable to vestibular dysfunction are representative of a problem with sensory integration.[77] Other potential causes include presyncopal lightheadedness, multisensory dizziness, and psychophysiologic dizziness.[75]

Balance is defined most simply as the ability to keep your body centered over your feet.[76] This is accomplished by coordinating inputs from the vestibular, visual, and proprioceptive systems. The underlying anatomy is complex and involves the semicircular canals, otolithic organs, and vestibular nerves peripherally, as well as the vestibular nuclei centrally. To provide coordination between these areas there are neural connections between the vestibular, oculomotor, and proprioceptive systems.[78] Disruption to any of these systems or their integration may result in a disturbance in balance. Common causes of dizziness/balance disorders include benign paroxysmal positional vertigo (BPPV), migraine-associated dizziness, or Meniere disease.[78] Potential etiologies can be divided in three broad categories, BPPV, a central vestibular problem (e.g., injury to vestibular nucleus), or a peripheral problem (e.g., injury to semicircular canals).[75] Medications, visual impairments, and mental health issues, such as anxiety, may also cause reports of dizziness and balance dysfunction by affecting any of these categories.[76] In addition, influence on balance may also come from outside of the three primary systems. For example, in 2008 Register-Mihalik et al. described a correlation between posttraumatic headache and balance deficits.[79]

Evaluation for dizziness and/or balance deficits is typically dependent on history and physical examination. A thorough history is crucial for separating potential causes of dizziness/balance deficits as described earlier. Important elements include history of trauma, triggers that exacerbate symptoms, headache, history of potentially ototoxic medications, as well as family and dietary history. The physical examination centers on vestibular testing and should be tailored to the patient.[78] Further evaluation may include videoelectronystagmography, rotary chair, posture platform, and the sensory organization test battery.[78]

Treatment of a balance disorder or dizziness starts with addressing potential nonvestibular causes, such as blood pressure or anxiety. Afterward, multiple medications may be trialed acutely, including systemic corticosteroids, meclizine, diazepam, vasodilators, and antihistamines.[78] BPPV can be addressed with the Dix-Hallpike maneuver, and vestibular rehabilitation can help with the reintegration of the various symptoms.[43,75]

CONCLUSION

Persons who have TBI are at risk for a unique set of medical complications. Recognizing individual risk factors for complications and screening at appropriate recovery intervals for the complications is a critical component of rehabilitative care. Early recognition by treating clinicians allows for early treatment to minimize the impact on functional outcome. Treatment of neurologic complication should be tailored to the patients' needs and functional goals.

REFERENCES

1. Whyte J, Nakase-Richardson R. Disorders of consciousness: outcomes, comorbidities, and care needs. *Arch Phys Med Rehabil.* 2013;94(10):1851–1854. https://doi.org/10.1016/j.apmr.2013.07.003.
2. Fisher RS, Blum DE, DiVentura B, et al. Seizure diaries for clinical research and practice: limitations and future prospects. *Epilepsy Behav.* 2012;24(3):304–310. https://doi.org/10.1016/j.yebeh.2012.04.128.
3. Haltiner AM, Temkin NR, Dikmen SS. Risk of seizure recurrence after the first late posttraumatic seizure. *Arch Phys Med Rehabil.* 1997;78(8):835–840.

4. Ritter AC, Wagner AK, Fabio A, et al. Incidence and risk factors of posttraumatic seizures following traumatic brain injury: a traumatic brain injury model systems study. *Epilepsia.* 2016;57(12):1968–1977. https://doi.org/10.1111/epi.13582.

5. Englander J, Bushnik T, Duong TT, et al. Analyzing risk factors for late posttraumatic seizures: a prospective, multicenter investigation. *Arch Phys Med Rehabil.* 2003;84(3):365–373. https://doi.org/10.1053/apmr.2003.50022.

6. Mazzini L, Cossa FM, Angelino E, Campini R, Pastore I, Monaco F. Posttraumatic epilepsy: neuroradiologic and neuropsychological assessment of long-term outcome. *Epilepsia.* 2003;44(4):569–574. https://doi.org/10.1046/j.1528-1157.2003.34902.x.

7. Harrison-Felix C, Pretz C, Hammond FM, et al. Life expectancy after inpatient rehabilitation for traumatic brain injury in the United States. *J Neurotrauma.* 2015;32(23):1893–1901. https://doi.org/10.1089/neu.2014.3353.

8. Carney N, Totten AM, O'Reilly C, Ullman JS, Hawryluk GW, Bell MJ, Bratton SL, Chesnut R, Harris OA, Kissoon N, Rubiano AM, Shutter L, Tasker RC, Vavilala MS., Wilberger J, Wright DW, Ghajar J. *Neurosurgery.* 2017 Jan 1;80(1):6–15. https://doi.org/10.1227/NEU.0000000000001432.

9. White JR, Walczak TS, Leppik IE, et al. Discontinuation of levetiracetam because of behavioral side effects: a case-control study. *Neurology.* 2003;61(9):1218–1221. https://doi.org/10.1212/01.WNL.0000091865.46063.67.

10. Binnie C. Modern electroencephalography: its role in epilepsy management. *Clin Neurophysiol.* 1999;110(10):1671–1697. https://doi.org/10.1016/S1388-2457(99)00125-X.

11. Greenwald B, Lombard LA, Watanabe TK. Managing sleepiness after traumatic brain injury. *PM R.* 2011;3(5):480–485. https://doi.org/10.1016/j.pmrj.2011.04.010.

12. Viola-Saltzman M, Watson NF. Traumatic brain injury and sleep disorders. *Neurol Clin.* 2012;30(4):1299–1312. https://doi.org/10.1016/j.ncl.2012.08.008.

13. Ouellet M-C, Morin CM. Fatigue following traumatic brain injury: frequency, characteristics, and associated factors. *Rehabil Psychol.* 2006;51(2):140–149. https://doi.org/10.1037/0090-5550.51.2.140.

14. Adrian C. *Medical Management of Adults with Neurologic Disabilities.* Demos Medical Publishing; 2008.

15. Larson EB, Zollman FS. The effect of sleep medications on cognitive recovery from traumatic brain injury. *J Head Trauma Rehabil.* 2010;25(1):61–67. https://doi.org/10.1097/HTR.0b013e3181c1d1e1.

16. Xu G-Z, Li Y-F, Wang M-D, Cao D-Y. Complementary and alternative interventions for fatigue management after traumatic brain injury: a systematic review. *Ther Adv Neurol Disord.* 2017;10(5):229–239. https://doi.org/10.1177/1756285616682675.

17. Jin H, Wang S, Hou L, et al. Clinical treatment of traumatic brain injury complicated by cranial nerve injury. *Injury.* 2010;41(9):918–923.

18. Hammond FM, Masel T. Cranial nerve disorders. In: Nathan D, Zasler MD, Douglas I, et al., eds. *Brain Injury Medicine.* 2nd ed. Demos Medical Publishing; 2012.

19. Patel P, Kalyanaraman S, Reginald J, et al. Post-traumatic cranial nerve injury. *Indian J Neurotrauma.* 2005;2(1):27–32. https://doi.org/10.1016/S0973-0508(05)80007-3.

20. Sabates NR, Gonce MA, Farris BK. Neuro-ophthalmological findings in closed head trauma. *J Neuro-Ophthalmol.* 1991;11(4):273.

21. Keane JR. Neuro-ophthalmic signs and symptoms of hysteria. *Neurology.* 1982;32(7):757–762. https://doi.org/10.1212/WNL.32.7.757.

22. Backonja M-M. Use of anticonvulsants for treatment of neuropathic pain. *Neurology.* 2002;59(5 suppl 2):S14–S17. https://doi.org/10.1212/WNL.59.5_suppl_2.S14.

23. Keane JR, Baloh RW. Posttraumatic cranial neuropathies. *Neurol Clin N Am.* 1992;10(4):849–867.

24. Greenwald BD, Kapoor N, Singh AD. Visual impairments in the first year after traumatic brain injury. *Brain Inj.* 2012;26(11):1338–1359. https://doi.org/10.3109/02699052.2012.706356.

25. Ciuffreda KJ, Kapoor N, Rutner D, Suchoff IB, Han ME, Craig S. Occurrence of oculomotor dysfunctions in acquired brain injury: a retrospective analysis. *Optometry.* 2007;78(4):155–161. https://doi.org/10.1016/j.optm.2006.11.011.

26. Kapoor N, Ciuffreda KJ. Vision disturbances following traumatic brain injury. *Curr Treat Options Neurol.* 2002;4(4):271–280. https://doi.org/10.1007/s11940-002-0027-z.

27. Suchoff IB, Kapoor N, Ciuffreda KJ, Rutner D, Han E, Craig S. The frequency of occurrence, types, and characteristics of visual field defects in acquired brain injury: a retrospective analysis. *Optometry.* 2008;79(5):259–265. https://doi.org/10.1016/j.optm.2007.10.012.

28. Mazzini L, Campini R, Angelino E, Rognone F, Pastore I, Oliveri G. Posttraumatic hydrocephalus: a clinical, neuroradiologic, and neuropsychologic assessment of long-term outcome. *YAPMR.* 2003;84(11):1637–1641. https://doi.org/10.1053/S0003-9993(03)00314-9.

29. Poca MA, Sahuquillo J, Mataró M, Benejam B, Arikan F, Báguena M. Ventricular enlargement after moderate or severe head injury: a frequent and neglected problem. *J Neurotrauma.* 2005;22(11):1303–1310. https://doi.org/10.1089/neu.2005.22.1303. http://online.liebertpub.com/doi/abs/10.1089/neu.2005.22.1303.

30. Guyot LL, Michael DB. Post-traumatic hydrocephalus. *Neurol Res.* 2000;22(1):25–28. https://doi.org/10.1080/01616412.2000.11741034.

31. De Bonis P, Pompucci A, Mangiola A, Rigante L, Anile C. Post-traumatic hydrocephalus after decompressive craniectomy: an underestimated risk factor. *J Neurotrauma.* 2010;27(11):1965–1970. https://doi.org/10.1089/neu.2010.1425.

32. Weintraub AH, Gerber DJ, Kowalski RG. Posttraumatic hydrocephalus as a confounding influence on brain injury rehabilitation: incidence, clinical characteristics, and outcomes. *Arch Phys Med Rehabil.* 2017;98(2):312–319. https://doi.org/10.1016/j.apmr.2016.08.478.

33. Schultz BA, Bellamkonda E. Management of medical complications during the rehabilitation of moderate-severe traumatic brain injury. *Phys Med Rehabil Clin N Am*. 2017;28(2):259–270. https://doi.org/10.1016/j.pmr.2016.12.004.

34. Vedantam A, Yamal J-M, Hwang H, Robertson CS, Gopinath SP. Factors associated with shunt-dependent hydrocephalus after decompressive craniectomy for traumatic brain injury. *J Neurosurg*. 2017:1–6. https://doi.org/10.3171/2017.1.JNS162721.

35. Chen H, Yuan F, Chen S-W, et al. Predicting posttraumatic hydrocephalus: derivation and validation of a risk scoring system based on clinical characteristics. *Metab Brain Dis*. 2017;69:270. https://doi.org/10.1007/s11011-017-0008-2.

36. Katz RT, Brander V, Sahgal V. Updates on the diagnosis and management of posttraumatic hydrocephalus. *Am J Phys Med Rehabil*. 1989;68(2):91–96.

37. Gao F, Liu F, Chen Z, Hua Y, Keep RF, Xi G. Hydrocephalus after intraventricular hemorrhage: the role of thrombin. *J Cereb Blood Flow Metab*. 2014;34(3):489–494. https://doi.org/10.1038/jcbfm.2013.225.

38. Banizs B. Dysfunctional cilia lead to altered ependyma and choroid plexus function, and result in the formation of hydrocephalus. *Development*. 2005;132(23):5329–5339. https://doi.org/10.1242/dev.02153.

39. Xiong G, Elkind JA, Kundu S, et al. Traumatic brain injury-induced ependymal ciliary loss decreases cerebral spinal fluid flow. *J Neurotrauma*. 2014;31(16):1396–1404. https://doi.org/10.1089/neu.2013.3110.

40. Chen Q, Feng Z, Tan Q, et al. Post-hemorrhagic hydrocephalus: recent advances and new therapeutic insights. *J Neurol Sci*. 2017;375:220–230. https://doi.org/10.1016/j.jns.2017.01.072.

41. Kammersgaard LP, Linnemann M, Tibæk M. Hydrocephalus following severe traumatic brain injury in adults. Incidence, timing, and clinical predictors during rehabilitation. *NeuroRehabilitation*. 2013;33(3):473–480. https://doi.org/10.3233/NRE-130980.

42. Kiefer M, Unterberg A. The differential diagnosis and treatment of normal-pressure hydrocephalus. *Dtsch Arztebl Int*. 2012;109(1–2):15–25; quiz 26. https://doi.org/10.3238/arztebl.2012.0015.

43. Blumenfeld H. Cerebellum. In: *Neuroanatomy through Clinical Cases*. Sinauer Associates Incorporated; 2010.

44. American Congress of Rehabilitation Medicine, Brain Injury-Interdisciplinary Special Interest Group, Disorders of Consciousness Task Force, Seel RT, Sherer M, et al. Assessment scales for disorders of consciousness: evidence-based recommendations for clinical practice and research. *Arch Phys Med Rehabil*. 2010;91(12):1795–1813. https://doi.org/10.1016/j.apmr.2010.07.218.

45. Missori P, Miscusi M, Formisano R, et al. Magnetic resonance imaging flow void changes after cerebrospinal fluid shunt in post-traumatic hydrocephalus: clinical correlations and outcome. *Neurosurg Rev*. 2006;29(3):224–228. https://doi.org/10.1007/s10143-006-0027-7.

46. Wen L, Wan S, Zhan RY, et al. Shunt implantation in a special sub-group of post-traumatic hydrocephalus—patients have normal intracranial pressure without clinical representations of hydrocephalus. *Brain Inj*. 2009;23(1):61–64. https://doi.org/10.1080/02699050802635265.

47. Chen Z, Yang Y, Chen G, Wang M, Song W. Impact of ventriculoperitoneal shunting on chronic normal pressure hydrocephalus in consciousness rehabilitation. *J Rehabil Med*. 2014;46(9):876–881. https://doi.org/10.2340/16501977-1856.

48. Ishikawa M, Oowaki H, Matsumoto A, Suzuki T, Furuse M, Nishida N. Clinical significance of cerebrospinal fluid tap test and magnetic resonance imaging/computed tomography findings of tight high convexity in patients with possible idiopathic normal pressure hydrocephalus. *Neurol Med Chir (Tokyo)*. 2010;50(2):119–123. https://doi.org/10.2176/nmc.50.119.

49. Marmarou A, Bergsneider M, Klinge P, Relkin N, Black PM. The value of supplemental prognostic tests for the preoperative assessment of idiopathic normal-pressure hydrocephalus. *Neurosurgery*. 2005;57(3 suppl):S17–S28. Discussion ii–v.

50. Lesniak MS, Clatterbuck RE, Rigamonti D, Williams MA. Low pressure hydrocephalus and ventriculomegaly: hysteresis, non-linear dynamics, and the benefits of CSF diversion. *Br J Neurosurg*. 2002;16(6):555–561. https://doi.org/10.1080/ibjn20.v016.i06.

51. De Bonis P, Mangiola A, Pompucci A, Formisano R, Mattogno P, Anile C. CSF dynamics analysis in patients with post-traumatic ventriculomegaly. *Clin Neurol Neurosurg*. 2013;115(1):49–53. https://doi.org/10.1016/j.clineuro.2012.04.012.

52. Daou B, Klinge P, Tjoumakaris S, Rosenwasser RH, Jabbour P. Revisiting secondary normal pressure hydrocephalus: does it exist? A review. *Neurosurg Focus*. 2016;41(3):E6. https://doi.org/10.3171/2016.6.FOCUS16189.

53. Oder GTW. Outcome after shunt implantation in severe head injury with post-traumatic hydrocephalus. *Brain Inj*. 2009;14(4):345–354. https://doi.org/10.1080/026990500120637.

54. Denes Z, Barsi P, Szel I, Boros E, Fazekas G. Complication during postacute rehabilitation: patients with posttraumatic hydrocephalus. *Int J Rehabil Res*. 2011;34(3):222–226. https://doi.org/10.1097/MRR.0b013e328346e87d.

55. Smith G, Pace J, Scoco A, et al. Shunt devices for neuro-intensivists: complications and management. *Neurocrit Care*. 2017;23(suppl 1):1–11. https://doi.org/10.1007/s12028-016-0366-3.

56. Hutchinson PJ, Kolias AG, Timofeev IS, et al. Trial of decompressive craniectomy for traumatic intracranial hypertension. *N Engl J Med*. 2016. https://doi.org/10.1056/NEJMoa1605215.

57. Halani SH, Chu JK, Malcolm JG, et al. Effects of cranioplasty on cerebral blood flow following decompressive craniectomy: a systematic review of the literature. *Neurosurgery*. 2017. https://doi.org/10.1093/neuros/nyx054.

58. Beauchamp KM, Kashuk J, Moore EE, et al. Cranioplasty after postinjury decompressive craniectomy: is timing of the essence? *J Trauma Acute Care Surg.* 2010;69(2):270–274. https://doi.org/10.1097/TA. 0b013e3181e491c2.

59. Ashayeri K, Jackson EM, Huang J, Brem H, Gordon CR. Syndrome of the trephined: a systematic review. *Neurosurgery.* 2016;79(4):525–534. https://doi.org/10.1227/NEU.0000000000001366.

60. Krauss J, Jankovic J. Movement disorders after traumatic brain injury. In: Nathan D, Zasler MD, Douglas I, et al., eds. *Brain Injury Medicine.* 2nd ed. Demos Medical Publishing; 2012.

61. Krauss JK, Jankovic J. Head injury and posttraumatic movement disorders. *Neurosurgery.* 2002;50(5):927–939. Discussion 939–940.

62. O'Suilleabhain P, Dewey RB. Movement disorders after head injury: diagnosis and management. *J Head Trauma Rehabil.* 2004;19(4):305–313.

63. Lee MS, Rinne JO, Ceballos-Baumann A, Thompson PD, Marsden CD. Dystonia after head trauma. *Neurology.* 1994;44(8):1374–1378.

64. Blackman JA, Patrick PD, Buck ML, Rust RS. Paroxysmal autonomic instability with dystonia after brain injury. *Arch Neurol.* 2004;61(3):321–328. https://doi.org/10.1001/archneur.61.3.321.

65. Krauss JK, Tränkle R, Kopp KH. Posttraumatic movement disorders after moderate or mild head injury. *Mov Disord.* 1997;12(3):428–431. https://doi.org/10.1002/mds.870120326.

66. Jang SH, Kwon HG. Injury of the dentato-rubro-thalamic tract in a patient with mild traumatic brain injury. *Brain Inj.* 2015;29(13–14):1725–1728. https://doi.org/10.3109/02699052.2015.1075170.

67. Stahl SM. Depression and bipolar disorders. In: *Stahl's Essential Psychopharmacology.* Cambridge University Press; 2013.

68. van Rooijen DE, Geraedts EJ, Marinus J, Jankovic J, van Hilten JJ. Peripheral trauma and movement disorders: a systematic review of reported cases. *J Neurol Neurosurg Psychiatry.* 2011;82(8):892–898. https://doi.org/10.1136/jnnp.2010.232504.

69. Pedemonte C, Pérez Gutiérrez H, González E, Vargas I, Lazo D. Use of onabotulinumtoxinA in post-traumatic oromandibular dystonia. *J Oral Maxillofac Surg.* 2015;73(1):152–157. https://doi.org/10.1016/j.joms.2014.07.027.

70. Buxbaum LJ, Ferraro MK, Veramonti T, et al. Hemispatial neglect: subtypes, neuroanatomy, and disability. *Neurology.* 2004;62(5):749–756. https://doi.org/10.1212/01.WNL.0000113730.73031.F4.

71. McKenna K, Cooke DM, Fleming J, Jefferson A, Ogden S. The incidence of visual perceptual impairment in patients with severe traumatic brain injury. *Brain Inj.* 2009;20(5):507–518. https://doi.org/10.1080/02699050600664368.

72. Chen P, Ward I, Khan U, Liu Y, Hreha K. Spatial neglect hinders success of inpatient rehabilitation in individuals with traumatic brain injury: a retrospective study. *Neurorehabil Neural Repair.* 2016;30(5):451–460. https://doi.org/10.1177/1545968315604397.

73. Azouvi P, Jacquin-Courtois S, Luauté J. Rehabilitation of unilateral neglect: evidence-based medicine. *Ann Phys Rehabil Med.* 2017;60(3):191–197. https://doi.org/10.1016/j.rehab.2016.10.006.

74. Chen P, Chen CC, Hreha K, Goedert KM, Barrett AM. Kessler Foundation Neglect Assessment Process uniquely measures spatial neglect during activities of daily living. *Arch Phys Med Rehabil.* 2015;96(5):869–876.e1. https://doi.org/10.1016/j.apmr.2014.10.023.

75. Maskell F, Chiarelli P, Isles R. Dizziness after traumatic brain injury: overview and measurement in the clinical setting. *Brain Inj.* 2006;20(3):293–305. https://doi.org/10.1080/02699050500488041.

76. Peterson M, Greenwald BD. Balance problems after traumatic brain injury. *Arch Phys Med Rehabil.* 2015;96:379–380. https://doi.org/10.1016/j.apmr.2013.06.012.

77. Franke LM, Walker WC, Cifu DX, Ochs AL, Lew HL. Sensorintegrative dysfunction underlying vestibular disorders after traumatic brain injury: a review. *J Rehabil Res Dev.* 2012;49(7):985–994. https://doi.org/10.1682/JRRD.2011.12.0250.

78. Chandrasekhar SS. The assessment of balance and dizziness in the TBI patient. *NeuroRehabilitation.* 2013;32(3):445–454. https://doi.org/10.3233/NRE-130867.

79. Register-Mihalik JK, Mihalik JP, Guskiewicz KM. Balance deficits after sports-related concussion in individuals reporting posttraumatic headache. *Neurosurgery.* 2008;63(1):76–80; discussion 80–82. https://doi.org/10.1227/01.NEU.0000335073.39728.CE.

CHAPTER 5

Assessment and Management of Military and Veteran Traumatic Brain Injury

JOEL SCHOLTEN, MD • LINDA M. PICON, MCD, CCC-SLP • GEOFFREY GRAMMER, MD

The assessment and management of military and veteran traumatic brain injury (TBI) follow the general guidelines for the management of TBI for civilians with some unique caveats. Although combat-related TBI is often associated with brain injury in military service members, the Defense and Veterans Brain Injury Center (DVBIC) reports that more than 80% of all TBIs diagnosed in the active duty population are reported in garrison and not during conflict.[1]

A TBI sustained in a war zone can be complicated by combat operations hindering access to care, potential risk of injury to emergency responders, prolonged transportation to definitive care, and the unique injury patterns due to the mechanism of injury, particularly blast. Combat-related TBI may be associated with significant psychological trauma, which can confound the evaluation and treatment[2] for service members and veterans. We separate mild from moderate to severe TBI in our discussion given clinical differences between these two groups.

MODERATE AND SEVERE TRAUMATIC BRAIN INJURY

Combat Care and Medical Evacuation

Service members injured in a deployed setting are often in austere environments that are remote from traditional medical care. The military has established a system of care to account for these conditions, with emphasis on reducing mortality and morbidity and maximizing readiness.

The first line of care in a deployed environment starts with first aid. All military service members deploying to a combat environment are trained in basic first aid and brain injury awareness. Deployed service members are given first aid kits, which are required gear on all missions. The goal of first aid remains rapid stabilization of wounds until definitive care can be obtained. The next level of care is provided by unit medics or corpsmen, who are usually embedded with their units and accompany service members on the battlefield. Although there are different levels of competency and training, all line medics and corpsman receive extensive training on field assessment and care that exceeds civilian emergency medical technician requirements. These specialized personnel receive training specific to brain injury assessment and field management. If service members require more than basic field care, they are transported to an established medical facility, which, depending on the injury, locale, and combat environment, can vary from a basic field station to a formal Combat Area Support Hospital with surgical capability. Transport to and between medical facilities may involve ground ambulance, rotary wing, and fixed wing travel and often exceeds transport times usually observed in civilian care. If patients cannot be treated and returned to duty with deployed medical assets, they are evacuated to fixed medical facilities outside of the combat area of operations. Transitions back to the continental United States may involve layovers in overseas military treatment facilities (MTFs) where more robust surgical, imaging, and laboratory capabilities allow for further stabilization before transoceanic flights are attempted.

On arrival to the continental United States, patients travel via ground ambulance from the airport to one of the major military medical centers. These facilities have full medical capability for definitive care where comprehensive psychological, cognitive, and physical effects of brain injury can be assessed and early interventions established. TBI consult teams, comprising multiple disciplines, evaluate patients and incorporate their recommendations into part of a greater polytrauma treatment plan. While in care at military medical treatment facilities, patients and their families receive support through medical case management and through warrior transition units (WTUs) specifically designed around complex care management, friends and family services, and reintegration efforts.

Rehabilitative Care in Veteran Affairs

Following medical stabilization and initiation of rehabilitation at the MTF, service members requiring further acute inpatient rehabilitation are provided the option to obtain rehabilitation at a private rehabilitation facility using their insurance benefits or at one of the Department of Veteran Affairs (VA) rehabilitation centers. Transferring these injured service members from an MTF to a VA rehabilitation facility following a deployment-related TBI can be medically complex, and significant efforts are invested to ensure a smooth and safe transition. VA liaisons, nurse and social work case managers, are embedded in MTFs to work with the Department of Defense (DoD) treatment teams to assist in conveying all necessary medical and psychosocial information to the receiving VA rehabilitation team. DoD and VA teams connect either by phone or videoconference to meet and discuss treatment plans and highlight the unique medical and rehabilitative details for the individual patient. Enhanced communication between teams minimizes the risk of error during the transition as well as provides assurance to the service members' family that care will remain integrated and cohesive.

These transitions are extremely complex, owing to both the distance traveled and degree of medical complexity, and care must be seamless and coordinated. VA Liaisons provide a final review to ensure that all necessary medical information, including radiologic studies, medication lists, and isolation status if necessary, is included with the patient for the medical transport. In addition, the Liaison oversees the final nurse-to-nurse report to provide a failsafe means to transmit care needs for the transition. The receiving VA rehabilitation team performs an updated medical and functional assessment on arrival using information provided by their DoD counterparts in an effort to seamlessly promote ongoing rehabilitation.

DoD and VA coined the term "Polytrauma" during the early stages of the post-9/11 conflicts to describe the complex injury pattern seen in injured service members commonly from blast exposure. These injuries were frequently secondary to improvised explosive devices and included a traumatic brain injury as well as injuries to

multiple other organ systems. To meet the needs of this cohort with complex injuries, VA enhanced its existing centers providing traumatic brain injury rehabilitation established in 1992 and redesignated them polytrauma rehabilitation centers (PRCs).[3] Medical rehabilitation at the PRC is similar to that in the private sector; however, the length of stay is determined by rehabilitation needs rather than limitations imposed by a third-party payer. Family members often travel with their injured service member and stay on the VA campus at a Fisher House.

The basic concepts of TBI rehabilitation in the inpatient PRC setting are no different than those in the civilian setting; however, several unique differences in the active duty/veteran population have been described. VA has been collaborating with the Health and Human Services TBI Model Systems since 2010 and has developed a similar longitudinal database to allow comparison of this unique active duty service member and veteran cohort with other specialized TBI rehabilitation centers.[4] Analysis of this rich dataset has just begun, and some early findings show significant differences between the two cohorts. For instance, the rehospitalization rate in the first year after acute rehabilitation is much higher for veterans when compared with civilians.[5] Future studies will allow better understanding of the differences of the military and veteran cohort following TBI. These findings are essential for VA to incorporate into its clinical practice management for longer-term TBI case, as VA adopts management of TBI in a chronic disease framework.[6,7] VA has established Polytrauma Network Sites (PNS) to serve as regional hubs to oversee TBI care for the region and assist an additional 90 local polytrauma support clinic teams and the approximately 30 VA medical centers that do not have a fully staffed outpatient TBI rehabilitation team.

In addition, the five PRCs have a Polytrauma Transitional Residential Program (PTRP) colocated at their site to provide longer-term rehabilitation for service members and veterans to successfully integrate back into the community. These programs have provided enhanced rehabilitation programming for individuals just completing acute inpatient rehabilitation as well as individuals with prior injuries struggling with community integration. Length of stay in these programs has been approximately 60 days and efforts focus on return to work, driving, and independent living.[8]

Discharge disposition after a PRC or PTRP rehabilitation stay is based on the needs of the individual as well as input from the service member's command. Many are placed on convalescent leave followed by return to duty or assignment to a WTU where they continue rehabilitation efforts and a determination is made regarding ability to return to duty or separation from service.

Behavioral Health Issues

Patients with moderate to severe brain injuries can suffer from behavioral health consequences that impede care, interfere with rehabilitation, and subvert community reintegration. Although a full review of the behavioral health consequences exceeds the scope of this chapter, there are many considerations unique to military service members. Combat-related TBI can occur in the context of significant traumatic events often with flash combat exposures, such as roadside bombs. Service members must negotiate comprehension of the events leading to their injury within their individual existential framework. Discovery of a fellow unit member's injury or death can further complicate focus on recovery. Any impairments of sensorium or cognition can limit mobilization of psychological resiliency during rehabilitation.

The impact of transporting the injured across the globe to reach definitive care facilities should not be underestimated. Medical evacuation over uneven terrain or through turbulent air assets can add to physical pain and suffering. Transitioning between geographic locales across time zones and through multiple medical facilities can be uncomfortable, disorientating, and anxiety provoking. Reuniting with friends and family usually does not occur until safe arrival at a garrison treatment facility, depriving patients of key social support early in their medical journey. The entire experience from point of injury to arrival at definitive care is not one that lends itself to comfort or consolidation and is unique to the military combat experience.

Recovery from polytrauma with brain injury, with or without disorders of consciousness, can be associated with bouts of delirium and agitation. Military service members may find themselves regaining self-awareness with their last recollections being from the battlefield. Perceived threats of a continuing battle, delusions of enemy capture, or residual valance of combat are some examples that can complicate reconstructive and rehabilitative recovery.

Moderate to severe brain injury can result in behavioral disturbances resulting from poor impulse control, cognitive deficits, affective dysregulation, and other neuropsychological sequela. Although acute management of maladaptive behaviors and symptoms is essential to promote recovery and

reintegration, it is the longer-term consequences that may increase the risk of marital demise, unemployment, substance abuse, financial ruin, or criminal activity. The unstructured home environment is more amenable to mechanisms of misconduct than a controlled hospital or rehabilitation environment, which may lead to recognition and care only after irreparable psychosocial consequences. This phenomenon can be more pronounced in the military population. Command oversight of patients and the structure of units supporting service members in medical care limit access to opportunities for misconduct and provides early recognition and intervention when these events do occur. This oversight does not continue once a service member leaves the military, and what may have been assessed as adequate behavioral and emotional control may destabilize on return to the civilian community. To predict this potential liability, it is essential that patients with moderate to severe injury be formally evaluated in a variety of community settings, with variable stimuli and access to the litany of services that make up the social fabric. With early assessment and intervention in those unable to demonstrate mastery of an unstructured environment, it is hoped that the psychosocial causalities of brain injury can be mitigated before subsequent harm has been acquired.

Community Reintegration

Successful community reintegration is the ultimate objective of TBI rehabilitation and care. In the case of mild or uncomplicated forms of brain injury, return to normal activity typically occurs within a few weeks or months. For those who sustain more complicated forms of TBI and may even require hospitalization, the recovery trajectory is substantially more complex, as discussed in previous sections of this chapter. Like civilians, service members and veterans with moderate and severe TBI may face years of residual disability and care needs that interfere with successful return to work, school, and social roles.

Planning for community reentry begins at the onset of acute rehabilitation, which is typically offered at a VA PRC. The individualized rehabilitation plans developed by an interdisciplinary team in collaboration with the service members/veterans and their family include a mutually agreed upon postrehabilitation destination. Services provided during the acute rehabilitation stay facilitate the long-term goal of successful reintegration into the desired community environment and life roles. Programs in the Polytrauma System of Care described earlier, such as the five inpatient Polytrauma

Transitional Rehabilitation Programs[8] and outpatient services provided at the PNS throughout the nation, provide comprehensive, specialized treatments (e.g., assistive technology laboratories, driver's training, adapted sports, vocational rehabilitation) to enable successful community reintegration. The National Intrepid Center of Excellence and the Intrepid Spirit sites throughout the Military Health System also offer integrated TBI rehabilitation and mental health service options to achieve optimal patient well-being.[9] A number of support programs are available to enable veterans to live in their communities after TBI, such as the VA Caregiver Program, and they offer training, respite, and mental health support and, in some cases, financial assistance to those who care for the most severely injured in the community. In addition, VA provides adapted housing grants, prosthetic services, and home health and extended community care services to facilitate living at home for those with service-connected disabilities.

Despite the availability of programs and services, community reintegration, which may include independent living, return to employment, volunteering or school, social participation, and activities such as cooking, shopping, and driving, remains challenging for most. In numerous reports of civilian TBI, difficulties in community reintegration, such as unemployment and inability to resume driving, among others, persist years after TBI and limit independence, psychological well-being, and quality of life after reentry into the community.[10,11] In the military population, multiple challenges and unresolved problems are commonly reported related to post-TBI community reintegration, specifically in community transportation, managing money and paying bills, and independence in housekeeping, shopping, and cooking.[12]

McGarity and colleagues[13] also describe community reintegration as problematic for veterans and active duty service members with a history of mild TBI or with moderate/severe TBI. Importantly, they describe comorbidities unique to this military population at 1-year follow-up that further inhibit full reintegration into the community and that may have implications for rehabilitation programming and long-term follow-up. In their study sample of 154 service members and veterans with mild or moderate/severe TBI, most with moderate/severe TBIs depended on others for driving and use of public transportation, had more employment restrictions when they were employed, and were less likely to participate in social and community activities 1 year after discharge from inpatient rehabilitation. Residual cognitive or physical impairments, in some cases both, resulted in these difficulties and are well-known predictors of community reintegration challenges across civilian and military groups with disabilities. Interestingly, a subset with history of military-related mild TBI (mTBI) who received time-limited inpatient rehabilitation also was dependent on others for transportation, had some employment restriction (e.g., required assistive technologies), and demonstrated reduced social participation 1 year after reentering their communities. Depressive and post-traumatic stress disorder (PTSD) symptoms and cognitive complaints were associated with reported problems in transportation, employment, and social participation in this mTBI cohort. Others also have reported that returning to and sustaining competitive employment in the first year after TBI is lower in service members and veterans than in the general population.[14] Those with the most challenges returning to school or competitive employment were more severely injured, as can be expected (e.g., poorer cognitive and physical functioning), and also experienced a greater degree of mental health symptoms, such as PTSD, depression, and general anxiety.[10,11]

These findings highlight the importance of early integration of TBI rehabilitation, vocational rehabilitation, and mental health services in transitional programs and after community reentry. Access to programs, services, and assistive technologies that support return to the school environment (in clinics or through veteran student programs in colleges and universities) may also be of benefit. Furthermore, there is a need for establishing focused long-term monitoring of needs and services accessed to mitigate community reentry challenges that may themselves lead to worsening mental health outcomes over time. In this regard, the VA offers a nationwide system of mental health care integrated with rehabilitation and primary care models with a focus on holistic long-term care for polytrauma/TBI and related comorbidities that is unparalleled in the community.[15] VA and DoD also lead clinical and research programs to help guide the services that promote successful reintegration into desired roles.

Service members and veterans report postdeployment difficulty participating in community activities and in relationships,[16] but those difficulties along with low satisfaction with life can linger for at least a year after community reentry, likely much longer, for those who sustain TBI.[13,17] In civilian and military groups alike, relationship dynamics change (friends, family, work) and isolation can set in.[18] Stevens et al.

report that among service members and veterans who were married at the time of injury, who were younger participants with less severe injuries, who had fewer years of education, and who had a preinjury history of mental health treatment were most likely to divorce within 2 years of discharge from inpatient rehabilitation. On the other hand, service members and veterans with severe TBI who were married at the time of injury tended to stay married. Although relationship status does not change for most according to Stevens and colleagues, isolation and disconnectedness also can occur to a couple or family unit as a whole. They highlight the potential benefits of marital or couples therapy for some during the follow-up trajectory, and we further stress the importance of therapies and support services for caregivers and families, including children.

In addition to long-term healthcare, rehabilitation, and support services provided across DoD and VA, building relationships with local community agencies is critical to increase access to resources in general, and to mitigate the decreased participation in leisure activity, specifically, reported by service members and veterans with TBI as they reenter their own communities.[19] Community partner agreements made with VA and DoD that provide grants, support programs, and extended services through nonprofit service organizations have been extremely beneficial for service members, veterans, caregivers, and families reentering the community. One such example is the VA Adaptive Sports Program, which has created partnerships with national organizations in local communities to promote sports activities, such as martial arts, golfing, boating, biking, basketball, and therapeutic riding, among many others, all adapted to the individual needs of the service member or veteran. In addition to special events such as the National Wheelchair Games, and the winter and summer (seasonal) sports clinics, adapted sports programs offered through VA and community partners provide opportunities for developing wellness and community connectedness.

Strengthening community reintegration means not only preparing service members and veterans for successful return to preinjury or desired roles but also supporting and sustaining them in the community in which they choose to live. It is the responsibility of providers, researchers, family members, caregivers, and service members and veterans themselves to support and encourage those with ongoing needs to remain engaged in care and community activities. Interventions such as life coaching or motivational interviewing may facilitate engagement and follow through in the community

by promoting awareness and increasing personal ownership. Long-term monitoring and follow-up as indicated by a provider can optimize community reentry outcomes and prevent problems from developing. Services should be provided based on the individual characteristics and needs of the service member or veteran, but research should continue to look for latent and preventable problems years after community reentry, as well as the types of services and doses that most support sustained success.

MILD TRAUMATIC BRAIN INJURY

The assessment and management of mTBI is challenging in civilian medical practices, and several unique factors compound this issue in the context of TBI sustained during active duty military service. Screening and treatment programs have been implemented in both agencies to promote early identification and management.

Mild Traumatic Brain Injury Screening and Assessment in Department of Defense

The DoD has regulations and recommendations for the assessment and management of mTBI in a deployed setting. Fundamental to the process is the requirement for screening of brain injury based on exposure to any incident where an injury may have occurred.[20] Screening is triggered when any service member is in a vehicle associated with a blast event, collision, or rollover, within 50 m of a blast (inside or outside) or sustains a direct blow to the head. Screening can also occur if command directed, such as, but not limited to, repeated exposures. Service members meeting these incident-based criteria are referred to a medic or healthcare provider for a formal assessment and treatment using standardized clinical tools.

The DVBIC developed the Concussion Management Algorithm (CMA) to assist providers managing mTBI in the deployed setting and provide decision points that recommend referral requirements, level of care needs, and recovery interventions. There are three algorithms within the CMA, one for the medic/corpsman, one for the initial provider, and one for MTFs with neuroimaging capabilities. The CMA begins with the recognition of red flags suggesting more severe injury that would warrant immediate escalation of care. Each algorithm has recommendations for education, rest, and reassessment, concluding with a return to duty, further treatment, or referral to a higher level of care.

The Military Acute Concussion Evaluation (MACE) is used within the CMA to collect descriptive data to support documentation that eases appropriate severity classification and assesses postinjury symptoms, cognitive deficits, and neurologic signs. The CMA and the MACE work synergistically to guide medics and healthcare providers in performing standardized clinical assessments and management for mTBI. Service members are required to participate in baseline cognitive assessment within 12 months of deployment using the DoD-designated neurocognitive assessment instrument, the Automated Neuropsychological Assessment Metrics. As part of the CMA, neurocognitive reassessment following a diagnosis of concussion in the deployed setting serves to inform return to duty decisions.

The Progressive Return to Activity (PRA) clinical suite is used by military providers to guide recovery after mTBI, both in the deployed and nondeployed setting. There are two versions of the PRA, one for primary care and the other for rehabilitation medicine. The PRA gives recommendations for six levels of escalating activity starting with rest and concluding with unrestricted activity, with graduation between stages predicated upon the absence of symptoms. This offers time for recovery and minimizes risk of reinjury or overexposure.

For patients with persistent symptoms after a concussion, The DoD and VA released clinical practice guidelines (CPGs) in 2016.[21] Treatment recommendations and clinical management algorithms are provided using the evidenced-based literature. The spectrum of medical disciplines is included in the guidelines reflecting requirements for multidisciplinary management that is often required for this subset of postconcussion patients.

Through the use of these clinical support tools, providers at all levels can appropriately address patient needs across a variety of medical environments. These tools have been made available through the DVBIC website (https://dvbic.dcoe.mil/) as well as through direct provider education.

Mild Traumatic Brain Injury Screening and Assessment in VA

VA implemented TBI screening in April 2007 for all veterans separating from DoD after September 11, 2001, following frequent reports of concussion due to blast exposure during deployment. A four-question screen was developed by DoD, VA, and academia subject matter experts (SMEs) to identify veterans with possible TBI, leading to a comprehensive TBI evaluation (CTBIE) by a TBI specialist.[22] The CTBIE is a templated note embedded in the electronic medical record that guides the clinician through a clinical interview to collect information regarding the trauma and review current symptoms through collection of the Neurobehavioral Symptom Inventory (NBSI). Following the CTBIE a definitive diagnosis is provided along with an individualized treatment plan.

Analysis of the VA's TBI screening and evaluation process has demonstrated that approximately half of those completing an evaluation receive a TBI diagnosis and that this cohort reports a high number of symptoms. Using the NBSI, a self-reported 22-item symptom measurement, most veterans endorse 21 of 22 symptoms, highlighting the need for an individualized approach to care.[23]

For those who have sustained a TBI and require ongoing rehabilitation an individualized rehabilitation and community reintegration (IRCR) plan of care is developed. The IRCR templated note helps rehabilitation teams ensure that common areas of functional difficulty following TBI are addressed. In addition, the Mayo Portland adaptability inventory (MPAI) participation subscale (M2PI) is the recommended metric for teams to use to determine if veterans are making progress in their rehabilitation efforts.[24] The MPAI measures functional participation in areas that individuals with a history of brain injury may have difficulty, including self-care skills, transportation, location, and money management.

Mild Traumatic Brain Injury Clinical Management

DoD and VA have jointly developed mTBI CPG utilizing a rigorous review of the available scientific literature to provide evidence-based direction to mTBI providers. These guidelines are not intended to regulate policy or standard of care for mTBI in the Departments, but rather to inform clinical decisions at critical points in the assessment and treatment. VA and DoD SMEs from neurology, mental health, primary care, pharmacy, and rehabilitation, among others, developed practice recommendations guided by key questions chosen for their relevance to clinical management of mTBI and potential to inform practice. CPG recommendations were rated or graded on the relative strength of published evidence, considering implications to the service member or veteran (e.g., benefits, values) and to the systems of care (resource use, feasibility). CPGs recommend for or against a practice or service being provided, and based on the strength of the current evidence. The mTBI CPG advises the care of service members, veterans, and National Guard and Reserve components eligible for care in VA and DoD who present for care and are 8 days post injury and beyond. The injury must be the result of an external force that resulted in alteration or loss of consciousness, based on the DoD definition of TBI.[25] Emergency evaluation of concussion and management of moderate, severe, and penetrating TBI are outside the scope of the mTBI CPG.

The first VA/DoD CPG for the management of mTBI or concussion in Primary Care was published in 2009. Given the limited body of evidence available, an update to the systematic literature review was completed through 2015 and an updated CPG was published in early 2016. In addition to four new recommendations the 2016 CPG replaced, amended, or carried forward most elements of the 2009 CPG. As in the 2009 version, there was insufficient evidence to make strong recommendations for or against any given practice across patients and settings for many recommendations. The CPG includes discussion sections, and in those cases, it offers practice suggestions based on the best available evidence and group consensus. The 2016 version arbitrarily extended the postinjury periods offered in 2009 to capture the chronicity of symptom presentation of this cohort, sometimes months or years after injury. Based on group consensus, the term "Patient with a history of mTBI" was chosen over "Patient with TBI," to better align with the current state of the science on (clinical) diagnosis of mTBI.

The 2016 CPG is organized into 2 algorithms and 23 evidence-based recommendations. The algorithms outline sequential steps at each critical juncture in the management of mTBI within a VA or DoD primary care or concussion care setting. Specifically, the algorithms highlight evaluations, interventions, treatments, referrals, and follow-up recommendations appropriate at both the initial presentation and at later time periods when managing chronic symptomatology. The algorithm for initial presentation systematically guides the provider through a clinical evaluation of TBI, including indicators (red flags) for urgent conditions that may require immediate attention. It assists in identification of symptoms by providing a list of the most frequently reported postconcussion symptoms and informs the next steps pertinent for management in deployed and nondeployed settings. Once functionally limiting symptoms and attributes are identified at the initial presentation, the algorithm for symptom management takes the primary care provider through a series of steps to assess, evaluate, and educate.

A symptom-driven approach in the primary care setting provides the framework for management of mTBI in the CPG. As in the 2009 version, strong emphasis was placed on the early identification and management of co-occurring conditions that may contribute to new or persisting symptoms, or to misattribution of symptoms. Interventions for coexisting mental health disturbances, pain, substance use disorders, and sleep difficulties should be implemented as a first step of any treatment regime. Also carried forward from the 2009 CPG, education about positive expectations of recovery and empowering patients through self-management techniques are essential components of early intervention. Focused evaluation of current symptoms, symptom attributes, exacerbating conditions, and functional limitations guide treatment for the first 30–90 days, followed by referral to TBI specialists for refractory symptoms. For persistent symptoms that remain functionally limiting, the CPG algorithm suggests engaging case managers with primary care to reinforce education, interventions, and available resources.

CPG recommendations were divided into four categories: (1) diagnosis and assessment, (2) co-occurring conditions, (3) treatment, and (4) setting of care. Each section provides graded, evidence-based guidance for treatments and services that should be considered. Under the symptom management appendix, the CPG also provides suggested guidance for symptom-based interventions, as well as dosing and timing, when available. One such example is the recommendation for management of posttraumatic headache, which suggests nonpharmacologic and pharmacologic options for acute pain (including head, face, and neck) and prevention of tension- and migraine-like headaches. Recommendations in support of symptom management where the evidence is emerging provide a caveat for short-term, functional goal-oriented treatment trials by TBI specialists, in the absence of evidence to recommend a type and dosage (e.g., recommendations for management of dizziness and disequilibrium, and cognitive and sensory complaints).

Other recommendations suggest "against" performing a procedure or providing a service. For example, updated review of the literature provided compelling evidence for the SME group to strongly recommend against adjusting management and outcome prognosis based on the mechanism of injury. Unlike the complex pathology associated with moderate and severe TBI, the potentially unique effects of blast or other potentially concussive mechanisms of injury are unknown, in particular, any associated pathophysiology. In the absence of such findings, treatment and prognosis remained driven by clinical examination in the 2016 CPG and the provider is cautioned against etiology-based management.

The 2016 CPG is not a prescriptive tool. Besides evidence-based recommendations, it places emphasis on the benefits of education, the patient-provider therapeutic alliance, setting positive expectations of recovery, and promoting self-management as part of the overall health and well-being of the service member and veteran with a history of mTBI. It acknowledges the potential need for long-term primary care monitoring for latent problems and comorbid conditions and the benefits of the case management model in primary care to encourage and support. The final step in the mTBI CPG algorithms and the goal of the CPG is the successful return to work/duty/school and participation in community, family, and society roles. The 2016 VA/DoD CPG for the Management of Concussion/mTBI and summary tools are publicly available at www.healthquality.va.gov.[21]

The management of veterans with a history of mTBI includes the challenges of addressing not only multiple symptoms but also multiple comorbid conditions. Comorbidities of pain and PTSD are common in outpatient VA TBI clinics and have been coined the "polytrauma clinical triad."[26] Development of an individualized treatment plan is essential owing to the complexities of the overlapping symptoms and potential contributions from each diagnosis. Team communication between the various healthcare providers involved in the individualized plan and the veteran and their family may also be challenging but necessary to deliver patient-centered care. Further analysis of VHA healthcare utilization data reveals 73% of all post-9/11 veterans accessing VA for healthcare with a history of TBI in fiscal year 2014 also carried a diagnosis of PTSD and 56% carried a diagnosis of both PTSD and pain.[27] This further highlights the need for individualized interdisciplinary care delivered in close collaboration with mental health providers.

CONCLUSION

The assessment and management of military and veteran TBI involves the same principles for the civilian population with a few notable caveats. Deployment-related blast injury has resulted in more complex injury patterns and highlighted the need for enhanced care for TBI in the DoD and VA. Both agencies have invested resources to establish systems of care to identify and provide adequate treatment for veterans and service members with traumatic brain injury. Efforts to improve and standardize mTBI diagnosis and treatment include the development of CPGs utilizing available scientific evidence. Delivery of an individualized rehabilitation plan of care is essential because of the complexities of symptom presentation and co-occurring diagnosis, including the polytrauma clinical triad of TBI, PTSD, and pain.

REFERENCES

1. Defense and Veterans Brain Injury Center. *DoD Worldwide Numbers for TBI*; 2017. http://dvbic.dcoe.mil/dod-worldwide-numbers-tbi.
2. Soble JR, Silva MA, Vanderploeg RD, et al. Normative data for the neurobehavioral symptom inventory (NSI) and post-concussion symptom profiles among TBI, PTSD, and nonclinical samples. *Clin Neuropsychol.* 2014;28(4):614–632. https://doi.org/10.1080/13854046.2014.894576.
3. *VA Polytrauma System of Care Handbook*; 2013. https://www.va.gov/optometry/docs/VHA_Handbook_1172_01_Polytrauma_System_of_Care.pdf.
4. Lamberty GJ, Nakase-Richardson R, Farrell-Carnahan L, et al. Development of a traumatic brain injury model system within the Department of Veterans Affairs polytrauma system of care. *J Head Trauma Rehabil.* 2014;29(3):E1–E7. https://doi.org/10.1097/HTR.0b013e31829a64d1.
5. Tran J, Hammond F, Dams-O'Connor K, et al. Rehospitalization in the first year following veteran and service member TBI: a VA TBI model systems study. *J Head Trauma Rehabil.* 2017. https://doi.org/10.1097/HTR.0000000000000296.
6. Masel BE, DeWitt DS. Traumatic brain injury: a disease process, not an event. *J Neurotrauma.* 2010;27(8):1529–1540. https://doi.org/10.1089/neu.2010.1358.
7. Malec JF, Hammond FM, Flanagan S, et al. Recommendations from the 2013 Galveston brain injury conference for implementation of a chronic care model in brain injury. *J Head Trauma Rehabil.* 2013;28(6):476–483. https://doi.org/10.1097/HTR.0000000000000003.
8. Duchnick JJ, Ropacki S, Yutsis M, Petska K, Pawlowski C. Polytrauma transitional rehabilitation programs: comprehensive rehabilitation for community integration after brain injury. *Psychol Serv.* 2015;12(3):313–321. https://doi.org/10.1037/ser0000034.
9. *National Intrepid Center of Excellence 2016 Annual Report*; 2017. http://www.wrnmmc.capmed.mil/NICoE/SiteAssets/NICoE_Annual_Report_2016.pdf.
10. Shames J, Treger I, Ring H, Giaquinto S. Return to work following traumatic brain injury: trends and challenges. *Disabil Rehabil.* 2007;29(17):1387–1395. https://doi.org/10.1080/09638280701315011.
11. Winter L, Moriarty HJ, Short TH. Self-reported driving difficulty in veterans with traumatic brain injury: its central role in psychological well-being. *PM R.* 2017. https://doi.org/10.1016/j.pmrj.2017.01.007.

12. Nakase-Richardson R. Development of the TBI rehabilitation needs survey for veterans and service members in post-acute stages of TBI. *Arch Phys Med Rehabil.* 2016;97(10):e127–e128. https://doi.org/10.1016/j.ampr.2016.08.398.

13. McGarity S, Barnett SD, Lamberty G, et al. Community reintegration problems among veterans and active duty service members with traumatic brain injury. *J Head Trauma Rehabil.* 2017;32(1):34–45. https://doi.org/10.1097/HTR.0000000000000242.

14. Dillahunt-Aspillaga C, Nakase-Richardson R, Hart T, et al. Predictors of employment outcomes in veterans with traumatic brain injury: a VA traumatic brain injury model systems study. *J Head Trauma Rehabil.* 2017. https://doi.org/10.1097/HTR.0000000000000275.

15. Sigford BJ. "To care for him who shall have borne the battle and for his widow and his orphan" (Abraham Lincoln): the Department of Veterans Affairs polytrauma system of care. *Arch Phys Med Rehabil.* 2008;89(1):160–162. https://doi.org/10.1016/j.apmr.2007.09.015.

16. Sayer NA, Noorbaloochi S, Frazier P, Carlson K, Gravely A, Murdoch M. Reintegration problems and treatment interests among Iraq and Afghanistan combat veterans receiving VA medical care. *Psychiatr Serv Wash DC.* 2010;61(6):589–597. https://doi.org/10.1176/ps.2010.61.6.589.

17. Gause LR, Finn JA, Lamberty GJ, et al. Predictors of satisfaction with life in veterans after traumatic brain injury: a VA TBI model systems study. *J Head Trauma Rehabil.* 2017. https://doi.org/10.1097/HTR.0000000000000309.

18. Stevens LF, Lapis Y, Tang X, et al. Relationship stability after traumatic brain injury among veterans and service members: a VA TBI model systems study. *J Head Trauma Rehabil.* 2017;32(4):234–244. https://doi.org/10.1097/HTR.0000000000000324.

19. Daggett VS, Bakas T, Buelow J, Habermann B, Murray LL. Needs and concerns of male combat veterans with mild traumatic brain injury. *J Rehabil Res Dev.* 2013;50(3):327–340.

20. Department of Defense. *Department of Defense Instruction 6490.11;* 2012. http://usaisr.amedd.army.mil/cpgs/DODI_6490.11_Policy_Guidance_for_Mgmt_of_Mild_Traumatic_Brain_Injury_or_Concussion_in_the_Deployed_Setting.pdf.

21. Department of Veteran Affairs. *VA/DoD Clinical Practice Guidelines;* 2016. http://www.healthquality.va.gov/policy/index.asp.

22. Department of Veteran Affairs. *Screening and Evaluation of Traumatic Brain Injury in Operation Enduring Freedom, Operation Iraqi Freedom, and Operation New Dawn Veterans;* 2017. https://www.va.gov/vhapublications/ViewPublication.asp?pub_ID=5376.

23. Scholten JD, Sayer NA, Vanderploeg RD, Bidelspach DE, Cifu DX. Analysis of US Veterans Health Administration comprehensive evaluations for traumatic brain injury in Operation Enduring Freedom and operation Iraqi Freedom Veterans. *Brain Inj.* 2012;26(10):1177–1184. https://doi.org/10.3109/02699052.2012.661914.

24. Malec JF. The Mayo-Portland participation index: a brief and psychometrically sound measure of brain injury outcome. *Arch Phys Med Rehabil.* 2004;85(12):1989–1996.

25. Woodson J. *Traumatic Brain Injury: Updated Definition and Reporting.* Health.mil; 2015. https://health.mil/Military-Health-Topics/Conditions-and-Treatments/Physical-Disability/Traumatic-Brain-Injury?type=Policies#RefFeed.

26. Lew HL, Otis JD, Tun C, Kerns RD, Clark ME, Cifu DX. Prevalence of chronic pain, posttraumatic stress disorder, and persistent postconcussive symptoms in OIF/OEF veterans: polytrauma clinical triad. *J Rehabil Res Dev.* 2009;46(6):697–702.

27. Taylor B. *Fiscal Year 2014 VA Utilization Report for Iraq and Afghanistan War Veterans Diagnosed with TBI;* 2015. https://www.polytrauma.va.gov/TBIReports/FY14-TBI-Diagnosis-HCU-Report.pdf.

CHAPTER 6

Assessment and Management of Sports Concussion

KATHLEEN R. BELL, MD • ROBERT RINALDI, MD • NYAZ DIDEHBANI, PhD

INTRODUCTION

Sports participation for children and adults alike has long been perceived and demonstrated to be beneficial in many ways. Organized sports can help children develop social connectedness, team building skills, and leadership skill and improve problem-solving and decision-making skills.[1] In addition, sports participation and regular physical activity in children and adults have been demonstrated to help combat many chronic health conditions, including childhood obesity, coronary artery disease, type 2 diabetes, and stroke.[1-3] It is estimated that on an annual basis in the United States, up to 44 million children and adolescents participate in organized sports and close to 170 million adults participate in regular physical activity.[4] With this involvement comes an increased risk for injury, including traumatic brain injury (TBI) and specifically sports-related concussion (SRC). As such, there has been a growing interest among those involved in sport (e.g., managers, athletic trainers, participants) and healthcare professionals on how to better assess and manage SRC. This chapter summarizes the present understanding of the pathophysiology of concussions, current recommendations regarding the initial assessment of SRC, and recommendations for the management of SRC-related somatic and cognitive complications.

EPIDEMIOLOGY OF SPORTS-RELATED CONCUSSION

The epidemiology of SRC is not clearly delineated in the literature. However, multiple studies have begun to define some consistent trends. It is estimated that in the United States, up to 3.8 million athletes sustain an SRC per year.[5] Although the incidence of SRC is similar among high school athletes and collegiate athletes, there are far more high school athletes than collegiate athletes, creating a much larger healthcare issue in the adolescent population. In a prospective study enrolling 7513 high school athletes and 1392 collegiate athletes, Marshall et al.[6] reported an incidence rate of 26.1 concussions per 100,000 athlete exposures, with an overall risk of 1.8 per 100 athletes. Among the seven sports assessed, nearly two-thirds of concussions occurred in football. This figure is in accordance with other recent sport-specific epidemiologic study results. Wasserman et al.[7] demonstrated that across 25 collegiate sports the percentage of concussions incurred during practices was very similar to those incurred during competition (46.8% vs. 53.2%). This raises the consideration of the need to advance appropriate medical management not only during competition but also during practices, especially given the much larger frequency of practices compared with games.

Presenting symptoms have also been shown to be relatively consistent across sports. Headache is the most prevalent complaint (87%–92%), with dizziness (69%–77%), feeling "in a fog" (62%), and difficulties concentrating (52%–58%) being other common complaints.[6,7] Factors that seem to be predictive of impaired cognitive function after concussion include a history of previous concussions, number and duration of postconcussion symptoms, and younger age. Although present evidence is limited, factors that may be predictive of an increased risk for postconcussion symptoms include being an adult female, longer duration of on-field cognitive changes and postinjury memory impairments, and showing generalized decreased cognitive function post injury.[8]

Time to resolution of symptoms differs from time to return to play. Although it varies between individual athletes, evidence suggests that high school athletes have a longer mean symptom resolution time than do collegiate athletes. Overall across all levels of play resolution of symptoms takes from a few days to a few weeks, with most athletes demonstrating resolution of symptoms within 7–10 days.[9] Return to play has been shown to occur within 7–13 days for most athletes across multiple sports, with data trends showing a general prolongation of that time over the past 5–10 years.[7,9] This progressive prolongation in return to play may likely be due to improved symptom monitoring and more conservative management of the part of athletic trainers and healthcare professionals.

PATHOPHYSIOLOGY OF SPORTS-RELATED CONCUSSIONS

A concussion results from a biomechanical force to the brain that results in a pathophysiologic response at the neurotransmitter level. The acceleration and deceleration of these forces on the neuronal structures initiates a neurometabolic cascade as described by Giza and Hovda.[10] The disruption at the neuronal level includes neurotransmitter dysregulation, metabolic mismatch, axonal stretching, neuroinflammation, and changes in cerebral blood flow (CBF).

Neurotransmitter Dysregulation

Immediately following a concussion, there is an efflux of potassium by voltage-gated channels and influx of sodium and calcium.[10] The efflux of intracellular potassium causes neuronal depolarization, creating a feedback loop of continued increase in extracellular potassium, depolarization, and neurotransmitter release. Glutamate is released, which promotes potassium efflux, stimulates receptors, and induces ligand-gated potassium channels. The binding of glutamate to the *N*-methyl-D-aspartate receptors creates hyperexcitability with an increase in intracellular calcium and unrestricted depolarization.[10,11]

Metabolic Mismatch and Need for Energy

As excitatory neurotransmitters are released, intracellular calcium accumulates in the mitochondria, which can damage cells and possibly cause cell death.[11] The massive depolarization resulting from dysregulation of the neurotransmitters creates an imbalance as the mitochondria attempts to meet the energy demands of the cell. This in turn leads to hyperglycolysis increasing lactate in the cell, which can then result in cerebral edema.[10-12]

Diffuse Axonal Injury

Forces can also damage microstructural parts such as dendrites, axons, and astrocytic processes. Axons are especially vulnerable to biomechanical stretch because of damage to neurofilaments and microtubules. Stretching of the axons can disrupt axonal transport, isolate the synapse, affect metabolism, damage the cytoskeleton as calcium builds up, and possibly disconnect the axon.[12-14] Stretching of the white matter has been associated with cognitive impairment[15] and with more vulnerability following repeat injuries.[16] Imaging techniques such as diffusion tensor imaging (DTI) have become more prominent in assessing white matter damage in individuals with concussion.[12,17]

Neuroinflammation

It is known that severe TBI leads to an inflammatory response, but recent research also indicates neuroinflammation in mild TBI.[18] Neuroinflammation results from abnormal metabolism within hours of the concussion,[19] which can increase the permeability of the blood-brain barrier and affect CBF.[20] CBF is tied to neuronal acidity and glucose metabolism. Thus CBF can be drastically altered when there is a mismatch in metabolism or increase in glycolysis.[10,21]

Pathophysiology and Symptoms

Giza and Hovda[12] hypothesized several links of post-TBI pathophysiology to clinically observable symptoms. They proposed that the immediate influx of ions following a concussion may result in migraine headaches, photophobia, and phonophobia. They also suggested a link between the energy demand on the mitochondria and an increased vulnerability to repeated injuries. Axonal injury and disrupted neurotransmission may affect cognition primarily in slowed processing. Finally, protease activation, damaged cytoskeleton, and cell death may contribute to chronic atrophy and persistent symptoms.

SIDELINE ASSESSMENT AND MANAGEMENT

The initial diagnoses and management of an acute SRC begins on the field once a concussion is suspected. Athletes may be removed from play once they encounter a significant blow to the head or when their behavior appears to deviate from the baseline. The sideline assessment allows for a brief evaluation for a suspected concussion and does not necessarily provide a definitive diagnosis of a head injury.[22,23]

The most critical goal of an initial evaluation of a suspected head injury is to assess severe life-threatening injuries. Athletes with severe observable signs, such as loss of consciousness, ataxia, tonic posturing, post-traumatic seizures, or severe signs of spinal cord injury, must be removed immediately and taken to the emergency room. It is important to note that most injured athletes do not demonstrate obvious signs of a concussion but should be removed from play and evaluated if one is suspected.[22]

Although there is no one diagnostic assessment or set of markers for diagnosis of an SRC, a multifactorial approach to sideline assessment is often used. The parts of a sideline assessment may include self-reported and observable symptoms, balance tests, oculomotor tests, neurologic examination, mental status examination, and cognitive tests.[23] Symptoms are frequently divided into physical symptoms, such as headaches, dizziness, motor impairment, poor balance, and impaired reflexes; cognitive symptoms, such as impaired memory and attention and slowed processing; emotional symptoms, such as irritability, nervousness, or sadness; and sleep disturbances.[22] A cognitive evaluation may include measures of attention, processing speed, and memory, whereas a neurologic examination may include an evaluation of oculomotor function and assessment of cranial nerve function. Many of the above-mentioned symptoms can be evaluated rather quickly and informally, but formal standardized assessments have been developed and are recommended.

The Standardized Concussion Assessment Tool, fifth edition (SCAT5), revised in 2017 following the Berlin Concussion Conference, is widely used and accessible for use by healthcare providers to assess an SRC.[22] The SCAT5 can be used for ages 13 years and older, and the pediatric version (child SCAT5)[24] can be used for children 12 years and under. The SCAT5 includes the Maddocks questions, Glasgow Coma Scale, a cervical spine screen, a symptom checklist, a neurologic screen, a balance test, and a cognitive screen. The Maddocks questions measure orientation specifically related to the sporting venue. Research has shown that standard orientation questions asking about person, place, and time are not as reliable within the context of a sporting event.[22] The Glasgow Coma Scale measures the severity of the head injury by measuring observable eye, verbal, and motor responses. The cervical spine assessment also examines observable spine and neck responses. The balance assessment is a modified Balance Error Scoring System (BESS, described later), which asks the athlete to stand as still as possible in three different stances for 20 s with eyes closed (errors are counted for each stance).[25] The cognitive screen is the Standardized Assessment of Concussion (SAC) and assesses orientation, immediate and delayed memory, and concentration.[26]

The SAC is a brief screener that includes orientation questions, immediate and delayed verbal memory, attention, and working memory. The SAC has good sensitivity and specificity with normative data.[27] However, research has indicated significant differences between males and females, which warrant the need for gender norms.[28,29]

Other standardized measures include several self-report symptom scales, including the Post-Concussion Symptoms Scale, revised, which consists of 21 self-reported statements referencing common postconcussion symptoms. Each item on the scale is rated on a 7-point Likert scale ranging from 0 to 6. The Rivermead Post-Concussion Symptoms Questionnaire a 16-item self-report measure of symptom severity. Postconcussion symptom inventory (PCSI) has forms for ages 5–17 years, ranging from 13 to 26 items depending on age. It also includes a 26-item parent/teacher scale and measures cognitive, emotional, sleep, and physical symptoms. The interrater reliability for the PCSI ranges from moderate to high (0.65–0.89), and internal consistency was high for total scales (0.80–0.90).[30]

The use of a visual scanning screen, the King-Devick test (K-D test), has also been performed on the sideline. During the K-D test, athletes read numbers across three test cards or on a computer-based application as quickly as they can without making errors. Time to completion and errors are documented for each of the three test cards. The goal is to detect impairment in eye movements, attention, and language.[31]

Although the above tests are some of the more commonly used tools in sideline assessment, there is a constant flow of new measures for concussion evaluation, each claiming to be the most sensitive measure. It is important to note that not all measures are created equal and that not one assessment will provide definitive diagnoses. The goal of the sideline assessment is to use a brief measure to assess whether or not a concussion occurred and to make the appropriate referral for a more comprehensive medical evaluation and follow-up.

CLINICAL ASSESSMENT AND MANAGEMENT
History and Physical Examination
As with all injury evaluations, the injury history can be helpful in establishing both the presence and severity of injury and establishing a baseline for measuring recovery. Information regarding the mechanism of injury, age, sex, sport and position played, presence or absence of documented loss of consciousness or

How do you feel currently? Please circle a number for each of the symptoms listed below.

Current symptoms	None	Mild		Moderate		Severe	
Headache	0	1	2	3	4	5	6
Pressure in head	0	1	2	3	4	5	6
Neck pain	0	1	2	3	4	5	6
Nausea/vomiting	0	1	2	3	4	5	6
Dizziness	0	1	2	3	4	5	6
Blurred vision	0	1	2	3	4	5	6
Balance problems	0	1	2	3	4	5	6
Sensitivity to light	0	1	2	3	4	5	6
Sensitivity to noise	0	1	2	3	4	5	6
Feeling slowed down	0	1	2	3	4	5	6
Feeling "in a fog"	0	1	2	3	4	5	6
"Don't feel right"	0	1	2	3	4	5	6
Difficulty concentrating	0	1	2	3	4	5	6
Difficulty remembering	0	1	2	3	4	5	6
Fatigue or low energy	0	1	2	3	4	5	6
Confusion	0	1	2	3	4	5	6
Drowsiness	0	1	2	3	4	5	6
More emotional	0	1	2	3	4	5	6
Irritability	0	1	2	3	4	5	6
Sadness	0	1	2	3	4	5	6
Nervous or anxious	0	1	2	3	4	5	6
Trouble falling asleep (if applicable)	0	1	2	3	4	5	6

Total number of symptoms	of 22
Symptom severity score	of 132
Do your symptoms get worse with physical activity?	Y N
Do your symptoms get worse with mental activity?	Y N
If 100% is feeling perfectly normal, what percent of normal do you feel?	

FIG. 6.1 Post-Concussion Symptom Scale (from SCAT5).

altered awareness, and preinjury baseline testing scores should be obtained. It is useful to ask directed questions regarding symptoms and symptom severity, most commonly using the Post-Concussion Symptom Score (Fig. 6.1) from the SCAT5.[32] In addition, one should obtain a history of previous concussions, the severity of previous concussions, and the amount of time for recovery from previous concussions. History regarding prior learning disability, neurologic diagnoses, or mental health syndromes may be helpful in directing management and evaluating recovery.

Although the physical examination should include the athlete's specific complaints, a neurologic examination (including cranial nerves, muscle strength, cognition, sensation, reflexes, balance, and coordination) and a comprehensive musculoskeletal examination of the head, face, neck, and shoulder girdle should be completed to determine subtle findings and possible contributors to accompanying conditions. Funduscopic examination to rule out papilledema may reveal signs of increased intracranial pressure. There are aspects of the history and physical examination that may warrant additional neuroimaging or frequent clinical reevaluations (Box 6.1).

Clinical Testing

There is no single test that can support the diagnosis of concussion, and overreliance on comparison with baseline testing may be perilous. There are a few commonly used tests for evaluating physical function after concussion that can be helpful in diagnosis and in following recovery to assist in deciding on activity recommendations. Balance testing using a normed test such as the BESS is helpful for repeated testing and requires only a foam pad and a stopwatch.[33] The K-D test is a computer-based test that combines visual movement and tracking, attention, and language that has alternate test forms and can also be repeated for evaluating recovery.[34]

Children and adolescents with sports-related injuries who present with a higher symptom score, regardless of symptom distribution, are slower to recover.[35] Although females may have higher symptom scores after concussion, they may report higher levels of symptoms before concussion as well, rendering this clinically insignificant.[36]

Neuroimaging

Neuroimaging modalities commonly considered in the evaluation of TBIs and SRC include both structural and functional studies. Structural studies typically considered include computed tomography (CT) and magnetic resonance imaging (MRI). Advanced functional studies include DTI, functional MRI, MR spectroscopy, positron emission tomography, single-photon emission CT, perfusion CT, and transcranial Doppler sonography (TCD). These studies may be of particular interest in the evaluation of SRC when the initial structural studies are normal, although the evidence supporting the indications for their use is limited.[37–39] The use of neuroimaging in the evaluation of the patient should be predicated on the point in time post injury the assessment is being done, the neurologic status of the patient, and the phase of recovery that the individual patient is in. In the acute phase of recovery (first 24–96 h) following an SRC, noncontrast CT structural imaging is typically used to identify any potential underlying skull fractures or intracranial bleeds. Noncontrast CT of the brain is recommended for patients with a loss of consciousness or posttraumatic amnesia following SRC if one or more of the following are present: headache, vomiting, deficits in short-term memory, physical evidence of trauma above the clavicle, posttraumatic seizures, GCS less than 15, focal neurologic deficits, or coagulopathy.[40] There exist established clinical

guidelines (the Canadian Head CT Rule and the New Orleans Head CT Criteria) that can aid in determining who would most benefit from CT imaging in the acute setting.[40] The use of MRI scans in the acute setting is generally warranted if there is neurologic deterioration of the patient.[40] The use of functional imaging in the acute setting is generally not indicated.[38,39] However, studies have demonstrated a high sensitivity and specificity of TCD in the acute phase of recovery for predicting neurologic outcome and the risk of neurologic deterioration, suggesting a possible role for TCD as an adjunct imaging tool in that setting.[41,42] Although there is some evidence suggesting value in the use of functional imaging to determine brain dysfunction during the chronic phase of recovery in light of normal structural imaging, the clinical application and role of these modalities remain unclear.[38] There are no published clinical guidelines regarding the use of structural or functional neuroimaging in the subacute (up to 3 months post injury) or chronic phases (>3 months post injury) of recovery.

New Approaches

Although there are weekly reports on the association of various biomarkers with concussion or mild TBI, there are no serum or cerebrospinal fluid biomarkers that have the required sensitivity and specificity required for diagnosis. Relatively small studies have reported that S100 calcium-binding protein β (S100B) and ubiquitin C-terminal hydrolase-L1 were elevated compared with controls and preseason level at a fair discrimination level in collegiate and high school athletes.[43–45] There is early evidence that serum neurofilament light might distinguish players with prolonged symptoms.[46] Electroencephalographic (EEG) recordings, event-related potentials, and EEG network recordings have all been investigated without reliable identification of concussion.[47,48] A number of investigators are exploring the use of autonomic phenomenon and heart rate variability as a potential noninvasive diagnostic method.[49,50] Reports of successful use of clinical concussion using a telemedicine robot has established feasibility of using this method, although a full investigation has not been completed.[51]

MANAGEMENT OF POSTCONCUSSION SYMPTOMS

Although most individuals with an SRC fully recover within 7–10 days, there is a subset of individuals who continue to experience ongoing somatic and cognitive symptoms. The most commonly reported persistent symptoms include headache, fatigue and sleep difficulties, dizziness and balance problems, neck pain, and cognitive disruption.[52] Emphasis should be placed on the early recognition and management of these complaints to reduce the long-term disability and improve overall quality of life.

Posttraumatic Headache

Posttraumatic headaches (PTHs) comprise the most common physical complaint after concussion. The International Classification of Headache Disorders, 3, has criteria for both acute (resolving within 3 months) and persistent headache (lasting more than 3 months) after moderate to severe brain injury and mild brain injury (as well as criteria for headache following whiplash). According to these criteria, a PTH must begin with 7 days of the injury, regaining consciousness, or the discontinuation of medications that might mask such a headache. No specific characteristics of PTHs are noted in these criteria. There has been little characterization of sport-related PTH. Generally after concussion, although headache is common in general population samples, headaches arising after trauma occur in 54%–69% and cumulatively in 91% of those with mild TBI and in 71% of those with moderate to severe TBI.[53,54] Risk factors for the occurrence of PTH include a history of preinjury headache syndrome, female sex, younger age, and family history of headache.[53] Pain after concussion, especially headache pain, can be chronic, with 33%–58% complaining of pain lasting more than 3 months.[53-55] Higher symptom scores on the SCAT3 are associated with more persisting PTH in athletes, although scores indicate lower severity of headache in athletes than for others with postconcussion symptoms.[56] Other comorbidities may affect the severity or chronicity of headache post concussion. Young athletes with concussion and headache presented with higher depression and anxiety scores.[57] In fact, the incidence of depression increases over the first year after TBI for those with headache.[58] PTH may also affect cognition. Athletes with postconcussion headaches perform worse on neurocognitive testing than those without, especially those meeting criteria for migraine headache.[59]

The underlying cause of the high incidence of PTH remains unclear, and mechanisms for migraine in general are still being elucidated. Migraine headache is associated with cortical spreading depression and subsequent depression of electrical activity and release of multiple peptides and inflammatory agents causing excitation of meningeal nociceptors and the trigeminoneurovascular system.[60-62] Cortical spreading depression has also been associated with concussion.[63] A likely candidate for regulating this process is calcitonin gene–related peptide, a widely distributed vasoactive neuropeptide.[60,64] The release of calcitonin gene–related peptide is associated with increased sensory activity, vasodilation, and neurogenic inflammation.[64] Interestingly, animal models have demonstrated that cortical spreading depression also decreases the efficiency of the glymphatic system in removing solutes from cerebrospinal fluid during sleep, which may account in part for continued inflammation that results in chronification of postconcussion migraine headaches.[65]

Some controversy exists regarding the classification of PTH. Large, prospective studies of the general population, mostly injured in motor vehicle crashes and falls, would indicate that most PTHs meet the criteria for migraine or migraine variant headaches.[66] Symptom analysis in child athletes supports this classification as well.[67] However, it would be unreasonable not to closely evaluate the athlete for musculoskeletal injury that could result in occipital neuralgia or cervicogenic headache.[68]

There is little literature that specifically discusses the management of PTHs in adult or child athletes, and controversy remains about when to return to play with persistent headache.[69-73] However, it is reasonable to treat acute PTH with hydration, over-the-counter nonsteroidal antiinflammatory drugs for 3–5 days, ice packs, rest, and, rarely, limited use of opioids. Acute headaches with migraine characteristics may respond to the use of triptans. Athletes with persistent headache should be reexamined for possible musculoskeletal triggers. Lifestyle changes should be examined: sufficient sleep, use of caffeine or other pain medications causing rebound headache, and ocular dysfunction may all affect headache persistence. In addition, evaluation for comorbid disorders such as depression or anxiety is useful. There is no guidance on return to play for athletes with persistent headache. It is doubtful that headaches persisting for longer than 3 months in athletes with no other findings are associated with physiologic changes that are likely to be worsened by physical activity, and early studies indicate some improvement in symptoms for those who return to physical activity.[74,75]

Cervical and Vestibular Dysfunction

The sudden acceleration-deceleration forces involved in concussive trauma can lead to concomitant "whiplash-type" injury to the cervical spine. Isolated cervical injuries and concussion can share similar symptoms, and therefore it is necessary to assess the cervical spine and musculature for injury in the concussed athlete who is having persistent symptomatology. Prolonged symptoms including headache, dizziness, postural control deficits, blurred vision, vertigo, poor concentration, and memory deficits have all been shown to occur in isolated whiplash injuries[76–78] as well as in isolated concussion. Leddy et al. demonstrated that, based on symptom reports alone, discrimination between physiologic postconcussion syndrome and cervicogenic/vestibular postconcussion syndrome was not possible.[79] Proposed mechanisms for cervicogenic-based symptoms following whiplash-type injuries include upper cervical afferent dysfunction leading to referred pain and headache symptoms, aberrant reflex pathways between cervical afferents and brainstem structures associated with balance leading to cervicogenic balance deficits, and postural stability deficits due to disturbances in the cervicocollic, cervicoocular, and cervicovestibular reflex pathways.[78,80] Other vestibular-related etiologies for dizziness and balance impairment can include benign positional vertigo secondary to dislodgement of calcium crystals into the semicircular canal, labyrinthine concussions, perilymphatic fistulas, and direct trauma to other components of the vestibular system.

A careful physical examination of the cervical spine and cervical musculature, including comprehensive neurologic, skeletal, and biomechanical evaluations, is therefore important in the patient with prolonged symptoms and/or cervical pain, as management of whiplash-related cervical injuries and cervical dysfunction differs considerably from the management of concussion-related symptoms. Attention should be paid to possible associated injuries, including cervical fractures, annular tears, and soft tissue and cervical ligamentous injuries during the assessment. Based on identified pathology and pain generators, beneficial management strategies for cervical-related injuries and dysfunction can include manual therapy, cervical spine mobilization and stretching, cold and/or heat modality applications, soft tissue injections, acupuncture, and massage.[80] Pharmacologic treatment commonly includes the use of muscle relaxants, although in many patients they can be cognitively sedating and therefore should be used with caution and monitored appropriately.

A thorough evaluation of both the oculomotor and vestibuloocular systems (VOS), as well as balance, is likewise important in patients with prolonged, refractory symptomatology that includes dizziness, vertigo, or balance dysfunction. Assessment of the oculomotor system should include evaluations of ocular alignment and range of motion, smooth pursuit, saccades, and vergence (convergence and divergence). Common bedside testing of the VOS includes the head thrust and head shake tests, the dynamic visual acuity test, and the vestibular/ocular motor screen. Advanced VOS testing with a rotary chair can assess for slow and high-velocity head rotation responses and can assess both peripheral and central elements of the VOS. Balance can be measured with metrics such as the BESS or through more formal testing via force plate assessment. The mainstay of treatment for dizziness and vestibular disorders is initiation of a comprehensive vestibular rehabilitation program focused on central nervous system adaptation and compensation for vestibular dysfunction.[81,82] In addition, short-term use of vestibular suppressant medications can be considered for the acute management of symptoms. The most commonly utilized medications include anticholinergics (scopolamine), antihistamines (meclizine and promethazine), and benzodiazepines.

Sleep Disorders and Fatigue

Although complaints of poor sleep and fatigue are common, the severity and functional implications of these conditions are often more severe after TBI. There is little literature that specifically addresses this problem in athletes. Those athletes with premorbid sleep difficulties are more likely to have neurocognitive and other symptoms after concussion and may be a marker for slow recovery.[83] However, for concussion in children, complaints of impaired sleep were prominent and associated with prolonged recovery.[84,85] Interestingly, a small study by Gosselin on concussed and nonconcussed athletes did not demonstrate any differences on polysomnagraphic recordings for parameters related to sleep but did suggest that there were differences in wakefulness between the two.[86]

Fatigue has not been found to correlate particularly well with sleep disorders in studies using polysomnography, and often self-report is at odds with evidence of sleep.[87] It is felt that fatigue may be a disorder of wakefulness or may have a number of other contributory factors involved. Comorbid conditions such as depression or stress disorder may increase the perception of fatigue and sleep disorder.[88] One case report documented a young athlete with persisting postconcussion symptoms after several concussions, including fatigue, who was found to have isolated growth hormone deficiency with borderline diabetes insipidus, which resolved with treatment.[89] It is important to remember as well that many "vague" symptoms such as fatigue can occur in a large percentage of nonconcussed children; in one large baseline study, 50% of boys and 67% of girls reported fatigue.[90] A factor analysis of the Post-Concussion Symptom Scale highlighted that combinations of factors or differences in factor loading from baseline to post concussion in youth athletes resulted in an elevation of a global cognitive-fatigue-migraine cluster within the week after concussion that differed from a sleep-arousal symptom factor.[91] The management of concussion-related fatigue can include both nonpharmacologic and pharmacologic approaches, depending on the underlying cause. Nonpharmacologic management strategies include instituting routine physical activity, such as aquatic and aerobic-based exercise, with the goal of improving physical well-being; education focusing on fatigue management strategies and energy conservation measures; addressing sleep abnormalities; and addressing contributing psychological factors. Studies assessing the efficacy of nonpharmacologic treatment approaches have been mostly limited and inconclusive.[92] Pharmacologic treatment options that have been objectively assessed for efficacy include modafinil, oral creatine, donepezil, and methylphenidate. Of these, only methylphenidate showed significant, dose-dependent benefit in the treatment of mental fatigue.[92]

Cognitive Dysfunction

Postinjury neuropsychological evaluation is not required for all athletes, but it may be helpful in return-to-life decisions (play, learn, work) following an SRC. Studies indicate adverse effects on cognition within the first 24 h of a concussion, with gradual improvement for most individuals within 4 weeks.[93,94] Common cognitive deficits following a concussion include poor attention, concentration, slowed processing, and memory deficits.[95] Many schools administer on-site computerized neurocognitive testing, such as the Immediate Post-Concussion Assessment and Cognitive Testing, Axon Sports, or Concussion Vital Signs, which offer a brief cognitive evaluation. These tools, if administered properly and reviewed by a licensed neuropsychologist, can provide useful information to the concussion management team in regards to cognitive functioning. However, athletes with persistent symptoms that affect daily function should be referred for a full neuropsychological examination to help determine appropriate rehabilitation and/or treatment.[96] Assessing and treating an SRC early on helps speed up recovery and prevent repeat injuries. The impact of repetitive head injuries on cognition in prolonged recovery has

demonstrated mixed results, with some linking repetitive head injuries with poor cognitive outcome and others reporting no such link. In addition, research has indicated an increased risk for neurodegenerative disorders later in life.[97] For example, epidemiologic studies have demonstrated an association between severe TBI and later development of Alzheimer disease,[98] but the link for milder head injury and concussions has not been established.

Behavior and mood changes following an SRC may include irritability, sleep disturbances, anxiety, and other emotional distress. Although these signs may occur at high frequency following an SRC, they are often transient and below the threshold for a clinical diagnoses of depression or anxiety. Research has shown that increases in depressive symptomology following an SRC are similar in athletes with orthopedic injuries and are often short lived.[99] Thus these changes in mood tend to be nonspecific, possibly associated with responses to significant life stressors, and/or may be exacerbated by premorbid conditions.[98] Some research has indicated that the number of concussions is linked with greater depressive symptoms in later life,[100,101] but further evaluation of the long-term effects on mood is needed. Therefore continued assessment of mood is necessary, with referral for therapy or medication management as needed during the recovery process.

Recovery of an athlete following an SRC varies depending on postinjury symptoms. For youth and college athletes, return to school is the first priority followed by return to social activities, including sports. Fortunately, most postconcussion symptoms return to baseline within a few weeks of injury, which allows the athlete to integrate back into the normal daily routine at school, home, and/or work. For an athlete in school, integration back to school may be difficult depending on the amount of missed assignments or tests. Common school-related difficulties[102,103] include difficulty paying attention, trouble learning new material, multitasking, following multistep directions, organizing, and taking longer to complete assignments. Guidelines have been established for a gradual return to learn typically within a week of the injury, and accommodations are recommended for those students who have not fully recovered within a week (Table 6.1).[103] A formal 504 plan can be set up through the school for students requiring short-term accommodations.[104,105] School accommodations depend on the symptoms and functional impairment of the student. These accommodations may include shorter assignments, repetition of material, extended time on assignments, rest breaks, preferred seating to decrease distractions, shorter days,

TABLE 6.1
Return to Learn Guidelines

Stage	Activity
Limited home activities	Engage in typical home activities (reading, electronic use) for brief periods (5- to 15-min increments) as long as symptoms do not increase
Limited school activities	Homework and other cognitive activities outside the classroom gradually increasing time spent on the activities
Part-time school	Gradual integration to school for partial days with accommodations as needed (frequent breaks, reduced noise/light, increase time on assignments)
Full-time school	Increase to full day to school as long as symptoms do not increase with continued accommodations as needed
Full return without accommodations	Resume full school days without accommodations and catch up with school work

later start time, and limited exposure to noise and light. Gradual return to school typically incorporates a four- to six-stage plan that ranges from no school, to gradually extending length of school day from 1 to 3 h, to full day with breaks and accommodations as needed. Similar difficulties and accommodations may follow reintegration to work depending on postconcussion symptoms. Employers may need to make accommodations that include rest breaks, limited computer use, limited noise and light, shorter workdays, and extension on assignments.

Return to play is also typically based on a gradual six-stage plan with increased physical exertion at each stage.[22,105] The athlete is often encouraged to rest 1–2 days during the first stage and then gradually increase from light aerobic exercise (walk, swim, stationary bike) to sport-specific exercise, to noncontact drills, to full practice, and then return to play. The athlete proceeds through each stage only in the absence of symptoms. Over the last decade, the recommendations of rest versus physical activity has changed, with an emphasis on limited rest and more emphasis on a gradual increase in physical exertion with the goal of getting athletes back to their typical daily routine as quickly as possible.[22]

Athletes may also have difficulty integrating back into social life, especially if they were restricted from practices, school, or work. They may feel isolated and may need support from the sports team or a healthcare professional on the emotional adjustment. Integration may also need to be gradual, such as limiting overstimulation from noise and/or light and social outings may need to be in smaller groups initially as symptoms resolve.[104–106]

Overall, most symptoms remit within 4 weeks of the injury but can persist in a subsample of individuals. Although it is difficult to predict those individuals at greater risk, a number of factors have been loosely associated with prolonged recovery, including genetics, preexisting conditions, and repeat injuries.[22]

PERSISTING POSTCONCUSSION SYNDROME

Makdissi has published a systematic review of persisting postconcussion complaints associated with SRC.[107] This syndrome is diagnosed when symptoms continue outside the normal range of time during which symptoms are bothersome, usually 2–3 weeks in adults and 4 weeks in children. There is no specific description; symptoms may vary (headache, dizziness, fatigue, cognitive complaints, sleep disorder, irritability, or emotionality) and are often comorbid with other disorders such as depression or painful injuries. Often, higher initial symptom scores predict the persistence of symptoms.[108] Treatment is generally aimed at the specific bothersome symptoms but is usually combined with strategies to reactivate the patient and improve the sense of control over the situation. Usually these patients are best treated in a multidisciplinary setting with good communication among providers. In addition, evaluation of exercise intolerance and physical examination may reveal a treatable disorder; activation and the positive resulting effects are particularly useful to engage on with the patient to improve tolerance.[109]

REFERENCES

1. Clark W. Kid's sports. *Can Soc Trends*. 2008;85(3):54–61.
2. Tremblay MS, Willms JD. Is the Canadian childhood obesity epidemic related to physical activity. *Int J Obes*. 2003;27:1100–1105.
3. Watson KB, Frederick GM, Harris CD, Carlson SA, Fulton JE. U.S. adults participation in specific activities: behavioral risk factor surveillance system - 2011. *J Phys Act Health*. 2015;12(suppl 1):S3–S10.

4. Daneshvar DH, Nowinski CJ, McKee AD, Cantu RC. The epidemiology of sport-related concussion. *Clin Sports Med.* 2011;30:1–17.

5. Langlois JA, Rutland-Brown W, Wald MM. The epidemiology and impact of traumatic brain injury: a brief overview. *J Head Trauma Rehabil.* 2006;21(5):375–378.

6. Marshall SW, Guskiewicz KM, Shankar V, McCrea M, Cantu RC. Epidemiology of sports related concussion in seven US high school and collegiate sports. *Inj Epidemiol.* 2015;2(1):13.

7. Wasserman EB, Kerr ZY, Zuckerman SL, Covassin T. Epidemiology of sports-related concussions in National Collegiate Athletic Association athletes from 2009-2010 to 2013-2014. *Am J Sports Med.* 2015;44(1):226–233.

8. Cancelliere C, Hincapie CA, Keightly M, et al. Systemic review of prognosis and return to play after sport concussion: results of the International Collaboration on Mild Traumatic Brain Injury Prognosis. *Arch Phys Med Rehabil.* 2014;95(3 suppl 2):S210–S229.

9. Williams RM, Puetz TW, Giza CC, Broglio SP. Concussion recovery time among high school and collegiate athletes: a systemic review and meta-analysis. *Sports Med.* 2015;45(6):893–903.

10. Giza CC, Hovda DA. The neurometabolic cascade of concussion. *J Athl Train.* 2001;36(3):228–235.

11. Steenerson K, Starling AJ. Pathophysiology of sports-related concussion. *Neurol Clin.* 2017;35(3):403–408.

12. Giza CC, Hovda DA. The new neurometabolic cascade of concussion. *Neurosurgery.* 2014;75(suppl 4):S24–S33.

13. Buki A, et al. Preinjury administration of the calpain inhibitor MDL-28170 attenuates traumatically induced axonal injury. *J Neurotrauma.* 2003;20(3):261–268.

14. von Reyn CR, et al. Calpain mediates proteolysis of the voltage-gated sodium channel alpha-subunit. *J Neurosci.* 2009;29(33):10350–10356.

15. Prins ML, et al. Repeat traumatic brain injury in the juvenile rat is associated with increased axonal injury and cognitive impairments. *Dev Neurosci.* 2010;32(5–6):510–518.

16. Longhi L, et al. Temporal window of vulnerability to repetitive experimental concussive brain injury. *Neurosurgery.* 2005;56(2):364–374.

17. Barkhoudarian G, Hovda DA, Giza CC. The molecular pathophysiology of concussive brain injury – an update. *Phys Med Rehabil Clin N Am.* 2016;27(2):373–393.

18. Israelsson C, et al. Distinct cellular patterns of upregulated chemokine expression supporting a prominent inflammatory role in traumatic brain injury. *J Neurotrauma.* 2008;25(8):959–974.

19. Loane DJ, Byrnes KR. Role of microglia in neurotrauma. *Neurotherapeutics.* 2010;7(4):366–377.

20. Habgood MD, et al. Changes in blood-brain barrier permeability to large and small molecules following traumatic brain injury in mice. *Eur J Neurosci.* 2007;25(1):231–238.

21. Maugans TA, et al. Pediatric sports-related concussion produces cerebral blood flow alterations. *Pediatrics.* 2012;129(1):28–37.

22. McCrory P, et al. Consensus statement on concussion in sport-the 5th international conference on concussion in sport held in Berlin, October 2016. *Br J Sports Med.* 2017. https://doi.org/10.1136/bjsports-2107-097699.

23. Patricios J, et al. What are the critical elements of sideline screening that can be used to establish the diagnosis of concussion? A systematic review. *Br J Sports Med.* 2017. https://doi.org/10.1136/bjsports-2016-097441.

24. Davis GA, et al. The child sport concussion assessment tool 5th edition (child SCAT5). *Br J Sports Med.* 2017. https://doi.org/10.1136/bjsports-2017-097492.

25. Guskiewicz KM, Ross SE, Marshall SW. Postural stability and neuropsychological deficits after concussion in collegiate athletes. *J Athl Train.* 2001;36(3):263–273.

26. Barr WB, McCrea M. Sensitivity and specificity of standardized neurocognitive testing immediately following sports concussion. *J Int Neuropsychol Soc.* 2001;7(6):693–702.

27. McCrea M. Standardized mental status testing on the sideline after sport-related concussion. *J Athl Train.* 2001;36(3):274–279.

28. Barr WB. Neuropsychological testing of high school athletes – preliminary norms and test-retest indices. *Arch Clin Neuropsychol.* 2003;18(1):91–101.

29. Tommasone BA, McLeod TCV. Contact sport concussion incidence. *J Athl Train.* 2006;41(4):470–472.

30. Sady MD, Vaughan CG, Gioia GA. Psychometric characteristics of the postconcussion symptom inventory in children and adolescents. *Arch Clin Neuropsychol.* 2014;29(4):348–363.

31. Leong DF, et al. The King-Devick test for sideline concussion screening in collegiate football. *J Optom.* 2015;8(2):131–139.

32. Echemendia RJ, Meeuwisse W, McCrory P, et al. The sport concussion assessment tool 5th edition (SCAT5): Background and rationale. *Br J Sports Med.* 2017;51(11):848–850.

33. Riemann BL, Guskiewicz KM. Effects of mild head injury on postural stability as measured through clinical balance testing. *J Athl Train.* 2000;35(1):19–25.

34. Galetta KM, Brandes LE, Maki K, et al. The King-Devick test and sports-related concussion: study of a rapid visual screening tool in a collegiate cohort. *J Neurol Sci.* 2011;309(1–2):34–39.

35. Howell DR, O'Brien MJ, Beasley MA, Mannix RC, Meehan 3rd WP. Initial somatic symptoms are associated with prolonged symptom duration following concussion in adolescents. *Acta Paediatr.* 2016;105(9):e426–e432.

36. Brown DA, Elsass JA, Miller AJ, Reed LE, Reneker JC. Differences in symptom reporting between males and females at baseline and after a sports-related concussion: a systematic review and meta-analysis. *Sports Med.* 2015;45(7):1027–1040.

37. Gardner AJ, Tan CO, Ainslie PN, et al. Cerebrovascular reactivity assessed by transcranial Doppler ultrasound in sport-related concussion: a systematic review. *Br J Sports Med.* 2014;0:1–7.

38. Eierud C, Craddock RC, Fletcher S, et al. Neuroimaging after mild traumatic brain injury: review and meta-analysis. *Neuroimage Clin.* 2014;4:283–294.

39. Wintermark M, Sanelli PC, Anzai Y, Tsiouris AJ, Whitlow CT. Imaging evidence and recommendations for traumatic brain injury: advanced neuro- and neurovascular imaging techniques. *Am J Neuroradiol.* 2015;36:E1–E11.

40. Jagoda AS, Bazarian JJ, Bruns JJ, et al. Clinical policy: neuroimaging and decision making in adult mild traumatic brain injury in the acute setting. *Ann Emerg Med.* 2008;52:714–748.

41. Bouzat P, Almeras L, Manhes P, et al. Transcranial Doppler to predict neurologic outcome after mild to moderate traumatic brain injury. *Anesthesiology.* 2016;125:346–354.

42. Bouzat P, Oddo M, Payen J. Transcranial Doppler after traumatic brain injury: is there a role? *Curr Opin Crit Care.* 2014;20:153–160.

43. Meier TB, Nelson LD, Huber DL, Bazarian JJ, Hayes RL, McCrea MA. Prospective assessment of acute blood markers of brain injury in sport-related concussion. *J Neurotrauma.* 2017;34.

44. McCrea M, Meier T, Huber D, et al. Role of advanced neuroimaging, fluid biomarkers and genetic testing in the assessment of sport-related concussion: a systematic review. *Br J Sports Med.* 2017;51(12):919–929.

45. Kulbe JR, Geddes JW. Current status of fluid biomarkers in mild traumatic brain injury. *Exp Neurol.* 2016;275(Pt 3):334–352.

46. Shahim P, Zetterberg H, Tegner Y, Blennow K. Serum neurofilament light as a biomarker for mild traumatic brain injury in contact sports. *Neurology.* 2017;88(19):1788–1794.

47. Broglio SP, Moore RD, Hillman CH. A history of sport-related concussion on event-related brain potential correlates of cognition. *Int J Psychophysiol.* 2011;82(1):16–23.

48. Broglio SP, Williams R, Lapointe A, et al. Brain network activation technology does not assist with concussion diagnosis and return to play in football athletes. *Front Neurol.* 2017;8:252.

49. Abaji JP, Curnier D, Moore RD, Ellemberg D. Persisting effects of concussion on heart rate variability during physical exertion. *J Neurotrauma.* 2016;33(9):811–817.

50. Senthinathan A, Mainwaring LM, Hutchison M. Heart rate variability of athletes across concussion recovery milestones: a preliminary study. *Clin J Sport Med.* 2017;27(3):288–295.

51. Vargas BB, Shepard M, Hentz JG, Kutyreff C, Hershey LG, Starling AJ. Feasibility and accuracy of teleconcussion for acute evaluation of suspected concussion. *Neurology.* 2017;88(16):1580–1583.

52. Makdissi M, Cantu RC, Johnston KM, McCrory P, Meeuwisse WH. The difficult concussion patient: what is the best approach to investigation and management of persistent (>10 days) postconcussive symptoms? *Br J Sports Med.* 2013;47:308–313.

53. Lucas S, Hoffman JM, Bell KR, Dikmen S. A prospective study of prevalence and characterization of headache following mild traumatic brain injury. *Cephalalgia.* 2014;34(2):93–102.

54. Hoffman JM, Lucas S, Dikmen S, et al. Natural history of headache after traumatic brain injury. *J Neurotrauma.* 2011;28(9):1719–1725.

55. Nampiaparampil DE. Prevalence of chronic pain after traumatic brain injury: a systematic review. *JAMA.* 2008;300(6):711–719.

56. Begasse de Dhaem O, Barr WB, Balcer LJ, Galetta SL, Minen MT. Post-traumatic headache: the use of the sport concussion assessment tool (SCAT-3) as a predictor of post-concussion recovery. *J Headache Pain.* 2017;18(1):60.

57. Bell KR, Vargas BB, Wilmoth K, et al. Poster 265 relationship between severe headache and elevated depression and anxiety scores after sports-related concussion. *PM R.* 2016;8(9S):S246.

58. Lucas S, Smith BM, Temkin N, Bell KR, Dikmen S, Hoffman JM. Comorbidity of headache and depression after mild traumatic brain injury. *Headache.* 2016;56(2):323–330.

59. Mihalik JP, Stump JE, Collins MW, Lovell MR, Field M, Maroon JC. Posttraumatic migraine characteristics in athletes following sports-related concussion. *J Neurosurg.* 2005;102(5):850–855.

60. Wang Y, Tye AE, Zhao J, et al. Induction of calcitonin gene-related peptide expression in rats by cortical spreading depression. *Cephalalgia.* 2016 Nov 9.

61. Ayata C, Lauritzen M. Spreading depression, spreading depolarizations, and the cerebral vasculature. *Physiol Rev.* 2015;95(3):953–993.

62. Karatas H, Erdener SE, Gursoy-Ozdemir Y, et al. Spreading depression triggers headache by activating neuronal Panx1 channels. *Science.* 2013;339(6123):1092–1095.

63. Lauritzen M, Dreier JP, Fabricius M, Hartings JA, Graf R, Strong AJ. Clinical relevance of cortical spreading depression in neurological disorders: migraine, malignant stroke, subarachnoid and intracranial hemorrhage, and traumatic brain injury. *J Cereb Blood Flow Metab.* 2011;31(1):17–35.

64. Russo AF. Calcitonin gene-related peptide (CGRP): a new target for migraine. *Annu Rev Pharmacol Toxicol.* 2015;55:533–552.

65. Schain AJ, Melo-Carrillo A, Strassman AM, Burstein R. Cortical spreading depression closes paravascular space and impairs glymphatic flow: implications for migraine headache. *J Neurosci.* 2017;37(11):2904–2915.

66. Lucas S, Hoffman JM, Bell KR, Walker W, Dikmen S. Characterization of headache after traumatic brain injury. *Cephalalgia.* 2012;32(8):600–606.

67. Heyer GL, Young JA, Rose SC, McNally KA, Fischer AN. Post-traumatic headaches correlate with migraine symptoms in youth with concussion. *Cephalalgia.* 2016;36(4):309–316.

68. Zasler ND. Sports concussion headache. *Brain Inj.* 2015;29(2):207–220.

69. Lucas S. Headache management in concussion and mild traumatic brain injury. *PM R*. 2011;3(10 suppl 2): S406–S412.

70. Watanabe TK, Bell KR, Walker WC, Schomer K. Systematic review of interventions for post-traumatic headache. *PM R*. 2012;4(2):129–140.

71. Seifert T. Post-traumatic headache therapy in the athlete. *Curr Pain Headache Rep*. 2016;20(6):41.

72. Conidi FX. Interventional treatment for post-traumatic headache. *Curr Pain Headache Rep*. 2016;20(6):40.

73. Kacperski J, Arthur T. Management of post-traumatic headaches in children and adolescents. *Headache*. 2016;56(1):36–48.

74. Thomas DG, Apps JN, Hoffmann RG, McCrea M, Hammeke T. Benefits of strict rest after acute concussion: a randomized controlled trial. *Pediatrics*. 2015;135(2): 213–223.

75. Grool AM, Aglipay M, Momoli F, et al. Association between early participation in physical activity following acute concussion and persistent postconcussive symptoms in children and adolescents. *JAMA*. 2016;316(23):2504–2514.

76. Endo K, Ichimaru K, Komagata M, et al. Cervical vertigo and dizziness after whiplash injury. *Eur Spine J*. 2006;15:886–890.

77. Treleaven J. Dizziness, unsteadiness, visual disturbances, and postural control: implications for the transition to chronic symptoms after a whiplash trauma. *Spine*. 2011;36(25 suppl):S211–S217.

78. Marshall CM, Vernon H, Leddy JJ, Baldwin BA. The role of the cervical spine in post-concussion syndrome. *Phys Sportsmed*. 2015:1–11. https://doi.org/10.1080/0091384 7.2015.1064301. Early Online.

79. Leddy JJ, Baker JG, Merchant A, et al. Brain or strain? Symptoms alone do not distinguish physiologic concussion from cervical/vestibular injury. *Clin J Sport Med*. 2015;25(3):237–242.

80. Cheever K, Kawata K, Tierney R, Galgon A. Cervical injury assessments for concussion evaluation: a review. *J Athl Train*. 2016;51(12):1037–1044.

81. Wallace B, Lifshitz J. Traumatic brain injury and vestibulo-ocular function: current challenges and future prospects. *Eye Brain*. 2016;8:153–164.

82. Tapia RN, Eapen BC. Rehabilitation of persistent symptoms after concussion. *Phys Med Rehabil Clin N Am*. 2017;28:287–299.

83. Sufrinko A, Pearce K, Elbin RJ, et al. The effect of preinjury sleep difficulties on neurocognitive impairment and symptoms after sport-related concussion. *Am J Sports Med*. 2015;43(4):830–838.

84. Eisenberg MA, Meehan 3rd WP, Mannix R. Duration and course of post-concussive symptoms. *Pediatrics*. 2014;133(6):999–1006.

85. Kostyun RO, Milewski MD, Hafeez I. Sleep disturbance and neurocognitive function during the recovery from a sport-related concussion in adolescents. *Am J Sports Med*. 2015;43(3):633–640.

86. Gosselin N, Lassonde M, Petit D, et al. Sleep following sport-related concussions. *Sleep Med*. 2009;10(1):35–46.

87. Ponsford JL, Ziino C, Parcell DL, et al. Fatigue and sleep disturbance following traumatic brain injury–their nature, causes, and potential treatments. *J Head Trauma Rehabil*. 2012;27(3):224–233.

88. Fogelberg DJ, Hoffman JM, Dikmen S, Temkin NR, Bell KR. Association of sleep and co-occurring psychological conditions at 1 year after traumatic brain injury. *Arch Phys Med Rehabil*. 2012;93(8):1313–1318.

89. Langelier DM, Kline GA, Debert CT. Neuroendocrine dysfunction in a young athlete with concussion: a case report. *Clin J Sport Med*. 2017;27.

90. Hunt AW, Paniccia M, Reed N, Keightley M. Concussion-like symptoms in child and youth athletes at baseline: what is "typical"? *J Athl Train*. 2016;51(10):749–757.

91. Kontos AP, Elbin RJ, Schatz P, et al. A revised factor structure for the post-concussion symptom scale: baseline and postconcussion factors. *Am J Sports Med*. 2012; 40(10):2375–2384.

92. Cantor JB, Ashman T, Bushnik T, et al. Systematic review of interventions for fatigue after traumatic brain injury model: a NIDRR traumatic brain injury model systems study. *J Head Trauma Rehabil*. 2014;29(6):490–497.

93. Broglio SP, Puetz TW. The effect of sport concussion on neurocognitive function, self-report symptoms and postural control: a meta-analysis. *Sports Med*. 2008;38(1):53–67.

94. Belanger HG, Vanderploeg RD. The neuropsychological impact of sports-related concussion: a meta-analysis. *J Int Neuropsychol Soc*. 2005;11(4):345–357.

95. Tapia RN, Eapen BC. Rehabilitation of persistent symptoms after concussion. *Phys Med Rehabil Clin N Am*. 2017;28(2):287–299.

96. Cicerone KD, et al. Evidence-based cognitive rehabilitation: updated review of the literature from 2003 through 2008. *Arch Phys Med Rehabil*. 2011;92(4):519–530.

97. Hart J, et al. Neuroimaging of cognitive dysfunction and depression in aging retired National Football League players: a cross-sectional study. *JAMA Neurol*. 2013;70(3):326–335.

98. McAllister T, McCrea M. Long-term cognitive and neuropsychiatric consequences of repetitive concussion and head-impact exposure. *J Athl Train*. 2017;52(3): 309–317.

99. Roiger T, Weidauer L, Kern B. A longitudinal pilot study of depressive symptoms in concussed and injured/nonconcussed National Collegiate Athletic Association Division I student-athletes. *J Athl Train*. 2015; 50(3):256–261.

100. Didehbani N, et al. Depressive symptoms and concussions in aging retired NFL players. *Arch Clin Neuropsychol*. 2013;28(5):418–424.

101. Kerr ZY, et al. Nine-year risk of depression diagnosis increases with increasing self-reported concussions in retired professional football players. *Am J Sports Med*. 2012;40(10):2206–2212.

102. Sady MD, Vaughan CG, Gioia GA. School and the concussed youth: recommendations for concussion education and management. *Phys Med Rehabil Clin N Am.* 2011;22(4):701–719. ix.

103. Iverson GL, Gioia GA. Returning to school following sport-related concussion. *Phys Med Rehabil Clin N Am.* 2016;27(2):429–436.

104. Halstead ME, et al. Returning to learning following a concussion. *Pediatrics.* 2013;132(5):948–957.

105. McNeal L, Selekmen J. Guidance for return to learn after a concussion. *NASN Sch Nurse.* 2017;32(5):310–316.

106. Master CL, et al. Importance of 'return-to-learn' in pediatric and adolescent concussion. *Pediatr Ann.* 2012; 41(9):1–6.

107. Makdissi M, Schneider KJ, Feddermann-Demont N, et al. Approach to investigation and treatment of persistent symptoms following sport-related concussion: a systematic review. *Br J Sports Med.* 2017;51(12): 958–968.

108. Heyer GL, Schaffer CE, Rose SC, Young JA, McNally KA, Fischer AN. Specific factors influence postconcussion symptom duration among youth referred to a sports concussion clinic. *J Pediatr.* 2016;174:33–38.e32.

109. Leddy J, Baker JG, Haider MN, Hinds A, Willer B. A physiological approach to prolonged recovery from sport-related concussion. *J Athl Train.* 2017;52(3): 299–308.

CHAPTER 7

Pediatric Traumatic Brain Injury

DAVID CANCEL, MD, JD • RUTH ALEJANDRO, MD, FAAPMR

Pediatric traumatic brain injury (TBI) represents a special subset within brain injury medicine. As stated in 1972 by Dr. Anthony Raimondi, pediatric neurosurgeon: "Children are not little adults. Infants are not little children. Newborns are not little infants."[1,2] This truism applies especially to pediatric TBI, which has become a pressing public health concern worldwide, including the United States.[3,4]

In this chapter, aspects of care in children with a TBI are compared and contrasted to those of the adult TBI population. These differences are evident from the epidemiologic characteristics, mechanisms of injury, and the neuroanatomic and pathophysiologic responses that make pediatric TBI so distinct from adult TBI. Within the pediatric population, variations in age, gender, and social influences also account for challenges not faced by adult patients. Issues of plasticity and the impact of pediatric TBI on brain recovery are briefly addressed to further recognize the "silent epidemic" that many of the less severe TBI survivors face when reintegrating into their families and communities (i.e., educational and other social activities).[5,6] This chapter also addressed rehabilitation efforts in various aspects of pediatric TBI: cognition and arousal, spasticity, medical complications, rehabilitation strategies, outcome measures, and transition to adult care.

A 2010 consensus statement generated by an international working group defined TBI as "…an alteration in brain function, or other evidence of brain pathology, caused by an external force."[7] TBI is a subset of acquired brain injury (ABI), which is defined as an injury to the brain, which is not hereditary, congenital, degenerative, or induced by birth trauma.[8] This underscores the fact that patients with a TBI have had some prior measure of normative development.

Unlike adult patients with TBI, the child with a brain injury faces maturational challenges specific to the pediatric population. These challenges are a result of the various stages of development inherent to childhood and adolescence. The adult patient has already matured and strives to regain lost function, whereas children have the additional challenge of trying to acquire an entirely new set of age-appropriate skills. These skills are necessary to reach the next appropriate stage of development. This creates a broad spectrum of developmental needs that must be accounted for throughout maturation. These elements can involve physical, educational, emotional, and psychosocial aspects of care. In addition, the care of the brain-injured child by default requires the involvement of family and caregivers, as children legally lack decision-making capacity. Parents and children in turn depend on medical, social, and academic institutions to assist in helping the child grow and develop.

These overlapping layers of support are critical to the development of the child. Research over the past several decades has recognized that the developing brain is inherently different than the adult brain in both anatomy and physiology. These differences are largely based on various stages of development in the immature brain and are adversely affected by injury.[9] Within this subsection of the pediatric TBI population, there exist further divisions in group characteristics. Newborns can be classified as ranging from birth to 27 days of age. Infants and toddlers range from 28 days to 2 years of age, whereas preschool children range from 2 to 5 years. School-aged children are from 5 to 12 years, and adolescents range from 12 to 18 years of age.

This subgrouping is a vital characteristic of pediatric TBI, as injury disrupts the normal stages of growth required for full maturation of the developing brain. Development in a typical child relies upon linking cognitive and physical abilities. It is essentially the function of all children to learn by exploring. Through play and exploration gross and fine motor abilities are acquired, cause and effect is learned, social interaction is promoted, and language is attained. An interruption in the process of cognitive maturation has implications on physical development, which in turn further impedes cognitive growth. A lack of proper treatment can not only lead to developmental delays but also result in the failure to ever reach these critical milestones. An additional factor is that, maturation, both physically and cognitively, can occur rapidly during critical periods of childhood. A disruption during these stages of development can further magnify disability.

The long-term sequelae for TBI survivors can affect all spheres of function (cognitive-linguistic, physical, educational, behavioral, and social) and identity (child, sibling, student, peer) and ultimately lead to permanent developmental disabilities.[10-12] Outcomes following a pediatric TBI must therefore be understood in a developmental context to better address deficits that may arise long after injury, when new developmental processes are emerging and/or existing developmental demands increase.[13,14]

Because of the lifelong developmental implications of pediatric TBI, it is generally agreed that the fundamental aim of managing TBI is to avoid brain injury.[15,16] Prevention of primary injury has been effective using various proactive strategies and programs. Parental education on prevention of child abuse,[17] helmets for bicyclists,[18] use of seatbelts and infant/toddler car seats,[19] and other programs have been effective in limiting the devastating long-term effects of TBI. Efforts over the last 20 years have generated an increased amount of research on the effectiveness of interventions and outcomes in pediatric TBI.[20] But to continue addressing the current "silent epidemic" of pediatric TBI, greater efforts are needed at the federal, state, city, and public health levels to understand the magnitude of this condition. To better understand the scope of pediatric TBI, the epidemiologic characteristics of brain injury in children must first be examined.

EPIDEMIOLOGY OF PEDIATRIC TRAUMATIC BRAIN INJURY

TBI is a leading cause of death and disability in pediatric trauma, representing the most common type of nondegenerative ABI in children.[3,21-23] According to records from the Centers for Disease Control (CDC), the rate of TBI-related visits, hospitalizations, and deaths entering via the emergency department (ED) within the United States during 2013 were distributed throughout extremes of age within the general population. The largest affected groups were infants, adolescents, and the elderly.[24]

The effects of TBI are devastating across all age groups, but in pediatric TBI, outcomes manifest differently compared with adults.[25] Consideration of the developmental stage of the child at the time of injury should also be kept in mind, as the causes of TBI for each pediatric subgroup varies. It is important to note that this same pattern of age-related mechanism of injury variation is also found in pediatric burn injuries. The most common cause of TBI in infants and toddlers, up to age 4 years, is from abusive head trauma (AHT)

secondary to child abuse and fire-related injuries.[3,26-28] In children with TBI under the age of 10 years the most common cause of TBI are transport-related accidents (passenger, bicyclist, pedestrian), falls, and assaults. Altogether, these account for more than 50% of TBIs in this age group. For those over the age of 10 years the most common cause of TBI is from sporting events[29,30] and motor vehicle crashes, reflecting the child's decision-making skills and behavior at the time of injury.[29]

Regardless of the age distribution, TBI remains a major health burden for the pediatric population in the United States. It is estimated that TBI affects over 680,000 children annually.[3,31] Retrospective US estimates of pediatric TBI-associated hospitalization rates revealed 50,658 TBI-related hospitalizations and a hospitalization rate of 70 cases per 100,000/year for most age groups. In the 15- to 17-year age group, there was a hospitalization rate of 125 cases per 100,000/year.[32] Population estimates of the yearly incidence of pediatric TBI range from 200 to over 500 per 100,000 persons, with variations existing across age and gender groups.[33,34] Upon reviewing the existing epidemiologic data, the reader must keep in mind that these estimates fail to include patients who did not access care through the ED or failed to receive care at all. CDC data reveal a total of 2.8 million persons with TBI across all ages: 2.5 million patients accessed the ED, 282,000 were hospitalized, and there were approximately 56,000 deaths.[25] Many patients, however, do not access care through the ED. Some patients are cared for by Veteran's Administration hospitals, private physicians, and urgent care centers. Other patients self-medicate, do not seek treatment, or fail to recognize the signs of a brain injury. These considerations are especially relevant because caregivers may fail to recognize these symptoms in children. This point is especially troubling in that children rely on their caregivers to recognize their injuries and seek treatment on their behalf. Because these patients are not documented in CDC statistics, the true occurrence of TBI, especially mild TBI (mTBI), is unknown.[35]

Because of this gap in knowledge, more research is needed on determining the true morbidity and mortality in pediatric TBI. Further complicating statistical assessments is the heterogeneity of pediatric TBI owing to age and developmental variation. Factors that also present epidemiologic challenges include lack of uniformity in defining what criteria constitutes injury, varying age in patient study selection, and multiple sources of data collection. Of the children who do present to the hospital for medical care, approximately 80%–90% have mild injuries.[36,37] Kraus noted that the rate of morbidity in survivors of pediatric TBI reflected that 75%–95% had good recovery, 10% had moderate disability, 1%–3% had severe disability, and less than 1% remained in a persistent vegetative state.[34] A study by Annegers in 1983 found that 1 in every 30 newborns before the age of 16 years sustain a TBI,[38] highlighting a pressing public health problem that is still underrecognized today.

People with TBIs have mortality rates that positively correlate with the severity of their brain injury. In severe pediatric TBI the mortality rate varies from 12% to 62%. In moderate TBI the mortality rate is 4%, whereas mTBI has a rate of less than 1%. Among children and adolescents, 40%–50% of traumatic deaths include a TBI.[34] The presence of serious concomitant injuries contributes to greater morbidity, including longer hospitalization, increased infections, fewer ventilator-free days, and a higher level of care required on discharge from the hospital.[39]

Although most statistical measures document patient mortality, pediatric TBI also adversely affects families, communities, and the general economy. It is estimated that 145,000 children and adolescents are living with lasting TBI sequelae affecting their cognitive, physical, and/or behavioral health.[40] In the United States, utilization of hospital resources by children less than 17 years of age with TBI-associated hospitalization accounts for more than $1 billion annually, with $2 billion annually for motor vehicle crash–related injuries in those 20 years and younger.[33,41]

In determining risk factors for pediatric TBI, statistical data such as age, gender, premorbid history, injury characteristics, family/psychosocial factors, developmental stage, and access to rehabilitation play a role in risk for injuries and recovery outcomes. Unique developmental and noninjury characteristics should be taken into consideration at all stages of recovery and rehabilitation treatment of pediatric patients with TBI. This knowledge in turn assists in optimizing recovery and managing the long-term consequences found in all pediatric TBI severities, of which mTBIs suffer the least in comparison.[42] Although most statistical measures document patient mortality, pediatric TBI also adversely affects families, communities, and the general economy. It is estimated that 145,000 children and adolescents are living with lasting TBI sequelae affecting their cognitive, physical, and/or behavioral health.[40] In the United States, utilization of hospital resources by children less than 17 years of age with TBI-associated hospitalization accounts for more than $1 billion annually, with $2 billion annually for motor vehicle crash–related injuries in those 20 years and younger.[32,41]

The following are the risk factors and relevant statistical data often associated with pediatric TBI.

Age

Children between the ages of 0–4 and 15–19 years had the highest estimated annual rates of TBI-related emergency room visits.[3,43,44] By the age of 10 years, 16% of children suffer at least one head injury necessitating medical care.[45] Children under the age of 2 years have a mortality rate of 50% and worse outcomes compared with children over 14 years. Children over the age of 14 years have a 14% mortality rate. This age group has a greater association with sporting injuries, leading to milder insults.[46] Most children under 18 years experience sports-related concussions.[47] In a retrospective study by Guerrero et al., children were found to have the highest incidence of mTBIs from "falls," motor vehicle–related causes, and being "struck by an object."[48] More severe injuries at younger ages are also characteristic of "high-risk" patients post-TBI.[49] In children under the age of 8 years with brain injuries compared with older children and adolescents, numerous studies show that poorer cognitive and academic outcomes are worse in the younger age group.[50,51] Barnes et al. noted that children injured before 6 1/2 years of age scored lower on word decoding compared with older patients and that children injured at 9 years or earlier had lower reading comprehension scores compared with those injured after 9 years of age.[52]

Gender

In comparing the relative risk of injury, males and females are not equally at risk for sustaining a TBI. Crowe et al. found that the relative risk for TBI is equal between both genders below age 2 years.[29] This relative risk for injury changes throughout childhood and adolescence. In school-aged children, males are more than twice more likely than girls for sustaining a TBI.[35] In adolescence, this mortality risk increases to a ratio of 4:1.[38] This increased risk has been linked to higher activity levels and exploratory behavior in boys.[53] In relation to sports, female athletes have higher concussion rates than their male counterparts when comparing similar sports activities.[54,55] In nonsports settings, work-related claims within a university system found that females have a higher incidence of concussion compared with males.[56] This finding may be related to reporter bias between genders, as females may be more willing to report and discuss the impact of an injury on their health.[57] Anatomic and physiologic factors include head and neck strength differences, with women having less head-neck mass and neck girth to absorb impact and acceleration forces.[58]

Premorbid History of Child and Family Environment

Psychosocial factors in families of TBI survivors changes relative to the age of the child. In very young survivors the psychosocial context and home environment are challenged with greater stress factors. Examples include single-parent homes, limited financial means, poor coping skills, psychiatric/psychological difficulties, and fewer family resources.[59-62] The end result is poor supervision and parental neglect.[63] In older children the preinjury cognitive profile, often associated with hyperactivity and attentional deficits, may be a risk factor.[64,65] In a 1992 study by Dicker, there was a 50% rate of premorbid learning disabilities or poor academic performance in individuals who suffered an mTBI.[66] These risk factors increase the likelihood of TBI and can also play an important role for recovery.[40,67] In a study by Ponsford et al., children who suffered an mTBI and presented to an ED were followed at 1 week and 3 months post injury. Those with postconcussive symptoms at week 1 improved by 3 months post injury. On the other hand, 17% of children with persisting residual deficits were identified as having preexisting conditions. These included previous head injury; hyperactivity; learning, behavioral, psychiatric, and neurologic conditions; and family difficulties.[68] Similar findings have been reproduced in other studies.[69,70]

Injury Characteristics

Other injury characteristics that predict poorer neurobehavioral outcomes include lower initial Glasgow Coma Scale (GCS) score, longer duration in impaired consciousness, increased duration of return to GCS score of 15 or posttraumatic amnesia (PTA) resolution (these scales are described later), and abnormal pupillary responses.[71-73] Predictive neuroimaging findings include bilateral brain edema, multiple and/or diffuse brain lesions, decreased brain volumes, and increased ventricular size.[71,74-78]

MEASUREMENT, PATHOPHYSIOLOGY, AND CLASSIFICATION OF TRAUMATIC BRAIN INJURY

The classification of pediatric TBI severity involves the integration of acute injury measurement scales and understanding the pathophysiology and mechanisms of injury. These can often be used to classify injury severity as mild, moderate, or severe. In turn, understanding the pathophysiology and mechanisms of injury can help the practitioner determine eventual outcome measures.

Measurement Scales in Pediatric Traumatic Brain Injury

The most commonly used measurement scales are the GCS, Loss of Consciousness (LOC), and PTA scales. The GCS was developed to evaluate the level of consciousness for patients with TBI.[79] It yields total scores from 3 to 15 whereby the lowest score indicates a greater impairment of consciousness. Three components evaluated in the GCS are eye opening, motor response, and verbal response. The total scores from each of these components are then used in the GCS classification system to delineate a "mild" injury (scores 13–15), "moderate" injury (scores 9–12), and "severe" injury (scores 3–8).[80] The duration of LOC and PTA are often used in combination with GCS scores.[81] LOC describes the time frame of loss of consciousness/coma. PTA is generally characterized by a loss of memory for events surrounding the injury, disorientation, confusion, and significant cognitive impairment.

The classification system for grading TBI severity often combines all three sets of scores. A "mild" score is defined by GCS score from 13 to 15, less than 30 min of LOC, and less than 24 h of PTA. "Moderate" is defined by GCS between 9 and 12, 30 min to 24 h LOC, and greater than 1 but less than 7 days of PTA. "Severe" is characterized by GCS from 3 to 8, LOC greater than 24 h, and PTA over 7 days. The chart depicting the TBI classification from Brasure et al. is given in Table 7.1.[82]

Despite frequent use of the GCS in the pediatric population, this scale does not take into consideration the developmental phases and challenges facing the pediatric population. The GCS works well for patients aged 5 years and above, but below this age there are considerable limitations in its application for

---

TABLE 7.1

Selected Criteria Used in Classifying Injury Severity in Traumatic Brain Injury

	Mild	Moderate	Severe
Glasgow Coma Scale	13–15	9–12	3–8
Loss of Consciousness	0–30 min	30 min–24 h	>24 h
Posttraumatic Amnesia	<24 h	>1 and <7 days	>7 days

From Brasure M, Lamberty GJ, Sayer NA, et al. *Multidisciplinary Postacute Rehabilitation for Moderate to Severe Traumatic Brain Injury in Adults.* Rockville, MD: Agency for Healthcare Research and Quality (US); 2012. (Comparative Effectiveness Reviews, No. 72.) https://www.ncbi.nlm.nih.gov/books/NBK99000/.

the pediatric population.[83] To address these limitations with the adult GCS for children, various pediatric coma scales have been designed.[84–93]

PTA assessment in children also has limitations compared with that in adults. The Galveston Orientation and Amnesia Test (GOAT) is a measure of orientation and attention used in adults to assess resolution of PTA.[94] The Children's Orientation and Amnesia Test (COAT) is used for children 3–15 years of age and considers the developmental level when assessing patients (discussed later in the chapter).[95]

Pathophysiology of the Developing Pediatric Brain

In addition to differences in measures of injury, there are significant pathophysiologic, neuroanatomic, and maturational vulnerabilities that distinguish pediatric injuries from those of adults.

Age-related neuroanatomic differences can include neurologic differences such as immature nerve cell myelination, increased cerebral water content and blood volume, decreased brain atrophy following injury, increased blood-brain permeability, enhanced diffusion of excitotoxic neurotransmitters, and impaired autoregulation following injury. Anatomic differences include a larger head to body ratio, decreased skull absorption of mechanical forces, and dependence on weaker neck musculature and ligamentous connections rather than bony structures. In addition, immature cognitive skills and behavior can contribute to a child's vulnerability to injury and can explain unfavorable outcomes in certain cases.[96–105]

This is not to imply that differences in age and development alone contribute to the vulnerabilities that distinguish pediatric from adult TBI. Complex, multifactorial contributions such as injury characteristics also play a role in pediatric TBI. It is worth noting that there are also non-injury-related influences such as premorbid functioning, age and health of parent/caregiver, family dynamics and psychiatric history, minority and socioeconomic status, and access to rehabilitation resources.[50,59,61,106–109] These can all have an impact on pediatric TBI survivors.

Classification of Pediatric Traumatic Brain Injury

TBI can be classified as a penetrating head injury (PHI) or closed head injury (CHI). Ten percent of all TBIs are PHI that can be caused by a knife, bullet, or hard object that damages the skull and dura, typically leading to focal pathology.[110] In adults, 30%–42% of patients have a greater incidence of focal injury than do children

at 15%–20%.[111] Focal neurologic deficits and posttraumatic epilepsy are also more prevalent in PHI overall compared with CHI.

Unlike adults, most pediatric TBI occur by CHI. A CHI may include skull fracture with an intact dural layer. It is important to note, however, that the absence of a skull fracture does not necessarily correlate with a less injured brain. Pediatric skulls have a pliable capacity that allows for a lower risk for fracture but can still be associated with significant underlying structural damage to the brain. In one study, skull fractures were absent in approximately 20% of fatal pediatric cases.[112]

Properties of the pediatric brain tissue and pediatric skull also play an important role in defining the underlying TBI. As suggested by biomechanical studies, infant brain tissue is mostly composed of axons. As children mature, increased myelination of astrocytes and oligodendrocytes decreases the "stiffness" of the brain tissue.[95,113] Another important aspect in the biomechanics of brain injury correlates with the age of the injured skull. Because skull thickness varies with age, the developing skull is thinner than an adult skull. In addition, an infant's unfused cranial sutures allows for increased cranial deformation compared with an adult.[114]

Mechanisms of Injury

Pediatric TBI typically produces more generalized brain injury, and the injury severity typically correlates with the extent of damage. Tissue destruction occurs via a complex array of immediate pathologic, biochemical, and physiologic changes. These changes are followed by secondary effects associated with inflammatory responses and other systemic reactions. The numerous mechanisms involved in brain damage are generalized into two phases of injury mechanisms. *Primary injury* is when brain damage occurs at the time of initial impact. *Secondary injury* consists of the physiologic processes set in motion hours to days to weeks or even longer periods after the primary injury.[115]

Primary injury

In primary injury the pathophysiology of direct brain damage results from acceleration-deceleration forces with or without skull fractures leading to contusions, coup-contrecoup injuries, cranial nerve injuries, and diffuse axonal injuries (DAIs). Brain injury can occur from jolting of the brain against the skull and/or shearing forces on the brain caused by a direct contact and/or indirect contact via acceleration-deceleration forces. The latter type is more common in pediatric TBI and more commonly caused by motor vehicle accidents associated with high-velocity acceleration-deceleration forces.[116–118]

Different types of inertial forces are involved in TBI: translational forces that undergo rapid movement typically in the sagittal direction about the brain's center of gravity located in the pineal region of the brain and upper brainstem[119] and rotational forces defined as those that undergo rapid acceleration-deceleration about the brain's center of gravity. Independent of impact forces, frontal temporal lobes situated over bony surfaces of the skull make the brain tissue vulnerable to contusions in the inferior frontal and anterior temporal lobes.[120] These specific contusions are widely recognized in producing an increased risk for cognitive and behavioral symptoms, or frontal lobe syndrome, often seen in TBI.[121] Impact of the head against another object can cause focal brain injury under the skull at the site of impact (coup) and at the site on the opposite side of the head (contrecoup).[122]

Movement of the head and neck on forceful impact results in angular acceleration forces, a combination of translational and rotational acceleration. Angular acceleration forces, the most damaging mechanism of the inertial forces, can occur with noncontact forces, such as an AHT. Angular acceleration forces are more often correlated with subdural hematomas (SDHs) and DAI. DAI is associated with greater LOC, respiratory apnea, and lower cerebral blood flow, especially in children.[112] Not surprisingly, significant long-term functional disabilities are correlated with DAI. DAI is a common characteristic of TBI, resulting in diffuse microscopic damage typically along gray and white matter boundaries and midline structures of the brain, namely, brainstem, superior cerebellar peduncles, fornices, corpus callosum, periventricular regions, and internal capsule.[123] Shearing forces that result from these types of inertial forces can cause tearing and stretching of axons at the cellular level. Typically, shearing forces occur in the patients with most severe TBI who do not survive.[124]

Current research models now propose that the mechanical forces on the pediatric brain do not necessarily cause a shearing effect. Instead, they initiate a progressive neuropathologic process that damages underlying cytoskeletal elements of the neuron, which then progresses to cellular damage and/or death.[125,126] Also associated with this cellular injury is delicate vasculature injury resulting in the deposition of hemosiderin, an iron-laden residue of hemorrhagic blood. Magnetic resonance imaging (MRI) of subacute and chronic brain injuries can detect residual hemosiderin. In pediatric cases, several studies have correlated the density and location of these microhemorrhagic

residuals to neuropsychological outcomes.[127,128] Forces exerted by rotation of the brain is greater at the surface and weaker in the deeper parts of the brain. Neuroimaging reveals more cortex injury in mTBI and both cortex and deeper types of injury in severe TBI.[129] In cases of severe TBI, axonal damage has been noted to be greater in the longer fiber tracts (i.e., corpus callosum).[120]

Secondary injury

Secondary injuries are the indirect effect of brain trauma, and children are more prone to secondary injuries. These can present through a number of altered regulatory mechanisms: increased intracranial pressure (ICP), cerebral edema (i.e., vasogenic or cytogenic edema), hypoxia due to decreased cerebral perfusion pressure, decreased cerebral blood flow in conjunction with increased metabolic demands, inflammation, and vasospasm. In addition, excitotoxicity from the increased release of neurotransmitters leads to greater neuronal damage, free radical and oxidative damage, cell receptor-mediated dysfunction, and calcium or other intracellular ion-mediated cell damage.[130–132] Intracranial hemorrhage (epidural, subdural, and intracerebral hematomas) is also a mechanism for secondary injuries, albeit more common in adults. On the other hand, increased ICP and cerebral edema are two major complications in secondary injury that are also noted to be more common in children.[133] Secondary injuries have been found to be predictive of poor outcome but are potentially preventable given appropriate and timely medical intervention.

Both primary and secondary brain damage can lead to increased ICP, which in turn adds to the vicious cycle of secondary brain damage via a positive feedback loop. An increased ICP further leads to a decrease in cerebral perfusion pressures, ischemia, edema, herniation, and possibly death. About 43% of children showing impaired cerebral autoregulation during the first week of a severe pediatric TBI are found to have a poorer outcome on a 6-month GCS follow-up.[102] As described earlier, a decreased cerebral blood flow with an increased metabolic demand leads to an increased risk for hypoxemia and hypotension. Mass effect from cerebral edema and intracranial hemorrhage can lead to midline shift and/or herniation of the brain. Cerebral edema is a common secondary brain injury and frequent cause of demise in patients with severe TBI.[134] Hydrocephalus, a treatable cause of secondary brain damage, can occur remotely post injury and can be detected when patients have a plateaued progress or regression in the rehabilitation phase of their care.

Attempts have been put forth to improve outcomes, based on the revised 2012 Brain Trauma Foundation

Guidelines. Recommendations include minimizing the risk of increased ICP, hypoxia, hypotension, fever, and medical stabilization. The result is that the new guidelines are considerably more focused on therapies for improvements in outcomes.[135,136]

Brain damage in TBI is a summation of the effects of multiple primary and secondary mechanisms that generally result in diffuse rather than focal patterns of damage, especially in pediatric patients with CHI. Cerebral atrophy and ventricular enlargement is commonly observed in neuroimaging of severe CHI survivors years later. The developing brains of the pediatric group respond differently to trauma than adults, with more susceptibility to hypoxic-ischemic insults, hypotension, posttraumatic swelling, and diffuse injuries.[105] Despite the similarities in brain injury mechanisms reviewed, individual differences with varying complex patterns of neuromuscular and neuropsychological impairments are evident in all patients with TBI.[137]

ABUSIVE HEAD TRAUMA—FORMERLY SHAKEN BABY SYNDROME

AHT is a unique feature of pediatric TBI and merits a separate section in this chapter. Statistically, child abuse is the major cause of TBI in the youngest pediatric subgroups. TBI in infants and toddlers results in higher incidences of morbidity and mortality than those seen in older children. This is mostly attributed to a significant incidence of AHT.[26,27,138,139] In 2009 the American Academy of Pediatrics officially recommended a change in terminology to AHT following advances in the pathologic mechanisms involved this specific type of TBI.[140] This change was important for both research and clinical translation, and also from a medicolegal perspective. AHT typically occurs in response to episodes of prolonged inconsolable crying, which is age appropriate for infants.[141,142] Risk factors for AHT included male gender, younger age (peak incidence at 3 months), younger mother (less than 21 years of age), and multiparity.[140,143] Studies estimate an incidence of 16–33 cases per 100,000 children per year in the first 2 years of life, at least 1200 seriously injured infants, and at least 80 deaths each year.[144] Other US estimates indicate that 50%–80% of head injury–related deaths in infants and toddlers result from abuse.[140] Significant disability of nearly 66% and a mortality rate ranging from 13% to 35% are reported in clinical studies.[140,145–147]

Biomechanical factors involved in the pathologic mechanism leading to AHT have been investigated. A well-known study by Prange directly measured the rotational velocities experienced by an anthropomorphic surrogate ("dummy infant") during vigorous non-impact shakes, inflicted impacts, and short-distance falls. Results revealed that vigorous shaking compared with a 1-ft fall onto concrete produced smaller acceleration forces compared with inflicted impacts (combining shaking and impact mechanisms). Inflicted impacts produced the largest acceleration forces, even when compared with other factors such as a 5-ft fall onto concrete. These inertial forces alone are associated with an increased likelihood of diffuse injury, traumatic axonal injury, and SDH, so it is even more devastating to an infant brain when impact forces are factored in.[148,149] Infants are also more likely to sustain more severe diffuse lesions than older children. Because infants have open fontanelles, softer skulls with poorer impact absorption, weaker neck muscles, and relatively large heads, they were more likely than older children to sustain a TBI due to abuse rather than a localized impact.[150]

The initial symptoms of AHT may be nonspecific (i.e., altered state of consciousness, seizures, vomiting, breathing difficulty, apnea, increasing head circumference, failure to thrive, and delayed development), and the traumatic event is not easily disclosed.[143,147,151,152] This highly vulnerable group of infants and toddlers and survivors of inflicted brain damage demonstrate unique features compared with other TBIs. Characteristically, noncontrast brain CT findings reveal SDH associated with diffuse and multiple hemorrhages, interhemispheric or posterior fossa location, and extension over the convexity of the brain. The patients often also have serious secondary complications, such as hypotension and hypoxia. Subdural and retinal hemorrhage (most common findings) and multiple fractures of varying ages raise suspicion in this age group. Investigations into observed periods of apnea have attributed these to the shaking/whiplash mechanism leading to cervical hyperextension and flexion leading to stretching injuries at the craniocervical junction. Axonal damage occurs at the junction of the corticospinal tracts and cervical cord roots.[153,154] A 3-year retrospective study assessing the utility of MRI in the evaluation of AHT also found a significant relationship with hypoxic-ischemic brain injuries (HIBIs), and 81% with HIBI also had a high incidence of cervical spine injuries.[155]

As noted previously, worse outcomes are noted in children under 2 years of age.[3,139] Survivors of AHT suffer damage that limits their experience-dependent learning and gene-environment–based interactions.[156,157] A small, prospective, longitudinal study of early childhood TBI, by Ewing-Cobbs et al., followed the intelligence quotient (IQ) and academic outcomes an average of 6 years post TBI. Results of TBI survivors with moderate and severe injuries, afflicted before the age of 6 years, revealed that nearly 50% of these children had IQ levels below the 10th percentile and experienced academic failure or transition to self-contained special education classrooms.[74] AHT survivors and their sequelae demonstrate the crucial need for continuing special education and rehabilitation services.

Common impairments specific to this very young AHT survivors include sensory-motor deficits, cognitive-linguistic deficits, increased risk of epilepsy, cortical blindness, learning disabilities, and behavioral deficits. These survivors face a prolonged course of brain development in which their impairments may not appear until academic challenges surface.[158]

MILD TRAUMATIC BRAIN INJURY AND CONCUSSION

Another distinct subset of pediatric TBI involves concussion, considered a form of mTBI. Although concussion and mTBI are not unique to pediatric TBI and the topic is reviewed elsewhere in this textbook, certain aspects of clinical classification of mTBI in children are worth noting.

A consensus statement generated at the fourth International Conference on Concussion in Sport in 2012 affirmed the following definition of concussion: "Concussion is a brain injury and is defined as a complex pathophysiologic process affecting the brain, induced by traumatic biomechanical forces." Other common features that also help define concussive head injury are the following: (1) may be caused by a forceful impact to the head and/or trunk of the body; (2) is considered a functional disturbance rather than a structural injury; (3) typically resolves with 1–2 weeks; (4) may or may not include neurologic impairment with the LOC.[159]

A large percentage of ED visits from 2001 to 2005 revealed that 65% of children within the age of 14–19 years had concussions in a group of athletes with overall age 8–19 years.[160] A study on the total annual healthcare expenditures from 1997 to 2000 for mTBI-related services for children 1–18 years old who were not hospitalized averaged $77.9 million.[161] As reviewed earlier in this chapter, age-related patterns revealed that older children suffered most TBIs from sports activities. Males involved in contact sports, such as rugby, American football, ice hockey, and lacrosse, have a higher incidence of mTBI and concussion. Females involved in soccer, lacrosse, and field hockey have a higher risk of concussion.[162,163] It has been estimated that more than 375,000 children and adolescents are diagnosed with minor head injury in the outpatient setting.[164]

Although the diagnosis and treatment of concussion and postconcussive symptoms are beyond the scope of this chapter and addressed elsewhere in this textbook, there have been challenges to the idea of physical rest in the immediate postinjury period until concussive symptoms have resolved. In a 2016 prospective, multicenter cohort study of 3063 school-aged children, Grool et al. determined that participants who engaged in early physical activity had a lower risk of postconcussive symptoms than those with no physical activity. Given the relatively high number of children with mTBI and concussions, future study in this area is warranted.[165]

REHABILITATION IN PEDIATRIC TRAUMATIC BRAIN INJURY

The acute medical care of TBI is discussed elsewhere in this text. Acute medical management of TBI, however, can often incorporate many of the principles and rehabilitation strategies discussed later. The following sections address common issues pertaining to the treatment of pediatric brain injury in the rehabilitation setting. The initial stages of rehabilitation can involve pharmacologic management for cognition and arousal. Medications and interventional techniques may be used to control spasticity and prevent the formation of contractures. Medical complications may develop during the acute rehabilitation stage, and selected medical issues are addressed. Finally, therapeutic rehabilitation strategies and outcome measures are presented to help guide treatment plans beyond the acute rehabilitation phase of care. These children often face the inevitable transition into adult TBI care.

PHARMACOLOGIC INTERVENTIONS FOR COGNITION AND AROUSAL

The following are selected medications that have been used and/or studied in the treatment of disorders of consciousness and cognition, sleep disorder, and dysautonomia in pediatric TBI. As mentioned earlier in this chapter, the physiologic changes that take place during maturation play a role in the selection of medications in pediatric TBI. Unlike in adults, neuronal density and the secretion of neurotransmitters vary throughout childhood.[166] These maturational factors may affect the efficacy of pharmacologic interventions to improve recovery after pediatric TBI. There is a need for additional research on the timing of pharmacologic interventions and in determining age-related outcomes with certain drugs.

Amantadine

The mechanism of amantadine is unclear. Amantadine seems to act as a direct antagonist at the N-methyl-D-aspartate (NMDA) receptor of the cell and indirectly as a dopamine agonist.[167] Amantadine has been shown to improve arousal, attention, and drive in adult patients with posttraumatic disorders of consciousness.[168] Clinical trials have shown success in a retrospective, case-controlled study involving 54 patients.[169] Another pilot study of five patients in a randomized, double-blind, placebo-controlled cross-over trial also yielded benefit, with no significant disruption in sleep.[170] Similar to adult studies, pediatric trials noted adverse effects of vomiting, agitation, and lowering of the seizure threshold.[169,171] These effects were noted to be dose dependent and reversible.[169] Dosing parameters for children under 16 years have been set at a starting dose of 4 mg/kg/day or 300 mg/day, up to 6 mg/kg/day or 400 mg/day.[170] In children over 16 years, starting doses have been listed at 100 mg two times a day (BID) for 14 days; the dose was increased to 150 mg BID and then to 200 mg BID.[171] There were no adverse effects of hypertonia and spasticity, which were noted in adult trials, whereas hallucinations were a significant adverse effect in the pediatric group.[169,171] For patients with renal dysfunction, dosing may need to be adjusted.[172]

Melatonin

Melatonin is produced in the pineal gland and mediated through the suprachiasmatic nucleus of the hypothalamus in response to dim light, is synthesized from serotonin in a circadian manner, and regulates the sleep-wake cycle. Receptors for melatonin are distributed throughout both the central and peripheral nervous systems. In cases of a disruption in sleep patterns the exogenous administration of melatonin has been postulated to help reset the sleep-wake cycle.[173] Currently, however, clinical trials have not demonstrated significant benefit with melatonin and melatonin receptor agonists in adults.[167,174]

There have been a few studies determining the effectiveness of melatonin in children. One study noted benefit among patients with autism, but the results were limited and contained numerous confounding factors that make interpretation of data difficult.[175] In a study involving children with chronic sleep deprivation, an effective dose of melatonin in the pediatric population was proposed by Van Geijlswijk IM et al.,

with a proposed dosage of 0.05 mg/kg given at the onset of dim light and again at bedtime.[176]

Beyond its role in the regulation of sleep, melatonin has been proposed to play a neuroprotective role in TBI. Melatonin seems to have antioxidant, antiinflammatory, antiischemic, and cell membrane–stabilizing properties that aid in recovery following brain injury.[177] Adult patients with TBI have been shown to have lower levels of melatonin production in the evening hours, indicating a disruption of the circadian regulation of melatonin synthesis. These were believed to reflect the neural response to injury.[178] Similar to adults, children also report difficulties with sleep after TBIs, even months after their injuries.

In contrast to adult patients, pediatric brain-injured patients may secrete more, not less, melatonin in the acute stages of brain injury. In a 2017 study, Marseglia L et al. demonstrated increased levels of melatonin in traumatic brain-injured patients.[179] This was a follow-up to a 2013 study in which critically ill children were noted to have higher levels of melatonin, among them traumatic brain-injured patients. The researchers theorized that the elevated melatonin levels may be a response to counteract the elevated oxidative stress associated with their critically ill state.[180] In the 2017 study the traumatic brain-injured patients were noted to have higher serum melatonin than their critically ill nontraumatic brain-injured counterparts, likely reflecting a response to oxidative stress or inflammation due to the head injury.[179] Given the limited research and lack of demonstrated benefit in clinical trials, melatonin at this time cannot be recommended in pediatric TBI. More research is needed to demonstrate the clinical benefits of this medication.

Atomoxetine

Atomoxetine has been proposed as a medication to improve cognition in TBI, based on animal models.[181] Atomoxetine was originally considered only as a norepinephrine reuptake inhibitor, but it has been efficacious and tolerated in children and adolescents with attention deficit hyperactivity disorder (ADHD).[182] The benefit of atomoxetine is that it is a nonstimulant drug.[183] It is believed to act at the locus coeruleus, improving attention and arousal. In a 2014 randomized controlled trial in adults with TBI by Ripley et al., results did not indicate any benefit in attention or arousal. The main reported adverse effects were insomnia and dry mouth (although small increases in blood pressure are possible with atomoxetine). Limitations of the study included a short length of trial time (2 weeks), variability among participants, time from injury, and difficulty in determining adequate outcome measures. Researchers speculated that, although there may be benefit with atomoxetine, there may need to be a longer trial time on the medication and different outcome measures.[184] Atomoxetine has also been found to act as an NMDA receptor antagonist.[185,186] This finding indicates that atomoxetine could still play a role in the treatment of pediatric TBI, especially given its proven tolerance in children. Weight-based dosing guidelines in children less than 70 kg with ADHD start at 0.5 up to 1.4 mg/kg/day. For children more than 70 kg the starting dose is 40 up to 100 mg/day.[187]

MEDICATIONS FOR DYSAUTONOMIA

Bromocriptine

Bromocriptine is a dopamine D2 agonist that exerts its effect on the corpus striatum and hypothalamus. There have been case reports documenting successful treatment of resistant central hyperthermia with bromocriptine.[188,189] A 2017 prospective trial by Munakomi et al. studied 36 patients (including three children), demonstrating benefit with bromocriptine in overall recovery from TBI. Inclusion criteria included minimally conscious state and hemodynamic stability, with exclusion criteria including autonomic instability. In children, doses were given at 3.75 mg/day.[190] In adults, bromocriptine has also been studied to determine its benefits in treating attention deficit, but there did not seem to be any cognitive improvement when using the medication.[191]

Morphine

Morphine is a centrally acting opioid analgesic[192] and has been used for autonomic instability, and its benefit has been demonstrated in case reports. In particular, intravenous morphine can be considered an option in cases in which other drugs such as clonidine and propranolol may cause hypotension or autonomic instability has been resistant to other medications.[193,194] There are no standardized dosing guidelines for the use of morphine for dysautonomia. For analgesia, weight-based guidelines for patients less than 50 kg recommend 0.05 mg/kg, with a maximum initial dose of 1–2 mg every 2–4 h as needed. The maximum dose in infants is 2 mg/dose. In children aged 1–6 years the maximum dose is 4 mg/dose, from 7 to 12 years 8 mg/dose, and in adolescents 10 mg/dose. For children more than 50 kg the initial recommended dose is 2–5 mg every 2–4 h as needed, with a lower dose range for opioid-naive patients.[195]

β-Adrenergic Receptor Antagonists

The use of β-blockers, such as propranolol, in the treatment of autonomic instability has been documented in the literature. The benefit is thought to lie in the slowing of the catecholamine-induced catabolic state and decreased cerebral metabolism. In a 2008 review article by Tran, there seemed to be benefit to the use of β-blockers in TBI, either alone or in combination with other medications such as clonidine. This benefit was also seen in studies with children, although none of the trials were prospective studies.[196] In a 2012 prospective randomized clinical trial, propranolol was given in combination with clonidine with benefit in TBI, with a study range starting at 16 years of age.[197] A 2017 retrospective study by Pozzi et al. found benefit to a combination of propranolol and diazepam.[198] A 2017 review by Alali again noted the benefit of β-blockers in TBI but called for more trials to determine standardized dosing recommendations and to compare efficacy among other forms of β-blockers.[199] Current guidelines for pediatric dosing of propranolol for hypertension has been recommended at a starting dose of 1–2 mg/kg/day divided BID or three times a day (TID), with a maximum dose of up to 640 mg/day.[200,201]

Clonidine

As mentioned earlier, clonidine has effects on spasticity as a second-line medication. Clonidine exerts its effect by increasing the presynaptic inhibition of motor neurons. Clonidine has been studied in the treatment of sympathetic hyperactivity in TBI and has been used in combination with β-blockers for acute treatment of TBI.[201] Although there are no established guidelines on the use of clonidine for dysautonomia, current fixed dosing guidelines for hypertension in children over 12 years of age start at 0.2 mg/day, with a maximum dose of 2.4 mg/day.[201] For weight-based dosing the starting dose is 5–10 mcg/kg/day given BID or TID, with a maximum of 25 mcg/kg/day up to 0.9 mg/day.[200]

Gabapentin

In its role as a medication for autonomic instability, gabapentin has been shown to be effective in a case series of six patients with TBI in whom standard treatments were ineffective. The subjects were in their late teens and early twenties. Doses ranged from 300 mg BID or TID up to 600 mg TID. The authors speculated that the effect of the drug may simply be treating neuropathic pain in the subjects, but this could not account for the stereotypical dysautonomic response patterns.[202]

PHARMACOLOGIC INTERVENTIONS FOR THE TREATMENT OF SPASTICITY

Unlike in adults the effects of spasticity on children have a direct impact on future growth and development. Spasticity and increased tone can lead to impaired muscle and bone development, skeletal deformity, pain, and abnormal future growth. Treatment goals for spasticity in the pediatric brain-injured child not only include goals for improving gross and fine motor function but also seek to improve positioning, comfort, and ease of care and decrease the need for surgical intervention in a growing child.[203] As in adults, spasticity treatment addresses systemic and focal impairments in mobility. Medications are further tailored to the patient's physical condition, level of consciousness, and cognition. Unlike in adults, spasticity management in pediatric patients must also incorporate future physical and developmental stages, which can affect the timing of these interventions. In the systemic management of spasticity, oral medications can act centrally or at the level of the muscle cells. The choice of medications for spasticity can therefore adversely affect cognitive recovery after TBI, which has an impact on learning and socialization, critical to normal development in a child. Interventional procedures can attempt to deliver medications directly to the central or peripheral nervous system; others directly target the muscle tissue. These focal treatments can be administered separately or in conjunction with surgical interventions.

ORAL MEDICATIONS FOR SPASTICITY

There are four major drugs used in the treatment of spasticity, which exert their effects systemically. The most common centrally acting medications in the treatment of spasticity are baclofen, tizanidine, and benzodiazepines. In children the most common adverse effect of centrally acting medications is sedation, which is often a consideration in infants and younger school-aged children. Peripherally, dantrolene is commonly used to avoid these adverse effects. Clonidine and gabapentin are second-line drugs, whereas cannabidiol and tolperisone are currently under investigation as alternatives to traditional medications. See Table 7.2 for a listing of these medications.

Baclofen

Baclofen has been widely used in the pharmacologic treatment of spasticity in children[204] and is administered in both oral and intrathecal formulations. In the oral formulation, baclofen crosses the blood-brain barrier and acts centrally as a $GABA_B$ receptor agonist at the level of the spinal cord, blocking polysynaptic and monosynaptic afferent neuronal transmission.[205] Adverse effects include sedation and fatigue. There have also been reports of baclofen associated with an increased or new-onset seizure activity.[203,206] Because of potential hepatotoxicity, there is a need to monitor liver function.[207] Owing to the adverse effect of sedation with the use of oral baclofen, treatment of spasticity in brain injury must be weighed against the potential for impeding recovery in the acute stages, especially with memory and attention deficits.[208]

The typical starting dose of baclofen in children is recommended at 2.5 mg/day, titrated up to a maximum of 20–60 mg/day.[209] Other recommendations have listed the starting dose of baclofen at 5–10 mg/day in three divided doses for children over 2 years of age, with a maximum dose of 40 mg/day in children from 2 to 7 years of age and 60 mg/day in children 8 years of age or older.[210] Other sources have suggested higher maximum doses for various age groups, with maximum doses for children over 8 years old as high as 80–200 mg per day.[211] In infants the starting dose has been documented as low as 0.36 mg/kg/day.[203] In neonates, there have been case reports of 0.5 mg/kg/day divided in four doses.[212]

Abrupt discontinuation of oral or intrathecal baclofen (ITB) may cause withdrawal. Common symptoms are increased spasticity, seizures, hyperthermia, and altered mental status. The most severe complication is rhabdomyolysis and multiorgan failure.[205] Treatment of withdrawal usually involves reinstitution of oral baclofen.[213]

Tizanidine

Tizanidine is a centrally acting α_2-adrenergic agonist that has been used in the treatment of spasticity in cerebral palsy and spinal cord injury. Tizanidine exerts its effect by increasing the presynaptic inhibition of motor neurons. Some common effects of tizanidine include sedation, drowsiness, hypotension, dizziness, and dry mouth. Because this drug is in the same imidazoline drug class as clonidine, it is often contraindicated in patients taking antihypertensives.[207] There is no definitive Food and Drug Administration dosing information on the use of tizanidine in the pediatric population.

There have, however, been studies on the use of tizanidine in children, and the suggested guidelines have varied in their recommended dosing. Palazon recommends a general dose of 1 mg/day in 18-month to 7-year-old children and 2 mg/day in 7- to 12-year-old children as initial doses. The maximum dose was listed

TABLE 7.2
Oral Medications for Spasticity

Medication	Mechanism of Action	Adverse Reactions	Dosing Parameters
Baclofen	Central: $GABA_B$ receptor agonist at the level of the spinal cord, blocking polysynaptic and monosynaptic afferent neuronal transmission	Common adverse effects include sedation and fatigue Reports of increased or new-onset seizure activity Need to monitor liver function	Usually listed at 2.5 mg/day, titrated up to a maximum of 20–60 mg/day (Scheinberg) Also can give 5–10 mg/day in three divided doses for children over 2 years of age, with a maximum dose of 40 mg/day in children from 2 to 7 years of age and 60 mg/day in children 8 years or older (Milla) Maximum doses for children over 8 years old as high as 80–200 mg per day (Lubsch) In infants, can have a starting dose as low as 0.36 mg/kg/day (Hansel) In neonates, as low as 0.5 mg/kg/day divided into four doses (Moran)
Tizanidine	Central: α_2-Adrenergic agonist increasing the presynaptic inhibition of motor neurons	Common effects include sedation, drowsiness, hypotension, dizziness, and dry mouth Contraindicated in patients taking antihypertensives	Starting dose: 1 mg/day in 18-month to 7-year-old children 2 mg/day in 7- to 12-year-old children Maximum dose 9–12 mg/day. Children older than 12 years—adult dosing (Palazon) For weight-based dosing 0.1–0.2 mg/kg/day divided into two or three doses. (Palazon citing Tanaka) 1 mg at bedtime for children under 10 years 2 mg at bedtime for children 10 years or more Maintenance dose 0.3–0.5 mg/kg/day divided four times daily (Patel)
Benzodiazepines	Central: Inhibitory effect at both the spinal cord and supraspinal levels by mediating $GABA_A$ receptors	Sedation Less commonly ataxia, urinary retention, constipation, and hypersalivation	Diazepam: 0.2–0.8 mg/kg/day, divided into three or four doses (Delgado)

Drug	Mechanism	Adverse effects	Dosing
Dantrolene	Peripheral: Inhibits release of calcium at the sarcoplasmic reticulum	Weakness, gastrointestinal symptoms (vomiting and diarrhea) The most serious adverse effect is hepatotoxicity with features of acute hepatitis	Starting dose 0.5 mg/kg twice daily (Patel) Maximum dose ranges up to 12 mg/kg/day (Chung)
Clonidine	Central: α_2 Adrenergic agonist increasing the presynaptic inhibition of motor neurons	Common effects include sedation, drowsiness, hypotension, dizziness, and dry mouth Contraindicated in patients taking antihypertensives	0.05 mg per day, increased by 0.05 mg weekly to a maximum of 0.3 mg/day (Edgar) 0.4 mg/day and a recommended maximum dosage of 1.8 mg/day (Lubsch)
Gabapentin	Central: Inhibits presynaptic glutamate release by modulating calcium channels	Sedation, dizziness, and ataxia	5 mg/kg/day divided into three doses for term infants (Edwards) 10.2 mg/kg/day, with maximum doses up to 25.5 mg/kg/day divided into three doses (Sacha) 40 mg/kg/day divided into three doses for children between 1 month and 5 years of age Starting dose 30 mg/kg/day divided into three doses with older children (Haig)
Cannabinoids	Central: CB-1 receptors in brain and spinal cord Peripheral: CB-2 receptors mostly in the peripheral nervous system Regulates glutamate excitotoxicity, intracellular calcium accumulation, and cellular apoptosis	Vomiting and restlessness	Data not established in children
Tolperisone	Central: Inhibits afferent nociceptive input to the spinal cord	Asthenia and sleepiness	Data not established in children

at 9–12 mg/day. Children older than 12 years had a dosing recommendation similar to that of adults. For weight-based dosing, there was a reference to an earlier study by Tanaka, at 0.1–0.2 mg/kg/day divided into two or three doses.[214] On the other hand, other sources cite starting at 1 mg at bedtime for children under 10 years and 2 mg for children 10 years or more. Maintenance dose was listed at 0.3–0.5 mg/kg/day divided four times daily.[215] Certain properties of tizanidine make this a potential alternative to baclofen. Unlike with baclofen, there are no concerns over potential seizure activity in patients and the adverse effect of dry mouth can be considered a benefit in patients who have problems with oral secretions.

Benzodiazepines

Benzodiazepines produce an inhibitory effect at both the spinal cord and supraspinal levels by mediating $GABA_A$ receptors. The result is presynaptic inhibition and a reduction of monosynaptic and polysynaptic reflexes. Diazepam is the most commonly given benzodiazepine at a dose of 0.2–0.8 mg/kg/day, divided into three or four doses. Sedation is the most common adverse effect, and it is often recommended to help with sleep.[204,207] Ataxia, urinary retention, constipation, and hypersalivation are also encountered.[216] Clonazepam, with a longer half-life, is another benzodiazepine that can also be given.[207]

Dantrolene

Dantrolene is often used as monotherapy, and it exerts its effect outside the central nervous system, directly at the muscle. This feature commonly makes dantrolene a viable choice when avoiding sedation. Dantrolene uncouples the excitation and contraction of muscle by inhibiting the release of calcium at the level of the sarcoplasmic reticulum.[207] Side effects included weakness and gastrointestinal symptoms (vomiting and diarrhea). The most serious adverse effect is hepatotoxicity with features of acute hepatitis,[217] although no cases have been reported in children.[204] Although studies have attempted to establish the safety of a low dose of dantrolene (under 200 mg) with some success,[218] there have been prior cases of hepatotoxicity under 150 mg doses.[217] Doses in children start at 0.5 mg/kg twice daily.[215] Maximum doses range up to 12 mg/kg/day.[216] Although dantrolene had been used as the first-line treatment for spasticity, some sources have cited dantrolene as a second-line or adjuvant medication in the treatment of refractory spasticity[207] and it has been cited as being effective in combination with diazepam.[204]

Second-line medications are often useful in combination with traditional medications in the treatment of spasticity. They can be used to avoid the adverse effects of adding another first-line medication or exert an additional beneficial effect on the patient's condition. Other times they have been given as monotherapy in refractory cases.

Clonidine

In the same imidazoline class as tizanidine, clonidine is a centrally acting α_2 adrenergic agonist that works by increasing the presynaptic inhibition of motor neurons. Some common effects of clonidine include hypotension, sedation, and dry mouth. It is contraindicated in patients taking antihypertensives.[207] Sources have cited a starting dose of 0.05 mg per day, increased by 0.05 mg weekly to a maximum of 0.3 mg/day.[219] Other sources have listed the average maintenance dosage of 0.4 mg/day and a recommended maximum dosage of 1.8 mg/day.[211] Clonidine also has the additional benefit of use in the treatment of sympathetic hyperactivity in TBI, making this a useful drug in the acute stages of pediatric TBI.[197]

Gabapentin

Gabapentin has been used mainly in the treatment of epilepsy and neuropathic pain and has been shown to inhibit presynaptic glutamate release by modulating calcium channels. It has a structure similar to that of GABA, without binding to those specific receptors. Gabapentin has been more often studied and used in the treatment of spasticity in spinal cord injury and multiple sclerosis.[220] Because of its effectiveness with neuropathic pain, it is often prescribed in patients who have both spasticity and neuropathy.[207] It has the adverse effects of sedation, dizziness, and ataxia.[221]

There are no significant data on the use or effectiveness of gabapentin for spasticity in children. In adults the administration dose has been listed starting at 400 mg TID, up to an effective dose of 1200 mg TID.[220,222,223] Sedation did not seem to be a significant adverse effect in the doses studied.[222,223] There is, however, research on the use of gabapentin for pain in infants, with doses starting as low as 5 mg/kg/day divided into three doses for term infants.[224] Other sources recommend an average starting dose of 10.2 mg/kg/day, with maximum doses up to 25.5 mg/kg/day divided into three doses.[225] Haig et al. recommend starting doses for children between 1 month and 5 years of age at 40 mg/kg/day divided into three doses. With older children the starting dose was set at 30 mg/kg/day divided into three doses. A higher dose in smaller children was attributed to physiologic differences of drug absorption between age groups.[226] The utility of gabapentin may lie in its use in patients with both epilepsy and spasticity.[227]

In comparing traditional medications, there is insufficient evidence that one medication has a greater effect than another in spasticity management.[228,229] In effect, practitioners must consider their choice of medication based on the side-effect profile and adverse effects, cost, accessibility, and ease of administration in customizing pharmacologic treatment. In the use of second-line or adjuvant medications, the clinical condition of the patient and additional clinical benefits must be considered in the choice of medication.

The following are additional drugs that are currently under investigation and that hold promise in the treatment of spasticity, based on limited success in adult trials. There are currently no established guidelines for the use of these medications in adults and therefore none in the pediatric population.

Cannabinoids

Cannabinoids have been studied in the management of spasticity secondary to multiple sclerosis and paraplegia. In the human body, cannabinoid receptors known as CB-1 are concentrated in the brain and spinal cord, whereas most CB-2 receptors are located in the peripheral nervous system. Activation of the CB-1 and CB-2 receptors is thought to have some effect on spasticity, but study results have been mixed. The American Academy of Neurology recommends future research with randomized controlled studies to determine the efficacy of cannabinoids.[230] A 2017 article by Kuhlen et al. demonstrated improvement in the treatment of drug-resistant spasticity with the use of tetrahydrocannabinol oil (dronabinol) with doses ranging from 0.08 to 1.0 mg/kg/day. Side effects were vomiting and restlessness.[231] In a 2015 review article, Whiting et al. determined that, although cannabinoids were associated with improvement in spasticity, the results did not reach a statistically significant level.[232] Nonetheless, experimental models suggest that cannabinoids may play a role in the treatment of perinatal brain injuries. It is believed that the early administration of cannabidiol may have a neuroprotective effect in patients.[233] Animal models have demonstrated that the endocannabinoid system has an endogenous neuroprotective effect that can help regulate glutamate excitotoxicity, intracellular calcium accumulation, and cellular apoptosis. At this time the lack of published data precludes fully recommending the use of cannabinoids for medicinal purposes in pediatrics, including epilepsy.[234]

Tolperisone

Tolperisone is another medication that has received more attention in the treatment of spasticity. It is a centrally acting muscle relaxant and exerts its effect by inhibiting afferent nociceptive input to the spinal cord, attenuating spinal reflexes and inhibiting descending reticulospinal projections.[235] In a study involving adult patients with spasticity of spinal origin, tolperisone was considered superior to baclofen in terms of efficacy and safety. The dosage was studied at 150–450 mg/day until up to 600 mg/day. Unlike other medications for spasticity, tolperisone has no substantial affinity to cholinergic, serotonergic, dopaminergic, or adrenergic receptors in the central nervous system. The most common adverse effects were asthenia and sleepiness.[236] This would potentially avoid the sedating effects and withdrawal risk seen in other centrally acting spasticity medications. Although its clinical benefit has not been widely studied, the nonsedating effect of tolperisone would make it a promising medication for the treatment of spasticity in brain-injured children.

INTERVENTIONAL MEDICATIONS FOR SPASTICITY

In lieu of oral pharmacotherapy, medications to treat spasticity can be injected around or within nerve and muscle tissue or administered intrathecally into the spinal cord. Often indicated for focal spasticity, these options can avoid the use of sedating medications. Listed in the following sections are medications used during interventional procedures for spasticity, including some that are less commonly used or are under investigation. When treating children, there is a greater concern for fear of injection and tolerance to pain than with adults. Interventional procedures can be a traumatic experience for both the patient and the family. Although most injection procedures can be done using topical analgesia to decrease pain and trauma, an alternative is to perform the injection under sedation. Sedation procedures often carry their own risks and benefit but can help control behavior and allow safer completion of a procedure. This is often the case with children younger than 6 years and those with developmental delays. Risks of sedation procedures include depression of respiratory drive, loss of patency of the airway, and loss of protective reflexes, increasing the risk for aspiration.[237] Some procedures require anesthesia and surgical intervention. Others can be performed in a clinic setting using anatomic localization, electrical stimulation, ultrasound imaging, or a combination of these techniques. Table 7.3 lists these interventional medications.

TABLE 7.3
Interventional Medications for Spasticity

Medication	Mechanism of Action	Adverse Reactions	Dosing Parameters
Botulinum toxin	Blocks transmission of neurotransmitter acetylcholine from the presynaptic nerve terminal at the neuromuscular junction	Most commonly localized pain and excessive weakness	For Botox: 10 units/kg/leg Dose not to exceed 400 units For Dysport: For unilateral injections: 10–15 units/kg, with a total dose not to exceed 15 units/kg or 1000 units, whichever is lower. For bilateral injections: guidelines are set at 20–30 units/kg, with a total dose not to exceed 30 units/kg or 1000 units, whichever is lower
Intrathecal baclofen	$GABA_B$ receptor agonist, blocking polysynaptic and monosynaptic afferent neuronal transmission	Mechanical and dose-related complications can occur	Titration based on clinical symptoms
Alcohol	Destruction of peripheral nerves via protein denaturation, axonal degeneration, and fibrosis of the surrounding microvasculature	Injection site pain, dysesthesia, and hypotension	50% dilution
Phenol	Destruction of peripheral nerves via protein denaturation, axonal degeneration, and fibrosis of the surrounding microvasculature	Injection site pain, dysesthesia, and hypotension	3% dilution
Hyaluronidase	Decreases viscosity of the extracellular matrix of muscle tissue	Allergic reaction Procedural reactions	Trial concentration 150 IU in 1 mL diluted with saline in 1:1 ratio

Botulinum Toxin

Botulinum toxin is approved for the treatment of focal spasticity.[215] The most commonly used formulation is OnabotulinumtoxinA ("Botox"), approved for the treatment of spasticity in adults within the United States.[238] Only AbobotulinumtoxinA ("Dysport") is approved for use in lower limb spasticity in children.[239] The only pediatric approved use of OnabotulinumtoxinA is for the treatment of blepharospasm (children 12 years or older) and cervical dystonia (children 16 years or older). All other uses of botulinum toxin are considered "off-label". Other botulinum toxin formulations (Myobloc and Xeomin) are approved only for the treatment of adults.[240,241]

Botulinum toxin exerts its effect at the presynaptic terminal of the neuromuscular junction, preventing the release of the neurotransmitter acetylcholine from the presynaptic nerve terminal.[207] Adverse events include localized pain and excessive weakness.[204] More severe adverse events can include respiratory failure and systemic weakness.[242] Studies on the adverse events of botulinum toxin in children with relation to body weight have been conflicting, and guidelines have changed over the years.[243] Current guidelines for AbobotulinumtoxinA recommend 10 units/kg/leg.[239] The recommended off-label use for OnabotulinumtoxinA ("Botox") varies depending on the specific muscle being injected. The total off-label dosing recommendation has ranged from 12–16 units/kg to 15–22 units/kg.[242,243] Current guidelines from the manufacturer have set a maximum dose of 400 units given in 3-month intervals.[238] For Dysport, manufacturer guidelines are set for unilateral or bilateral injections. For unilateral injections, guidelines are set at 10–15 units/kg, with a total dose not to exceed 15 units/kg or 1000 units, whichever is lower. For bilateral injections, guidelines are set at 20–30 units/kg, with a total dose not to exceed 30 units/kg or 1000 units, whichever is lower.[239]

Intrathecal Baclofen

ITB is approved for the treatment of general spasticity and has the same mechanism of action as its oral formulation. The benefit of ITB lies in the reduced concentration of medication needed to exert its effect. To provide enough effective medication to cross the blood-brain barrier, escalating doses of the oral formulation are needed. Eventually the adverse effect of sedation outweighs the benefit of reduced tone. In other circumstances the dose of baclofen cannot be titrated high enough orally to provide effective relief. The dose of ITB has been estimated at 100–1000 times smaller than the dose for oral baclofen.[229] ITB has been approved for spasticity of central origin in patients 4 years or older. It is considered "off-label" in children younger than 4 years. For pediatric TBI, it is recommended that ITB be considered no less than 1 year after injury.[244] Contraindications include hypersensitivity to oral baclofen.[245]

With regards to the delivery of ITB, there is no standardized technique for the actual ITB pump implant procedure.[246] Most pediatric pumps are implanted subfascially, whereas adult pumps are implanted subdermally. In addition, the complication rate of ITB implantation seems to be higher in children than in adults.[244,247] Mechanical complication rates vary from 4% to 24%, whereas infectious complications range from 5% to 26%.[244] Common complications of ITB can also include dose-related causes (overdose or withdrawal) and implant malfunction.[246] There also seems to be an increased incidence of infection in patients with gastrostomy tube placement.[248] Treatment of withdrawal includes administration of oral baclofen at a starting dose of 10–20 mg every 6 h based on patient tolerance and effectiveness. Recommended adjunctive medications for ITB withdrawal can also include benzodiazepines and cyproheptadine, a serotonin agonist.[249]

Neurolysis With Alcohol/Phenol

A less costly alternative in the management of spasticity is the use of alcohol and phenol, which effect neurolysis through the destruction of peripheral nerves. At concentrations over 50% in alcohol and 3% in phenol, the result is protein denaturation, axonal degeneration, and fibrosis of the surrounding microvasculature.[250] Procedures can be performed using electrical stimulation, ultrasound, or a combination of both. The most commonly injected nerves included the obturator nerve and sciatic branches to the hamstrings and adductor magnus. Adverse events include injection site pain, dysesthesia, and hypotension.[251] Alcohol and phenol have an advantage over botulinum toxin in decreased cost and reduction in number of injections

per year. The effect of the medication can last for at least 6 months. To parents, this can be an attractive alternative to the more frequent botulinum toxin injections. Neurolysis can also be combined with botulinum toxin administration in a single-event, multilevel chemoneurolysis procedure. With this approach, a greater number of muscles can be targeted during a single procedure.[252] Neurolysis is reserved for the proximal nerves, and botulinum toxin can be used for distal or smaller musculature.[48,49]

Hyaluronidase

In one case series, hyaluronidase has been used off-label in the treatment of upper limb spasticity of cerebral origin, with improved active and passive joint range of motion. The hyaluronidase enzyme hydrolyzes hyaluronan (hyaluronic acid), a glycosaminoglycan found in muscle. Hyaluronic acid has been implicated in muscle shortening after cerebral injury, through an increased viscosity of the extracellular matrix. Hyaluronidase decreases the viscosity of the extracellular matrix, with improved movement within the muscle tissue. This also avoids the use of sedating medications or ones that would weaken muscle tissue. In a 2016 study by Raghavan et al., the treatment was well tolerated and remained effective at least 3 months after follow-up. Of the 20 patients in the study, 6 were children 10–15 years of age.[253] Further studies are needed to explore whether hyaluronidase can provide an alternative to current procedural treatments.

SELECTED MEDICAL COMPLICATIONS IN PEDIATRIC TRAUMATIC BRAIN INJURY

Similar to adults, children with TBI often have medical complications secondary to their underlying brain injury. The following are selected medical issues frequently encountered in pediatric TBI. Although similar complications exist in the adult brain-injured population, there can be distinct differences in the frequency, management, and outcomes in pediatric TBI.

Heterotopic Ossification

Heterotopic ossification (HO) is defined as the formation of mature, lamellar bone in nonosseous tissue and often occurs between the muscle and the joint capsule.[254] The underlying mechanisms for HO are still not fully understood. Overall the incidence of HO among patients with TBI can range from 11% to 73.3%,[255] whereas clinically relevant HO can vary from 10% to 23%.[256] For those who sustain a brain injury, the hips, elbows, and knees are the most commonly involved areas in the development of HO.[257] This process, however, can occur in any region of the body. One case report has documented the occurrence of HO in the calvarium of an 18-year-old patient with TBI following a bilateral craniectomy.[258]

The incidence of HO in children seems to be lower than that in adults, with serum alkaline phosphatase levels that were within normal ranges in patients under 17 years of age.[259] Risk factors that contribute to the formation of HO have been studied, including severity of brain injury. In a 2007 study, Simonsen et al. noted a higher incidence of HO among the more severe cases, in patients with fractures, and among women. Gender differences were attributed to humeral and hormonal factors mediating the formation of HO. The youngest patient in this retrospective study was 16 years of age.[255] The presence of autonomic instability can also be a risk factor and may be predictive of HO. In a 2007 study, Hendricks et al. demonstrated that, although DAI, spasticity, and systemic infection were associated with an increased risk of HO, only autonomic instability had both positive and negative predictive values with regard to the risk of developing HO.[260] In 2000 Kluger et al. concluded that a persistent vegetative state was also a risk factor for HO, independent of the etiology for the vegetative state.[259]

Symptoms of HO can include pain, warmth, and swelling in the affected area. Caution must be taken in individuals who sustain a concurrent spinal cord injury, as these patients may not report pain in the affected region.[257] In adults, treatment with nonsteroidal anti-inflammatory drugs (NSAIDs) and bisphosphonates is the standard of care.[257,261]

NSAIDs, such as indomethacin, have been recommended at doses of 1–2 mg/kg/day given in divided doses. The maximum daily dosage should not exceed 3 mg/kg/day or 150–200 mg/day, whichever is less. There have been some reported cases of interaction with β-adrenergic receptor antagonists, leading to a blunting of the antihypertensive effect of these medications.[256] Salicylates have also been recommended at a daily dose of 60 mg/kg over 6 weeks. As with all NSAIDs, care must be taken with renal dosing.

In children with TBI the use of bisphosphonates has not been well studied. Although there seems to be benefit to the use of bisphosphonates, there are insufficient data on the long-term effects of their use. There are concerns over the long half-life of bisphosphonates, unknown teratogenic effect, and impact on growing bone. They have been recommended in patients who have a significantly low bone mineral density and are at high risk of fractures or those with disabling bone pain.[262] In other pediatric populations taking bisphosphonates, short-term use has instead been advised.[263]

Rehabilitation goals with HO include rest and immobilization in the initial acute phase, followed by active assisted range-of-motion exercises. Surgical excision should be considered for large lesions, when the origin or insertion of a muscle is involved and when the function of a joint is severely impaired.[264] Excision can be considered at least 1 year after bone maturation.[259]

Venous Thromboembolism

In children the incidence of venous thromboembolism (VTE) related to trauma is significantly lower than in adults. The overall estimated incidence of VTE in pediatric patients is as high as 0.4% compared with adult patients with trauma at 0.9%.[265] In pediatric patients, VTE was associated with older age, surgery, blood transfusion, mechanical ventilation, greater severity of injury, and lower GCS score in patients with brain injury.[266] In addition, children aged 16–21 years seemed to have a greater risk for being diagnosed with a VTE compared with children aged 0–12 years.[267] In adults the decision to use anticoagulation following a TBI should be made based on whether the risks outweigh the benefits. Although prophylaxis seems to be safe among patients at low risk of progression of a previous hemorrhage or development of a new bleed, current studies have not yet reached a consensus on prophylactic anticoagulation in adults.[268] Although current guidelines do not recommend VTE prophylaxis in pediatric patients, there is at least one study suggesting prophylaxis in children based on an additive points scale to provide a VTE prediction score. The score incorporated the GCS, intensive care unit admission, patient age, gender, intubation, and fracture risk as elements that separately, or in combination, could guide the type of prophylaxis, mechanical or chemical, that a patient would require.[269]

Psychological and Behavioral Difficulties

In the adult population, patients with severe TBI may demonstrate significant emotional and behavioral problems in adjustment compared with mTBI groups. These difficulties have an impact on successful physical rehabilitation, vocational skills, and community reintegration.[270] Similar to adults, psychological and behavioral difficulties can also occur in children following a TBI. In children, difficulties with behavior and adjustment can not only affect these aforementioned domains but also have greater consequences for younger children undergoing development in language, learning, and other areas of cognition. Studies have demonstrated that up to half of brain-injured children have psychological or behavioral problems, prompting the need for clinicians to monitor for difficulties in adjustment and socialization with pediatric TBI. Problems with attention deficit, hyperactivity, irritability, aggressiveness, emotional lability, and oppositional behavior are all commonly seen in children following TBI.[271,272]

In the case of mTBI, there is evidence that some of the traits seen in patients were premorbid behavioral conditions that placed children at risk for mTBI, prompting the need for clinicians to further investigate a patient's preinjury history in assessing post-TBI status.[273] TBI has been associated with both premorbid and postinjury ADHD.[274] Previous studies have documented a rate of premorbid ADHD ranging from 10% to 22% of patients having TBI, with Max et al.[64] citing premorbid ADHD as a risk factor for TBI. This theory has been challenged for its small sample size, severity of injury in patients with TBI, and inclusion of an orthopedic control group, with Adeyemo et al.[275] theorizing that there is instead a stronger link between TBI and the subsequent development of ADHD. Max et al. have also documented patients with TBI developing ADHD,[64] and in a 2016 retrospective study in Taiwan, Yang et al. documented a higher ADHD risk for children with TBI than that of the general population.[276] Nonetheless, behavioral problems in pediatric TBI lead to difficulties across a spectrum of cognitive and social domains, with a need for strengthening self-awareness and self-control skills.[271]

Depression seems to occur less frequently in children than in adults.[271] In a 2017 study by Rhine et al. on posttraumatic stress following TBI, there was an association found between depression and elevated posttraumatic stress.[277] Serotonergic antidepressants and cognitive behavioral interventions seem to have the best preliminary evidence for treating depression following TBI.[278] In a 2015 Cochrane review of nonpharmacologic treatments for TBI, Gertler et al. were unable to determine any compelling evidence in support of any particular intervention that would inform clinical practice. Only six studies met the inclusion criteria, with a total of 334 adult participants. Nonpharmacologic treatments included cognitive behavioral therapy, exercise, and transcranial magnetic stimulation (TMS). Only one study mentioned minor, transient adverse events from repetitive TMS. There were no studies meeting the inclusion criteria that had participants under the age of 18 years, although researchers included pediatric treatments in their analysis.[279]

Endocrine Dysfunction

Endocrine dysfunction has been studied in adult TBI. In the pediatric population, there are limited data on this topic. Selected endocrine dysfunction in the pediatric population includes deficiencies in growth hormone (GH), gonadotropin releasing hormone (GnRH), and cortisol and diabetes insipidus (DI). Overall, there is a lack of consensus regarding pediatric guidelines for endocrine stimulation testing. Hormone assays, diagnostic criteria, and time from injury are not standardized when diagnosing endocrine dysfunction following TBI. In addition, there may be drugs used in the acute stage that can affect neuroendocrine function. The most common endocrine deficiency seems to be GH deficiency (varies from 2% to 57% of cases), followed by GnRH deficiency (4%–37%).[280] In a prospective study of 31 children with TBI by Kaulfers et al., 74% of patients had endocrine dysfunction within the first 12 months post injury, with 29% of patients having endocrine dysfunction at 12 months post injury. In this study, precocious puberty was the most common endocrine deficiency.[281] Precocious puberty is a unique feature of pediatric TBI, requiring GnRH agonist therapy to slow the progression of puberty.[280] Deficiency in GnRH has lifelong implications in that early discovery and treatment can directly have an impact on growth and development.[282] Permanent DI is rarely reported after TBI in children. Low serum cortisol is also inversely associated with severity of injury.[280] In a 2006 review article, Acerini et al. noted that 100% of 21 case reports cited evidence of pituitary deficiency, with no clear pattern about which type of injury was predictive of causing hypopituitarism. Low serum cortisol and DI seemed to be associated with a greater likelihood of hypopituitarism.[282] Current guidelines recommend that endocrine surveillance occurs at 6 and 12 months after TBI.[280]

Epilepsy

As in the case of adults, posttraumatic seizures and epilepsy are known complications of TBI.[283] These complications can have long-term developmental effects. Difficulties in learning and behavioral problems can have a cognitive and social impact in children. With severe cases of posttraumatic epilepsy, there can be a slow and progressive deterioration in psychomotor abilities.[284]

Posttraumatic seizures can be classified as early (occurring within 7 days of injury) or late (occurring more than 7 days after injury).[285] An estimated 5%–21% of children experience posttraumatic seizures, whereas 32%–40% develop a recurrence of seizures.[286] The development of posttraumatic epilepsy has been associated with younger age, severity of injury, and nonaccidental trauma.[283,287] An association with immediate seizures has not been found.[286] Other risk factors also include subdural hemorrhage, prehospital hypoxia, and impact seizures.[287] In a 2017 prospective study of 191 patients with mTBI, Keret et al. noted that posttraumatic seizures in mTBI were also predictive of posttraumatic epilepsy. Other risk factors within the study noted that the length of hospitalization was an indirect measure of severity of injury and was associated with a greater risk of posttraumatic epilepsy. Contrary to prior studies, Keret et al. did not find an association with age and the development of posttraumatic epilepsy.[286]

The decision to use seizure prophylaxis is still controversial. Similar to that of adults, the American Academy of Neurology and the Brain Trauma Foundation Guidelines for children with severe TBI recommend the use of phenytoin for the prevention of early posttraumatic seizures, but there is no indication for the use of antiepileptic medications for late posttraumatic seizures.[283,285] In adults, seizure prophylaxis in the first week after injury is advised but should not continue after the first week because of lack of additional benefit, unless posttraumatic seizures develop. These same standards have been applied to children.[285,288–290]

Although guidelines have been set on the administration of mediations, there are no set guidelines on the timing and choice of medication, which has led to variations in drugs (e.g., fosphenytoin vs. phenytoin), timing of administration, and use of multiple medications.[291] Levetiracetam has been proposed as an alternative choice because of its safety profile and lack of requisite serum levels.[283,291] In a 2016 review, Yang et al. did not find any difference in terms of efficacy or adverse effects with levetiracetam over phenytoin with regard to early or late seizure prophylaxis following TBI.[292]

Olfactory Dysfunction

Anosmia is a less studied sequela of TBI that may have a greater effect on the pediatric population than on the adult population. Changes in olfactory function in the adult population have been shown to affect diet, personal hygiene, and activities of daily living.[293] In children, this can be further extended to affect feeding and therefore growth and development. There is also an increased safety burden because of the inability to sense dangerous fumes or odors. In a 2014 review article by Bakker et al., 3%–58% of patients studied were noted to have olfactory dysfunction, with an association between injury severity and presence of olfactory

deficits.[293] In a 2016 prospective study, Bakker et al. noted that children with continued impairments after 9 months post injury were more likely to have ongoing deficits.[294]

Noninvasive Brain Stimulation for Neuronal Repair and Remodeling

Alternatives to pharmacologic interventions have been studied, and an area of recent interest has been noninvasive brain stimulation. Brain stimulation attempts to restore motor function by driving neural repair and brain remodeling.[295] There are generally two types of brain stimulation: TMS and transcranial current stimulation (tCS). TMS produces a magnetic field of sufficient magnitude and density to depolarize neurons and modulate cortical excitability beyond the duration of the length or train of stimulation.[296] Impulses can be delivered via single pulses or in repetitive trains of stimulation. tCS transmits either a direct (transcranial direct current stimulation or tDCS) or alternating current to regions of the brain to increase or decrease neuronal excitability.[297]

TMS has been tolerated in the pediatric population and has been studied in the treatment of pediatric conditions such as depression, stroke recovery, ADHD, epilepsy, and movement disorders.[297–299] Given that these are all potential sequelae of pediatric TBI, the use of electrical stimulation holds promise. There are, however, little data on pediatric TBI.[300] Lu et al. have proposed a theoretical benefit showing improvement in neuronal plasticity after TBI using rat models, but this has yet to be translated into human studies.[301] In contrast, in a 2015 review article, Dhaliwal et al. examined the application of electrical stimulation in adult TBI. Although there appeared to be improvements in cognitive and motor impairment, there was less compelling evidence for improvement in disorders of consciousness.[302] Common risks of electrical stimulation include pain or burning from electrode placement, headache, hearing loss, and induction of seizures. These risks appear to be less prevalent in the pediatric population.[299] Other less common risks include changes in hormone levels and neurotransmitter and autonomic activity, but these have not been studied well.[296]

REHABILITATION STRATEGIES IN PEDIATRIC TRAUMATIC BRAIN INJURY

There are different theories regarding recovery of function after brain injury; recovery of function through restitution or by substitution. Restitution of function is a result of the inherent mechanisms of healing and physiologic recovery. Substitution refers to reorganization or compensation in the recovery of function. In the acute phase, these two processes seem to overlap. After 6 months, substitution is considered to be the underlying mechanism of recovery. This process is similar for both children and adults.[303]

As previously mentioned, the rehabilitation of children with a TBI is distinguished from that of adults by the presence of developmental considerations. These factors are therefore incorporated into the rehabilitation program, guiding treatment and offering insight into short- and long-term outcomes. The developmental timing of a brain injury often dictates the rehabilitation goals and therapy strategies for each child. Ranging from feeding strategies in an infant to executive functioning in a teenager, functional goals vary across different age groups. For the very young, this means a set of goals that are constantly shifting and changing to meet the needs of their developmental landscape.

In children whose development is incomplete, a disruption of emerging motor and cognitive skills place future skills and learning at risk, as each new milestone is dependent on the previous one.[304] The potential for recovery depends on the interaction of internal and externally factors that have been found to be predictive of recovery. Age, preinjury factors, and severity of injury have all been considered to be predictive of functional outcome following TBI.[304–306] In addition, the family environment must also be considered in determining rehabilitation goals and outcomes.[305,307] In a 2016 study, Ryan et al. noted that children with more severe TBI had social problems, which significantly increased from 12 to 24 months post injury, with the proximal family environment and coping mechanisms playing a role in determining long-term social problems.[308] A comprehensive rehabilitation program is therefore designed to facilitate neurologic recovery, provide alternative strategies to compensate for functional deficits, and promote or maximize functional/social independence. The eventual goal is reintegration into the community with the aid of appropriate services, if needed.[304,309]

In the acute care of a patient with pediatric TBI, treatment is similar to that of adults. Passive range-of-motion exercises, standing programs, splinting, and serial casting are often done to prevent contracture formation and reduce spasticity.[227] Reintegration of vestibular, ocular, and proprioceptive feedback mechanisms can improve motor skills and coordination.[309] Postural control and positioning tolerance can be done at the bedside even in the most severely involved patients. These treatments are supplemented by pharmacotherapy to improve arousal and cognition and reduce spasticity. These treatments can often begin before the acute rehabilitation admission, upon which time short- and long-term goals are addressed for each child. These evaluations can be made using standardized assessment tools such as the Functional Independence Measure for Children (WeeFIM) and Pediatric Evaluation of Disability Inventory (PEDI), allowing progress to be tracked and periodic reassessment of goals.

Short-term goals, especially during the acute rehabilitation process, are based on clinical presentation and are often patient specific. In an infant, these can include feeding strategies and verbal communication, the development of bimanual skills, or promoting the transition from crawling to standing, then cruising to walking. In older children, these goals shift to improve school-age functional abilities and community reintegration. Speech therapy may be needed for aphasia or dysarthria. Occupational therapy can address cognitive rehabilitation, graphomotor abilities, play skills, and self-care. Physical therapy may be needed for strengthening weakened muscle groups and ambulation (both in balance and correcting abnormal gait patterns). Bracing may be needed to provide corrective alignment of the joints, reduce tone, prevent deformity, and normalize gait patterns. Neuropsychological testing can help elucidate specific areas of cognitive deficit. In the older child, memory, vocational skills, and activities of daily living may also be the focus of therapy. Long-term goals are often assessed in the outpatient setting and are designed to promote the continued acquisition of age-appropriate developmental milestones and cognitive abilities.

Another aspect of pediatric TBI rehabilitation that receives little attention is dysphagia, noted in up to 3.8%–5.3% of patients studied.[310] In the case of children with severe TBI, dysphagia has been documented to be as high as 68% of patients studied.[311] The effects of feeding disorder in pediatric TBI include poor growth and development in a child with increased metabolic demands secondary to their brain injury and increased risk for aspiration.[310] Associated risk factors for dysphagia include an increased length of hospital stay, length of ventilation, and duration of supplemental feeding.[312] Compensatory feeding strategies are often used, ranging from food texture and liquid consistency modification to oromotor strategies and head positioning techniques. If there is a prognosis for improvement, recovery time is variable. For children with more common diffuse cortical injuries, a return to a normal diet can typically occur in less than 12 weeks post injury. With more severe injuries, recovery may take up to 1 year.[310]

REHABILITATION OUTCOME MEASURES IN PEDIATRIC TRAUMATIC BRAIN INJURY

The use of meaningful outcome measures to predict recovery provides valuable information for parents, clinicians, and researchers. Although some of the instruments used to predict recovery are derived from adult scales, there have been assessment tools designed specifically for children. These instruments are used to predict outcomes based on injury severity and on functional performance and are further used to predict risk factors and outcomes among different patient populations.

Glasgow Outcome Scale Extended Peds

Designed to predict outcome measures from infancy to adulthood, the Glasgow Outcome Scale Extended (GOS-E) Peds is modeled after the Glasgow Outcome Scale (GOS) and has been shown to correlate with the GOS in predicting functional outcome after TBI. The GCS and the GOS-E-Peds provide an easily obtained level of consciousness based on visual, motor, and verbal responses used for clinical assessment and prognosis.[313] In adults the GCS is predictive of a number of functional outcome variables at short- and long-term follow-up after TBI. In severe injuries, correlation of the GOS-E Peds with other outcome measures was moderate to high, reaching statistical significance for measures of learning, impulsivity, and overall hyperactivity. Researchers have shown that the GOS-E Peds is an improvement over the GOS as a valid measure of overall outcome of infants, toddlers, and younger children.[314]

Children's Orientation and Amnesia Test

The COAT is an objective, standardized means of assessing PTA and cognitive functioning in children and adolescents from 3 to 15 years in the early stages of recovery from TBI. As noted earlier in this chapter, the COAT is derived from the GOAT. PTA has been determined to be useful for predicting short- and long-term outcome after pediatric TBI.[313,315] The COAT is composed of 16 items that assess general orientation, temporal orientation, and memory.[316]

Time to Follow Commands

Time to Follow Commands (TFCs) is defined as the interval in days from injury until the individual followed simple verbal commands twice within a 24-h period.[313] In a 2017 study, Davis et al. demonstrated the utility of TFC in predicting functional outcome after pediatric TBI as measured by the GOS-E Peds. They further postulated that using the TFC and also the TFC + PTA added statistically significant predictive power above and beyond the GCS.[317]

Both in the acute rehabilitation setting and longitudinally, the two most common outcome measures for children are the WeeFIM and the PEDI. Both have been used to assess children with TBI.

Functional Independence Measure for Children

The WeeFIM is an adaptation of the Functional Independence Measure (FIM) used in adults. The WeeFIM was originally designed to be used in children from 6 months to 7 years of age without disabilities and older children and adolescents with developmental disabilities. It has been further expanded to include children up to 18 years of age, allowing the WeeFIM to interface with the adult FIM.[318] The WeeFIM describes performance in three domains: self-care (eight items), mobility (five items), and cognition (five items). Higher WeeFIM scores on admission were associated with shorter length of stay and higher discharge scores. Similarly, a shorter time from injury to rehabilitation admission was associated with shorter stay and higher discharge scores.[319] The WeeFIM is used by a trained and licensed practitioner and can take 10–20 min to administer.[318,320]

Pediatric Evaluation of Disability Inventory

The PEDI is designed as a method of assessing functional performance in the domains of self-care (73 items), mobility (59 items), and social function (65 items). There are an additional 20 questions based on caregiver assistance.[321] The PEDI was designed for use in children aged 6 months to 7.5 years with physical limitations or a combination of physical and cognitive limitations. It can also be used in older children with developmental disabilities. The PEDI can take from 30 min to an hour to administer, and no specific training is required to administer the PEDI.[318,320] A computer-adaptive test form of the PEDI, known as the PEDI-CAT, has also been developed. The goal of the computerized test version is to minimize the number of items administered using a computer algorithm but still allow the clinician to obtain an estimate of functioning. The PEDI-CAT also seeks to expand the age range of the PEDI up to 21 years.[321]

In a 2001 study, Ziviani et al. compared the utility of the WeeFIM and PEDI in children with TBI. Although both the PEDI and WeeFIM had high interrater reliability, there were distinct differences. The WeeFIM seemed to be a good global and time-efficient measure of functional ability, whereas the PEDI seemed to be more

TABLE 7.4
Comparison of the WeeFIM and PEDI Assessment Scales

Scale	Cost	Items	Time	Age Range	Transition to Adult Scales	Credentialing Required
WeeFIM	Expensive	18	10–20 min	6 months–21 years	Yes	Yes
PEDI	Inexpensive	217	30–60 min	6 months–7.5 years	No	No

PEDI, Pediatric Evaluation of Disability Inventory; *WeeFIM*, Functional Independence Measure for Children.

detailed and could translate well into individual treatment goals.[318] Another notable difference is that the PEDI is more cost-effective than the WeeFIM.[318,320] In a 2017 review, Williams et al. compared the suitability of the WeeFIM and the PEDI as outcome measures in TBI. All of the accepted studies were either retrospective case series or cohort studies. Williams considered the WeeFIM a more reliable measurement tool because of the presence of greater ceiling effects noted in the PEDI. This conclusion, however, may have been confounded by multiple studies in the review that emanated from a single rehabilitation center using the PEDI. Interestingly, most trials utilized multiple services to administer the WeeFIM and PEDI, including on admission and discharge, making interrater reliability another confounding factor in the review. However, neither PEDI nor WeeFIM take into account injury severity and medical complications in their assessments.[320] Table 7.4 lists a comparison of the WeeFIM and PEDI.

Beyond the generally accepted outcome measures, studies have also focused on determining factors that would be predictive of longitudinal neurologic and functional recovery. Catroppa et al. studied outcomes and predictors of functional recovery 5 years after injury in children aged 2–7 years. Investigators collected data on adaptive, behavioral, and social variables via parental questionnaires; children were tested on intellectual and educational skills. One of the predictors of long-term outcome in these areas seemed to be the severity of injury.[322] Statistical models have also been introduced to determine outcomes in pediatric brain injury, with a checklist of negative predictors, such as preexisting cognitive deficits, injury severity, and intubation predicting physical and cognitive disabilities. In a 2005 study, Wechsler et al. noted that the likelihood of cognitive impairment was increased by factors of 3.2 and 5.8 in children obtunded or comatose on arrival at an acute care facility. By developing a clinician checklist tool, providers in the acute care setting would better determine which patients benefit from long-term inpatient rehabilitative care.[323]

In a 2009 meta-analysis, Babikian and Asarnow provided a summary on neurocognitive outcomes after pediatric TBI. Data were grouped across age, postinjury intervals, and severity of injury. Researchers noted the lack of well-defined and discrete groups indicating severity of injury, standardized time points post injury, and age groups, limiting their analysis. In mTBI, most studies found no statistically significant lasting effects on neurocognitive functioning. Patients with moderate TBI were noted to have deficits in intellectual functioning and attention even 2 years post injury compared with controls. Members of the severe TBI group continued to have impairments across neurocognitive domains. They seemed to fall farther behind their age-related peers over time, which may have been related to their younger age at time of injury. Overall, the domains that appeared most sensitive to TBI across groups were intellectual functioning, processing speed, attention, and verbal memory. The domains showing the most recovery included intellectual functioning and processing speed.[324]

Fay et al. investigated longitudinal patterns of functional deficits in children with moderate to severe TBI compared with children with orthopedic injuries. Although results showed that a substantial proportion of children with moderate to severe injury had relatively few functional deficits during recovery, a significant number of children with severe TBI demonstrated neuropsychological, behavioral, adaptive, and academic deficits over 4 years post injury. These children were at risk for persistent deficits years after recovery. Children with better premorbid functioning seemed to have a greater chance of recovery over time, whereas those with a significant premorbid history were more likely to have negative impact from their injury.[325]

In addition to the severity of injury and premorbid history, race has also been found to be a predictor of recovery in TBI. In a 2006 study, Haider et al. noted that black children with a TBI were more likely to have greater severity of injury, higher likelihood of discharge to an inpatient facility, and increased odds of having functional deficits at discharge.[326] In a 2015 cohort study, Jimenez et al. noted that Hispanic and non-Hispanic black children had lower discharge functional cognitive scores compared with non-Hispanic white children. Younger age, lower admission functional independence scores, and Medicaid insurance were associated with lower functional cognitive independence at discharge. Non-Hispanic black children were also noted to have significantly lower scores in all areas that were measured. For Hispanic children, there was also a greater likelihood of being treated in nonpediatric rehabilitation facilities.[327]

TRANSITION TO ADULT CARE

Eventually the pediatric patient must transition to adult care. This transition can often be difficult and needs to occur in stages. Self-management skills, trust in adult care, interdisciplinary cooperation, and family/social support systems have been recognized as factors in the successful transition to adult services. In addition, education and involvement of the patient's goals and experiences during the process have been associated with a more successful transition to adult care.[312,328] Gender differences may also play a role in transition of care, as the process may be experienced differently by male and female patients. In one study of patients with TBI, Lindsay et al. noted that, although both male and female study participants had experienced a similar transition process and availability of care, there were differences between genders. Males had less reliance upon relational factors such as family involvement and social support compared with females. Although the sample size of participants was small (four women, six men), their experiences were similar to those in other patient populations.[329]

CONCLUSION

There are multiple features that distinguish the treatment of children with brain injury from that of adults. From epidemiologic characteristics to physiologic differences, treatment strategies to outcome measures, pediatric TBI poses unique challenges not seen in adults. Comprehensive, team-based care led by a brain injury specialist can provide the best outcome for these children, our most vulnerable patients.

REFERENCES

1. Raimondi AJ. *Pediatric Neuroradiology.* 1972.
2. Shea KM, Alonzo C, Amitai Y, et al. *Children Are Not Little Adults: Children's Health and Environment – WHO Training Package for the Health Sector* July 2008 Version; 2008.
3. Faul M, Xu L, Wald MM, Coronado VG. *Traumatic Brain Injury in the United States: Emergency Department Visits, Hospitalizations and Deaths 2002-2006.* Atlanta, GA: Centers for Disease Control and Prevention, National Center for Injury Prevention and Control; 2010. CDC Report: https://www.cdc.gov/traumaticbraininjury.
4. Dewan MC, Mummareddy N, Wellons JC, Bonfield CM. Epidemiology of global pediatric traumatic brain injury: qualitative review. *World Neurosurg.* 2016;91:497–509.
5. Savage RG, DePompei R, Tyler J, Lash M. Pediatric traumatic brain injury: a review of pertinent issues. *Pediatr Rehabil.* 2005;8(2):92–103.
6. Langlois JA, Marr A, Mitchko J, Johnson RL. Tracking the silent epidemic and educating the public: CDC's traumatic brain injury-associated activities under the TBI act of 1996 and the Children's Health Act of 2000. *J Head Trauma Rehabil.* 2005;20(3):196–204.
7. Menon DK, Schwab K, Wright DW, et al. Position statement: definition of traumatic brain injury. *Arch Phys Med Rehabil.* 2010;91:1637–1640.
8. Brain Injury Association of America (BIAUSA). *What Is the Difference Between Acquired Brain Injury and Traumatic Brain Injury?* http://www.biausa.org/FAQRetrieve.aspx?ID=43913.
9. Dosman CF, Andrews D, Goulden KJ. Evidence-based milestones ages as a framework for developmental surveillance. *Paediatr Child Health.* 2012;17(10):561–568.
10. Jaffe KM, Polissar NL, Fay GC, Liao S. Recovery trends over three years following pediatric traumatic brain injury. *Arch Phys Med Rehabil.* 1995;76:17–26.
11. Yeates KO, Swift EE, Taylor HG, et al. Short- and long-term social outcomes following pediatric traumatic brain injury. *J Int Neuropsychol Soc.* 2004;10:412–426.
12. Anderson V, Brown S, Hewitt H, Hoile H. Educational, vocational, psychosocial and quality of life outcomes for adult survivors of childhood traumatic brain injury. *J Head Trauma Rehabil.* 2009;24(5):303–312.
13. Chevignard M, Toure H, Brugel DG, Poirier J, Laurent-Vannier A. A comprehensive model of care for rehabilitation of children with acquired brain injuries. *Child Care Health Dev.* 2010;36(1):31–43.
14. Ewing-Cobbs L, Prasad MR, Landry SH, Kramer L, DeLeon R. Executive functions following traumatic brain injury in young children: a preliminary analysis. *Dev Neuropsychol.* 2004;26:487–512.
15. Nguyen VQC, Cruz TH, McDeavitt JT. Traumatic brain injury and the science of injury control. State-of-the-art-reviews. *PM R.* 2001:213–227.
16. Committee on Injury, Violence, and Poison Prevention, Durbin DR. Child passenger safety. *Pediatrics.* 2011;127(4):788–793.

17. Dias MS, Smith K, DeGuehery K, Mazur P, Li V, Shaffer ML. Preventing abusive head trauma among infants and young children: a hospital-based, parent education program. *Pediatrics.* 2005;115(4).

18. Kaushnik R, Krisch I, Schroeder DR, Flick R, Nemergut ME. Pediatric bicycle-related head injuries: a population-based study in a county without a helmet law. *Inj Epidemiol.* 2015;2(1):16.

19. Elliott MR, Kallan MJ, Durbin DR, Winston FK. Effectiveness of child safety seats vs seat belts in reducing risk for death in children in passenger vehicle crashes. *Arch Pediatr Adolesc Med.* 2006;160(6):617–621.

20. Thurman DJ, Alverson C, Dunn KA, et al. Traumatic brain injury in the United States: a public health perspective. *J Head Trauma Rehabil.* 1999;14:602–615.

21. Rutland-Brown W, Langlois JA, Thomas KE, Xi YL. Incidence of traumatic brain injury in the United States, 2003. *J Head Trauma Rehabil.* 2006;21:544–548.

22. Summers CR, Ivins B, Schwab KA. Traumatic brain injury in the United States: an epidemiological overview. *Mt Sinai J Med.* 2009;76:105–110.

23. Anderson V, Catroppa C, Morse S, Haritou F, Rosenfeld J. Functional plasticity or vulnerability after early brain injury? *Pediatrics.* 2005;116(6):1374–1382.

24. National Center for Injury Prevention and Control. Traumatic brain injury-related emergency department visits, hospitalizations, and deaths – United States, 2007 and 2013. Atlanta, GA: Department of Health and Human Services, Centers for Disease Control and Prevention. *MMWR Surveill Summ.* 2017;66(No.SS-9):1–16. https://doi.org/10.15585/mmwr.ss6609a1.

25. Koepsell TD, Rivara FP, Vavilala MS, et al. Incidence and descriptive epidemiologic features of traumatic brain injury in King County, Washington. *Pediatrics.* 2001;128:946–954.

26. Adelson PD, Kochanek PM. Head injury in children. *J Child Neurol.* 1998;13:2–15.

27. Holloway M, Bye A, Moran K. Non-accidental head injury in children. *Med J Aust.* 1994;160:786–789.

28. Keenan HT, Bratton SL. Epidemiology and outcomes of pediatric traumatic brain injury. *Dev Neurosci.* 2006;28:256–263.

29. Crowe L, Babl F, Anderson V, Catroppa C. The epidemiology of paediatric head injuries: data from a referral centre in Victoria, Australia. *J Paediatr Child Health.* 2009;45(6):346–350.

30. Langlois JA, Rutland-Brown W, Thomas KE. *Traumatic Brain Injury in the United States: Emergency Department Visits, Hospitalizations, and Deaths.* Atlanta, GA: Centers for Disease Control and Prevention, National Center for Injury Prevention and Control; 2006.

31. Langlois JA, Rutland-Brown W, Thomas KE. The incidence of traumatic brain injury among children in the United States: differences by race. *J Head Trauma Rehabil.* 2005;20:229–238.

32. Schneier AJ, Shields BJ, Hostetler SG, et al. Incidence of pediatric traumatic brain injury and associated hospitalization resource utilization in the United States. *Pediatrics.* 2006;118:483–492.

33. Kraus JF. Epidemiological features in brain injury in children: occurrence, children at risk, causes and manner of injury, severity and outcomes. In: Broman SH, Michels ME, eds. *Traumatic Head Injury in Children.* New York, NY: Oxford University Press; 1995:22–39.

34. Tate RL, McDonald S, Lulham JM. Incidence of hospital-treated traumatic brain injury in an Australian community. *Aust N Z J Public Health.* 1998;22:419–423.

35. Sosin DM, Sniezek JE, Thurman DJ. Incidence of mild and moderate brain injury in the United States, 1991. *Brain Inj.* 1996;10:47–54.

36. Lescohier I, DiScala C. Blunt trauma in children: causes and outcomes of head versus intracranial injury. *Pediatrics.* 1993;91:721–725.

37. Cassidy JD, Carroll LJ, Peloso PM, et al. Incidence, risk factors, and prevention of mild traumatic brain injury: results of the WHO Collaborating Centre Task Force on mild traumatic brain injury. *J Rehabil Med.* 2004;43:28–60.

38. Annegers JF. The epidemiology of head trauma in children. In: Shapiro K, ed. *Pediatric Head Trauma.* Mount Kisco, NY: Futura; 1983:1–10.

39. Stewart TC, Alharfi IM, Fraser DD. The role of serious concomitant injuries in the treatment and outcome of pediatric severe traumatic brain injury. *J Trauma Acute Care Surg.* 2013;75(5):836–842.

40. Zaloshnja E, Miller T, Langlois JA, Selassie AW. Prevalence of long-term disability from traumatic brain injury in the civilian population of the United States, 2005. *J Head Trauma Rehabil.* 2008;23:394–400.

41. Gardner R, Smith GA, Chany AM, Fernandez SA, McKenzie LB. Factors associated with hospital length of stay and hospital charges among children in the United States. *Arch Pediatr Adolesc Med.* 2007;161(9):889–895.

42. Ylvisaker M, Feeney T. Executive functions, self-regulation, and learned optimism in paediatric rehabilitation: a review and implications for intervention. *Pediatr Rehabil.* 2002;5:51–70.

43. *Brain Injury in Children.* Brain Injury Association of America. http://libguides.gwumc.edu/c.php?g=27773&p=170272.

44. Bazarian JJ, McClung J, Shah MN, Cheng YT, Flesher W, Kraus J. Mild traumatic brain injury in the United States, 1998-2000. *Brain Inj.* 2005;19(2):85–91.

45. Barlow KM, Crawford S, Stevenson A, Sandhu SS, Belanger F, Dewey D. Epidemiology of postconcussion syndrome in pediatric mild traumatic brain injury. *Pediatrics.* 2010;126(2):e374–e381.

46. Michaud LJ, Rivara FP, Grady MS, Reay DT. Predictors of survival and severe disability after severe brain injury in children. *Neurosurgery.* 1992;31:254–264.

47. Halstead ME, Walter KD, Council of Sports Medicine and Fitness. Sports-related concussions in children and adolescents. *Pediatrics.* 2010;126(3):597–615.

48. Guerrero JL, Thurman DL, Sniezek JE. Emergency department visits associated with traumatic brain injury: United States, 1995-1996. *Brain Inj*. 2000;14(2):181–186.

49. Anderson V, Moore C. Age at injury as a predictor following pediatric head injury: a longitudinal perspective. *Child Neuropsychol*. 1995;1(3):187–202.

50. Taylor HG, Alden J. Age-related differences in outcomes following childhood brain insults: an introduction and overview. *J Int Neuropsychol Soc*. 1997;3:1–13.

51. Verger K, Junque C, Jurado MA, et al. *Brain Inj*. 2000; 14(6):495–503.

52. Barnes MA, Dennis M, Wilkinson M. Reading after closed head injury in childhood: effects on accuracy, fluency, and comprehension. *Dev Neuropsychol*. 1999;15:1–24.

53. Lehr E. *Psychological Management of Traumatic Brain Injuries in Children and Adolescents*. Rockville, MD: Aspen; 1990.

54. Laker SR. Epidemiology of concussion and mild traumatic brain injury. *Phys Med Rehabil*. 2011;3(10 suppl 2): S354–S358.

55. Dick RW. Is there a gender difference in concussion incidence and outcomes? *Br J Sports Med*. 2009;43(suppl 1): i46–i50.

56. Saleh SS, Fuortes L, Vaughn T, Bauer E. Epidemiology of occupational injuries and illnesses in a university population: a focus on age and gender differences. *Am J Ind Med*. 2001;39(6):581–586.

57. Granito V. Psychological response to athletic injury: sex differences. *J Sports Behav*. 2002;25:243–259.

58. Tierney RT, Sitler MR, Swanik CB, Swanik KA, Higgins M, Torg J. Gender differences in head-neck segment dynamic stabilization during head acceleration. *Med Sci Sports Exerc*. 2005;37(2):272–279.

59. Anderson VA, Morse S, Klugg G, et al. Predicting recovery from head injury in young children: a prospective analysis. *J Int Neuropsychol Soc*. 1997;3:568–580.

60. Parslow RC, Morris KP, Tasker RC, Forsyth RJ, Hawley CA. Epidemiology of traumatic brain injury in children receiving intensive care in the U.K. *Arch Dis Child*. 2005;90:1182–1187.

61. Taylor HG, Drotar D, Wade SL, Yeates KO, Stancin T, Klein S. Recovery from traumatic brain injury in children: the importance of the family. In: Broman SH, Michel ME, eds. *Traumatic Head Injury in Children*. New York, NY: Oxford University Press; 1995:188–218.

62. Rivara JB, Jaffe KM, Fay GC, et al. Family functioning and injury severity as predictors of child functioning one year following traumatic brain injury. *Arch Phys Med Rehabil*. 1993;74:1047–1055.

63. Moyes CD. Epidemiology of serious head injuries in childhood. *Child Care Health Dev*. 1980;6(1):1–9.

64. Max JE, Lansing AE, Koele SL, et al. Attention deficit hyperactivity disorder in children and adolescents following traumatic brain injury. *Dev Neuropsychol*. 2004; 25(1–2):159–177.

65. Dalby PR, Obrutz JE. Epidemiological characteristics and sequelae of closed head-injured children and adolescents: a review. *Dev Neuropsychol*. 1991;7:35–68.

66. Dicker BG. Profile of those at risk for minor head injury. *J Head Trauma Rehabil*. 1992;7:83–91.

67. Anderson V, Northam E, Hendy J, Wrennal J. *Developmental Neuropsychology: A Clinical Approach*. Hove and New York: Taylor & Francis Psychology Press; 2001.

68. Ponsford J, WIllmott C, Rothwell A, et al. Cognitive and behavioral outcome following mild traumatic head injury in children. *J Head Trauma Rehabil*. 1999;14(4):360–372.

69. Asnarow RF, Satz P, Light R, Zaucha K, Lewis R, McCleary C. The UCLA study of mild closed head injuries in children and adolescents. In: Broman SH, Michel ME, eds. *Traumatic Head Injury in Children*. New York, NY: Oxford, University Press; 1995:117–146.

70. Brown G, Chadwick O, Shaffer D, Rutter M, Traub M. A prospective study of children with head injuries: III. Psychiatric sequelae. *Psychol Med*. 1981;11(1):63–78.

71. Massagli TL, Jaffe KM, Fay GC, Polissar NL, Liao S, Rivara JB. Neurobehavioral sequelae of severe pediatric traumatic brain injury: a cohort study. *Arch Phys Med Rehabil*. 1996;77:223–231.

72. Prasad MR, Ewing-Cobbs L, Swank PR, Kramer L. Predictors of outcome following traumatic brain injury in young children. *Pediatr Neurosurg*. 2002;36:64–74.

73. Woodward H, Winterbalther K, Donders J, Hackbarth R, Kuldanek A, Sanfilippo D. Prediction of neurobehavioral outcome 1-5 years after postpediatric traumatic head injury. *J Head Trauma Rehabil*. 1999;14:351–359.

74. Ewing-Cobbs L, Prasad MR, Kramer L, et al. Late intellectual and academic outcomes following traumatic brain injury sustained during early childhood. *J Neurosurg*. 2006;105:2887–2896.

75. Salorio CF, Slomine BS, Grados MA, Vasa RA, Christensen JR, Gerring JP. Neuroanatomic correlates of CVLT-C performance following pediatric traumatic brain injury. *J Int Neuropsychol Soc*. 2005;11:686–696.

76. Bonnier C, Marique P, Van Hout A, Potelle D. Neurodevelopmental outcome after severe traumatic brain injury in very young children: role for subcortical lesions. *J Child Neurol*. 2007;22:519–529.

77. Brenner T, Frier MC, Holoshouser BA, Burley, Ashwal S. Predicting neuropsychologic outcome after traumatic brain injury in children. *Pediatr Neurol*. 2003;28:104–114.

78. Serra-Grabulosa JM, Junque C, Verger K, Salgado-Pineda P, Maneru C, Mercader JM. Cerebral correlates of declarative memory dysfunctions in early traumatic brain injury. *J Neurol Neurosurg Psychiatr*. 2005;76:129–131.

79. Teasdale G, Jennett B. Assessment of coma and impaired consciousness: a practical scale. *Lancet*. 1974;2:81–84.

80. McDonald CM, Jaffe KM, Fay GC, et al. Comparison of indices of traumatic brain injury severity as predictors of neurobehavioral outcome in children. *Arch Phys Med Rehabil*. 1994;75(3):328–337.

81. Wagner AK, Arenth PM, Kwasnica CK, Rogers EH. Traumatic brain injury. In: Braddom RL, ed. *Physical Medicine and Rehabilitation*. 4th ed. Elsevier Health Sciences; 2011:1133–1175.

82. Brasure M, Lamberty GJ, Sayer NA, et al. *Multidisciplinary Postacute Rehabilitation for Moderate to Severe Traumatic Brain Injury in Adults*. Rockville, MD: Agency for Healthcare Research and Quality (US); 2012 (Comparative Effectiveness Reviews, No. 72.) https://www.ncbi.nlm.nih.gov/books/NBK99000/.

83. Kirkham FJ, Newton CRJC, Whitehouse W. Pediatric coma scales. *Dev Med Child Neurol*. 2008;50:267–274.

84. Simpson DA, Cockington RA, Hanieh A, Raftos J, Reilly PL. Head injuries in infants and young children: the value of the paediatric coma scale. Review of literature and report on a study. *Childs Nerv Sys*. 1991;7:183–190.

85. Holmes JF, Palchak MJ, MacFarlane T, Kupperman N. Performance of the pediatric glasgow coma scale in children with blunt head trauma. *Acad Emerg Med*. 2005;12(9):814–819.

86. Borgialli DA, Mahajan P, Hoyle JD, et al. *Acad Emerg Med*. 2016;23(8):878–884.

87. Gedit R. Head injury. *Pediatr Rev*. 2001;22:118–124.

88. Yager JY, Johnston B, Seshia SS. Coma scales in pediatric practice. *Am J Dis Child*. 1990;144:1088–1091.

89. Tatman A, Warren A, Williams A, Powel JE, Whitehouse W. Development of a modified paediatric coma scale in intensive care clinical practice. *Arch Dis Child*. 1997;77:519–521.

90. Reilly PL, Simpson DA, Spord R, Thomas L. Assessing the conscious level in infants and young children: a paediatric version of the Glasgow coma scale. *Childs Nerv Sys*. 1988;4:30–33.

91. Morray JP, Tyler DC, Jones TK, Stuntz JT, Lemire RJ. Coma scale for use in brain-injured children. *Crit Care Med*. 1984;12:1018–1020.

92. Raimondi AJ, Hirschauer J. Head injury in the infant and toddler. Coma scoring and outcome scale. *Childs Brain*. 1984;11:12–35.

93. James HE, Trauner DA. The Glasgow coma scale. In: James HE, Anas NG, Perkin RM, eds. *Brain Insults in Infants and Children: Pathophysiology and Management*. Orlando, Florida: Grune and Stratton Inc; 1985:179–182.

94. Zasler ND, Katz DI, Zafonte RD, Arciniegas DB, Bullock MR, Kreutzer JS, eds. *Brain Injury Medicine, 2nd Edition: Principles and Practice*. Demos Medical Publishing; 2012:587.

95. Ewing-Cobbs L, Levin HS, Fletcher JM, Miner ME, Eisenberg HM. The children's orientation and amnesia test: relationship to severity of acute head injury and to recovery of memory. *Neurosurgery*. 1990;27(5):683–691. Discussion 691.

96. Arbogast K, Marguiles S. A fiber-reinforced composite model of the viscoelastic behavior of the brainstem in shear. *J Biomech*. 1999;32:865–870.

97. Paus T, Zijdenbos A, Worsely K, et al. Structural maturation of neural pathways in children and adolescents: in vivo study. *Science*. 1999;283:1908–1911.

98. Giorgi A, Watkins KE, Douaud G. Changes in white matter microstructure during adolescence. *NeuroImage*. 2008;39:52–61.

99. Himwich HE. Early studies of the developing brain. In: Himwich W, ed. *Biochemistry of the Developing Brain*. vol. 1. New York, NY: Marcel Dekker Inc; 1973:2–20.

100. Muizelaar J, Marmarou A, DeSalles A, et al. Cerebral blood flow and metabolism in severely head injured children.1. Relationship with GCS, outcome, ICPA and PVI. *J Neurosurg*. 1989;71:63–71.

101. Udomphorn Y, Armstead WM, Vavilala MS. Cerebral blood flow and autoregulation after pediatric traumatic brain injury. *Pediatr Neurol*. 2008;38:225–234.

102. Katayama Y, Becker DP, Tamura T, Hovda DA. Massive increases in extracellular potassium and the indiscriminate release of glutamate following concussive brain injury. *J Neurosurg*. 1990;73:889–900.

103. Vavilala MS, Muangman S, Tontisirin N, et al. Impaired cerebral autoregulation and 6-month outcome in children with severe traumatic brain injury: preliminary findings. *Dev Neurosci*. 2006;28(4–5):348–353.

104. Bittigau P, Sifringer M, Pohl D, et al. Apoptotic neurodegeneration following head trauma is markedly enhanced in the immature brain. *Ann Neurol*. 1999;45:724–735.

105. Giza CC, Mink RB, Madikians A. Pediatric traumatic brain injury: not just little adults. *Curr Opin Crit Care*. 2007;13:143–152.

106. Ponsford J, Willmott C, Rothwell A, et al. Cognitive and behavioral outcome following mild traumatic brain injury in children. *J Int Neuropsychol Soc*. 1997;3:225.

107. Yeates KO, Taylor HG, Drotar D, et al. Pre-injury family environment as a determinant of recovery from traumatic brain injuries in school-age children. *J Int Neuropsychol Soc*. 1997;3:617–630.

108. DiScala C, Osberg S, Savage RC. Children hospitalized for traumatic brain injury: transition to post-acute care. *J Head Trauma Rehabil*. 1997;12:1–10.

109. Cronin AF. Traumatic brain injury in children: issues in community function. *Am J Occup Ther*. 2000;55:377–384.

110. Marr AL, Coronado VG, eds. *Central Nervous System Injury Surveillance Data Submission Standards – 2002*. Atlanta, GA: Centers for Disease Control and Prevention, National Center for Injury Prevention and Control; 2004.

111. Levin HS, Culhane KA, Mendelsohn D, et al. Cognition in relation to magnetic resonance imaging in head-injured children and adolescents. *Arch Neurol*. 1993;50(9):897–905.

112. Gennarelli T, Thibault L. Biomechanics of acute subdural hematoma. *J Trauma*. 1982;22:680–686.

113. Yamada H. *Strength of Biological Materials*. Baltimore: Williams and Wilkins Co; 1970.

114. Coats B, Marguiles SS. Material properties of human infant skull and suture at high rates. *J Neurotrauma*. 2006;23:1222–1232.

115. Graham DI, Gennarelli TA. Pathology of brain damage after head injury. In: Copper PR, Golfinos JG, eds. *Head Injury.* New York: McGraw-Hill; 2000:133–153.

116. Andriessen T, Jacobs B, Vos E. Clinical characteristics and pathophysiological mechanisms of focal and diffuse traumatic brain injury. *J Cell Mol Med.* 2010;14(10):2381–2392.

117. Feng Y, Abney T, Okamoto R, Pless R, Genin G, Bayly P. Relative brain displacement and deformation during constrained mild frontal head impact. *J R Soc Interf.* 2010;7(53):1677–1688.

118. Gaetz M. The neurophysiology of brain injury. *Clin Neurophysiol.* 2004;115:4–18.

119. Halliday AL. Pathophysiology. In: Marion DW, ed. *Traumatic Brain Injury.* New York: Thieme; 1999:29–38.

120. Graham DI. Neuropathology of head injury. In: Narayan RK, Wilberger Jr JE, Povlishock JT, eds. *Neurotrauma.* New York: McGraw-Hill; 1996:43–59.

121. Bigler ED. Anterior and middle cranial fossa in traumatic brain injury: relevant neuroanatomy and neuropathology in the study of neurophysiological outcome. *Neuropsychology.* 2007;21(5):515–531.

122. Adams JH, Mitchell DE, Graham DI, Doyle D. Diffuse brain damage of immediate impact type: its relationship to 'primary brain stem damage' in head injury. *Brain.* 1977;100(3):489–502.

123. Povlishock JT. Traumatically induced axonal injury in animals and humans: pathogenesis and pathobiological implications. *Brain Pathol.* 1992;2:1–12.

124. Li XY, Feng DF. Diffuse axonal injury: novel insights into detection and treatment. *J Clin Neurosci.* 2009;16:614–619.

125. Buki A, Povlishock JT. All roads lead to disconnection?-traumatic axonal injury revisited. *Acta Neurochir (Wien).* 2006;148:181–193.

126. Farkas O, Povlishock JT. Cellular and subcellular change evoked by diffuse traumatic brain injury: a complex web of change extending far beyond focal damage. *Prog Brain Res.* 2007;161:43–59.

127. Ashwal S, Babikian T, Gardner-Nichols J, et al. Susceptibility-weighted imaging and proton magnetic resonance spectroscopy in assessment of outcome after pediatric traumatic brain injury. *Arch Phys Med Rehabil.* 2006;87:S50–S58.

128. Scheid R, Walther K, Guthke T, et al. Cognitive sequelae of diffuse axonal injury. *Arch Neurol.* 2006;63:418–424.

129. Levin HS, Williams D, Crofford MJ, et al. Relationship of depth of brain lesions to consciousness and outcome after closed head injury. *J Neurosurg.* 1988;69:861–866.

130. Graham DI, Gennarelli TA, McIntosh TA. Trauma. In: Graham DI, Lantos PI, eds. *Greenfield's Neuropathology.* New York, NY: Arnold; 2002:823–898.

131. Greve MW, Zink BJ. Pathophysiology of traumatic brain injury. *Mt Sinai J Med.* 2009;76(2):97–104.

132. Chestnut RM, Marshall LF, Klauber MR, et al. The role of secondary brain injury in determining outcome from severe head trauma. *J Trauma.* 1993;34:216–222.

133. Kochanek PM, Clark RSB, Ruppel RA, et al. Biochemical, cellular, and molecular mechanisms in the evolution of secondary damage after severe traumatic brain injury in infants and children: lessons learned from the bedside. *Pediatr Crit Care Med.* 2000;1:4–19.

134. Plesnila N. Decompression craniectomy after traumatic brain injury: recent experimental results. *Prog Brain Res.* 2007;161:393–400.

135. Kochanek PM, Carney N, Adelson PD, Ashwal S, Bell MJ, et al. Guidelines for the acute medical management of severe traumatic brain injury in infants, children, and adolescents – second edition. *Peditr Crit Care Med.* 2012;13(suppl):S1–S82.

136. Bell MJ, Kochanek PM. Pediatric traumatic brain injury in 2012: the year with new guidelines and common data elements. *Crit Care Clin.* 2013;29(2):223–238.

137. Alexander MP. Traumatic brain injury. In: Benson DF, Blumer D, eds. *Psychiatric Aspects of Neurologic Disease.* New York: Grune & Stratton; 1982:219–249.

138. Keenan H, Bratton S. Epidemiology and outcomes of pediatric brain injury. *Dev Neurosci.* 2006;28(4–5):256–263.

139. Prange MT, Coats B, Duhiame AC, Margulies S. Anthropomorphic simulations of falls, shakes, and inflicted impacts in infants. *J Neurosurg.* 2003;99:143–150.

140. Parks S, Sugerman D, Xu L, Coronado V. Characteristics of non-fatal abusive head trauma among children in the USA, 2003-2008: application of the CDC operational case definition to national hospital inpatient data. *Inj Prev.* 2012;18:392–398.

141. Catherine N, Ko JJ, Barr RG. Getting the word out: advice on crying and colic in popular parenting magazines. *J Dev Behav Pediatr.* 2008;29:508–511.

142. Barr R. Crying behavior and its importance for psychosocial development in children. In: Tremblay RE, Boivin M, Peters RD, eds. *Encyclopedia on Early Childhood Development.* Montreal, QC: Centre of Excellence for Early Childhood Development and Strategic Knowledge Cluster on Early Childhood Development; 2006:1–10.

143. Keenan HT, Runyan DK, Marshall SW, et al. A population-based comparison of clinical and outcome characteristics of young children with serious inflicted and noninflicted traumatic brain injury. *Pediatrics.* 2004;114:633.

144. Narang S, Clarke J. Abusive head trauma; past, present, future. *J Child Neurol.* 2014;29(12):1747–1756.

145. Duhaime AC, Christian CW, Rorke LB, Zimmerman RA. Non-accidental head injury in infants-the "shaken-baby syndrome". *N Engl J Med.* 1998;338:1822.

146. Fanconi M, Lips U. Shaken baby syndrome in Switzerland: results of a prospective follow-up study, 2002-2007. *Eur J Pediatr.* 2010;169:1023–1028.

147. Sieswerda-Hoogendoorn T, Boos S, Spivack B, Bilo RA, van Rijn RR. Abusive head trauma part I: clinical aspects. *Eur J Pediatr.* 2012;171:415–423.

148. Margulies S, Thibault L, Gennarelli T. Physical model simulations of brain injury in the primate. *J Biomech.* 1990;23:823–836.

149. Miller R, Margulies S, Leoni M, et al. Finite element modeling approaches for predicting injury in an experimental model of severe diffuse axonal injury. In: *Proceedings of the 42nd Stapp Car Crash Conference, Warrendale, PA, Society of Automotive Engineers*; 1998:155–167.

150. Hahn YS, Chyung C, Barthel MJ, Bailes J, Flannery AM, McLone DG. Head injuries in children under 36 months of age. Demography and outcome. *Childs Nerv Syst.* 1988;4:34–40.

151. Duhaime AC, Alario AJ, Lewander WJ, et al. Head injury in very young children: mechanisms, injury types, and ophthalmologic findings in 100 hospitalized patients younger than 2 years of age. *Pediatrics.* 1992;90(2 Pt 1):179–185.

152. Christian CW, Committee on Child Abuse and Neglect, American Academy of Pediatrics. The evaluation of suspected child physical abuse. *Pediatrics.* 2015;135:e1337.

153. Geddes JF, Vowles GH, Hacksaw AK, et al. Neuropathology of inflicted head injury in children. II. Microscopic brain injury in infants. *Brain.* 2001;124(Pt 7):1299–1306.

154. Brennan L, Rubin DM, Christian CW, Duhaime AC, Mirchandani HG, Rorke-Adams LB. Neck injuries in young pediatric homicide victims. *J Neurosurg Pediatr.* 2009;3(3):232–239.

155. Kadom N, Khademian Z, Vezina G, Shalaby-Rana E, Rice A, Hinds T. Usefulness of MRI detection of cervical spine and brain injuries in the evaluation of abusive head trauma. *Pediatr Radiol.* 2014;44(7):839–848.

156. Tierney AL, Nelson CA. Brain development and the early role of experience in the early years. *Zero Three.* 2009;30(2):9–13.

157. Nelson CA, Zeanah CH, Fox NA, Marshall PJ, Smyke A, Guthrie D. Cognitive recovery in socially deprived young children: the Bucharest Early Intervention Project. *Science.* 2007;318:1937–1940.

158. Bonnier C, Nassogne MC, Evrard P. Outcome and prognosis of whiplash shaken infant syndrome; late consequences after a symptom-free interval. *Dev Med Child Neurol.* 1995;37:943–956.

159. McCrory P, Meeuwisse WH, Aubry M, et al. Consensus statement on concussion in sport: the 4th international conference on concussion in sport held in Zurich. *Br J Sports Med.* 2012;2013(47):250.

160. Bakhos LL, Lockhart GR, Myers R, Linakis JG. Emergency department visits for concussion in young athletes. *Pediatrics.* 2010;126(3):e550–e556.

161. Brener I, Harman JS, Kelleher KJ, Yeates KO. Medical costs of mild to moderate traumatic brain injury in children. *J Head Trauma Rehabil.* 2004;19(5):405–412.

162. Marar M, McIlvain NM, Fields SK, Comstock RD. Epidemiology of concussions among United States high school athletes in 20 sports. *Am J Sports Med.* 2012;40:747.

163. Pfister T, Pfister K, Hagel B, et al. The incidence of concussion in youth sports: a systematic review and meta-analysis. *Br J Sports Med.* 2016;50:292.

164. Mannix R, O'Brien MJ, Meehan WP 3rd. The epidemiology of outpatient visits for minor head injury:2005 to 2009. *Neurosurgery.* 2013;73:129.

165. Grool AM, Aglipay M, Momoli F, et al. Association between early participation in physical activity following acute concussion and persistent postconcussive symptoms in children and adolescents. *JAMA.* 2016;316(23):2504–2514. https://doi.org/10.1001/jama.2016.17396.

166. Carrey N, Kutcher S. Developmental pharmacodynamics: implications for child and adolescent psychopharmacology. *J Psychiatr Neurosci.* 1998;23(5):274–276.

167. Sateia MJ, Buysse DJ, Krystal AD, Neubauer DN, Heald JL. Clinical practice guideline for the pharmacologic treatment of chronic insomnia in adults: an American Academy of Sleep Medicine clinical practice guideline. *J Clin Sleep Med.* 2017;13(2):307–349. https://doi.org/10.5664/jcsm.6470.

168. Giacino JT, Fins JJ, Laureys S, Schiff ND. Disorders of consciousness after acquired brain injury: the state of the science. *Nat Rev Neurol.* 2014;10(2):99–114. https://doi.org/10.1038/nrneurol.2013.279.

169. Green LB, Hornyak JE, Hurvitz EA. Amantadine in pediatric patients with traumatic brain injury a retrospective, case-controlled study. *Am J Phys Med Rehabil.* 2004;83(12):893–897.

170. McMahon MA, Vargus-Adams JN, Michaud LJ, Bean J. Effects of amantadine in children with impaired consciousness caused by acquired brain injury: a pilot study. *Am J Phys Med Rehabil.* 2009;88(7):525–532. https://doi.org/10.1097/PHM.0b013e3181a5ade3.

171. Giacino JT, Whyte J, Bagiella E, et al. Placebo-controlled trial of amantadine for severe traumatic brain injury. *N Engl J Med.* 2012;366(9):819–826. https://doi.org/10.1056/NEJMoa1102609.

172. Aoki FY, Sitar DS. Clinical pharmacokinetics of amantadine hydrochloride. *Clin Pharmacokinet.* 1988;14(1):35–51.

173. Samantaray S, Das A, Thakore NP, et al. Therapeutic potential of melatonin in traumatic central nervous system injury. *J Pineal Res.* 2009;47:134–142. https://doi.org/10.1111/j.1600-079X.2009.00703.x.

174. Wilt TJ, MacDonald R, Brasure M, et al. Pharmacologic treatment of insomnia disorder: an evidence report for a clinical practice guideline by the American College of Physicians. *Ann Intern Med.* 2016;165:103–112. https://doi.org/10.7326/M15-1781.

175. Goldman SE, Adkins KW, Calcutt MW, et al. Melatonin in children with autism spectrum disorders: endogenous and pharmacokinetic profiles in relation to sleep. *J Autism Dev Disord.* 2014;44(10):2525–2535. https://doi.org/10.1007/s10803-014-2123-9.

176. Van Geijlswijk IM, van der Heijden KB, Egberts AC, Korzilius HP, Smits MG. Dose finding of melatonin for chronic idiopathic childhood sleep onset insomnia: an RCT. *Psychopharmacology.* 2010;212(3):379–391. https://doi.org/10.1007/s00213-010-1962-0.

177. Maldonado MD, Murillo-Cabezas F, Terron MP, et al. The potential of melatonin in reducing morbidity-mortality after craniocerebral trauma. *J Pineal Res.* 2007;42(1):1–11.

178. Shekleton JA, Parcell DL, Redman JR, Phipps-Nelson J, Ponsford JL, Rajaratnam SM. Sleep disturbance and melatonin levels following traumatic brain injury. *Neurology.* 2010;74(21):1732–1738. https://doi.org/10.1212/WNL.0b013e3181e0438b.

179. Marseglia L, D'Angelo G, Manti S, et al. Melatonin secretion is increased in children with severe traumatic brain injury. *Int J Mol Sci.* 2017;18(5):1053. https://doi.org/10.3390/ijms18051053.

180. Marseglia L, Aversa S, Barberi I, et al. High endogenous melatonin levels in critically ill children: a pilot study. *J Pediatr.* 2013;162(2):357–360. https://doi.org/10.1016/j.jpeds.2012.07.019.

181. Reid WM, Hamm RJ. Post-injury atomoxetine treatment improves cognition following experimental traumatic brain injury. *J Neurotrauma.* 2008;25(3):248–256. https://doi.org/10.1089/neu.2007.0389.

182. Durell TM, Adler LA, Williams DW, et al. Atomoxetine treatment of attention-deficit/hyperactivity disorder in young adults with assessment of functional outcomes: a randomized, double-blind,placebo-controlled clinical trial. *J Clin Psychopharmacol.* 2013;33(1):45–54. https://doi.org/10.1097/JCP.0b013e31827d8a23.

183. Donnelly C, et al. Safety and tolerability of atomoxetine over 3 to 4 years in children and adolescents with ADHD. *J Am Acad Child Adolesc Psychiatr.* 2009;48(2):176–185. https://doi.org/10.1097/CHI.0b013e318193060e.

184. Ripley DL, Morey CE, Gerber D, et al. Atomoxetine for attention deficits following traumatic brain injury: results from a randomized controlled trial. *Brain Inj.* 2014;28(12):1514–1522. https://doi.org/10.3109/02699052.2014.919530.

185. Ludolph AG, Udvardi PT, Schaz U, et al. Atomoxetine acts as an NMDA receptor blocker in clinically relevant concentrations. *Br J Pharmacol.* 2010;160(2):283–291. https://doi.org/10.1111/j.1476-5381.2010.00707.x.

186. Udvardi PT, Föhr KJ, Henes C, et al. Atomoxetine affects transcription/translation of the NMDA receptor and the norepinephrine transporter in the rat brain – an in vivo study. *Drug Des Dev Ther.* 2013;7:1433–1446. https://doi.org/10.2147/DDDT.S50448.

187. http://pi.lilly.com/us/strattera-pi.pdf. (Product Packaging).

188. Natteru P, George P, Bell R, Nattanmai P, Newey CR. Central hyperthermia treated with bromocriptine. *Case Rep Neurol Med.* 2017;2017:1712083. https://doi.org/10.1155/2017/1712083.

189. Yu K-W, Huang Y-H, Lin C-L, Hong C-Z, Chou L-W. Effectively managing intractable central hyperthermia in a stroke patient by bromocriptine: a case report. *Neuropsychiatr Dis Treat.* 2013;9:605–608. https://doi.org/10.2147/NDT.S44547.

190. Munakomi S, Bhattarai B, Mohan Kumar B. Role of bromocriptine in multi-spectral manifestations of traumatic brain injury. *Chin J Traumatol.* 2017;20(2):84–86. https://doi.org/10.1016/j.cjtee.2016.04.009.

191. Whyte J, Vaccaro M, Grieb-Neff P, Hart T, Polansky M, Coslett HB. The effects of bromocriptine on attention deficits after traumatic brain injury: a placebo-controlled pilot study. *Am J Phys Med Rehabil.* 2008;87(2):85–99. https://doi.org/10.1097/PHM.0b013e3181619609.

192. Pergolizzi Jr JV, LeQuang JA, Berger GK, Raffa RB. The basic pharmacology of opioids informs the opioid discourse about misuse and abuse: a review. *Pain Ther.* 2017;6(1):1–16. https://doi.org/10.1007/s40122-017-0068-3.

193. Raithel DS, Ohler KH, Porto I, Bicknese AR, Kraus DM. Morphine: an effective abortive therapy for pediatric paroxysmal sympathetic hyperactivity after hypoxic brain injury. *J Pediatr Pharmacol Ther.* 2015;20(4):335–340. https://doi.org/10.5863/1551-6776-20.4.335.

194. Baguley IJ, Cameron ID, Green AM, Slewa-Younan S, Marosszeky JE, Gurka JA. Pharmacological management of Dysautonomia following traumatic brain injury. *Brain Inj.* 2004;18(5):409–417.

195. Berde CB, Sethna NF. Analgesics for the treatment of pain in children. *N Engl J Med.* 2002;347(14):1094–1103.

196. Tran TY, Dunne IE, German JW. Beta blockers exposure and traumatic brain injury: a literature review. *Neurosurg Focus.* 2008;25(4):E8. https://doi.org/10.3171/FOC.2008.25.10.E8.

197. Patel MB, McKenna JW, Alvarez JM, et al. Decreasing adrenergic or sympathetic hyperactivity after severe traumatic brain injury using propranolol and clonidine (DASH after TBI study): study protocol for a randomized controlled trial. *Trials.* 2012;13:177. https://doi.org/10.1186/1745-6215-13-177.

198. Pozzi M, Conti V, Locatelli F, et al. Paroxysmal sympathetic hyperactivity in pediatric rehabilitation: pathological features and scheduled pharmacological therapies. *J Head Trauma Rehabil.* 2017;32(2):117–124. https://doi.org/10.1097/HTR.0000000000000255.

199. Alali AS, Mukherjee K, McCredie VA, et al. Beta-blockers and traumatic brain injury: a systematic review, meta-analysis, and Eastern Association for the Surgery of Trauma guideline. *Ann Surg.* 2017. https://doi.org/10.1097/SLA.0000000000002286.

200. Kavey RE, Daniels SR, Flynn JT. Management of high blood pressure in children and adolescents. *Cardiol Clin.* 2010;28(4):597–607. https://doi.org/10.1016/j.ccl.2010.07.004.

201. National Institutes of Health, National Heart, Lung, and Blood Institute. *Expert Panel on Integrated Guidelines for Cardiovascular Health and Risk Reduction in Children and Adolescents* Clinical Practice Guidelines; 2011. http://www.nhlbi.nih.gov/guidelines/cvd_ped/peds_guidelines_full.pdf.

202. Baguley IJ, Heriseanu RE, Gurka JA, Nordenbo A, Cameron ID. Gabapentin in the management of dysautonomia following severe traumatic brain injury: a case series. *J Neurol Neurosurg Psychiatr.* 2007;78:539–541. https://doi.org/10.1136/jnnp.2006.096388.

203. Hansel DE, Hansel CR, Shindle MK, et al. Oral baclofen in cerebral palsy: possible seizure potentiation? *Pediatr Neurol.* 2003;29(3):203–206.

204. Delgado MR, Hirtz D, Aisen M, et al. Practice parameter: pharmacologic treatment of spasticity in children and adolescents with cerebral palsy (an evidence-based review): report of the Quality Standards Subcommittee of the American Academy of Neurology and the Practice Committee of the Child Neurology Society. *Neurology.* 2010;74(4):336–343. https://doi.org/10.1212/WNL.0b013e3181cbcd2f.

205. Pérez-Arredondo A, Cázares-Ramírez E, Carrillo-Mora P, et al. Baclofen in the therapeutic of sequele of traumatic brain injury: spasticity. *Clin Neuropharmacol.* 2016; 39(6):311–319.

206. Rush JM, Gibberd FB. Baclofen-induced epilepsy. *J R Soc Med.* 1990;83(2):115–116.

207. Chang E, Ghosh N, Yanni D, Lee S, Alexandru D, Mozaffar T. A review of spasticity treatments: pharmacological and interventional approaches. *Crit Rev Phys Rehabil Med.* 2013;25(1–2):11–22.

208. Simon O, Yelnik AP. Managing spasticity with drugs. *Eur J Phys Rehabil Med.* 2010;46(3):401–410.

209. Scheinberg A, Hall K, Lam LT, O'Flaherty S. Oral baclofen in children with cerebral palsy: a double-blind cross-over pilot study. *J Paediatr Child Health.* 2006;42(11):715–720.

210. Milla PJ, Jackson AD. A controlled trial of baclofen in children with cerebral palsy. *J Int Med Res.* 1977;5(6):398–404.

211. Lubsch L, Habersang R, Haase M, Luedtke S. Oral baclofen and clonidine for treatment of spasticity in children. *J Child Neurol.* 2006;21(12):1090–1092.

212. Moran L, Cincotta T, Krishnamoorthy K, Insoft RM. The use of baclofen in full-term neonates with hypertonia. *J Perinatol.* 2005;25:66–68. https://doi.org/10.1038/sj.jp.7211194.

213. Dario A, Tomei G. A benefit-risk assessment of baclofen in severe spinal spasticity. *Drug Saf.* 2004;27(11):799–818.

214. Palazón García R, Benavente Valdepeñas A, Arroyo Riaño O. Protocolo de uso de la tizanidina en la parálisis cerebral infantile [Protocol for tizanidine use in infantile cerebral palsy]. *An Pediatr (Barc).* 2008;68(5):511–515. [Article in Spanish].

215. Patel DR, Soyode O. Pharmacologic interventions for reducing spasticity in cerebral palsy. *Indian J Pediatr.* 2005;72:869. https://doi.org/10.1007/BF02731118.

216. Chung CY, Chen CL, Wong AM. Pharmacotherapy of spasticity in children with cerebral palsy. *J Formos Med Assoc.* 2011;110(4):215–222. https://doi.org/10.1016/S0929-6646(11)60033-8.

217. Wilkinson SP, Portmann B, Williams R. Hepatitis from dantrolene sodium. *Gut.* 1979;20(1):33–36.

218. Kim JY, Chun S, Bang MS, Shin HI, Lee SU. Safety of low-dose oral dantrolene sodium on hepatic function. *Arch Phys Med Rehabil.* 2011;92(9):1359–1363. https://doi.org/10.1016/j.apmr.2011.04.012.

219. Edgar TS. Oral pharmacotherapy of childhood movement disorders. *J Child Neurol.* 2003;18(suppl 1):S40–S49.

220. Gruenthal M, Mueller M, Olson WL, Priebe MM, Sherwood AM, Olson WH. Gabapentin for the treatment of spasticity in patients with spinal cord injury. *Spinal Cord.* 1997;35(10):686–689.

221. Rabchevsky AG, Kitzman PH. Latest approaches for the treatment of spasticity and autonomic dysreflexia in chronic spinal cord injury. *Neurotherapeutics.* 2011;8(2):274–282. https://doi.org/10.1007/s13311-011-0025-5.

222. Priebe MM, Sherwood AM, Graves DE, Mueller M, Olson WH. Effectiveness of gabapentin in controlling spasticity: a quantitative study. *Spinal Cord.* 1997;35(3):171–175.

223. Cutter NC, Scott DD, Johnson JC, Whiteneck G. Gabapentin effect on spasticity in multiple sclerosis: a placebo-controlled, randomized trial. *Arch Phys Med Rehabil.* 2000;81(2):164–169.

224. Edwards L, DeMeo S, Hornik CD, et al. Gabapentin use in the neonatal intensive care unit. *J Pediatr.* 2016;169:310–312. https://doi.org/10.1016/j.jpeds.2015.10.013.

225. Sacha GL, Foreman MG, Kyllonen K, Rodriguez RJ. The use of gabapentin for pain and agitation in neonates and infants in a neonatal ICU. *J Pediatr Pharmacol Ther.* 2017;22(3):207–211. https://doi.org/10.5863/1551-6776-22.3.207.

226. Haig GM, Bockbrader HN, Wesche DL, et al. Single-dose gabapentin pharmacokinetics and safety in healthy infants and children. *J Clin Pharmacol.* 2001;41(5):507–514.

227. Zafonte R, Elovic EP, Lombard L. Acute care management of post-TBI spasticity. *J Head Trauma Rehabil.* 2004;19(2):89–100.

228. Chou R, Peterson K, Helfand M. Comparative efficacy and safety of skeletal muscle relaxants for spasticity and musculoskeletal conditions: a systematic review. *J Pain Symptom Manage.* 2004;28(2):140–175.

229. Ertzgaard P, Campo C, Calabrese A. Efficacy and safety of oral baclofen in the management of spasticity: a rationale for intrathecal baclofen. *J Rehabil Med.* 2017;49(3):193–203. https://doi.org/10.2340/16501977-2211.

230. Koppel BS, Brust JC, Fife T, et al. Systematic review: efficacy and safety of medical marijuana in selected neurologic disorders: report of the Guideline Development Subcommittee of the American Academy of Neurology. *Neurology.* 2014;82(17):1556–1563. https://doi.org/10.1212/WNL.0000000000000363.

231. Kuhlen M, Hoell JI, Gagnon G, et al. Effective treatment of spasticity using dronabinol in pediatric palliative care. *Eur J Paediatr Neurol.* 2016;20(6):898–903. https://doi.org/10.1016/j.ejpn.2016.07.021.

232. Whiting PF, Wolff RF, Deshpande S, et al. Cannabinoids for medical use: a systematic review and meta-analysis. *JAMA.* 2015;313(24):2456–2473. https://doi.org/10.1001/jama.2015.6358.

233. Fernandez-Lopez D, Lizasoain I, Moro MA, et al. Cannabinoids: well-suited candidates for the treatment of perinatal brain injury. *Brain Sci.* 2013;3(3):1043–1059.

234. Campbell CT, Phillips MS, Manasco K. Cannabinoids in pediatrics. *J Pediatr Pharmacol Ther.* 2017;22(3):176–185. https://doi.org/10.5863/1551-6776-22.3.176.

235. Tekes K. Basic aspects of the pharmacodynamics of tolperisone, a widely applicable centrally acting muscle relaxant. *Open Med Chem J.* 2014;8:17–22. https://doi.org/10.2174/1874104501408010017.

236. Luo D, Wu G, Ji Y, et al. The comparative study of clinical efficacy and safety of baclofen vs tolperisone in spasticity caused by spinal cord injury. *Saudi Pharm J.* 2017;25(4):655–659. https://doi.org/10.1016/j.jsps.2017.04.041.

237. American Academy of Pediatrics, American Academy of Pediatric Dentistry, Coté CJ, Wilson S. Guidelines for monitoring and management of pediatric patients during and after sedation for diagnostic and therapeutic procedures: an update. *Pediatrics.* 2006;118(6):2587–2602. https://doi.org/10.1542/peds.2006-2780.

238. https://www.allergan.com/assets/pdf/botox_pi.pdf. (Product Packaging).

239. http://www.dysport.com/pdfs/Dysport_Medication_Guide.pdf. (Product Packaging).

240. https://www.accessdata.fda.gov/drugsatfda_docs/label/2000/botelan120800lb.pdf. (Product Packaging).

241. https://www.accessdata.fda.gov/drugsatfda_docs/label/2010/125360lbl.pdf. (Product Packaging).

242. Crowner BE, Torres-Russotto D, Carter AR, Racette BA. Systemic weakness after therapeutic injections of botulinum toxin a: a case series and review of the literature. *Clin Neuropharmacol.* 2010;33(5):243–247. https://doi.org/10.1097/WNF.0b013e3181f5329e.

243. Willis AW, Crowner B, Brunstrom JE, Kissel A, Racette BA. High dose botulinum toxin A for the treatment of lower extremity hypertonicity in children with cerebral palsy. *Dev Med Child Neurol.* 2007;49(11):818–822. https://doi.org/10.1111/j.1469-8749.2007.00818.x.

244. Woolf SM, Baum CR. Baclofen pumps: uses and complications. *Pediatr Emerg Care.* 2017;33(4):271–275. https://doi.org/10.1097/PEC.0000000000001090.

245. Saulino M, et al. Best practices for intrathecal baclofen therapy: patient selection. *Neuromodulation.* 2016;19(6):607–615. https://doi.org/10.1111/ner.12447.

246. Awaad Y, Rizk T, Siddiqui I, Roosen N, McIntosh K, Waines GM. Complications of intrathecal baclofen pump: prevention and cure. *ISRN Neurol.* 2012;2012:575168. https://doi.org/10.5402/2012/575168.

247. Vender JR, Hester S, Waller JL, Rekito A, Lee MR. Identification and management of intrathecal baclofen pump complications: a comparison of pediatric and adult patients. *J Neurosurg.* 2006;104(1 suppl):9–15.

248. Fjelstad AB, Hommelstad J, Sorteberg A. Infections related to intrathecal baclofen therapy in children and adults: frequency and risk factors. *J Neurosurg Pediatr.* 2009;4(5):487–493. https://doi.org/10.3171/2009.6.PEDS0921.

249. Saulino M, Anderson DJ, Doble J, et al. Best practices for intrathecal baclofen therapy: troubleshooting. *Neuromodulation.* 2016;19(6):632–641. https://doi.org/10.1111/ner.12467.

250. Kocabas H, Salli A, Demir AH, Ozerbil OM. Comparison of phenol and alcohol neurolysis of tibial nerve motor branches to the gastrocnemius muscle for treatment of spastic foot after stroke: a randomized controlled pilot study. *Eur J Phys Rehabil Med.* 2010;46(1):5–10.

251. Karri J, Mas MF, Francisco GE, Li S. Practice patterns for spasticity management with phenol neurolysis. *J Rehabil Med.* 2017. https://doi.org/10.2340/16501977-2239.

252. Ploypetch T, Kwon JY, Armstrong HF, Kim H. A retrospective review of unintended effects after single-event multi-level chemoneurolysis with botulinum toxin-a and phenol in children with cerebral palsy. *PM R.* 2015;7(10):1073–1080. https://doi.org/10.1016/j.pmrj.2015.05.020.

253. Raghavan P, Lu Y, Mirchandani M, Stecco A. Human recombinant hyaluronidase injections for upper limb muscle stiffness in individuals with cerebral injury: a case series. *EBioMedicine.* 2016;9:306–313. https://doi.org/10.1016/j.ebiom.2016.05.014.

254. Sakellariou VI, Grigoriou E, Mavrogenis AF, Soucacos PN, Papagelopoulos PJ. Heterotopic ossification following traumatic brain injury and spinal cord injury:insight into the etiology and pathophysiology. *J Musculoskelet Neuronal Interact.* 2012;12(4):230–240.

255. Simonsen LL, Sonne-Holm S, Krasheninnikoff M, Engberg AW. Symptomatic heterotopic ossification after very severe traumatic brain injury in 114 patients: incidence and risk factors. *Injury.* 2007;38(10):1146–1150.

256. https://www.accessdata.fda.gov/drugsatfda_docs/label/2009/018332s032lbl.pdf.

257. Aubut J-AL, Mehta S, Cullen N, Teasell RW, ERABI Group, Scire Research Team. A comparison of heterotopic ossification treatment within the traumatic brain and spinal cord injured population: an evidence based systematic review. *Neurorehabilitation.* 2011;28(2):151–160. https://doi.org/10.3233/NRE-2011-0643.

258. Vega RA, Hutchins L. Heterotopic ossification of the calvarium following bilateral craniectomies in traumatic brain injury. *Ochsner J.* 2017;17(1):118–120.

259. Kluger G, Kochs A, Holthausen H. Heterotopic ossification in childhood and adolescence. *J Child Neurol.* 2000;15(6):406–413.

260. Hendricks HT, Geurts AC, van Ginneken BC, Heeren AJ, Vos PE. Brain injury severity and autonomic dysregulation accurately predict heterotopic ossification in patients with traumatic brain injury. *Clin Rehabil.* 2007;21(6):545–553.

261. Sullivan MP, Torres SJ, Mehta S, Ahn J. Heterotopic ossification after central nervous system trauma: a current review. *Bone Joint Res.* 2013;2(3):51–57. https://doi.org/10.1302/2046-3758.23.2000152.

262. Boyce AM, Tosi LL, Paul SM. Bisphosphonate treatment for children with disabling conditions. *PM R.* 2014;6(5):427–436. https://doi.org/10.1016/j.pmrj.2013.10.009.

263. Eghbali-Fatourechi G. Bisphosphonate therapy in pediatric patients. *J Diabetes Metab Disord*. 2014;13:109. https://doi.org/10.1186/s40200-014-0109-y.

264. Sferopoulos NK, Anagnostopoulos D. Ectopic bone formation in a child with a head injury: complete regression after immobilisation. *Int Orthop*. 1998;21(6):412–414. https://doi.org/10.1007/s002640050197.

265. Leeper CM, Vissa M, Cooper JD, Malec LM, Gaines BA. Venous thromboembolism in pediatric trauma patients: ten-year experience and long-term follow-up in a tertiary care center. *Pediatr Blood Cancer*. 2017;64(8). https://doi.org/10.1002/pbc.26415. Epub 2017 January 9.

266. Yen J, Van Arendonk KJ, Streiff MB, et al. Risk factors for venous thromboembolism in pediatric trauma patients and validation of a novel scoring system: the risk of clots in kids with trauma (ROCKIT score). *Pediatr Crit Care Med*. 2016;17(5):391–399. https://doi.org/10.1097/PCC.0000000000000699.

267. Van Arendonk KJ, Schneider EB, Haider AH, Colombani PM, Stewart FD, Haut ER. Venous thromboembolism after trauma: when do children become adults? *JAMA Surg*. 2013;148(12):1123–1130. https://doi.org/10.1001/jamasurg.2013.3558.

268. Shen X, Dutcher SK, Palmer J, et al. A systematic review of the benefits and risks of anticoagulation following traumatic brain injury. *J Head Trauma Rehabil*. 2015;30(4):E29–E37. https://doi.org/10.1097/HTR.0000000000000077.

269. Connelly CR, Laird A, Barton JS, et al. A clinical tool for the prediction of venous thromboembolism in pediatric trauma patients. *JAMA Surg*. 2016;151(1):50–57. https://doi.org/10.1001/jamasurg.2015.2670.

270. Hanks RA, Temkin N, Machamer J, Dikmen SS. Emotional and behavioral adjustment after traumatic brain injury. *Arch Phys Med Rehabil*. 1999;80(9):991–997.

271. Poggi G, Liscio M, Adduci A, et al. Psychological and adjustment problems due to acquired brain lesions in childhood: a comparison between post-traumatic patients and brain tumour survivors. *Brain Inj*. 2005;19(10):777–785.

272. Pastore V, Colombo K, Villa F, et al. Psychological and adjustment problems due to acquired brain lesions in pre-school-aged patients. *Brain Inj*. 2013;27(6):677–684. https://doi.org/10.3109/02699052.2013.775482.

273. Peterson RL, Connery AK, Baker DA, Kirkwood MW. Preinjury emotional-behavioral functioning of children with lingering problems after mild traumatic brain injury. *J Neuropsychiatr Clin Neurosci*. 2015;27(4):280–286. https://doi.org/10.1176/appi.neuropsych.14120373.

274. Keenan HT, Hall GC, Marshall SW. Early head injury and attention deficit hyperactivity disorder: retrospective cohort study. *BMJ*. 2008;337:a1984. https://doi.org/10.1136/bmj.a1984.

275. Adeyemo BO, Biederman J, Zafonte R, et al. Mild traumatic brain injury and ADHD: a systematic review of the literature and meta-analysis. *J Atten Disord*. 2014;18(7):576–584. https://doi.org/10.1177/1087054714543371.

276. Yang LY, Huang CC, Chiu WT, Huang LT, Lo WC, Wang JY. Association of traumatic brain injury in childhood and attention-deficit/hyperactivity disorder: a population-based study. *Pediatr Res*. 2016;80(3):356–362. https://doi.org/10.1038/pr.2016.85.

277. Rhine T, Cassedy A, Yeates KO, Taylor HG, Kirkwood MW, Wade SL. Investigating the connection between traumatic brain injury and posttraumatic stress symptoms in adolescents. *J Head Trauma Rehabil*. 2017. https://doi.org/10.1097/HTR.0000000000000319.

278. Fann JR, Hart T, Schomer KG. Treatment for depression after traumatic brain injury: a systematic review. *J Neurotrauma*. 2009;26(12):2383–2402. https://doi.org/10.1089/neu.2009.1091.

279. Gertler P, Tate RL, Cameron ID. Non-pharmacological interventions for depression in adults and children with traumatic brain injury. *Cochrane Database Syst Rev*. 2015;(12):CD009871. https://doi.org/10.1002/14651858.CD009871.pub2.

280. Reifschneider K, Auble BA, Rose SR. Update of endocrine dysfunction following pediatric traumatic brain injury. *J Clin Med*. 2015;4(8):1536–1560. https://doi.org/10.3390/jcm4081536.

281. Kaulfers AM, Backeljauw PF, Reifschneider K, et al. Endocrine dysfunction following traumatic brain injury in children. *J Pediatr*. 2010;157(6):894–899. https://doi.org/10.1016/j.jpeds.2010.07.004.

282. Acerini CL, Tasker RC, Bellone S, Bona G, Thompson CJ, Savage MO. Hypopituitarism in childhood and adolescence following traumatic brain injury: the case for prospective endocrine investigation. *Eur J Endocrinol*. 2006;155(5):663–669.

283. Ostahowski PJ, Kannan N, Wainwright MS, et al. Variation in seizure prophylaxis in severe pediatric traumatic brain injury. *J Neurosurg Pediatr*. 2016;18(4):499–506.

284. Holmes GL. Effects of seizures on brain development: lessons from the laboratory. *Pediatr Neurol*. 2005;33(1):1–11. Epub 2005 April 13.

285. Bratton SL, Chestnut RM, Ghajar J, et al. Guidelines for the management of severe traumatic brain injury. XIII. Antiseizure prophylaxis. *J Neurotrauma*. 2007;24(suppl 1):S83–S86.

286. Keret A, Bennett-Back O, Rosenthal G, et al. Posttraumatic epilepsy: long-term follow-up of children with mild traumatic brain injury. *J Neurosurg Pediatr*. 2017;20(1):64–70. https://doi.org/10.3171/2017.2.PEDS16585.

287. Liesemer K, Bratton SL, Zebrack CM, Brockmeyer D, Statler KD. Early post-traumatic seizures in moderate to severe pediatric traumatic brain injury: rates, risk factors, and clinical features. *J Neurotrauma*. 2011;28(5):755–762. https://doi.org/10.1089/neu.2010.1518.

288. Chen JW, Ruff RL, Eavey R, Wasterlain CG. Posttraumatic epilepsy and treatment. *J Rehabil Res Dev*. 2009;46(6):685–696.

289. Verellen RM, Cavazos JE. Post-traumatic epilepsy: an overview. *Therapy.* 2010;7(5):527–531. https://doi.org/10.2217/THY.10.57.

290. Chang BS, Lowenstein DH, Quality Standards Subcommittee of the American Academy of Neurology. Practice parameter: antiepileptic drug prophylaxis in severe traumatic brain injury: report of the Quality Standards Subcommittee of the American Academy of Neurology. *Neurology.* 2003;60(1):10–16. https://doi.org/10.1212/01.WNL.0000031432.05543.14.

291. Nita DA, Hahn CD. Levetiracetam for pediatric posttraumatic seizure prophylaxis. *Pediatr Neurol Briefs.* 2016;30(3):18. https://doi.org/10.15844/pedneurbriefs-30-3-1.

292. Yang Y, Zheng F, Xu X, Wang X. Levetiracetam versus Phenytoin for seizure prophylaxis following traumatic brain injury: a systematic review and meta-analysis. *CNS Drugs.* 2016;30(8):677–688. https://doi.org/10.1007/s40263-016-0365-0.

293. Bakker K, Catroppa C, Anderson V. Olfactory dysfunction in pediatric traumatic brain injury: a systematic review. *J Neurotrauma.* 2014;31(4):308–314. https://doi.org/10.1089/neu.2013.3045.

294. Bakker K, Catroppa C, Anderson V. Recovery of olfactory function following pediatric traumatic brain injury: a longitudinal follow-up. *J Neurotrauma.* 2016;33(8):777–783. https://doi.org/10.1089/neu.2015.4075.

295. Clayton E, Kinley-Cooper SK, Weber RA, Adkins DL. Brain stimulation: neuromodulation as a potential treatment for motor recovery following traumatic brain injury. *Brain Res.* 2016;1640(Pt A):130–138. https://doi.org/10.1016/j.brainres.2016.01.056.

296. Rossi S, Hallett M, Rossini PM, Pascual-Leone A, The Safety of TMS Consensus Group. Safety, ethical considerations, and application guidelines for the use of transcranial magnetic stimulation in clinical practice and research. *Clin Neurophysiol.* 2009;120(12):2008–2039. https://doi.org/10.1016/j.clinph.2009.08.016.

297. Krishnan C, Santos L, Peterson MD, Ehingera M. Safety of noninvasive brain stimulation in children and adolescents. *Brain Stimul.* 2015;8(1):76–87. https://doi.org/10.1016/j.brs.2014.10.012.

298. Rubio B, Boes AD, Laganiere S, Rotenberg A, Jeurissen D, Pascual-Leone A. Noninvasive brain stimulation in pediatric ADHD: a review. *J Child Neurol.* 2016;31(6):784–796. https://doi.org/10.1177/0883073815615672.

299. Frye RE, Rotenberg A, Ousley M, Pascual-Leone A. Transcranial magnetic stimulation in child neurology: current and future directions. *J Child Neurol.* 2008;23(1):79–96. https://doi.org/10.1177/0883073807307972.

300. Chung MG, Lo WD. Noninvasive brain stimulation: the potential for use in the rehabilitation of pediatric acquired brain injury. *Arch Phys Med Rehabil.* 2015;96(4 suppl):S129–S137. https://doi.org/10.1016/j.apmr.2014.10.013.

301. Lu H, Kobilo T, Robertson C, Tong S, Celnik P, Pelleda G. Transcranial magnetic stimulation facilitates neurorehabilitation after pediatric traumatic brain injury. *Sci Rep.* 2015;5:14769. https://doi.org/10.1038/srep14769.

302. Dhaliwal SK, Meek BP, Modirrousta MM. Non-invasive brain stimulation for the treatment of symptoms following traumatic brain injury. *Front Psychiatr.* 2015;6:119. https://doi.org/10.3389/fpsyt.2015.00119.

303. Catroppa C, Anderson V. Planning, problem-solving and organizational abilities in children following traumatic brain injury: intervention techniques. *Pediatr Rehabil.* 2006;9(2):89–97.

304. Haley, et al. Pediatric rehabilitation and recovery of children with traumatic injuries. *Pediatr Phys Ther.* 1992;4(1):24–30.

305. Dumas HM, et al. Functional recovery in pediatric traumatic brain injury during inpatient rehabilitation. *Am J Phys Med Rehabil.* 2002;81(9):661–669.

306. Prasad MR, Swank PR, Ewing-Cobbs L. Long-term school outcomes of children and adolescents with traumatic brain injury. *J Head Trauma Rehabil.* 2017;32(1):E24–E32. https://doi.org/10.1097/HTR.0000000000000218.

307. Taylor HG, et al. Influences on first-year recovery from traumatic brain injury in children. *Neuropsychology.* 1999;13(1):76–89.

308. Ryan NP, et al. Longitudinal outcome and recovery of social problems after pediatric traumatic brain injury (TBI): contribution of brain insult and family environment. *Int J Dev Neurosci.* 2016;49:23–30. https://doi.org/10.1016/j.ijdevneu.2015.12.004.

309. Popernack ML, Gray N, Reuter-Rice K. Moderate-to-severe traumatic brain injury in children: complications and rehabilitation strategies. *J Pediatr Health Care.* 2015;29(3):e1–e7. https://doi.org/10.1016/j.pedhc.2014.09.003.

310. Morgan AT. Dysphagia in childhood traumatic brain injury: a reflection on the evidence and its implications for practice. *Dev Neurorehabil.* 2010;13(3):192–203. https://doi.org/10.3109/17518420903289535.

311. Morgan A, Ward E, Murdoch B, Kennedy B, Murison R. Incidence, characteristics, and predictive factors for dysphagia after pediatric traumatic brain injury. *J Head Trauma Rehabil.* 2003;18(3):239–251.

312. Morsa M, et al. Factors influencing the transition from pediatric to adult care: a scoping review of the literature to conceptualize a relevant education program. *Patient Educ Couns.* 2017; pii: S0738-3991(17)30306-3. https://doi.org/10.1016/j.pec.2017.05.024.

313. Suskauer SJ, Slomine BS, Inscore AB, Lewelt AJ, Kirk JW, Salorio CF. Injury severity variables as predictors of WeeFIM scores in pediatric TBI: time to follow commands is best. *J Pediatr Rehabil Med.* 2009;2(4):297–307.

314. Beers SR, et al. Validity of a pediatric version of the Glasgow outcome scale-extended. *J Neurotrauma.* 2012;29(6):1126–1139. https://doi.org/10.1089/neu.2011.2272.

315. Briggs R, Birse J, Tate R, Brookes N, Epps A, Lah S. Natural sequence of recovery from child post-traumatic amnesia: a retrospective cohort study. *Child Neuropsychol.* 2016;22(6):666–678. https://doi.org/10.1080/09297049.2015.1038988.

316. Iverson GL, Iverson AM, Barton EA. The children's orientation and amnesia test: educational status is a moderator variable in tracking recovery from TBI. *Brain Inj.* 1994;8(8):685–688.

317. Davis KC, Slomine BS, Salorio CF, Suskauer SJ. Time to follow commands and duration of post-traumatic amnesia predict GOS-E Peds scores 1–2 years after TBI in children requiring inpatient rehabilitation. *J Head Trauma Rehabil.* 2016;31(2):E39–E47. https://doi.org/10.1097/HTR.0000000000000159.

318. Ziviani J, Ottenbacher KJ, Shephard K, Foreman S, Astbury W, Ireland P. Concurrent validity of the functional independence measure for children (WeeFIM) and the pediatric evaluation of disabilities inventory in children with developmental disabilities and acquired brain injuries. *Phys Occup Ther Pediatr.* 2001;21(2–3):91–101.

319. Rice SA, Blackman JA, Braun S, Linn RT, Granger CV, Wagner DP. Rehabilitation of children with traumatic brain injury: descriptive analysis of a nationwide sample using the WeeFIM. *Arch Phys Med Rehabil.* 2005;86(4):834–836.

320. Williams KS, Young DK, Burke GAA, Fountain DM. Comparing the WeeFIM and PEDI in neurorehabilitation for children with acquired brain injury: a systematic review. *Dev Neurorehabil.* 2017:1–9. https://doi.org/10.1080/17518423.2017.1289419.

321. Dumas HM, Fragala-Pinkham MA, Haley SM, et al. Item bank development for a revised pediatric evaluation of disability inventory (PEDI). *Phys Occup Ther Pediatr.* 2010;30(3):168–184. https://doi.org/10.3109/01942631003640493.

322. Catroppa C, et al. Outcome and predictors of functional recovery 5 years following pediatric traumatic brain injury (TBI). *J Pediatr Psychol.* 2008;33(7):707–718. https://doi.org/10.1093/jpepsy/jsn006.

323. Wechsler B, et al. Functional status after childhood traumatic brain injury. *J Trauma.* 2005;58(5):940–949. Discussion 950.

324. Babikian T, Asarnow R. Neurocognitive outcomes and recovery after pediatric TBI: meta-analytic review of the literature. *Neuropsychology.* 2009;23(3):283–296. https://doi.org/10.1037/a0015268.

325. Fay TB, Yeates KO, Wade SL, Drotar D, Stancin T, Taylor HG. Predicting longitudinal patterns of functional deficits in children with traumatic brain injury. *Neuropsychology.* 2009;23(3):271–282. https://doi.org/10.1037/a0014936.

326. Haider AH, et al. Black children experience worse clinical and functional outcomes after traumatic brain injury: an analysis of the National Pediatric Trauma Registry. *J Trauma.* 2007;62(5):1259–1262. Discussion 1262–1263.

327. Jimenez N, Osorio M, Ramos JL, Apkon S, Ebel BE, Rivara FP. Functional independence after inpatient rehabilitation for traumatic brain injury among minority children and adolescents. *Arch Phys Med Rehabil.* 2015;96(7):1255–1261. https://doi.org/10.1016/j.apmr.2015.02.019.

328. Hislop J, et al. Views of young people with chronic conditions on transition from pediatric to adult health services. *J Adolesc Health.* 2016;59(3):345–353. https://doi.org/10.1016/j.jadohealth.2016.04.004.

329. Lindsay S, et al. Gender and transition from pediatric to adult health care among youth with acquired brain injury: experiences in a transition model. *Arch Phys Med Rehabil.* 2016;97(suppl 2):S33–S39. https://doi.org/10.1016/j.apmr.2014.04.032.

CHAPTER 8

Geriatric Traumatic Brain Injury

WILLIAM ROBBINS, MD • DAVID X. CIFU, MD

INTRODUCTION

As the population ages, the number of older adults (65 years and older) who sustain a traumatic brain injury (TBI), who survive the injury, who are hospitalized, and who require rehabilitation care will increase, representing a significant opportunity for the field of brain injury medicine. Importantly, TBI in older adults typically results in a high morbidity, need for longer rehabilitation (either skilled nursing facility [SNF] or inpatient rehabilitation facility [IRF]) care, and poorer outcomes when compared with younger individuals.[1-3]

EPIDEMIOLOGY

The incidence of TBI in older adults has doubled in the past 20 years, and that increase is greatest for individuals aged 83–90 years.[1] Adults 75 years and older have the highest rates of TBI-related hospitalization and death. Although individuals 65 years or older represent only 10% of all patients with TBI, they account for 50% of TBI-related deaths.[2] In these elders, TBI is responsible for more than 80,000 emergency department visits each year, and three-quarters of these visits result in hospitalization. In addition, the TBI-related fatality rate among adults over age 65 years is more than twice as high as that among adults 20–44 years of age.[3]

Falls are by far the leading cause of TBI annually in the older population, with the risk of falls increasing with age. Approximately one-third of the adult population over the age of 65 years will fall each year, and this rate increases to one-half of the adult population over the age of 80 years. In 2013 the total cost of fall injuries was 34 billion dollars, with the financial toll for older adult falls expected to increase as the population ages, reaching 67.7 billion dollars by 2020.[4] The risk of falls can be stratified as depicted in Box 8.1. The next most common causes of TBI in older adults are motor vehicle incidents, pedestrian-vehicle incidents, violent trauma, and sports-related injury (including falls from bicycles).[1]

PATHOPHYSIOLOGY OF THE AGING BRAIN AND PATHOLOGY

The volume and weight of the brain declines with age at a rate of around 5% per decade after age 40 years, with the rate of decline increasing with age, particularly over age 70 years.[5,6] Moreover, the dura adheres more tightly to the skull with age. These factors lead to greater shearing forces on the bridging veins when the skull sustains even a low-velocity impact (e.g., ground-level fall), increasing the chance of a subdural hematoma. The prefrontal cortex, hippocampus, cerebellum, and temporal lobe are the most affected, whereas the occipital lobe is the least. Men and women may also differ, with frontal and temporal lobes most affected in men and the hippocampus and parietal lobes in women.[7,8]

In terms of neurotransmitters, dopamine levels decline by around 10% per decade from early adulthood on. Factors resulting in decreased dopamanergic transmission include: dopaminergic pathways between the frontal cortex and the striatum decline with increasing age, levels of dopamine itself decline, synapses and receptors are reduced, and binding to receptors is reduced. Serotonin and brain-derived neurotrophic factor levels also fall with increasing age and may be implicated in the regulation of synaptic plasticity and neurogenesis in the adult brain.[9]

BOX 8.1
Fall Risk Stratification

1. Chronic
Neurologic/musculoskeletal disease, sensory impairment, dementia, medical condition

2. Short term
Episodic hypotension, acute illness, alcohol, medication effects

3. Activity related
Walking, climbing/descending stairs, climbing ladders

4. Environmental
Poor lighting, throw rugs, ill-fitting shoes, pets

Another factor to consider with regard to the aging brain and its cognitive performance is hormonal influence. It is known that sex hormones can affect cognitive processes in adulthood and that changes in sex hormones occur in aging, particularly in women at menopause. Glucose metabolism also declines with age, as well as cerebrovascular efficiency. Other physiologic factors include calcium dysregulation, mitochondrial dysfunction, and the production of reactive oxygen species.[10]

MECHANISM OF INJURY

Falls, which are typically low velocity (e.g., ground level), are more likely to cause focal injuries, such as subdural hematomas and focal contusions, with concomitant focal musculoskeletal injuries. Motor vehicle and pedestrian–motor vehicle injuries are the next most common cause of TBI in the older adult population, and these injuries are more likely high-velocity injury. Subdural hematomas are the most common significant intracranial injury with any etiology of injury in this age group owing to the increased susceptibility of the bridging veins to shearing forces.

Medications affecting hemostasis are a major source of secondary injury risk in older adults. Preinjury antiplatelet agents are associated with three times higher mortality among patients older than 50 years and intracranial bleeding progressed in 10% of elderly patients with TBI on clopidogrel.[11,12] Individuals on antiplatelet therapy are three times more likely to be discharged to long-term inpatient facilities and have 14 times higher mortality rate compared with those not on antiplatelets. Nearly 20% of elders admitted to a level 1 trauma center with head injury were on warfarin, reflecting the importance of impact of warfarin on management and outcome of head injuries.[13] Individuals over 55 years of age on warfarin presenting with minor head injuries were 2.7× more likely to suffer from intracranial hemorrhage.[14]

MILD TRAUMATIC BRAIN INJURY IN OLDER INDIVIDUALS

Mortality is greater among elders across all injury severities, including mild TBI. The diagnosis of mild TBI in older adults can be challenging if the patient's baseline cognitive function is unknown or if it is altered. Family members or caregivers who know the patient may be useful in establishing the injured older adult's baseline cognition. Elders with baseline cognitive deficits (even mild) may appear more altered in the alien emergency room environment. In older patients with mild TBI, there are higher rates of abnormal computed tomography (CT) findings unrelated to the new insult, which may or may not have clinically significant impact.[15] In one report, 14% of older adults seen in the emergency department with mild TBIs had an abnormal CT scan, and 20% of those required neurosurgical intervention.[16]

ACUTE CARE

As with all individuals, in older adults mortality can be reduced with rapid diagnosis and surgical intervention. In one study, overall survival and good recovery following craniotomy in elderly head injury was 30%–77%, with moderate TBI showing a better outcome than severe TBI.[17–21] Volume of traumatic Intra-cranial hemorrhage greater than 50 mL was associated with poor 1-year outcome.[22] Decompressive craniectomy did not show significant benefit in older patients after failing maximal medical treatment. At 1-year post decompressive craniectomy, 80% of elderly patients with severe TBI had poor outcome.[23] Although research suggests that outcomes after TBI are poor in many elderly patients, the option of palliative measures should be discussed with the surrogate decision maker in all cases.

REHABILITATION

Most studies report a poorer response to and outcome with aggressive rehabilitation in elders with TBI.[24,25] It has been found that older patients had significantly slower and more costly progress in rehabilitation and significantly lower rates of discharge home, as compared with a long-term care facility, after TBI.[24]

The immediate goal of rehabilitation is to prevent complications associated with the trauma, such as deep venous thrombosis, atelectasis, pneumonia, and the associated period of immobilization, such as joint contracture, cardiac debility, and skin breakdown; thus rehabilitation strategies should focus on a range of nursing, medical, physical, and cognitive strategies to optimize recovery and functional independence.[25]

Level of Rehabilitation Care

When determining the most appropriate setting for rehabilitation in older adults with TBI, several factors must be taken into consideration: premorbid functioning, premorbid cognitive limitations, the appropriate level of intensity of therapies, the ability of the individual to attend and comprehend, appropriateness of home discharge environment, the likelihood of return

TABLE 8.1 Funding Options for Rehabilitation Services								
	Acute Care Services	Acute Inpatient Rehabilitation	Subacute Care	SNF	Outpatient	Home Health Services	Day Rehabilitation	Day Care Services
Medicare	x	x	x	x	x	x		
Medicaid	x	x		x	x	x		Partial
Private	x	Some	x	Some	x	x	x	

SNF, skilled nursing facility.

to a community residential setting, the level of ongoing medical care needed, and available funding. Individuals who are functioning well below the previous baseline, can tolerate three or more hours of therapy daily, and have the appropriate supports to be discharged to the community are good candidates for an IRF admission. Individuals who cannot tolerate three hours of therapy daily or are unlikely to return to a residential community environment would best benefit from SNF-based rehabilitation care (i.e., require some skilled therapy services at least 5 days/week). If the patient does not require the medical and nursing care available in an IRF or SNF, is unable to tolerate transport several times weekly to a rehabilitation center, but is likely to make functional progress with rehabilitation and has a strong support system, then home health rehabilitation services are appropriate. In patients who are functioning at a level that does not allow return home but cannot tolerate or benefit from any intensity of therapy services and those requiring a more acute level of medical care, such as ongoing ventilator assistance or ongoing cardiac or pulmonary monitoring, a long-term acute care facility with less than five times a week therapy is an appropriate option. In addition, where available, age-appropriate residential programs for individuals with cognitive and/or behavioral dysfunction (e.g., Alzheimer Center) may be appropriate. Although many of these facilities are designed for older adults with chronic cognitive deficits (e.g., dementia), they provide a controlled and appropriately enriched environment, specially trained staff, access to rehabilitation therapies, and a focus on the interplay between medical issues and cognitive difficulties that would also benefit individuals with potentially transient limitations (e.g., TBI). Periodic reassessment of an elder's progress should be made to reassess appropriateness of therapy setting and intensity. Evaluation of funding sources should be done before patient admission at any level of rehabilitation care. Reimbursement for each level of care is outlined in Table 8.1.[26]

Behavior and Cognition

Dementia affects nearly 10% of community-dwelling adults over 65 years, and that percentage increases with advancing age.[27] TBI is one of the many etiologies of delirium and in some cases dementia. A 9-year, population-based study of elderly patients showed fall-related TBI predicts earlier onset of dementia.[28] It is important to ascertain premorbid cognitive function and mental capacity when predicting outcomes.

Hypoarousal and hypoattention are very common after TBI, especially in older adults. First-line treatments include reestablishing a normal sleep-wake cycle with appropriate sleep hygiene, minimizing sedative medications, and limiting excess external stimuli in the surrounding environment. Careful attention should be paid to sundowning in this population. Short-acting methylphenidate can be used in individuals without advanced coronary artery disease, and the results can be seen within several days. Carbidopa-levadopa may be used in individuals presenting with parkinsonian features, with onset within several weeks.

Depression is very common after TBI, with even higher rates in the elderly population.[29] When cognitive impairment is prevalent after TBI, especially in the elderly, it is commonly confused with the diminished ability for thinking and concentration seen in major depression. Therefore timely recognition and treatment of the depression is important to ensure the best possible outcomes. In one imaging study, using magnetic resonance imaging, findings suggested the possible role of frontotemporal lobe and basal ganglia pathology in depression after TBI.[30]

Special Senses
Hearing
Normal aging is associated with decline in auditory function. More than 90% of older persons with hearing loss have age-related sensorineural hearing loss, which is a gradual, symmetric loss of hearing

(predominantly of high frequencies) that is worse in noisy environments.[31] Hearing aids may not be readily available and are difficult to adjust in patients with cognitive and language deficits but should be reintroduced as soon as possible. It is important to limit excess background noise, engage the individual directly with eye contact, and, when necessary, use an alternative form of communication.

Vision

Vision declines with age, and age-related changes include decreased acuity and refractive power, increased intraocular pressure, and changes to the lens and cornea. Most older individuals wear some type of corrective lenses for near and distant vision. Because corrective lenses are often lost or damaged during the traumatic event and subsequent hospitalization, it is important to evaluate vision and replace lenses as soon as possible. Restarting glaucoma medication is important in this population.

Smell and taste

The olfactory nerve is the most common cranial nerve affected after TBI. Anosmia also affects taste and can lead to decreased appetite, which is an important factor in achieving adequate nutrition. Anosmia also can affect safety, as one may not be able to detect the smell of something burning or the odor of rotten food.

Medications

More than 90% of the patient population over the age of 65 years takes at least one prescription medication daily, most take two or more.[32] Moreover, in the acute care setting many medications may be added, which are no longer needed in the rehabilitation settings. A thorough medication review, based on the patient's home medication profile, should be performed on admission to the rehabilitation settings. Special consideration should be taken into maximizing cardiopulmonary function while minimizing polypharmacy to reduce fall risk. Common medications that are often used in older adults but may limit cognitive functioning or recovery include β-blockers, certain H_2 blockers, tricyclic antidepressants, benzodiazepine, sleep agents, antiemetics, and other centrally acting medications (Box 8.2).

Bowel and Bladder Continence

Maintaining bowel and bladder continence is important to both avoid disruption of the therapeutic day and optimize quality of life. Normal aging affects the bladder in many ways; older individuals with TBI are at an even greater risk for incontinence because of the inability to sense bladder fullness and suppression of

---

BOX 8.2
Common Medications That Can Impair Cognition in the Elderly

β-Blockers
Tricyclic antidepressants
Benzodiazepines anxiolytics
Sleep agents
Antiemetics
Certain H_2 blockers

---

the pontine micturition center. It is common for older individuals with a history of incontinence to limit liquid intake, so maintaining adequate hydration is paramount. Incontinence also increases the risk of skin breakdown and pressure ulcers. Older individuals are at higher risk for skin breakdown owing to immobility, decreased adipose tissue, and decreased skin turgor. It is important to perform frequent skin checks, maintain proper positioning in bed and in the wheelchair, and provide continuous education and support in regards to pressure relief.

PAIN

Acute pain from the trauma can be nociceptive, neuropathic, or visceral in nature. Older individuals have a higher likelihood of having a preexisting pain management condition. Proper analgesia should be achieved so the patient can fully participate in therapies while limiting the sedative and cognitive dulling side effects that are associated with many classes of pain medications. Also, the exploration of nonpharmaceutical modalities is paramount in this population to avoid polypharmacy.

ORTHOSTASIS

Orthostatic hypotension is common after trauma secondary to prolonged bed rest. In addition, older adults are more likely to have preexisting hypertension and cardiovascular disease. When posttraumatic hypertension is also present, additional blood pressure–lowering agents are often added during the acute care phase of recovery when the patient is more immobile. These factors increase the likelihood of orthostatic hypotension in this population. In addition to a thorough medication review, postural education, abdominal binders, and thromboembolic disease hose can be used. When nonpharmacologic intervention is inadequate, medications such as midodrine and Florinef may be used.

HYDROCEPHALUS

The elderly population is already at higher risk for developing hydrocephalus. Alterations in gait, urinary problems, and confusion may be attributed to the TBI itself, so there needs to be a high level of suspicion on this population.[33] A head CT may reveal enlarged ventricles. In the setting of a nonrevealing head CT, a bedside diagnostic lumbar puncture can be done if clinical suspicion is still high.

ETHICAL CONSIDERATIONS

Elder abuse is not uncommon, especially among those individuals with poor social support. Not only physical abuse but also emotional (e.g., neglect), financial, and emotional abuse are increasing.[34] Ongoing family education and evaluation of a patient's social support is fundamental throughout the rehabilitation process. In the event that the patient does not have capacity for medical and/or financial decision making, it is important to educate the family and provide guidance in appointment of a qualified decision maker who has the patient's best interest in mind.

AFTERCARE

Before discharge, proximity and quality of their support structure should be evaluated, as well as providing a thorough home evaluation to minimize fall risk and subsequent injury. Elder abuse is not uncommon in older adults with either preexisting or new-onset disability.

CONCLUSION

Caring for older adults with TBI presents many challenges and opportunities at all stages of the rehabilitation process. As the elderly population increases, so will the number of older individuals sustaining TBI and requiring rehabilitation services. Preventing TBI in the older adult by addressing modifiable risk factors, particularly fall prevention, is essential. Being able to understand and address the unique physiologic and psychological needs specific to this population is key in individualizing the rehabilitation plan of care therefore optimizing functional outcomes.

REFERENCES

1. Ramanathan DM, McWilliams N, Schatz P, et al. Epidemiological shifts in elderly TBI: 18-year trends in Pennsylvania. *J Neurotrauma*. 2011;29.
2. US Centers for Disease Control and Prevention. Incidence rates of hospitalization related to traumatic brain injury—12 states, 2002. *Morb Mortal Wkly Rep*. 2006;55(8):201–204.
3. Thompson HJ, McCormick WC, Kagan SH. Traumatic brain injury in older adults: epidemiology, outcomes, and future implications. *J Am Geriatr Soc*. 2008;54(10):1590–1595. https://www.ncbi.nlm.nih.gov/pmc/articles/PMC2367127/.
4. *Falls Prevention Facts*. NCOA; 2017. https://www.ncoa.org/news/resources-for-reporters/get-the-facts/falls-prevention-facts/.
5. Svennerholm L, Boström K, Jungbjer B. Changes in weight and compositions of major membrane components of human brain during the span of adult human life of Swedes. *Acta Neuropathol*. 1997;94:345–352.
6. Scahill R, Frost C, Jenkins R, et al. A longitudinal study of brain volume changes in normal ageing using serial registered magnetic resonance imaging. *Arch Neurol*. 2003;60:989–994.
7. Murphy D, DeCarli C, McIntosh A, et al. Sex differences in human brain morphometry and metabolism: an in vivo quantitative magnetic resonance imaging and positron emission tomography study on the effect of ageing. *Arch Gen Psychiatr*. 1996;53:585–594.
8. Compton J, Van Amelsoort T, Murphy D. HRT and its effect on normal ageing of the brain and dementia. *Br J Clin Pharmacol*. 2001;52:647–653.
9. Mattson M, Maudsley S, Martin B. BDNF and 5-HT: a dynamic duo in age-related neuronal plasticity and neurodegenerative disorders. *Trends Neurosci*. 2004;27:589–594.
10. Peters R. Ageing and the brain. *Postgrad Med J*. 2006;82:84–88. https://doi.org/10.1136/pgmj.2005.036665.
11. Ohm C, Mina A, Howells G, et al. Effects of antiplatelet agents on outcomes for elderly patients with traumatic intracranial hemorrhage. *J Trauma Inj Infect Crit Care*. 2005;58(3):518–522.
12. Wong DK, Lurie F, Wong LL. The effects of clopidogrel on elderly traumatic brain injured patients. *J Trauma*. 2008;65(6):1303–1308.
13. Lavoie A, Ratte S, Clas D, et al. Preinjury warfarin use among elderly patients with closed head injuries in a trauma center. *J Trauma Inj Infect Crit Care*. 2004;56(4):802–807.
14. Claudia C, Claudia R, Agostino O, et al. Minor head injury in warfarinized patients: indicators of risk for intracranial hemorrhage. *J Trauma*. 2011;70(4):906–909.
15. *Traumatic Brain Injuries in Older Adults*. https://www.aliem.com/2016/02/traumatic-brain-injuries-older-adults.
16. MRC C, Perel P, Arango M, et al. Predicting outcome after traumatic brain injury: practical prognostic models based on large cohort of international patients. *BMJ*. 2008;336(7641):425–429.
17. Munro PT, Smith RD, Parke TR. Effect of patients' age on management of acute intracranial haematoma: prospective national study. *BMJ*. 2002;325(7371):1001.
18. Mitra B, Cameron PA, Gabbe BJ, et al. Management and hospital outcome of the severely head injured elderly patient. *ANZ J Surg*. 2008;78(7):588–592.
19. Ushewokunze S, Nannapaneni R, Gregson BA, et al. Elderly patients with severe head injury in coma from the outset–has anything changed? *Br J Neurosurg*. 2004;18(6):604–607.

20. Wong GK, Graham CA, Ng E, et al. Neurological outcomes of neurosurgical operations for multiple trauma elderly patients in Hong Kong. *J Emerg Trauma Shock.* 2011;4(3):346–350.

21. Mohindra S, Mukherjee KK, Gupta R, et al. Continuation of poor surgical outcome after elderly brain injury. *Surg Neurol.* 2008;69(5):474–477.

22. Wong GK, Tang BY, Yeung JH, et al. Traumatic intracerebral haemorrhage: is the CT pattern related to outcome? *Br J Neurosurg.* 2009;23(6):601–605.

23. Pompucci A, De Bonis P, Pettorini B, et al. Decompressive craniectomy for traumatic brain injury: patient age and outcome. *J Neurotrauma.* 2007;24(7):1182–1188.

24. LeBlanc J, de Guise E, Gosselin N, Feyz M. Comparison of functional outcome following acute care in young, middle-aged and elderly patients with traumatic brain injury. *Brain Inj.* 2006;20(8):779–790.

25. Frankel JE, Marwitz JH, Cifu DX, Kreutzer JS, Englander J, Rosenthal M. A follow-up study of older adults with traumatic brain injury: taking into account decreasing length of stay. *Arch Phys Med Rehabil.* 2006;87(1):57–62.

26. Englander J, Cifu D, Tran T. The older adult. In: *Brain Injury Medicine.* New York, NY: Demos; 2007:321.

27. Bavishi S, Cifu D. Management of traumatic brain injury in the older adult. In: *Manual of Traumatic Brain Injury Medicine.* New York, NY: Demos; 2011:438.

28. Luukinen H, Viramo P, Herala M, et al. Fall-related brain injuries and the risk of dementia in elderly people: a population-based study. *Eur J Neurol.* 2005;12(2):86–92.

29. Menzel JC. Depression in the elderly after traumatic brain injury: a systematic review. *Brain Inj.* 2008;22(5):375–380.

30. Rao V, Munro CA, Rosenberg P, et al. Neuroanatomical correlates of depression in post traumatic brain injury: preliminary results of a pilot study. *J Neuropsychiatr Clin Neurosci.* 2010;22(2):231–235.

31. Yueh B, Shapiro N, MacLean CH, Shekelle PG. Screening and management of adult hearing loss in primary care: scientific review. *JAMA.* 2003;289(15):1976–1985.

32. Englander J, Cifu D, Tran T. The older adult. In: *Brain Injury Medicine.* New York, NY: Demos; 2007:320.

33. Lavine J, Flanagan SR. Traumatic brain injury in the elderly. In: *Brain Injury Medicine.* New York, NY: Demos; 2013:425.

34. Eapen B, Jaramillo C, Cifu D. Management of traumatic brain injury in the older adult. In: *Manual of Traumatic Brain Injury: Assessment and Management.* New York, NY: Demos; 2016:529–535.

CHAPTER 9

Anoxic Brain Injury

BILLIE A. SCHULTZ, MD

Prolonged lack or limited oxygen to the brain may result in an anoxic brain injury. This injury is referred in the literature as hypoxic, anoxic, anoxic-ischemic, or hypoxic-ischemic injury. For the purposes of this chapter, the injury is referred to as an anoxic brain injury.

Initially anoxic brain injury was described in 1945, in the setting of nitric oxide poisoning, and anoxic brain injury survivors were described as having decreased judgment, loss of insight, apathy, indifference, restlessness, and deficits of attention and memory.[1] Further characterization of behaviors post anoxic brain injury included "silly and childlike behavior" and "peculiar emotional changes."[2] As science has advanced, explanations of the underlying pathophysiology leading to these neurologic and behavioral changes have improved. Treatment has advanced, and rehabilitation needs have been addressed.

ETIOLOGY

Any event causing insufficient oxygenation to the brain can result in an anoxic brain injury. This can be secondary to an event affecting circulation, including hypotension, cardiac arrhythmias or arrest, and hypovolemia such as with massive blood loss. In addition, respiratory failure limits oxygen delivery to the brain parenchyma. Intrinsic pulmonary disease, suffocation, complications of anesthesia or drug use, drowning or cervical trauma affecting the airway, or impaired delivery of oxygen, such as with carbon monoxide poisoning, are potential causes.

EPIDEMIOLOGY

Most data available refer to anoxic injury in the setting of cardiac arrhythmia or arrest. In the United States, more than 700,000 people experience a myocardial infarction annually; of those only 114,000 die.[3] Sudden cardiac arrest is seen in the setting of myocardial infarction related to coronary artery disease, arrhythmias, and drug overdose. Approximately 85% of cardiac arrests occur outside the hospital.[4] Out of hospital arrests occur at residence, public settings, and nursing homes.[3] Previously, survival was poor for out-of-hospital cardiac arrests, making it a target for practice change.

Much emphasis has been placed on prehospital care for sudden cardiac arrest, including availability of automated external defibrillators (AEDs), training in compression-only cardiopulmonary resuscitation (CPR), emergency and 911 awareness, and first responder training. Recent data show that 26.4% of persons sustaining an out-of-hospital cardiac arrest survive to hospital admission, with 10% surviving till dismissal. This has improved survival to hospital discharge, with estimates showing improvements from 6% to 10% from 2005 to 2012, respectively.[4]

Also noted in the same data was a trend to less neurologic disability, with previous estimates of 6.9% of all persons surviving cardiac arrest having a good or moderate cerebral performance (defined as being independent with activities of daily living [ADLs] and able to work in a competitive or sheltered environment).[5]

PATHOPHYSIOLOGY

The brain is very susceptible to ischemia. This is due to its high metabolic demands needing a continuous supply of circulating blood replenishing oxygen and glucose. Certain areas of the brain are more susceptible. These include the hippocampus (CA1 subfield-Sommer sector), cerebellar Purkinje cells, pyramidal neurons in neocortex 3, 5, and 6, superior brainstem structures, subcortical structures (basal ganglia, thalamus, amygdala), and vascular watershed areas. Watershed areas include the anterior border zone between the anterior (ACA) and middle cerebral arteries (MCA), the posterior border zone between the MCA and posterior cerebral artery (PCA), and the internal border zone between the MCA superficial branches and the deep branches of the MCA/ACA.[6]

As with traumatic brain injury, anoxic injury results in both primary and secondary injuries. The primary injury in the setting of cardiac arrest occurs during the time of pulselessness and initial restoration of spontaneous circulation (defined as the reperfusion injury). The prolonged ischemia secondary to inadequate oxygenation and nutrient delivery results in "toxin accumulation, anoxic depolarization, loss of ion gradients, and disruption of blood brain barrier and glutamate release." During reperfusion, there is free radical formation, nitric oxide toxicity, and further glutamate release, excitotoxicity, reactive hyperemia, calcium shifts, and cerebral edema and microhemorrhages. A phenomenon called the "no-reflow" phenomenon also plays a role whereby despite restoration of blood flow there is still hypoperfusion at the microvascular level, possibly because of the above-mentioned events. Cumulatively, this results in cell death.[7–10] The secondary injury includes any ongoing ischemia, autoregulatory failure, cerebral hypoperfusion, blood-brain barrier breakdown/edema, seizures, oxidative injury, hyperpyrexia, and early care withdrawal.

EXAMINATION AND EVALUATION

Clinical presentation is heterogeneous, varying dependent on the duration of hypoxia, premorbid function, and the area of brain most affected. In severe cases, disordered consciousness is present. In those cases, a brain specialist, either neurology or rehabilitation, is often asked to follow up and assist with prognostication. The initial examination focuses on the brainstem reflexes, presence of generalized myoclonus, and motor responses to noxious stimuli. As this aids in prognostication, often the information gathered is synthesized to counsel families regarding continued care and expectations. Additional elements of an examination include range of motion and muscle tone and skin examination to ensure no secondary complications, such as skin integrity changes or contractures.

In conscious patients, cognitive assessment includes arousal/alertness, attention, processing speed, memory, judgment/reasoning, insight, planning/organization, and problem solving. Affect/behavioral examination assesses for agitation, emotional lability, abulia, depression, or anxiety. Cerebellar/fine motor testing evaluates for choreoathetosis and ataxia. Focal motor and sensory deficits and their effects on function should be evaluated.

Unique clinical sequelae can include:
1. Balint syndrome: oculomotor apraxia, optic ataxia, and simultangnosia due to bilateral parietooccipital damage from posterior watershed ischemia
2. "Man in a Barrel" syndrome: bilateral upper limb paresis with preserved lower limb function from watershed ischemia between the ACA and MCA

3. Paraparesis or tetraparesis from watershed spinal cord ischemia in upper/lower thoracic and lumbar regions
4. Cortical blindness from watershed ischemia near the PCA distribution
5. Akinetic rigid syndrome/parkinsonism
6. Amnestic syndrome from damage to the hippocampi
7. Lance-Adams syndrome otherwise known as chronic posthypoxic myoclonus. It manifests as a significant action myoclonus associated with ataxia.[11]

Further evaluation can include EEG monitoring and somatosensory evoked potentials (SSEPs). Once again, these can help with prognostication. As SSEPs are not affected by drugs, temperature, or acute metabolic derangements that can be seen in the comatose patient, they may play more of a role in prognostication compared with EEG results. Literature is available exploring it's use for prognostication; however, MRI with diffusion-weighted sequences can help determine the extent of the injury, with CT scan being less useful.[12,13] Ongoing interest in a serum Limited biomarker that can help prognostication continues. The most studied are neuron-specific enolase (NSE) and S100, but as a single result they are less helpful for prognostication.[13,14]

PROGNOSIS

During the acute period, providers and family members are interested in outcome, specifically good or bad outcome. In part, this is to allow conversation regarding end of life and organ donation or expected ongoing care needs. There are many studies summarizing the factors associated with a poor outcome, although the definition of poor outcome varies by study (Table 9.1).

Review of the literature shows that, on average 18%–22% of persons survive out-of-hospital ventricular fibrillation cardiac arrest to hospital dismissal,[16–18] although communities with automated electronic defibrillation (AED) devices available to all first responds have increased survivorship.[19]

TREATMENT

To help manage the primary brain injury, high-quality CPR is emphasized in addition to early defibrillation with the goal of return of spontaneous circulation as early as possible, minimizing the time without adequate oxygenation. About 3–4 min of arrest can be enough to cause neuronal changes, and it has been shown that within 10 min of blood flow cessation, the needed nutrients, including glucose, adenosine triphosphate, and phosphocreatine, are nearly depleted.[10] For

TABLE 9.1
Factors Associated With a Poor Outcome

Symptom	Time Frame
Anoxia duration	>8–10 min
Duration of CPR	>30 min
Myoclonic status epilepticus	Day 1
Absent pupillary or corneal reflexes	Days 1–3
Serum NSE >33 µg/L	Days 1–3 for patients with nontherapeutic hypothermia
Absent N20 responses on SSEP bilaterally	Days 1–3
Motor response extensor or none	Day 3 for patients with nontherapeutic hypothermia; possibly longer for therapeutic hypothermia patients
EEG with nonreactive background	
EEG with burst suppression and generalized epileptiform activity	
Loss of gray-white matter differentiation on head CT	
Widespread cortical restricted diffusion on brain MRI	

CPR, cardiopulmonary resuscitation; NSE, neuron specific enolase; SSEP, somatosensory evoked potential.
Data from Fugate JE, Wijdicks EF. Anoxic-ischemic encephalopathy. In: Flemming KD, Jones LK, ed. *Mayo Clinic Neurology Board Review: Clinical Neurology for Initial Certification and MOC.* 3rd ed. New York: Oxford University Press; 2015:35–38; Wijdicks EF, Hijdra A, Young GB, Bassetti CL, Wiebe S. Practice parameter: prediction of outcome in comatose survivors after cardiopulmonary resuscitation (an evidence-based review): report of the Quality Standards Subcommittee of the American Academy of Neurology. *Neurology.* 2006;67(2):203–210. https://doi.org/10.1212/01.wnl.0000227183.21314.cd; Zandbergen EG, Hijdra A, Koelman JH, et al. Prediction of poor outcome within the first 3 days of postanoxic coma. *Neurology.* 2006;66(1):62–68. https://doi.org/10.1212/01.wnl.0000191308.22233.88; Bouwes A, Binnekade JM, Kuiper MA, et al. Prognosis of coma after therapeutic hypothermia: a prospective cohort study. *Ann Neurol.* 2012;71(2):206–212. https://doi.org/10.1002/ana.22632.

this reason, much more emphasis has been placed on the improvement of chest compression rates and quality of compression.[20,21] The availability and use of AED devices has become more widespread and had a positive impact on survival after out-of-hospital cardiac arrest.[22]

The goals of secondary injury management are to maintain cerebral perfusion and oxygenation, seizure detection and treatment, edema management, early coronary revascularization, and to provide therapeutic cooling. Therapeutic cooling inhibits apoptosis and reduces free radical and excitatory neurotransmitter formation. Therapeutic cooling involves cooling patients to 32–34°C and maintaining this for 24 h. It has been shown to reduce mortality and improve neurologic outcomes in adults after cardiac arrest.[23,24]

In addition, other consultative services may be required in the acute setting depending on other systems injuries. There may be a need for dialysis, antiepileptic treatment, alteration or additions to cardiac medications, long-term respiratory support possibly including tracheostomy, and nutritional support. After long-term mechanical ventilation, vocal cord dysfunction can be seen. Also, weight loss,

deconditioning, and possibly critical illness neuropathy or myopathy can be seen depending on the time in a less responsive state. If high-quality CPR was administered, the patient may experience pain due to rib fractures.

REHABILITATION-SPECIFIC TREATMENT
TBI and anoxic brain injury have been compared and were found to be similar at the time of rehabilitation admission and dismissal when functional outcome measures were analyzed, including functional independence measure scores; however, anoxic brain injury trends toward more likely to dismiss to subacute rehabilitation and a shorter length of inpatient rehabilitation facility stay.[25-28] This is hypothesized because of a slower recovery curve. Most studies discuss the significant memory deficits that can persist years after the anoxic event.[25-29] Although patients surviving an anoxic brain injury have a slower recovery when compared with those with TBI, they have been shown to achieve significant gains and should be considered for acute inpatient rehabilitation.[30] There is limited evidence that non-cardiac-mediated anoxic brain injury

is associated with a greater cost and length of stay on acute rehabilitation when compared with cardiac etiology.[31]

Patients have been described as having disorders of consciousness, locked-in syndrome, cognitive deficits, behavioral changes, psychological disorders, movement disorders, spasticity, and changes in vision, balance, and gait. The physiatrist's role may include defining the level of consciousness by using tools such as the JFK Coma Recovery Scale.[32] Rehabilitation specialists also may consider medication trials to improve arousal, attention, agitation, and participation. Patients may have respiratory needs with or without tracheostomy and need for parenteral nutritional support. Family and patient education is necessary after this type of injury. Not only are there potential long-term sequelae from the hypoxic injury but also possible long-term medical complications/needs from the underlying etiology of the hypoxic event. In addition to medical providers, there may be a need for social work and rehabilitation psychology as the patient can experience anxiety related to the fear of a future event or shock for implanted device. This can cause patients to alter their behaviors and avoid physical exertion, which can negatively affect quality of life.

Rehabilitation medical management is individualized to the patient and is similar to that for most acquired brain injury. Spasticity and dystonia commonly occur after anoxic brain injury. A brain rehabilitation specialist is well equipped to manage this through medications, injections, bracing, casting, splinting, stretching, and intrathecal drug delivery systems. The most important element of spasticity management is determining goals of treatment with the patient, family, and care team. Not all spasticity requires treatment, as some patients utilize spasticity for transfers or ambulation. Potential goals of treatment include pain, positioning, functional limiting spasticity, and cosmesis. Initial treatment is typically conservative. Emphasis in the ICU setting on range of motion and positioning decreases future contractures, although no conclusive evidence supports use of this.[33] Systemic medication management can be effective but limited by adverse effects of the medications. Dantrolene works peripherally, whereas the other commonly used medications, baclofen, tizanidine, and diazepam, are centrally acting and more likely to cause sedation. Medical use of cannabis has become more accepted in the past decade for treatment of spasticity. Based on a meta-analysis published in 2015, there are limited studies on this topic with a trend toward improvement in spasticity not reaching statistical significance. The studies analyzed the broader category of spasticity and were mostly limited to multiple sclerosis (MS).[34] Targeted therapy with chemodenervation, either phenol or botulinum toxin, must be individualized to the patient. It can be an excellent choice when targeting specific muscles affected by spasticity or dystonia; however, for widespread spasticity/dystonia affecting all four limbs, the trunk, and cervical musculature, careful consideration needs to be made to muscle selection based on the patient-centric goals established for the treatment of the spasticity. In cases of more diffuse spasticity, intrathecal baclofen (ITB) can be an option. The timing of intrathecal drug delivery can be controversial, with some arguments against early placement. A small study analyzed patients following ITB pump implantation at a mean postinjury placement of 13.9 months. Scores assessing the level of disability were unchanged; however, modified Ashworth scores and pain decreased, whereas gait speed and motor skills improved.[35] A comparison of the use of ITB for spinal versus cortical etiology showed a significant difference in use of chemodenervation for upper extremity spasticity.[36] Dosing also varies among diagnoses that are treated with ITB. Patients with anoxic injury tend to require higher dosing than those with stroke. Also, nonambulators use higher dosing compared with ambulators, possibly because the ambulators use their tone for transfers and mobility.[37]

Myoclonus can be seen during the acute recovery period of anoxic brain injury but may also persist long term. One small study described patients after anoxic brain injury who developed action myoclonus. Persistent myoclonus was the only residual symptom in half the patients followed.[38] Myoclonus negatively affects function, including mobility, communication, and ability to perform ADLs. However, treatment is challenging, as many suggested treatments are sedating. Multiple antiepileptics and benzodiazepines have been used for management. First-line treatment includes clonazepam and valproic acid, with levetiracetam also shown to be beneficial in this setting.[39] One case report also shows success in managing post–anoxic brain injury myoclonus with a small dose of ITB.[40] Other movement disorders, including parkinsonism, dystonia, chorea, tics, athetosis, and tremor, can be seen after anoxic brain injury and can be debilitating. Development of the movement disorders may be delayed, with onset months to years after the initial anoxic insult.[41] The underlying etiology of the movement disorder development is often ascribed to the involvement of the basal ganglia, although other structural involvement includes the neocortex, hippocampus, cerebellum, striatum, substantia nigra, and globus pallidus.[39] As the basal ganglia can be involved, medications acting on the dopaminergic system, levodopa and dopamine agonists, have been used in the treatment. Neurosurgical treatments have been explored with less success, although bilateral thalamic deep brain stimulation is promising.[42]

BRAIN DEATH

Brain death, in the lay literature, is often used to describe any disorder of consciousness whereby the person does not respond to the environment; however, there is a very specific definition of brain death in the medical community. Brain death as defined by the Uniform Determination of Death Act (UDDA) is the "irreversible cessation of all functions of the entire brain, including the brain stem."[43] Typically the neurologist is asked to comment on brain death; however, if the neurologist is unavailable, a brain injury medicine specialist may be asked to comment.

The UDDA did include the caveat that the determination of death must be made with "accepted medical standards." However, this was not clearly defined and variability existed from state to state, with some requiring a second physician to concur, the need for specific physician qualifications, or religious exceptions. To standardize care, guidelines for determining brain death were published by the American Academy of Neurology (AAN) in 1995[44] and emphasized three clinical findings, coma with a known cause, absence of brainstem reflexes, and apnea. Despite publication of guidelines, practices varied depending on the institution.[45] Updated guidelines for the determination of brain death were published by the AAN in 2010 (Table 9.2).[46]

ETHICS AND ANOXIC BRAIN INJURY

Brain death is well defined as are the management recommendations. More controversy exists in patients with disorders of consciousness who are unable to express their wishes. A sequential approach is recommended.[47] First, the prognosis should be definitely established followed by a decision in the level of care. If there are differences between the decision maker's requests and the physician recommendations, the facilities ethics or legal team may get involved. The case of Terri Schiavo is an extreme example outlining the challenges of these decisions. The case demonstrates the concept of persistent vegetative state and the certainty that there will be no meaningful recovery. Despite the initial ruling in the case, ordering cessation of feeds in 2001, further hearings and legislature delayed final removal of the feeding

---

TABLE 9.2
Diagnosis of Brain Death

Prerequisites
Coma, irreversible with cause known
Neuroimaging explains coma
CNS depressant drug effect absent (if indicated toxicology screen; if barbiturates given, serum level < 10 μg/mL)
No evidence of residual paralytics (electrical stimulation of paralytics used)
Absence of severe acid-base, electrolyte, endocrine abnormality
Normothermia or mild hypothermia (core temperature >36°C)
Systolic blood pressure ≥100 mm Hg
No spontaneous respirations
Examination
Pupils nonreactive to bright light
Corneal reflex absent
Oculocephalic reflex absent (tested only if C-spine integrity ensured)
No facial movement to noxious stimuli at supraorbital nerve, temporomandibular joint
Gag reflex absent
Cough reflex absent to tracheal suctioning
Absence of motor response to noxious stimuli in all four limbs (spinally medicated reflexes are permissible)

Continued

TABLE 9.2 Diagnosis of Brain Death—cont'd
Apnea testing
Patient is hemodynamically stable
Ventilator adjusted to provide normocarbia ($PaCo_2$ 34–45 mm Hg)
Patient preoxygenated with 100% FiO_2 for >10 min to PaO_2 >200 mm Hg
Patient well-oxygenated with a PEEP of 5 cm of water
Provide oxygen via a suction catheter to the level of the carina at 6 L/min or attach T-piece with CPAP at 10 cm H_2O
Disconnect ventilator
Spontaneous respirations absent
Arterial blood gas drawn at 8–10 min, patient reconnected to ventilator
PCO_2 ≥60 mm Hg or 20 mm Hg rise from normal baseline value
OR:
Apnea test aborted
Ancillary testing (only one needs to be performed; to be ordered only if clinical examination cannot be fully performed owing to patient factors, or if apnea testing inconclusive or aborted)
Cerebral angiogram
99mTc-*HMPAO SPECT*
EEG
TCD examination
Time of death
Name of physician and signature

99mTc-HMPAO SPECT, 99mTc-hexamethylpropyleneamineoxime single-photon emission computed tomography; *CPAP*, continuous positive airway pressure; *PEEP*; *TCD*, transcranial Doppler.

tube until 2005.[48] The complexities of this case, played out for the media, illustrate the daily challenges in care and counseling for this patient population.

CONCLUSIONS

Anoxic brain injury is a highly heterogeneous process, in the underlying pathology, etiology, clinical manifestation, and rehabilitation needs. Care needs to be taken to individualize recommendations and treatment. Rehabilitation specialists are essential in the care of these patients, providing support, education, and functional management.

REFERENCES

1. Fletcher D. Personality disintegration incident to anoxia: observations with nitrous oxide anesthesia. *J Nerv Ment Dis*. 1945;102:392–403.
2. Steegmann AT. Clinical aspects of cerebral anoxia in man. *Neurology*. 1951;1(4):261–274.
3. Benjamin EJ, Blaha MJ, Chiuve SE, et al. Heart disease and stroke statistics-2017 update: a report from the American Heart Association. *Circulation*. 2017;135(10):e146–e603. https://doi.org/10.1161/cir.0000000000000485.
4. Chan PS, McNally B, Tang F, Kellermann A. Recent trends in survival from out-of-hospital cardiac arrest in the United States. *Circulation*. 2014;130(21):1876–1882. https://doi.org/10.1161/circulationaha.114.009711.
5. McNally B, Robb R, Mehta M, et al. Out-of-hospital cardiac arrest surveillance – cardiac arrest registry to enhance survival (CARES), United States, October 1, 2005–December 31, 2010. *Morb Mortal Wkly Rep*. 2011;60(8):1–19. Surveillance Summaries (Washington, DC: 2002).
6. Busl KM, Greer DM. Hypoxic-ischemic brain injury: pathophysiology, neuropathology and mechanisms. *NeuroRehabilitation*. 2010;26(1):5–13. https://doi.org/10.3233/nre-2010-0531.
7. Caine D, Watson JD. Neuropsychological and neuropathological sequelae of cerebral anoxia: a critical review. *J Int Neuropsychol Soc*. 2000;6(1):86–99.
8. Elmer J, Callaway CW. The brain after cardiac arrest. *Semin Neurol*. 2017;37(1):19–24. https://doi.org/10.1055/s-0036-1597833.

9. Sekhon MS, Ainslie PN, Griesdale DE. Clinical pathophysiology of hypoxic ischemic brain injury after cardiac arrest: a "two-hit" model. *Crit Care (Lond, Engl)*. 2017;21(1):90. https://doi.org/10.1186/s13054-017-1670-9.

10. Fugate JE, Wijdicks EF. Anoxic-ischmic encephalopathy. In: Flemming KD, Jones LK, eds. *Mayo Clinic Neurology Board Review: Clinical Neurology for Initial Certification and MOC*. 3rd ed. New York: Oxford University Press; 2015: 35–38.

11. Lance JW, Adams RD. The syndrome of intention or action myoclonus as a sequel to hypoxic encephalopathy. *Brain*. 1963;86:111–136.

12. Greer D, Scripko P, Bartscher J, et al. Clinical MRI interpretation for outcome prediction in cardiac arrest. *Neurocrit Care*. 2012;17(2):240–244. https://doi.org/10.1007/s12028-012-9716-y.

13. Wijdicks EF, Hijdra A, Young GB, Bassetti CL, Wiebe S. Practice parameter: prediction of outcome in comatose survivors after cardiopulmonary resuscitation (an evidence-based review): report of the Quality Standards Subcommittee of the American Academy of Neurology. *Neurology*. 2006;67(2):203–210. https://doi.org/10.1212/01.wnl.0000227183.21314.cd.

14. Zandbergen EG, Hijdra A, Koelman JH, et al. Prediction of poor outcome within the first 3 days of postanoxic coma. *Neurology*. 2006;66(1):62–68. https://doi.org/10.1212/01.wnl.0000191308.22233.88.

15. Bouwes A, Binnekade JM, Kuiper MA, et al. Prognosis of coma after therapeutic hypothermia: a prospective cohort study. *Ann Neurol*. 2012;71(2):206–212. https://doi.org/10.1002/ana.22632.

16. Atwood C, Eisenberg MS, Herlitz J, Rea TD. Incidence of EMS-treated out-of-hospital cardiac arrest in Europe. *Resuscitation*. 2005;67(1):75–80. https://doi.org/10.1016/j.resuscitation.2005.03.021.

17. Nichol G, Thomas E, Callaway CW, et al. Regional variation in out-of-hospital cardiac arrest incidence and outcome. *JAMA*. 2008;300(12):1423–1431. https://doi.org/10.1001/jama.300.12.1423.

18. Rea TD, Eisenberg MS, Sinibaldi G, White RD. Incidence of EMS-treated out-of-hospital cardiac arrest in the United States. *Resuscitation*. 2004;63(1):17–24. https://doi.org/10.1016/j.resuscitation.2004.03.025.

19. Bunch TJ, White RD, Smith GE, et al. Long-term subjective memory function in ventricular fibrillation out-of-hospital cardiac arrest survivors resuscitated by early defibrillation. *Resuscitation*. 2004;60(2):189–195. https://doi.org/10.1016/j.resuscitation.2003.09.010.

20. Cheskes S, Schmicker RH, Rea T, et al. The association between AHA CPR quality guideline compliance and clinical outcomes from out-of-hospital cardiac arrest. *Resuscitation*. 2017;116:39–45. https://doi.org/10.1016/j.resuscitation.2017.05.003.

21. Meaney PA, Bobrow BJ, Mancini ME, et al. Cardiopulmonary resuscitation quality: [corrected] improving cardiac resuscitation outcomes both inside and outside the hospital: a consensus statement from the American Heart Association. *Circulation*. 2013;128(4):417–435. https://doi.org/10.1161/CIR.0b013e31829d8654.

22. White RD, Asplin BR, Bugliosi TF, Hankins DG. High discharge survival rate after out-of-hospital ventricular fibrillation with rapid defibrillation by police and paramedics. *Ann Emerg Med*. 1996;28(5):480–485.

23. Mild therapeutic hypothermia to improve the neurologic outcome after cardiac arrest. *New Engl J Med*. 2002;346(8): 549–556. https://doi.org/10.1056/NEJMoa012689.

24. Arrich J, Holzer M, Havel C, Mullner M, Herkner H. Hypothermia for neuroprotection in adults after cardiopulmonary resuscitation. *Cochrane Database Syst Rev*. 2016;2:Cd004128. https://doi.org/10.1002/14651858.CD004128.pub4.

25. Cullen NK, Crescini C, Bayley MT. Rehabilitation outcomes after anoxic brain injury: a case-controlled comparison with traumatic brain injury. *PM R*. 2009;1(12):1069–1076. https://doi.org/10.1016/j.pmrj.2009.09.013.

26. Cullen NK, Weisz K. Cognitive correlates with functional outcomes after anoxic brain injury: a case-controlled comparison with traumatic brain injury. *Brain Inj*. 2011;25(1):35–43. https://doi.org/10.3109/02699052.2010.531691.

27. Fitzgerald A, Aditya H, Prior A, McNeill E, Pentland B. Anoxic brain injury: clinical patterns and functional outcomes. A study of 93 cases. *Brain Inj*. 2010;24(11):1311–1323. https://doi.org/10.3109/02699052.2010.506864.

28. Shah MK, Al-Adawi S, Dorvlo AS, Burke DT. Functional outcomes following anoxic brain injury: a comparison with traumatic brain injury. *Brain Inj*. 2004;18(2):111–117. https://doi.org/10.1080/0269905031000149551.

29. Mateen FJ, Josephs KA, Trenerry MR, et al. Long-term cognitive outcomes following out-of-hospital cardiac arrest: a population-based study. *Neurology*. 2011;77(15):1438–1445. https://doi.org/10.1212/WNL.0b013e318232ab33.

30. Shah MK, Carayannopoulos AG, Burke DT, Al-Adawi S. A comparison of functional outcomes in hypoxia and traumatic brain injury: a pilot study. *J Neurol Sci*. 2007;260(1–2):95–99. https://doi.org/10.1016/j.jns.2007.04.012.

31. Burke DT, Shah MK, Dorvlo AS, Al-Adawi S. Rehabilitation outcomes of cardiac and non-cardiac anoxic brain injury: a single institution experience. *Brain Inj*. 2005;19(9):675–680. https://doi.org/10.1080/02699050400024953.

32. Sawyer K, Callaway C, Wagner A. Life after death: surviving cardiac arrest—an overview of epidemiology, best acute care practices, and considerations for rehabilitation care. *Curr Phys Med Rehabil Rep*. 2017;5(1): 30–39.

33. Harvey LA, Katalinic OM, Herbert RD, Moseley AM, Lannin NA, Schurr K. Stretch for the treatment and prevention of contractures. *Cochrane Database Syst Rev*. 2017;1:Cd007455. https://doi.org/10.1002/14651858.CD007455.pub3.

34. Whiting PF, Wolff RF, Deshpande S, et al. Cannabinoids for medical use: a systematic review and meta-analysis. *JAMA*. 2015;313(24):2456–2473. https://doi.org/10.1001/jama.2015.6358.

35. Francisco GE, Hu MM, Boake C, Ivanhoe CB. Efficacy of early use of intrathecal baclofen therapy for treating spastic hypertonia due to acquired brain injury. *Brain Inj.* 2005;19(5):359–364.

36. Saval A, Chiodo AE. Intrathecal baclofen for spasticity management: a comparative analysis of spasticity of spinal vs cortical origin. *J Spinal Cord Med.* 2010;33(1):16–21.

37. Clearfield JS, Nelson ME, McGuire J, Rein LE, Tarima S. Intrathecal baclofen dosing regimens: a retrospective chart review. *Neuromodulation.* 2016;19(6):642–649. https://doi.org/10.1111/ner.12361.

38. Werhahn KJ, Brown P, Thompson PD, Marsden CD. The clinical features and prognosis of chronic posthypoxic myoclonus. *Mov Disord.* 1997;12(2):216–220. https://doi.org/10.1002/mds.870120212.

39. Lu-Emerson C, Khot S. Neurological sequelae of hypoxic-ischemic brain injury. *NeuroRehabilitation.* 2010;26(1):35–45. https://doi.org/10.3233/nre-2010-0534.

40. Birthi P, Walters C, Ortiz Vargas O, Karandikar N. The use of intrathecal baclofen therapy for myoclonus in a patient with Lance Adams syndrome. *PM R.* 2011;3(7):671–673. https://doi.org/10.1016/j.pmrj.2010.12.023.

41. Kuoppamaki M, Bhatia KP, Quinn N. Progressive delayed-onset dystonia after cerebral anoxic insult in adults. *Mov Disord.* 2002;17(6):1345–1349. https://doi.org/10.1002/mds.10260.

42. Ghika J, Villemure JG, Miklossy J, et al. Postanoxic generalized dystonia improved by bilateral Voa thalamic deep brain stimulation. *Neurology.* 2002;58(2):311–313.

43. Uniform Determination of Death Act. 12 Uniform Laws Annotated (U.L.A.). 589 (West 1993 and West Supp 1997).

44. Practice parameters for determining brain death in adults (summary statement). The Quality Standards Subcommittee of the American Academy of Neurology. *Neurology.* 1995;45(5):1012–1014.

45. Greer DM, Wang HH, Robinson JD, Varelas PN, Henderson GV, Wijdicks EF. Variability of brain death policies in the United States. *JAMA Neurol.* 2016;73(2):213–218. https://doi.org/10.1001/jamaneurol.2015.3943.

46. Wijdicks EF, Varelas PN, Gronseth GS, Greer DM. Evidence-based guideline update: determining brain death in adults: report of the Quality Standards Subcommittee of the American Academy of Neurology. *Neurology.* 2010;74(23):1911–1918. https://doi.org/10.1212/WNL.0b013e3181e242a8.

47. Young GB. Ethics in the intensive care unit with emphasis on medical futility in comatose survivors of cardiac arrest. *J Clin Neurophysiol.* 2000;17(5):453–456.

48. Perry JE, Churchill LR, Kirshner HS. The Terri Schiavo case: legal, ethical, and medical perspectives. *Ann Intern Med.* 2005;143(10):744–748.

CHAPTER 10

Neuropsychiatric Sequelae of Traumatic Brain Injury

SUZANNE MCGARITY, PHD • NATHALIE DIEUJUSTE, BA •
LISA A. BRENNER, PHD, ABPP • HAL S. WORTZEL, MD

INTRODUCTION

Neuropsychiatric sequelae of traumatic brain injury (TBI) include physical, cognitive, emotional, and behavioral symptoms that may affect functional ability and participation, both during and after the acute rehabilitation process. Although these neuropsychiatric domains tend to be discussed as distinct entities, co-occurring symptoms frequently result in complex clinical scenarios that create challenges for accurate diagnosis and treatment planning. Physical, cognitive, emotional, and behavioral symptoms interact with and influence one another, such that determining the etiology of any given neuropsychiatric presentation, and the most salient targets for treatment, requires careful evaluation. Hence, the assessment and treatment of those living with a history of TBI requires attending to the index TBI, as well as (1) the individual's preinjury neuropsychiatric status and psychosocial history and (2) the postinjury environment and co-occurring illnesses/injuries. Best practices for a comprehensive and thorough assessment of the emotional and behavioral disturbance associated with TBI include a neuropsychiatric interview and examination, augmented by collateral data (e.g., staff and family observations), as well as data from self-report and caregiver-based measures. Specific guidance regarding these components is beyond the scope of this chapter. For further information see *Textbook of Traumatic Brain Injury*[1] (Chapter 4. Neuropsychiatric Assessment), *Brain Injury Medicine* (Chapter 60. Neuropsychological Assessment and Treatment Planning),[2] and *Manual of Traumatic Brain Injury: Assessment and Management*.[3] As a general rule, assessment should be undertaken with the goal of identifying symptoms and psychosocial circumstances that, when targeted with evidence-based interventions, would be expected to yield functional gains. This chapter provides an overview of the more common emotional disturbances (i.e., depression, anxiety, mania, emotional dyscontrol, trauma and stressor-related disorders, and psychosis) and behaviors sequelae of TBI (apathy, disinhibition, and aggression).

EMOTIONAL DISTURBANCES

Depression

Depression is the most prevalent psychiatric condition reported among those living with a history of TBI.[4–6] Longitudinal studies report incidence rates from 25% to 52%, within the first year post injury. Some evidence suggests that damage to specific areas of the brain, such as the prefrontal cortices and basal ganglia, may increase the risk for depression.[4,7–9] Preinjury personal characteristics (e.g., history of psychiatric diagnosis [especially depression], low income, tendency to experience high levels of stress) and postinjury psychosocial factors (e.g., difficulty with adjustment to injury-based limitations and disability, unemployment) increase the risk for developing post-TBI depression.[4,7,8] Depression post injury will likely affect physical health, quality of life, and rehabilitation outcomes, making early detection and treatment important.

The differential diagnosis of depression in the subacute TBI setting can be particularly challenging, as many symptoms of depression are easily confused with other common conditions and circumstances observed among those recovering from acute injuries. For example, physical pain may result in tearfulness, poor appetite, and social withdrawal. In addition, observed or self-reported slow cognitive processing and impaired attention may be due to neuronal injury rather than a depressed state. Problems with fatigue and sleep disruption are common in a rehabilitation setting because of scheduling and medical monitoring activities. This high degree of overlap may lead to overdiagnosis of depression and unnecessary or premature treatment. Conversely, depression may be underdiagnosed secondary to patients with more severe brain injuries having a lack of awareness of symptoms or an inability to report their dysphoric emotions. During such periods, staff may inadvertently normalize clinically significant depression in the context of recent injury and illness, thereby missing opportunities for intervention.

TABLE 10.1
Pharmacologic Treatments for Depression in Persons With Traumatic Brain Injury

Category	Examples	Advantages	Disadvantages
Selective serotonin reuptake inhibitors (SSRIs)	• Sertraline • Fluoxetine • Escitalopram • Citalopram	• Relatively safe • Ease of use • May reduce comorbid anxiety, irritability, and impulsivity • Most have short half-lives • May reduce perceived somatic and cognitive symptoms	• Some potential for adverse effects and drug-drug interactions
Serotonin-norepinephrine reuptake inhibitors	• Venlafaxine • Duloxetine • Milnacipran	• May also produce analgesic affects	• Less evidence for efficacy versus SSRIs
Tricyclic antidepressants	• Amitriptyline • Desipramine	• Can offer rapid response	• May have intolerable side-effect profiles (e.g., seizures) • Potential interactions with other medications • Dangerous in overdose
Monoamine oxidase inhibitors	• Phenelzine • Moclobemide	• Similar to SSRIs with regard to benefits and adverse effects	• Similar to SSRIs with regard to adverse effects • Cognitive impairments may limit the ability to adhere to dietary restrictions
Other antidepressants	• Buproprion	• Sustained-release form may offer benefit	• May lower seizure threshold
Stimulants	• Methylphenidate	• May benefit amotivation, lethargy, attention, and processing speed	• May interfere with sleep • May contribute to anxiety or behavioral problems

The information and recommendations in this table have been adapted from Jorge and Arciniegas,[12,13] Warden et al.,[14] and Fann et al.[15]

Assessing for depression in post-acute rehabilitation settings ideally involves a combination of detection strategies, including both validated and standardized measures, such as the Beck Depression Inventory-II or Patient Health Questionnaire-9 and clinical interview to investigate[10,11] for hallmark features (pervasive sadness, anhedonia, and feelings of worthlessness and/or guilt). For nonverbal patients, behavioral observations, such as tearfulness, isolation, and disinterest, may serve as useful clues. As noted earlier, obtaining a preinjury history of psychiatric illnesses is also paramount.

For moderate to severe depression, pharmacologic interventions are appropriate. Table 10.1 provides the recommended pharmacologic agents used to treat depression in persons with TBI.[4,7] In cases of severe or refractory depression following TBI, electroconvulsive therapy may be considered.

For some, the treatment and management of post-TBI depression during the postacute period should include psychotherapeutic interventions. Although psychotherapeutic interventions can be effectively adapted to meet the needs of those with cognitive impairments, these interventions are not indicated for persons with current posttraumatic amnesia (PTA) or those with aphasic disorders that would prevent them from meaningfully participating in treatment protocols. Cognitive behavioral therapy (CBT) for depression targets the thought processes and behaviors that drive and maintain depressive episodes. CBT has been successfully adapted to meet the unique needs of patients with TBI[16–19] who present with depression. Adaptations for persons with TBI include emphasizing psychoeducation, extended session length to allow for repetition of information, and coping skills training for managing TBI symptoms.[20] For further information regarding

TABLE 10.2
Pharmacologic Treatments for Manic and Mixed Mood Sates in Persons With Traumatic Brain Injury

Medication	Advantages	Disadvantages
Valproate	• Less likely to adversely affect cognition compared with lithium and anticonvulsants • Can be used as antimania prophylaxis • Relatively tolerable	• May adversely affect cognition • May cause tremor, ataxia, and gait disturbances • Associated with weight gain and gastrointestinal symptoms
Lithium carbonate	• Evidence for efficacy in treatment of mixed mood states	• May adversely affect cognition • Associated with nausea, ataxia, tremor, and lethargy • Lowers seizure threshold • Narrow therapeutic window and need to monitor blood levels
Other anticonvulsants (e.g., carbamazepine, lamotrigine)	• Effective for the treatment of posttraumatic mania, hypomania, or mixed states	• May adversely affect cognition • May cause motor side effects • May cause cardiac or metabolic disturbance
Atypical antipsychotics (e.g., quetiapine, risperidone, olanzapine, ziprasidone, aripiprazole)	• Effective for the treatment of posttraumatic mania, hypomania, or mixed states	• May adversely affect cognition • May cause motor side effects • May cause cardiac or metabolic disturbance

The information and recommendations in this table have been adapted from Whelan-Goodinson et al.,[26] Fann and Jakupcak,[27] Jorge and Arciniegas,[28] and Cittolin-Santos et al.[29]

adapting psychological interventions for those with a history of TBI see the Ohio State University online training module entitled *Accommodating the Symptoms*[21] *of TBI*.

Mania, Hypomania, and Mixed Mood States

Posttraumatic mania, hypomania, and mixed mood states are relatively infrequent compared with depression. The limited research available suggests that rates range from 9% to 27%.[22,23] Factors contributing to the development of secondary mania included basopolar temporal lesions and injury to the right hemispheric limbic system.[22] One study suggests that family history of mood disorder is associated with mania after TBI.[24] As previously suggested, best practices for the diagnosis of emotional disturbances require careful clinical interviewing and noting the nature and timing of symptoms and concurrent behavioral disturbances. Key features of mania following TBI are the presence of *both* elevated/irritable mood and abnormally and persistently increased energy/activity. These symptoms must also be significant enough to cause impairment in daily functioning.

Mania and bipolar spectrum disorders diagnosed after TBI are typically treated in the same manner as idiopathic manic and mixed mood states,[12] with pharmacologic agents as the first-line intervention. Specific medications used to treat post-TBI manic symptoms and their respective advantages and disadvantages[7,12,25,26] are outlined in Table 10.2. To date, there is no clear guidance on specific psychotherapeutic approaches to treating mania or mixed mood states in persons with TBI. It is recommended that psychoeducation about bipolar disorders and appropriate coping skills be offered early in the course of rehabilitation by trained psychologists or mental health practitioners. In general, psychoeducational and psychotherapeutic approaches should model those used with treating idiopathic bipolar disorder.[7,12] Treatment recommendations for bipolar disorder can be found in the practice guidelines published by the American Psychiatric Association.[30]

Anxiety

Research suggests that anxiety disorders are the second most frequent psychiatric disorder diagnosed following TBI (after depression).[26,31] A meta-analysis of anxiety following brain injury reported that 11% of those living with a history of TBI were diagnosed with generalized anxiety disorder (GAD).[32] The analysis also revealed that 37% of all individuals studied reported symptoms

TABLE 10.3
Pharmacologic Treatments for Anxiety in Persons With Traumatic Brain Injury

Category	Examples	Advantages	Disadvantages
Selective serotonin reuptake inhibitors	• Sertraline • Fluoxetine • Escitalopram • Citalopram	• May be helpful in treating comorbid depression and anxiety • Relatively safe • Ease of use • May reduce comorbid anxiety, irritability, and impulsivity • Most have short half-lives • May reduce perceived somatic and cognitive symptoms	• Can cause initial activating effects leading to nonadherence or early discontinuation • Some potential for adverse effects and dug-drug interactions • Sexual side effects, sedation, and apathy possible at high doses
Anxiolytics	• Buspirone	• Useful for generalized anxiety symptoms	• Can lower seizure threshold
Benzodiazepines	• Lorazepam • Alprazolam • Diazepam • Clonazepam	• Useful in short-term treatment for acute anxiety	• Potential adverse effects on cognitive systems, which may be particularly problematic for those already experiencing cognitive impairment • May negatively affect motor systems • Can be habit forming • May cause rebound anxiety

The information and recommendations in this table have been adapted from Fann and Jakupcak[27] and Plantier and Luaute.[39]

of anxiety that surpassed predetermined clinically significant levels on the self-report measures (e.g., Hospital Anxiety Depression Scale,[33] Leeds Scale for the Self-assessment of Anxiety and Depression,[34] and the State Trait Anxiety Inventory[35]). Another investigation reported panic attacks being 5.8% more common among persons with TBI compared with members of the general population.[36] Evidence suggests that anxiety disorder rates following TBI are associated with TBI severity, as well as time since injury. For example, the meta-analysis previously described revealed that GAD is less common after mild injuries versus severe injuries (11% vs. 15%), and clinically significant self-reported anxiety was substantially more prevalent in cases of mild injury versus severe injury (53% vs. 38%). This study also described a "peak" of anxiety prevalence at 2–5 years post injury, suggesting that injured persons may be particularly vulnerable during this period.[32] Anxiety and depression often coexist in the general population and in brain-injured persons. Rates of GAD among patients with a history of TBI and depression have been reported to be as high as 41.2%.[37] Comorbid depression and anxiety warrant special consideration in choosing appropriate treatment (see later discussion).

As with depression, assessing for anxiety in post-acute rehabilitation settings should include a combination of detection strategies, such as psychometrically sound measures coupled with a clinical interview to obtain information about the specificity of the worry/concern, the temporal nature of the periods of worry, the content of the worry, and any associated physical symptoms. Furthermore, the worry/concern must exceed what most individuals would experience under similar circumstances.

The treatment and management for anxiety after TBI should involve evidence-based therapeutic approaches. CBT and motivational interviewing have been shown to be helpful.[19,38] Such treatments can be offered and incorporated into the rehabilitation setting or offered as part of a longer-term follow-up treatment plan. Medications are an important intervention for the treatment of moderate to severe anxiety following TBI and are listed in Table 10.3.[40] The ideal treatment approach to post-TBI anxiety is multimodal.[40,41] For example, patients may initially benefit from pharmacologic treatment for anxiety with the ultimate goal of tapering off such medications once psychotherapy has afforded a reduction in anxiety and an enhanced ability to deploy more long-term coping strategies.

Emotional Dyscontrol

Emotional dyscontrol involves a tendency toward unpredictable and rapidly fluctuating emotions and includes the conditions pathologic laughing and crying (PLC), affective lability, and irritability. PLC is also referred to as emotional incontinence or pseudobulbar affect and is observed as moment-to-moment spontaneous and excessive behavioral responses to mild or neutral stimuli. The emotional displays do not necessarily bear any relationship to the individual's internal emotional experience, either during or between the episodes. Affective lability, also referred to as emotional lability, involves the tendency to experience disproportionately intense bouts of emotion in response to meaningful personal or social stimuli. Posttraumatic irritability refers to impatience, anger, and loss of temper that is not related to another psychological or physical condition. Emotional dyscontrol is commonly observed first in the early stages of recovery after TBI. Symptoms are typically observed to be most severe during this time period[42] and therefore often require management in rehabilitation settings. Evidence suggests that PLC can occur in 5%–11% of patients with TBI during the first year post injury.[43,44] Affective lability rates in populations with TBI are widely variable and difficult to estimate, yet one study suggests rates as high as 33%–46% following severe TBI.[45,46] Posttraumatic irritability has been identified in 35%–71%[46,47] of brain-injured persons. Proper diagnosis of emotional dyscontrol following TBI requires serial observation of the affective/behavioral response. Emotional dyscontrol can be confused with symptoms of mood disorders, such as depression, irritable mania/hypomania, or mixed mood episode. Similarly, careful attention should be paid to the temporal relationship between overt and intense emotional responses and episodic increases in pain or trauma-related triggers. Recurring moment-to-moment instances of inappropriate emotional expression that do not provoke a persistent change in prevailing mood are the hallmark of a brain injury–related inability to regulate emotional responses. Persons exhibiting symptoms of emotional dyscontrol often feel embarrassed and report distress stemming from these affective displays.

The management of posttraumatic affective lability and irritability should start with nonpharmacologic approaches, particularly when symptoms range from mild to moderate and cognitive functioning is relatively intact.[48] Counseling, education, and/or psychotherapy to improve self-efficacy and self-regulation are appropriate initial treatment modalities. Modified group therapy has been shown to be effective at reducing the frequency of expressed and experienced anger post severe TBI.[49] Rehabilitation interventions that concurrently address emotional self-regulation and

functional cognitive performance are also supported in the literature.[50] Pharmacotherapy may be beneficial for patients exhibiting severe symptoms of emotional dyscontrol or for those who do not respond to psychological interventions. Selective serotonin reuptake inhibitors (SSRIs) are appropriate first-line choices in most instances. For PLC and affective lability, switching to, or augmenting with, methylphenidate, lamotrigine, valproate, or carbamazepine is appropriate when SSRIs prove ineffective. Case reports suggest that posttraumatic irritability may also respond favorably to valproate, carbamazepine, methylphenidate, quetiapine, aripiprazole, buspirone, or propranolol. Dextromethorphan-quinidine is another option for PLC, although the quinidine component creates considerable risk for drug-drug interactions.[48,51–57]

Trauma-Related Disorders

Biomechanical trauma (causing TBI) frequently co-occurs with emotional trauma. Hence, acute stress disorder (ASD) and posttraumatic stress disorder (PTSD) may develop after injury events, particularly the types of events that result in TBI (e.g., combat, assault). It is therefore necessary to be mindful of the signs and symptoms of ASD and PTSD in acute and post-acute rehabilitation settings so that injured persons are able to access treatment early on, giving them the best chance for recovery. Studies suggest that incidence rates of PTSD are higher for those with TBI compared with the general population.[58] Incidence rates of PTSD following TBI vary greatly by study and range from 3% to 59%.[58] This wide variability is thought to be the result of diverse manifestations of PTSD following TBI. In terms of observed course and development, some studies suggest that PTSD is most likely to develop in the first year post injury, particularly 6–12 months after injury, with rates remaining stable up to 2 years post injury and declining thereafter.[36]

For persons with TBI in subacute rehabilitation settings, time since injury may be less than 1 month. If an individual is exhibiting signs of a trauma-related disorder and it has been less than 1 month since injury, ASD is the appropriate diagnosis. Assessing and addressing ASD as early as possible is vital in preventing the development of PTSD. If symptoms have persisted longer than 1 month, the diagnosis of PTSD may be appropriate. However, to meet criteria, two hallmark features, reexperiencing and efforts to avoid thoughts or situations that trigger memories of the experience, must be present. Nightmares and flashbacks would certainly warrant further diagnostic evaluation via structured clinical interview and behavioral observation. Most other symptoms of PTSD overlap with other physical, psychiatric, and injury-related conditions (e.g., problems with sleep, irritability, memory, and concentration disorders).

Fortunately, there are evidence-based psychological interventions for PTSD that can be successfully adapted to meet the needs of persons with TBI. Research supports the efficacy of prolonged exposure and cognitive processing therapy for those living with TBI, with specific modifications to the protocol, such as extended session time and repeated education throughout treatment.[59–62] Treatment for PTSD after TBI should include psychoeducation about the deleterious effects of maladaptive coping strategies, such as isolation and substance/alcohol use. When formal PTSD treatments are not available in rehabilitation settings, other types of psychological interventions may prove beneficial for symptom management, such as stress management and relaxation training. However, although such methods facilitate engagement in other rehabilitation services, they do not result in full resolution of the PTSD disorder and specific evidence-based interventions targeting PTSD should be recommended as part of a long-term treatment plan. Pharmacologic treatment of PTSD includes the use of SSRIs. Other pharmacologic agents used to treat PTSD in populations with TBI include mood stabilizers, atypical antipsychotics, and other drugs such as propranolol[63,64]; however, no medication has demonstrated efficacy in treating PTSD that is comparable with the evidence-based psychological interventions described earlier. Prazosin has been successfully used to address nightmares related to PTSD, especially when combined with sleep hygiene instruction.[65]

Psychosis

Psychosis following TBI is relatively rare. Research suggests an incidence of 0.7%–9.8%.[66] Positive symptoms, such as delusions and hallucinations, are predominant in posttraumatic psychosis, whereas negative symptoms, such as blunted affect, are less common.[66] Auditory hallucinations are most common, followed by visual hallucinations, and then tactile hallucinations.[66] Similarly, varying types of delusions have been reported; common examples include paranoid, persecutory, reference, and grandiose delusions.[36,66] Studies suggest that injury location, specifically the hippocampus, can influence the risk for post-TBI psychosis. Prior head injuries, neurologic conditions or disorders, and genetic predispositions to psychosis have also been associated with posttraumatic psychosis.[67] Substance use, and more specifically cannabis use, before and

after TBI is associated with the onset and worsening of psychosis after injury.[68,69] Diagnosis of posttraumatic psychosis should incorporate assessment of any premorbid psychiatric conditions and substances/alcohol use. During the initial stages of recovery, symptoms of acute posttraumatic confusional state or PTA may mimic psychosis.[70]

Psychotic symptoms following TBI are almost always treated with pharmacologic interventions. If other comorbid conditions are driving psychotic symptoms, it is important to first address the underlying condition (e.g., hallucinations in the context of a medication-induced delirium). If psychotic symptoms do not resolve after this initial approach, if there are no underlying comorbid conditions, or if psychotic symptoms are severe and yielding substantial distress and/or behavioral disturbances, atypical antipsychotics are preferred (e.g., quetiapine, olanzapine, aripiprazole).[36]

BEHAVIORAL DISTURBANCES
Apathy

Post-TBI apathy is characterized by a state of diminished motivation. It can be described as a clinically significant decrease in goal-directed cognition, emotion, and/or behavior. It often co-occurs with other types of behavioral dyscontrol, as described later. Studies suggest that apathy occurs in 29%–50% of patients with severe TBI.[71–73] Damage to both the anterior cingulate-subcortical circuits and the lateral orbitofrontal-subcortical circuits can contribute to apathy and disinhibited behavior.[74] In such cases, impaired motivation and generalized disengagement is punctuated by periodic discrete episodes of inappropriate behavioral responses to environmental stimuli. Posttraumatic apathy can often be mistaken for a symptom of an underlying depressive disorder and as such requires careful consideration in differential diagnosis. True posttraumatic apathy that exists on its own must be differentiated from depression in that there is little to no significant experience of dysphoric emotion but rather a distinct and consistent decrease in thinking, feeling, and acting that is not related to changes in underlying mood.

There is very limited research on the treatment for apathy after TBI. Psychostimulants, including methylphenidate and dextroamphetamine, may increase goal-directed behavior. However, when apathy is paired with disinhibition or aggression, such treatments should be implemented with caution. Alternative options for the treatment of apathy post-TBI include amantadine, selegiline, and acetylcholinesterase inhibitors.[75] SSRIs are often prescribed when apathy is mistaken for depression and can exacerbate the problem, leading to a cycle whereby worsened apathy precipitates higher dosing, resulting in even more apathy.

Disinhibition

Disinhibition following TBI is defined as socially or contextually inappropriate nonaggressive verbal, physical, and sexual acts that reflect a lessening or loss of inhibitions and/or inability to appreciate social or cultural behavioral norms. In moderate to severe TBI, rates of disinhibition range from 12% to 32%.[48] Diagnosis must take into account cultural considerations, presence of pain conditions and associated pain behaviors, and presence of premorbid personality characteristics.

Behavioral analysis and behavior management strategies are particularly useful in the management of both disinhibition and aggression (described in more detail later). Providers in rehabilitation settings may develop specifically tailored behavior modification plans to address dysfunctional behaviors associated with disinhibition and aggression. Such plans are most successful when formulated using patient and family input to identify antecedents of the problematic behavior and best methods by which to modify or eliminate it (e.g., reinforcement of desired behavior vs. punishment for undesired behavior). Family and caregivers are also essential to implementing consistency, which is key to the success of any behavioral modification plan. Social skills training in an individual or group format may also prove beneficial.

Pharmacotherapy for posttraumatic disinhibition includes SSRIs as a first-line treatment. Alternative drugs used to treat this type of behavioral dyscontrol are anticonvulsants, including valproate, carbamazepine, and lamotrigine. When disinhibited behaviors center on sexual acts, antiandrogenic agents have been reported to be of benefit. Finally, atypical antipsychotics warrant consideration when patients do not respond to other approaches.

Aggression

Aggression is operationally defined as a specific set of verbal or behavioral outbursts directed at objects or people in the environment. Posttraumatic aggression incidence rates range from 15% to 51% in cases of severe TBI.[48] Frontal lobe lesions, especially those involving the lateral orbitofrontal circuit, are often associated with post-TBI aggression.[76] Evidence suggests that premorbid psychological factors, such as antisocial personality disorder, also contribute to the increased incidence of posttraumatic aggression.[77]

Aggressive behaviors are a significant challenge to providers in rehabilitation settings because they frequently interfere with rehabilitation efforts, disrupt social support networks, and may cause critical safety concerns. Moreover, effective management of behavioral disturbances often takes time and trial and error. This should be done before aggression leads to significant negative social and legal consequences, as these may compromise access to care.[78]

It is important to carefully quantify and qualify the frequency, nature, and severity of aggressive behavior. Without establishing a baseline, it can be very difficult to determine whether or not a given act represents a significant change from baseline or whether interventions are affording any benefit (or harm). Reduction in terms of frequency and severity is often a more realistic goal than elimination. Environmental and behavioral techniques should be offered either alone or in conjunction with pharmacotherapy. Such techniques include behavioral analysis and management. When specifically addressing aggressive behaviors, behavioral management strategies might include assertiveness training, differential reinforcement scheduling, social extinction, contingent observation, self-controlled time-out, overcorrection, and contingent restraint.

Medication management of acute post-TBI aggression warrants special consideration. Antipsychotics (preferably newer atypical agents) and benzodiazepines are the mainstays when the dangers attendant to acute aggression mandates rapid behavior control. Such treatment should be titrated and discontinued once the acute behavioral crisis has abated. Pharmacologic strategies for chronic post-TBI aggression are typically dictated by co-occurring symptoms and circumstances. For example, aggression precipitated by pain would warrant better pain control.

Chronic aggression occurring in association with depression or anxiety would warrant use of an SSRI, whereas aggression in association with mania or seizures would indicate a trial of an antiepileptic/mood stabilizer. Aggression associated with psychotic symptoms would suggest treatment with antipsychotics; atypical antipsychotics are preferred over typical antipsychotics (e.g., haloperidol) because of concern for treatment-induced akathisia and extrapyramidal side effects. In cases in which the above-mentioned pharmacologic interventions do not prove beneficial, other drug treatments warrant consideration, including lithium, buspirone, and β-adrenergic receptor agonists.[39]

CONCLUSION

It is imperative that persons who have sustained a TBI have the opportunity to fully engage in rehabilitative care as soon as possible after injury. To this end, effective management of neuropsychiatric sequelae following injury is of utmost importance. Early identification of symptoms, accurate diagnosis, and judicious use of interventions that maximizes therapeutic response while minimizing adverse effects will provide patients with the best chance of recovery and restoration of function.

REFERENCES

1. Arlinghaus KA, Pastorek NJ, Graham DP. Neuropsychiatric assessment. In: Silver JM, McAlister TW, Yudofsky SC, eds. *Textbook of Traumatic Brain Injury*. 2nd ed. Arlington, VA: American Psychiatric Association; 2011:55–72.
2. Hsu NH, Godwin EE, Shaaf KW, Smith SW, Taylor LA, Kreutzer JS. Neuropsychological assessment and treatment planning. In: Zasler ND, Katz DI, Zafonte RD, Arciniegas DB, Bullock MR, Kreutzer JS, eds. *Brain Injury Medicine: Principles and Practice*. 2nd ed. New York, NY: Demos Medical Publishing; 2012:1002–1020.
3. Zollman FS. *Manual of Traumatic Brain Injury Assessment and Management*. 2nd ed. New York, NY: Demos Medical Publishing; 2016.
4. Fann JR, Hart T, Schomer KG. Treatment for depression after traumatic brain injury: a systematic review. *J Neurotrauma*. 2009;26(12):2383–2402.
5. Fisher LB, Pedrelli P, Iverson GL, et al. Prevalence of suicidal behaviour following traumatic brain injury: longitudinal follow-up from the NIDRR traumatic brain injury model systems. *Brain Inj*. 2016;30(11):1311–1318.
6. Fann JR, Bombardier CH, Temkin NR, et al. Incidence, severity, and phenomenology of depression and anxiety in patients with moderate to severe traumatic brain injury. *Psychosomatics*. 2003;44:161.
7. Jorge RE, Arciniegas DB. Disorders of mood and affect. In: Arciniegas DB, Zasler ND, Vanderplog RD, Jaffee MS, eds. *Management of Adults with Traumatic Brain Injury*. Washington, DC: American Psychiatric Publishing; 2013:167–194.
8. Jorge RE, Robinson RG. Mood disorders. In: Silver JM, McAlister TW, Yudofsky SC, eds. *Textbook of Traumatic Brain Injury*. 2nd ed. Arlington, VA: American Psychiatric Association; 2011:179–181.
9. Cnossen MC, Scholten AC, Lingsma HF, et al. Predictors of major depression and posttraumatic stress disorder following traumatic brain injury: a systematic review and meta-analysis. *J Neuropsychiatr Clin Neurosci*. 2017;29(3):206–224.
10. Beck AT, Steer RA, Brown GK. *Beck Depression Inventory-II Manual*. 2nd ed. San Antonio, TX: Psychological Corp; 1996.
11. Fann JR, Bombardier CH, Dikmen S, et al. Validity of the patient health questionnaire-9 in assessing depression following traumatic brain injury. *J Head Trauma Rehabil*. 2005;20(6):501–511.
12. Jorge RE, Arciniegas DB. Mood disorders after TBI. In: Jorge RE, Arciniegas DB, eds. *Neuropsychiatry of Traumatic Brain Injury*. New York, NY: Elsevier; 2014:13–29.
13. Jorge RE, Arciniegas DB. Disorders of mood and affect. In: Arciniegas DB, Zasler ND, Vanderploeg RD, Jaffee MS, eds. *Management of Adults with Traumatic Brain Injury*. Arlington, VA: American Psychiatric Publishing; 2013:174–177.
14. Warden DL, Gordon B, McAllister TW, et al. Guidelines for the pharmacological treatment of neurobehavioral sequalae of TBI. *J Neurotrauma*. 2006;23(10):1468–1501.
15. Fann JR, Hart T, Schomer KG. Treatment for depression after traumatic brain injury: a systematic review. *J Neurotrauma*. 2009;26:2383–2402.
16. Liu ZQ, Zeng X, Duan CY. Neuropsychological rehabilitation and psychotherapy of adult traumatic brain injury patients with depression: a systematic review and meta-analysis. *J Neurosurg Sci*. 2017;62(1):24–35.
17. Anson K, Ponsford J. Evaluation of a coping skills group following traumatic brain injury. *Brain Inj*. 2006;20(2):167–178.
18. Tiersky LA, Anselmi V, Johnston MV, et al. A trial of neuropsychologic rehabilitation in mild-spectrum traumatic brain injury. *Arch Phys Med Rehabil*. 2005;86(8):1565–1574.
19. Ponsford J, Lee NK, Wong D, et al. Efficacy of motivational interviewing and cognitive behavioral therapy for anxiety and depression symptoms following traumatic brain injury. *Psychol Med*. 2016;46(5):1079–1090.
20. Rocky Mountain Mental Illness Research Education and Clinical Center (MIRECC). *Toolkit for Providers of Clients with Co-occurring TBI and Mental Health Symptoms*. https://www.mirecc.va.gov/visn19/tbi_toolkit/.
21. The Ohio State University College of Medicine. *Traumatic Brain Injury*. https://tbi.osu.edu/modules.
22. Jorge RE, Robinson RG, Starkstein SE, Arndt SV, Forrester AW, Geisler FH. Secondary mania following traumatic brain injury. *Am J Psychiatr*. 1993;150(6):916–921.
23. van Reekum R, Cohen T, Wong J. Can traumatic brain injury cause psychiatric disorders? *J Neuropsychiatr Clin Neurosci*. 2000;12(3):316–327.
24. Robinson RG, Boston JD, Starkstein SE, Price TR. Comparison of mania and depression after brain injury: causal factors. *Am J Psychiatr*. 1988;145(2):172–178.
25. Cittolin-Santos GF, Freeden JC, Cotes RO. A case report of mania and psychosis five months after traumatic brain injury successfully treated using olanzapine. *Case Rep Psychiatr*. 2017;2017:7541307.
26. Whelan-Goodinson R, Ponsford J, Johnston L, Grant F. Psychiatric disorders following traumatic brain injury: their nature and frequency. *J Head Trauma Rehabil*. 2009;24(5):324–332.
27. Fann JR, Jakupcak M. Anxiety disorders. In: Arciniegas DB, Zasler ND, Vanderploeg RD, Jaffee MS, eds. *Management of Adults with Traumatic Brain Injury*. Arlington, VA: American Psychiatric Publishing; 2013:195–211.

28. Jorge RE, Arciniegas DB. Mood disorders after TBI. In: Jorge RE, Arciniegas DB, eds. *Neuropsychiatry of Traumatic Brain Injury.* New York, NY: Elsevier; 2014:23–24.

29. Cittolin-Santos GF, Fredeen JC, Cotes RO. A case report of mania and psychosis five months after traumatic brain injury successfully treated using olanzapine. *Case Rep Psychiatr.* 2017;2017:7541307.

30. Practice guideline for the treatment of patients with bipolar disorder (revision). *Am J Psychiatr.* 2002;159(4 suppl): 1–50.

31. Albrecht JS, Peters ME, Smith GS, Rao V. Anxiety and posttraumatic stress disorder among Medicare beneficiaries after traumatic brain injury. *J Head Trauma Rehabil.* 2017;32(3):178–184.

32. Osborn AJ, Mathias JL, Fairweather-Schmidt AK. Prevalence of anxiety following adult traumatic brain injury: a meta-analysis comparing measures, samples and postinjury intervals. *Neuropsychology.* 2016;30(2): 247–261.

33. Zigmond AS, Snaith RP. The hospital anxiety and depression scale. *Acta Psychiatr Scand.* 1983;67(6):361–370.

34. Snaith RP, Bridge GW, Hamilton M. The Leeds scales for the self-assessment of anxiety and depression. *Br J Psychiatr.* 1976;128:156–165.

35. Spielberger CD, Gorsuch RL, Lushene RE. *Manual for the State-Trait Anxiety Inventory;* 1970.

36. Stefan A, Mathe JF, SOFMER Group. What are the disruptive symptoms of behavioral disorders after traumatic brain injury? A systematic review leading to recommendations for good practices. *Ann Phys Rehabil Med.* 2016; 59(1):5–17.

37. Jorge RE, Robinson RG, Starkstein SE, Arndt SV. Depression and anxiety following traumatic brain injury. *J Neuropsychiatr Clin Neurosci.* 1993;5(4):369–374.

38. Soo C, Tate R. Psychological treatment for anxiety in people with traumatic brain injury. *Cochrane Database Syst Rev.* 2007;(3):Cd005239.

39. Plantier D, Luaute J. Drugs for behavior disorders after traumatic brain injury: systematic review and expert consensus leading to French recommendations for good practice. *Ann Phys Rehabil Med.* 2016;59(1):42–57.

40. Fann JR, Jakupcak M. Anxiety disorders. In: Arciniegas DB, Zasler ND, Vanderploog RD, Jaffee MS, eds. *Management of Adults with Traumatic Brain Injury.* Washington, DC: American Psychiatric Publishing; 2013:195–212.

41. Mallya S, Sutherland J, Pongracic S, Mainland B, Ornstein TJ. The manifestation of anxiety disorders after traumatic brain injury: a review. *J Neurotrauma.* 2015;32(7): 411–421.

42. American Psychiatric Association DSM-5 Task Force. In: *Major or Mild Neurocognitive Disorder due to Traumatic Brain Injury.* American Psychiatric Association; 2013.

43. Tateno A, Jorge RE, Robinson RG. Pathological laughing and crying following traumatic brain injury. *J Neuropsychiatr Clin Neurosci.* 2004;16(4):426–434.

44. Zeilig G, Drubach DA, Katz-Zeilig M, Karatinos J. Pathological laughter and crying in patients with closed traumatic brain injury. *Brain Inj.* 1996;10(8):591–597.

45. Nakase-Thompson R, Sherer M, Yablon SA, Nick TG, Trzepacz PT. Acute confusion following traumatic brain injury. *Brain Inj.* 2004;18(2):131–142.

46. McKinlay WW, Brooks DN, Bond MR, Martinage DP, Marshall MM. The short-term outcome of severe blunt head injury as reported by relatives of the injured persons. *J Neurol Neurosurg Psychiatr.* 1981;44(6):527–533.

47. Deb S, Lyons I, Koutzoukis C. Neurobehavioural symptoms one year after a head injury. *Br J Psychiatr.* 1999;174:360–365.

48. Arciniegas DB, Wortzel HS. Emotional and behavioral dyscontrol after traumatic brain injury. *Psychiatr Clin North Am.* 2014;37(1):31–53.

49. Walker AJ, Nott MT, Doyle M, Onus M, McCarthy K, Baguley IJ. Effectiveness of a group anger management programme after severe traumatic brain injury. *Brain Inj.* 2010;24(3):517–524.

50. Cattelani R, Zettin M, Zoccolotti P. Rehabilitation treatments for adults with behavioral and psychosocial disorders following acquired brain injury: a systematic review. *Neuropsychol Rev.* 2010;20(1):52–85.

51. Kant R, Smith-Seemiller L, Zeiler D. Treatment of aggression and irritability after head injury. *Brain Inj.* 1998;12(8): 661–666.

52. Wroblewski BA, Joseph AB, Kupfer J, Kalliel K. Effectiveness of valproic acid on destructive and aggressive behaviours in patients with acquired brain injury. *Brain Inj.* 1997;11(1):37–47.

53. Azouvi P, Jokic C, Attal N, Denys P, Markabi S, Bussel B. Carbamazepine in agitation and aggressive behaviour following severe closed-head injury: results of an open trial. *Brain Inj.* 1999;13(10):797–804.

54. Kim E, Bijlani M. A pilot study of quetiapine treatment of aggression due to traumatic brain injury. *J Neuropsychiatr Clin Neurosci.* 2006;18(4):547–549.

55. Umene-Nakano W, Yoshimura R, Okamoto T, Hori H, Nakamura J. Aripiprazole improves various cognitive and behavioral impairments after traumatic brain injury: a case report. *Gen Hosp Psychiatr.* 2013;35(1):103.e7–103.e9.

56. Gualtieri CT. Buspirone: neuropsychiatric effects. *J Head Trauma Rehabil.* 1991;6(1):90–92.

57. Elliott FA. Propranolol for the control of belligerent behavior following acute brain damage. *Ann Neurol.* 1977; 1(5):489–491.

58. Halbauer JD, Ashford JW, Zeitzer JM, Adamson MM, Lew HL, Yesavage JA. Neuropsychiatric diagnosis and management of chronic sequelae of war-related mild to moderate traumatic brain injury. *J Rehabil Res Dev.* 2009;46(6): 757–796.

59. Ragsdale KA, Voss Horrell SC. Effectiveness of prolonged exposure and cognitive processing therapy for U.S. veterans with a history of traumatic brain injury. *J Trauma Stress.* 2016;29(5):474–477.

60. Chard KM, Schumm JA, McIlvain SM, Bailey GW, Parkinson RB. Exploring the efficacy of a residential treatment program incorporating cognitive processing therapy-cognitive for veterans with PTSD and traumatic brain injury. *J Trauma Stress.* 2011;24(3):347–351.

61. Wolf GK, Strom TQ, Kehle SM, Eftekhari A. A preliminary examination of prolonged exposure therapy with Iraq and Afghanistan veterans with a diagnosis of posttraumatic stress disorder and mild to moderate traumatic brain injury. *J Head Trauma Rehabil.* 2012;27(1):26–32.

62. Wolf GK, Kretzmer T, Crawford E, et al. Prolonged exposure therapy with veterans and active duty personnel diagnosed with PTSD and traumatic brain injury. *J Trauma Stress.* 2015;28(4):339–347.

63. McAllister TW. Psychopharmacological issues in the treatment of TBI and PTSD. *Clin Neuropsychol.* 2009;23(8):1338–1367.

64. Kennedy JE, Jaffee MS, Cooper DB. Posttraumatic stress disorder. In: Arciniegas DB, Zasler ND, Vanderplog RD, Jaffee MS, eds. *Management of Adults with Traumatic Brain Injury.* Washington, DC: American Psychiatric Publishing; 2013:213–238.

65. Bogdanov S, Naismith S, Lah S. Sleep outcomes following sleep-hygiene-related interventions for individuals with traumatic brain injury: a systematic review. *Brain Inj.* 2017;31(4):422–433.

66. Batty R, Rossell S, Francis A, Ponsford J. Psychosis following traumatic brain injury. *Brain Impair.* 2013;14(1):21–41.

67. Fujii DE, Ahmed I. Risk factors in psychosis secondary to traumatic brain injury. *J Neuropsychiatr Clin Neurosci.* 2001;13(1):61–69.

68. Rabner J, Gottlieb S, Lazdowsky L, LeBel A. Psychosis following traumatic brain injury and cannabis use in late adolescence. *Am J Addict.* 2016;25(2):91–93.

69. Jain S, Srivastava A. Frontal lobe abnormality and psychosis in traumatic brain injury and cannabis abuse. *ASEAN J Psychiatr.* 2017;18(1):21–24.

70. Wolkin A, Malaspina D, Perrin M, McAllister TW, Corcoran C. Psychotic disorders. In: Silver JM, McAlister TW, Yudofsky SC, eds. *Textbook of Traumatic Brain Injury.* 2nd ed. Arlington, VA: American Psychiatric Association; 2011:189–198.

71. Rao V, Spiro JR, Schretlen DJ, Cascella NG. Apathy syndrome after traumatic brain injury compared with deficits in schizophrenia. *Psychosomatics.* 2007;48(3):217–222.

72. Lane-Brown AT, Tate RL. Measuring apathy after traumatic brain injury: psychometric properties of the apathy evaluation scale and the frontal systems behavior scale. *Brain Inj.* 2009;23(13–14):999–1007.

73. Ciurli P, Formisano R, Bivona U, Cantagallo A, Angelelli P. Neuropsychiatric disorders in persons with severe traumatic brain injury: prevalence, phenomenology, and relationship with demographic, clinical, and functional features. *J Head Trauma Rehabil.* 2011;26(2):116–126.

74. Arciniegas DB, Silver JM. Psychopharmacology. In: Silver JM, McAlister TW, Yudofsky SC, eds. *Textbook of Traumatic Brain Injury.* 2nd ed. Arlington, VA: American Psychiatric Association; 2011:553–570.

75. Lane-Brown A, Tate R. Interventions for apathy after traumatic brain injury. *Cochrane Database Syst Rev.* 2009;(2):Cd006341.

76. Grafman J, Schwab K, Warden D, Pridgen A, Brown HR, Salazar AM. Frontal lobe injuries, violence, and aggression: a report of the Vietnam head injury study. *Neurology.* 1996;46(5):1231–1238.

77. Tateno A, Jorge RE, Robinson RG. Clinical correlates of aggressive behavior after traumatic brain injury. *J Neuropsychiatr Clin Neurosci.* 2003;15(2):155–160.

78. Wortzel HS, Arciniegas DB. A forensic neuropsychiatric approach to traumatic brain injury, aggression, and suicide. *J Am Acad Psychiatr Law.* 2013;41(2):274–286.

CHAPTER 11

Pharmacologic Management of the Patient With Traumatic Brain Injury

DAVID L. RIPLEY, MD, MS • SANGEETA DRIVER, MD, MPH •
RYAN STORK, MD • MITHRA MANEYAPANDA, MD

Medication management for individuals who have sustained a traumatic brain injury (TBI) remains one of the most confusing, challenging, and rewarding areas of medicine. The challenges associated with the management of these individuals is understandable; the human brain is perhaps the most complex and poorly understood structure in the universe. We are only beginning to appreciate the nuances of its function.

To add further complexity to the situation, no two injuries are exactly alike. Our current crude method of classification of brain injury into "mild, moderate, and severe" categories remains woefully inadequate. The challenges brought on by the complexity of this situation has manifest itself in the generally scant objective evidence to support the use of medications following brain injury. Because the situation is far more complex than "mild, moderate, and severe," and researchers continue to group together many individuals in the same category, the resulting output has been numerous failed trials and inadequate objective information to guide clinicians in "evidence-based practice."

Despite this, through careful observation and collection of a plethora of anecdotal information, as well as borrowing from experience in treatment and research into medical management of other neurologic conditions, some generalities can be gleaned. This chapter will focus on what is generally considered the standard of practice for medication administration in the rehabilitation of individuals following TBI.

PHILOSOPHY OF MEDICATION MANAGEMENT AFTER BRAIN INJURY: GENERAL GUIDELINES

There are some general concepts regarding medication management after TBI that are important to follow when possible. In today's medical care climate, with pressures placed on the pace of rehabilitation by our current reimbursement system, these concepts

are getting harder to follow. However, these guidelines should be followed whenever possible.

*It is more important what **not** to give than what **to** give*

Given the complexity of the brain, as well as the nuances associated with its injury, there is a strong argument to do nothing. Knowing that the brain will recover neurologically to a large degree without any medication, rehabilitation efforts should be focused on standard therapy and biological support. In fact, there may be more evidence regarding the potential harm that certain classes of medications may do to the recovering brain. Understanding the harmful impact that these medications may have, and avoiding these medications, may in the long run have more benefit to these patients than even administrating other ones.

Err on the side of cognition

Often, clinicians are faced with a choice between treating a condition associated with TBI and the potentially adverse consequences of the treatment. A perfect example of this is spasticity management. Therapy staff will often strongly encourage physicians to administer antispasticity medications in an attempt to improve some aspect of a patient's function. However, almost all of these medications have untoward cognitive side effects. Often, a choice must be made between *cognitive function* and *physical function*. When given this choice, directing your actions on improving cognitive function is usually preferred when caring for patients with brain injury.

Pick a direction and go with it

There are often patients who present with two or more competing problems, wherein treating one may worsen another. A clinician needs to avoid the temptation to place a patient on two different medications with competing pharmacologic mechanisms of action; for example, do not place a patient on both a pro- and an antidopaminergic medication at the same time. In these cases, *de duobus malis minus eligendum*—pick the lesser of two evils and go that direction. Additionally, the previous rule applies—err on the side of cognition. In many cases, *doing nothing* may be the most appropriate course of action.

One change at a time

It is best to start making one change and observing the effects before making another change, either adding or removing a medication or making dose adjustments.

Start low, go slow

This rule may be the most difficult to follow in today's fast-paced rehabilitation environment. However, following injury, nerve cells are lost, affecting the neurotransmitter levels and the presence of receptors and the nerves that they work on, making any medication administration effect potentially different from that in an uninjured brain. It is imperative to be judicious in the initial dosing of medication.

Observe the effects of your changes carefully

It is important to closely monitor the changes that each change has in the patient's cognitive and functional performance. Patients may exhibit effects from medication administration that will be unexpected.

Be willing to change direction if results necessitate it

Keep in mind that the injured brain may not respond to medications normally. Disrupted pathways, insufficient receptors, and breakdown of the blood-brain barrier are some of the many factors that may change the way the individual responds to medication administration. Carefully observe if the medication is having the intended effect, or in some cases, a different effect altogether. The astute clinician must be willing to change direction when the clinical circumstances require it.

COGNITION
Disorders of Consciousness and Hypoarousal

Recent research into disorders of consciousness (DOC) has resulted in an exponential increase in the understanding of this problem. There is now potential for cautious optimism where previously there was little to no hope for individuals with DOC following TBI. The findings in research on patients with DOC has led to treatments that are useful in individuals with hypoarousal and slowed cognitive processing speed following brain injury as well. Arousal is the foundation

upon which every other cognitive function in the brain rests. Therefore improving arousal is the most basic facet of improving cognitive function following TBI.

Amantadine is an antiviral agent with antiparkinsonian actions. Its mechanism of action is not fully understood, but it appears to increase dopamine availability in the central nervous system (CNS) and also acts as a weak *N*-methyl-D-aspartate (NMDA) antagonist. It has been shown to improve arousal in patients with moderate to severe TBI.[1] In a placebo-controlled trial of 184 patients in a vegetative or minimally conscious state 1–4 months from TBI, patients received for 4 weeks either amantadine or placebo while in the inpatient rehabilitation setting. Those in the treatment group had an increased rate of recovery as measured by the Disability Rating Scale (DRS) during the 4-week treatment period. Overall improvement in DRS was similar between the groups at 6 weeks.[2] In a placebo-controlled, crossover study of 35 subjects in the acute phase after TBI, a trend toward more rapid functional improvement was demonstrated during the 6-week amantadine treatment.[3]

Bromocriptine is a dopamine agonist at the dopamine type 2 receptor. It was noted to improve arousal in a small, retrospective chart review of five patients in vegetative state.[4] Bromocriptine may also have dual use as an agent to improve autonomic instability in individuals exhibiting dysautonomia in association with impaired level of arousal.

Levodopa/carbidopa has also been used in DOC. Levodopa is a precursor of dopamine. Carbidopa is a decarboxylase inhibitor that inhibits the peripheral conversion of levodopa to dopamine and increases the availability of levodopa in the CNS. Haig and Ruess reported the case of a 24-year-old man in a vegetative state 6 months after TBI who, within days of starting levodopa/carbidopa, became responsive and conversant.[5] Additionally, Matsuda et al. reported four cases of patients in persistent vegetative states and one case of a patient in a minimally conscious state who had improved responsiveness when levodopa was initiated for parkinsonian symptoms.[6,7] A prospective study of eight patients in the vegetative state for an average duration of 104 days after TBI showed improvement in consciousness, with seven patients recovering consciousness with incremental doses of levodopa.[8]

Modafinil is a CNS stimulant that promotes wakefulness through an unclear mechanism of action. In a recent small retrospective pilot study, modafinil was associated with improved arousal in patients with prolonged DOC.[9] The efficacy of modafinil for treating fatigue and excessive daytime sleepiness (EDS) in patients with chronic TBI has also been investigated. In a small placebo-controlled, double-blind pilot study, administration of modafinil for 6 weeks improved EDS, but not fatigue.[10] In contrast, a double-blind, placebo-controlled crossover trial of 53 patients with TBI at least 1 year postinjury found that modafinil (400 mg daily) had no significant effect on EDS or fatigue.[11]

Zolpidem is a nonbenzodiazepine sedative-hypnotic that acts as a γ-aminobutyric acid (GABA) agonist with preferential binding to the ω-1 receptor. Several case reports have reported a paradoxical increase in arousal with the use of zolpidem in patients with DOC.[12–21] A placebo-controlled, double-blind, single-dose, crossover study of 84 patients with DOC for at least 4 months found a temporary response in 4.8% of patients after a 10 mg dose of zolpidem. Responders could not be distinguished from nonresponders based on demographic or clinical features.[20] The temporary response may necessitate more frequent dosing to maintain arousal.

Methylphenidate is a CNS stimulant that increases dopamine and norepinephrine levels by blocking reuptake. Few studies have investigated its effect on improving arousal. Martin and Whyte performed a meta-analysis of a series of single-subject repeated crossover trials in 22 patients with DOC secondary to brain injury and found no significant effect of methylphenidate on responsiveness or command following.[22] However, another study demonstrated that individuals with severe TBI had shorter intensive care unit and total hospital lengths of stay.[23] The hypothesis behind this effect is that methylphenidate improved the level of arousal in individuals who received it, allowing them to progress more quickly. Methylphenidate is associated with numerous anecdotal reports of improved arousal and is frequently used in this setting by clinicians. However, clinicians must exercise caution with this medication early after injury because it may exacerbate autonomic dysfunction, particularly tachycardia and hypertension.

Additional dopaminergic agents that have been investigated in DOC include pramipexole and apomorphine. Patrick et al. performed a small randomized, double-blind trial with 10 children and adolescents who were treated with either pramipexole or amantadine. Both groups showed improvement, and there was no difference in arousal between the two medications.[24] In an open-label pilot study, subcutaneous apomorphine was continuously infused in eight patients in vegetative or minimally conscious state after TBI. Improvements were seen within 1 day to 1 month, and seven patients recovered consciousness.[25]

There have also been limited reports suggesting improvement in arousal in patients with DOC with intrathecal baclofen therapy.[26–28]

Attention and Processing Speed

Disorders of attention and processing speed are extremely common following brain injury. Impairments in attention and processing speed have effects on many downstream cognitive functions, such as memory and executive function. Attempts to treat attention problems are often a focus of clinicians trying to improve the overall cognitive function in individuals following brain injury. Most clinicians utilize medications that are typically used for attention disorders in other non-TBI populations. Unfortunately, despite much anecdotal evidence of efficacy, there is little objective evidence supporting the use of particular medications for attention problems following TBI.

Methylphenidate is probably the single medication most widely studied for use for various problems after TBI. Several studies have supported the use of methylphenidate to improve attention and/or processing speed after brain injury. In a randomized controlled trial of 34 patients with moderate to severe TBI in the postacute phase of recovery, 6 weeks of methylphenidate resulted in an increase in processing speed and attentiveness with some on-task behaviors.[29] In a randomized, crossover, double-blind study of 40 patients with moderate to severe TBI in the postacute phase, methylphenidate (0.3 mg/kg twice a day) demonstrated improvement in processing speed.[30] A smaller prospective multiple baseline design study demonstrated improved attention with methylphenidate in patients in the subacute phase of acquired brain injury.[31] Additionally, a randomized, placebo-controlled, double-blind trial in 23 patients in the subacute phase after complicated mild to moderately severe TBI showed an improvement in attention with 30 days of methylphenidate.[32]

Dextroamphetamine is another CNS stimulant that has been studied in patients with TBI with attentional impairments. In a single-subject double-blind, placebo-controlled crossover study, dextroamphetamine resulted in improved cognitive processing efficiency in a patient with TBI 5 years earlier.[33] A retrospective chart review of patients with severe TBI reported a positive effect on attention with dextroamphetamine.[34] Lisdexamfetamine dimesylate, a prodrug of dextroamphetamine, has recently been studied in the moderate to severe TBI population. A randomized, double-blind, placebo controlled crossover trial of 13 patients in the postacute phase of injury demonstrated improvement in sustained attention and working memory with lisdexamfetamine dimesylate.[35]

Donepezil is an acetylcholinesterase inhibitor that is commonly used in the treatment of Alzheimer disease. One randomized, placebo-controlled crossover trial of patients in the postacute period after TBI demonstrated improvement in attention with donepezil.[36] A smaller case series of patients with chronic TBI reported significant improvement in processing speed, learning, and divided attention with donepezil.[37]

Atomoxetine is a selective norepinephrine reuptake inhibitor used for the treatment of attention-deficit/hyperactivity disorder. There have been limited investigations for its use in TBI, but there is much anecdotal evidence supporting its efficacy for attention disorders following TBI.[38] One randomized, placebo-controlled, crossover trial of patients with chronic moderate to severe TBI with subjective attentional difficulties demonstrated no improvement in attention with 2 weeks of atomoxetine therapy.[39]

Bromocriptine is also a medication that has been used to treat attentional deficits following TBI. Like other medications, however, objective evidence is lacking. One double-blind, placebo-controlled, crossover pilot study investigating the effect of bromocriptine on attention in patients with moderate to severe TBI was conducted in the postacute period of recovery. No improvement in attention was found with bromocriptine treatment.[40]

Like other dopaminergic medications, amantadine has also been used for attention impairment. In a series of patients with frontal lobe dysfunction, improved attention with amantadine treatment was demonstrated.[41] Conversely, in a small double-blind, placebo-controlled, crossover trial of 10 patients with moderate to severe TBI in the subacute phase of recovery, amantadine demonstrated no effect on attention.[42]

Citicoline is available in the United States as a nutraceutical and has been used clinically outside the United States for many years for stroke and head trauma. A large, randomized, double-blind trial of 1213 patients with mild to severe TBI demonstrated no difference in attention, processing speed, memory, or functional status with 90 days of citicoline compared with placebo.[43]

Memory

Memory impairment is also very common following TBI with up to 80% found to have ongoing problems with memory following TBI.[44] This is frequently cited as one of the most "problematic" long-term issues following TBI.

The mainstay of treatment of memory disorder following TBI are the acetylcholinesterase inhibitors. These medications act by preventing the breakdown of acetylcholine in the synapse, making it more bioavailable. This effect is hypothesized to occur primarily in the hippocampus. Originally this effect was noted with physostigmine.[45,46] However, the effect is too short-acting to be practical for most patients. Donepezil is currently the most commonly used medication in this class, with most research evidence supporting its use. A randomized, placebo-controlled crossover trial demonstrated memory improvement in the postacute period after TBI with donepezil.[36] Notably, in the initial treatment group, improvements were sustained after the washout period and placebo phase, suggesting a carryover effect of donepezil. This effect has also been observed clinically. A smaller study using a single-subject research design also demonstrated improvement in memory with donepezil.[47] Similarly, a single-subject multiple baseline design study of three adolescents with severe TBI demonstrated improved memory with donepezil.[48]

Rivastigmine is another acetylcholinesterase inhibitor that has been studied in patients with TBI with persistent cognitive impairment. Objective evidence of efficacy, however, is lacking. In a large, randomized, double-blind, placebo-controlled trial of 157 patients with mild to severe TBI, no significant difference was found in cognition with rivastigmine treatment.[49] A posthoc analysis of more severely impaired patients found some significant improvements in the rivastigmine group. In a randomized, double-blind, placebo-controlled crossover trial of patients with mild to severe TBI, no significant improvement was found with rivastigmine treatment in the majority of computerized neuropsychologic tests. Significant improvement was also reported in subtraction test and 10- to 15-min vigilance test.[50]

Galantamine is another acetylcholinesterase inhibitor that has been utilized for memory dysfunction following TBI. No human subject trials have been performed, although anecdotal evidence suggests that it is effective. A rodent study demonstrated cognitive improvement following TBI.[51]

Memantine is an NMDA antagonist that is indicated for moderate to severe Alzheimer dementia. Anecdotal evidence suggests that it has efficacy for improving memory impairment in individuals with TBI. Although no human studies have been done for patients with TBI, rodent studies demonstrate evidence of neuroprotective effects following brain trauma.[52,53] Anecdotal reports indicate that some patients may have irritability and worsening behavior problems with memantine.

Ginkgo is a dietary supplement that is derived from the *Ginkgo biloba* tree and has been reported to have neuroprotective and cognition-enhancing proper-ties.[54,55] At this time no studies investigating its use in humans with TBI have been published.

Methylphenidate is often used to enhance general cognitive performance, including memory. Its mecha-nism is likely "upstream" improvements in atten-tion and processing speed rather than direct effect on memory function. However, in a double-blind, placebo-controlled trial, a single dose of methylphe-nidate (20 mg) resulted in significant improvement in working memory and visuospatial attention compared with placebo.[56] In contrast, two randomized controlled trials have reported no effect of methylphenidate on memory after TBI.[32,57]

Executive Functioning

There have been a limited number of studies investi-gating potential pharmacotherapies for executive dys-function after brain injury. One case study reported improvements in executive function in a patient 5 years post-TBI with amantadine. Further improve-ments were noted with the addition of levodopa/car-bidopa.[41] An open-label study of patients with chronic TBI reported significant improvements in executive function with amantadine treatment (400 mg daily). Positron emission tomography was performed on six of these patients and demonstrated increased left pre-frontal cortex glucose metabolism with treatment.[58]

Additionally, a randomized, double-blind, placebo-controlled crossover trial of patients with severe TBI demonstrated improvement in executive function with low-dose bromocriptine.[59]

Aphasia

The role of pharmacotherapies in the treatment of aphasia and communication impairments post-TBI has not been established. In patients with poststroke aphasia, several investigations have studied the effect of medications that augment catecholaminergic and cholinergic functions. Medications that may aid in the improvement of poststroke aphasia include done-pezil,[60,61] galantamine,[62] dextroamphetamine,[63,64] memantine,[65] and piracetam.[66–68] Studies of the effec-tiveness of bromocriptine and levodopa have been mixed (Table 11.1).[69–72]

Agitation

Agitation is a common occurrence following a TBI. Due to a lack of consensus on a singular definition, the incidence has been reported to range from 11% to 70% following a moderate to severe injury.[73,74] In 1997, a survey of the Brain Injury Special Interest Group of the American Academy of Physical Medicine and Rehabili-tation was conducted to determine national patterns of defining agitation.[75] Following this survey, a unify-ing definition for posttraumatic agitation was devised.

TABLE 11.1
Medications for Cognition

Problem	Medication	Dosing (Start/Max)	Common Side Effects	Comments
Hypoarousal	Amantadine	Start: 100 mg bid Max: 200 mg bid dose in the morning and at noon	Dizziness, insomnia, nausea	Contraindicated in preg-nancy, breastfeeding; likely epileptogenic
	Bromocriptine	Start: 2.5 mg bid Max: 10 mg bid Dose in the morning and noon	Nausea, constipation	Uncontrolled hyperten-sion, breast feeding, preeclampsia
	Levodopa/Carbidopa	Start: 50 mg/25 mg bid	Constipation, dizziness, orthostatic hypotension	Contraindicated in closed-angle glaucoma, MAOi therapy, mela-noma
	Zolpidem	Start: 5 mg daily Max dose for paradoxical arousal is unknown	Sedation	Only effective in select subpopulation with dis-order of consciousness
	Modafinil	Start: 100 mg bid Max: 200 mg bid Dose in the morning and at noon	Headache, nausea	

Continued

TABLE 11.1
Medications for Cognition—cont'd

Problem	Medication	Dosing (Start/Max)	Common Side Effects	Comments
Attention and processing speed	Methylphenidate	Start: 10 mg bid Max: 72 mg/day Various formulations	Anorexia, nausea, vomiting, insomnia	May worsen anxiety, glaucoma, contraindicated with MAOi therapy; concern for abuse
	Atomoxetine	Start: 18 mg daily Max: 100 mg daily	Xerostomia, nausea, insomnia	Closed-angle glaucoma, MAOi therapy, pheochromocytoma
	Dextroamphetamine	Start: 5 mg daily Max: 60 mg daily	Headache, irritability, insomnia, anorexia	Substance abuse, glaucoma, hyperthyroidism, MAOi therapy, arteriosclerosis
	Lisdexamfetamine	Start: 30 mg daily Max: 70 mg daily	Anorexia, insomnia, irritability, xerostomia	Contraindicated in MAOi therapy
Memory	Donepezil	Start: 5 mg daily Max: 10 mg daily	Diarrhea, insomnia, nausea, headache	
	Rivastigmine	Start: 1.5 mg bid Max: 6 mg bid	Diarrhea, nausea, vomiting, anorexia, dizziness	
	Galantamine	Start: 4 mg bid Max: 12 mg bid	Diarrhea, nausea, vomiting,	
	Memantine	Start: 5 mg daily Max: 10 mg bid	Headache, diarrhea, dizziness	Has been associated with increased irritability in TBI

bid, twice daily; *MAOi*, monoamine oxidase inhibitor; *Max*, maximum; *TBI*, traumatic brain injury.

Posttraumatic agitation was defined as "a subtype of delirium unique to survivors of a TBI in which the survivor is in the state of post-traumatic amnesia and there are excesses of behavior that include some combination of aggression, akathisia or inner restlessness that may manifest in motor activity, disinhibition, and/or emotional lability."[76]

Addressing posttraumatic agitation is a critical component of brain injury rehabilitation. The first step to accurate diagnosis and treatment is the identification of factors that may be contributing to or confounding the diagnosis such as pain, infections and metabolic derangements, atypical seizure activity, endocrine dysfunction such as hyperthyroidism, and drug or alcohol withdrawal.[77] Once such factors are corrected, environmental and behavioral modifications should be utilized as first-line treatment. Promoting good sleep patterns and sleep hygiene is of critical importance. In addition, minimizing sensory stimulation can help mitigate agitation. Examples include reducing ambient noise, dimming lights, and limiting the number of individuals

interacting with a patient to avoid overstimulation. For patients with akathisia, allowing freedom of movement through supervised ambulation or wheelchair mobility may help behavior. Physical restraints can worsen agitation and should be avoided whenever possible. If restraints are necessary due to patient safety concerns, less restrictive restraints such as bed enclosures, wheelchair wraparound belts, and soft mitts should be utilized. Finally, a structured behavioral plan may help in identifying precipitating behaviors and providing clinical staff with safe techniques for intervention.

Pharmacologic interventions may need to be utilized if a patient continues to be at risk for self-harm or causing harm to others despite environmental and behavioral modification. Certain classes of medications including typical antipsychotics and benzodiazepines should generally be avoided because of their potential to impair neurorecovery.[78,79] A 2006 Cochrane review found nonselective β-blockers such as propranolol to have the most evidence for treatment of posttraumatic agitation.[80] This medication also treats posttraumatic

TABLE 11.2
Medications for Agitation

Medication	Starting Dose	Common Side Effects	Comments
Propranolol	10 mg prn	Sedation, hypotension, bradycardia, orthostasis	Also helpful for dysautonomia
Trazodone	25 mg prn	Sedation, priapism	Avoid high doses
Valproic acid	125 mg bid	Hepatic impairment, sedation, weight gain, rash	
Carbamazepine	100 mg bid	Blood dyscrasias, Syndrome of Inappropriate AntiDiuretic Hormone Release (SIADH), hepatic impairment, rash	
Risperidone	0.5 mg prn	Sedation, akathisia, metabolic impairment	
Quetiapine	25 mg prn	Sedation, anticholinergic side effects	May result in confusion in elderly patients
Olanzapine	2.5 mg prn	Sedation, rash, metabolic impairment, weight gain, hypotension, dizziness	Available as injection; may have a paradoxical arousal effect at low doses
Ziprasidone	Oral 20 mg prn IM 10 mg prn	QT prolongation, hypotension, dizziness, electrolyte disturbance, metabolic changes, akathisia	
Buspirone	5 mg bid	Dizziness, nausea, headache, nervousness, light-headedness.	Contraindicated with MAOi
Amantadine	100 mg daily	Dizziness, insomnia, nausea	Contraindicated in pregnancy, breastfeeding; Is likely epileptogenic

bid, twice daily; *IM*, intramuscular; *MAOi*, monoamine oxidase inhibitor.

autonomic dysregulation and therefore serves as an ideal medication choice for patients with concurrent issues. Side effects to monitor for include hypotension and bradycardia. Trazodone, a commonly used sleep agent, may be effective in decreasing agitation and can be utilized in the inpatient rehabilitation setting as a first-line "as-needed" agent during episodes of increased agitation and is often the drug of choice of "experts" in the field of brain injury medicine.[81] Mood stabilizers such as valproic acid and carbamazepine can also be utilized. A retrospective study demonstrated decreased agitation within 1 week of valproic acid administration in over 90% of sampled patients.[82] Potential adverse effects may include medication toxicity, hepatotoxicity, and thrombocytopenia. In addition to valproic acid, studies have demonstrated the effectiveness of carbamazepine in treating posttraumatic agitation.[83,84] Potential adverse effects may include medication toxicity, renal failure, hyponatremia, and hematologic dysfunction. In addition, the possible teratogenic side effects of mood stabilizers must be considered with use in the female population. Atypical antipsychotics such as risperidone and quetiapine have also been utilized in the treatment of agitation. These agents are generally favored over typical antipsychotics given less dopamine blockade, which results in a safer side effect profile and less potential for extrapyramidal symptoms, and multiple studies suggesting impairment in neurologic and functional recovery with typical antipsychotics. Antidepressants such as selective serotonin reuptake inhibitors (SSRIs) have been reported to reduce post-TBI aggression and irritability.[85] In addition, buspirone, a serotonin 1A receptor partial agonist, may be useful in addressing agitation related to anxiety.[86] Interestingly, neurostimulants such as amantadine are increasingly being trialed for the treatment of posttraumatic agitation given that irritability and aggression may partially stem from slowed cognitive processing speed and the inability to effectively process sensory information (Table 11.2).[87,88]

SLEEP DISTURBANCE

Sleep disturbances have been reported in up to 70% of patients with TBI.[89] Regulating sleep is vital to cognitive recovery and is often the first point of intervention in the acute inpatient rehabilitation setting.

TBIs can result in a variety of sleep-wake disorders including insomnia, EDS, narcolepsy, sleep-related breathing disorders, and circadian rhythm sleep disorders

(CRSD). Insomnia is a common post-TBI sleep disorder, reported in 30%–60% of patients.[90] It is characterized by difficulty falling asleep or maintaining sleep. EDS has been reported in 14%–57% of patients[90] and is defined by the American Academy of Sleep Medicine as the inability to maintain wakefulness and alertness during the major waking episodes of the day. Of note, EDS must be differentiated from fatigue, which is a subjective lack of mental or physical energy. Narcolepsy is a less prevalent post-TBI sleep disorder, which involves poor control of sleep-wake cycles with rapid eye movement sleep intrusion into the wake state. Classically, it involves a tetrad of symptoms including EDS, cataplexy (a sudden and transient episode of muscle weakness), hypnagogic or hypnopompic hallucinations (visual or auditory perceptions upon falling or awakening from sleep), and sleep paralysis.[91] Sleep-related breathing disorders can occur following TBI and include obstructive sleep apnea caused by upper airway obstruction or central sleep apnea, which involves an intermittent neurologically mediated loss of respiratory effort. CRSD have also been reported following TBI and are defined as a mismatch between endogenous sleep-wake rhythms and the 24-h external light-darkness cycle. Often, melatonin secretion and body temperature are altered in CRSD.[90]

The diagnosis and treatment of post-TBI sleep disorders is a critical component of brain injury rehabilitation. The evaluation of sleep disturbances should first involve a comprehensive clinical interview. The interview should obtain key information related to pre- and postinjury patterns of sleep, sleep quality and quantity, the presence of EDS and daytime napping, and a review of systems to assess for other factors that may be contributing to the sleep disturbance. Such factors may include pain, mood disturbances, bowel and bladder dysfunction, movement disorders, medications, and the intake of other substances including caffeine, alcohol, and nicotine. In addition to the clinical interview, other subjective and objective measures may aid in diagnosis. Common subjective measures used include sleep diaries, sleep logs, and self-report questionnaires such as the Pittsburgh Sleep Quality Index and the Insomnia Severity Index for assessment of sleep quality and insomnia, the Epworth Sleepiness Scale for EDS, and the Morningness-Evening-ness or Sleep Timing Questionnaires for CRSD. Objective measures include polysomnography and actigraphy.

The treatment of post-TBI sleep disorders usually requires a multifactorial approach including both nonpharmacologic and pharmacologic interventions. First, environmental and behavioral changes should be instituted to promote sleep hygiene. This includes developing a regular sleep schedule, following a daily bedtime routine, creating a restful bedroom environment with minimal light and optimal temperature, avoiding late night screen time, minimizing daytime napping, engaging in daily exercise, and limiting evening caffeine, alcohol, and nicotine intake. Other nonpharmacologic treatments supported by the literature include cognitive behavioral therapy, acupuncture, and bright light therapy. Finally, Continuous Positive Airway Pressure (CPAP) should be utilized for the treatment of sleep-related breathing disorders such as obstructive sleep apnea.

Certain classes of sleep medications are generally avoided in the TBI population because of potential adverse effects. Benzodiazepines may impair neurologic recovery as noted in prior animal studies[92,93] and can cause daytime sedation and anterograde amnesia. Anticholinergic medications such as tricyclic antidepressants (TCAs) and diphenhydramine can have detrimental cognitive side effects and potentially lower the seizure threshold.[94]

Trazodone is often used to promote sleep maintenance following a TBI. At lower doses, it acts as an effective hypnotic agent by blocking 5-hydroxytryptamine (HT)2A receptors and H1 histamine and α1 adrenergic receptors.[95] Melatonin has also been utilized in the treatment of TBI-related sleep disturbances. A 2016 study found that patients with TBI showed 42% less melatonin production overnight compared with healthy controls,[96] and a preliminary trial found that the use of melatonin was associated with improved daytime alertness.[97] Ramelteon is a melatonin receptor agonist approved by the Food and Drug Administration for the treatment of insomnia with sleep onset abnormalities. Preliminary evidence from a double-blind placebo-controlled trial demonstrated improvements in total sleep time and some aspects of cognitive functioning following a 3-week trial of ramelteon.[98] Other nonbenzodiazepine agents such as zolpidem and eszopiclone have been utilized to promote sleep initiation and maintenance following a TBI, although there are little data describing its effectiveness in this patient population. Amitriptyline is often useful for sleep and concomitant headache, but cognitive impairment and anticholinergic side effects limit its usefulness. It is frequently used with success for individuals with mild TBI. Finally, mirtazapine may be considered for use in patients with concomitant mood and appetite disturbances (Table 11.3).

MOOD AND PSYCHIATRIC ISSUES

Patients who have sustained a TBI may exhibit a number of comorbid psychiatric issues during their recovery. In many cases, treatment is the same as it would be

TABLE 11.3
Medications for Sleep

Medication	Dosing (Start/Max)	Common Side Effects	Comments
Trazodone	Start: 25 mg Max: 200 mg Dose once at bedtime	Sedation, priapism	Higher doses may result in antihistaminic effects
Melatonin	Start: 2 mg Max: unknown	Drowsiness	Timing of dosing is important
Ramelteon	Start: 8 mg Max: 8 mg	Depression, hallucinations, somnambulation, amnesia, hypogonadism	
Zolpidem	Start: 5 mg Max: 10 mg	Somnambulation, dizziness, headache	
Eszopiclone	Start: 1 mg Max: 3 mg	Behavior change, headache, unpleasant taste	Caution with liver impairment
Amitriptyline	Start: 25 mg Max: 150 mg	Anticholinergic side effects, worsening confusion	Avoid with moderate to severe TBI
Mirtazapine	Start: 15 mg Max: 45 mg	Suicidality, orthostatic hypotension, dizziness, weight gain, hepatic impairment	Case reports of agranulocytosis, contraindicated with MAOis

MAOis, monoamine oxidase inhibitors; *TBI,* traumatic brain injury.

for idiopathic psychiatric issues, with some reservations based on the need to keep in mind the concepts of neuroplasticity and recovery. Many psychotropic medications have adverse effects on neurologic and functional recovery, which must be kept in mind.

A review was conducted of psychotropic medications used for patients following moderate to severe TBI in an inpatient rehabilitation setting.[99] In a sample of 2130 patients, the most frequently administered medications were narcotic analgesics (72% of sample), followed by antidepressants (67%), anticonvulsants (47%), anxiolytics (33%), hypnotics (30%), stimulants (28%), antipsychotics (25%), and antiparkinson agents (25%). This study indicated that the use of psychotropic medications increased, rather than decreased, during the course of rehabilitation. Males and more severely impaired individuals tended to receive more psychotropic medications than other groups.

Depression

As many as 90% of individuals who have sustained brain injury will experience a transient episode of depression,[100] making it the most common mood disorder following TBI. In one study, 42% of patients referred for rehabilitation following TBI met the *Diagnostic and Statistical Manual of Mental Disorders* (Fourth Edition) criteria for major depression.[101] In a 15-year follow-up, approximately 1% of individuals with TBI will commit suicide.[102] Antidepressant medications, therefore, are some of the most commonly prescribed medications in post-TBI care.[99]

There is general consensus among clinicians who care for individuals with TBI that antidepressant medications, particularly the SSRIs, facilitate neurologic recovery following TBI. However, objective evidence to support this is lacking, and in fact, one study demonstrated longer lengths of stay in inpatient rehabilitation for individuals who were prescribed antidepressants during their rehab stay.[103]

In general, because of their favorable side effect profile, and general lack of cognitive side effects, SSRIs are considered the drug class of choice for depression following TBI. There are several medications in this class. Sertraline, citalopram, and escitalopram are preferred because of better side effect profiles, quicker onset of action, and less sedation than other medications in this class, such as fluoxetine and paroxetine. This class has the added benefit of a secondary indication for anxiety as well.

The newer, serotonin-norepinephrine reuptake inhibitors (SNRIs) are also considered effective choices for depression. Medications in this class include duloxetine and venlafaxine. These medications have the added benefit of being effective treatments for neuropathic pain.

TABLE 11.4
Medications for Depression

Medication	Dosing (Start/Max)	Common Side Effects	Comments
Sertraline	Start: 50 mg daily Max: 200 mg daily	Nausea, diarrhea, tremor, decreased libido	Contraindicated with MAOis, monitor for serotonin syndrome
Citalopram	Start: 20 mg daily Max: 40 mg daily	QT prolongation, nausea, dizziness, decreased libido	Contraindicated with MAOis, monitor for serotonin syndrome
Escitalopram	Start: 10 mg daily Max: 20 mg daily	Suicide risk, nausea, diarrhea, insomnia, decreased libido	Contraindicated with MAOis, monitor for serotonin syndrome
Paroxetine	Start: 20 mg daily Max: 50 mg daily	Asthenia, sweating, nausea, diarrhea, decreased appetite, somnolence, dizziness, tremor, dry mouth, decreased libido	Contraindicated with MAOis, monitor for serotonin syndrome
Fluoxetine	Start: 20 mg daily Max: 60 mg daily	Unusual dreams, decreased libido, anorexia, tremor	Contraindicated with MAOis, monitor for serotonin syndrome
Amitriptyline	Start: 25 mg daily Max: 200 mg daily	Anticholinergic, sedation, confusion, seizures, confusion, ataxia, tremors, peripheral neuropathy, dizziness, weakness, fatigue, headache, paralytic ileus, hyperpyrexia, urinary retention, constipation, blurred vision, mydriasis, dry mouth	Acceptable for use in mild TBI, avoid in moderate to severe TBI; after prolonged administration, abrupt cessation of treatment may produce nausea, headache, and malaise
Duloxetine	Start: 40 mg daily Max: 120 mg divided daily	Nausea, dry mouth, somnolence, fatigue, constipation, decreased appetite, sweating	Contraindicated with MAOis and narrow angle glaucoma
Venlafaxine	Start: 75 mg daily Max: 225 mg divided daily	Hypertension, insomnia, nervousness, dizziness	Contraindicated with MAOis and narrow-angle glaucoma; avoid use in myasthenia gravis

MAOis, monoamine oxidase inhibitors; *TBI*, traumatic brain injury.

TCAs are considered acceptable choices for depression following TBI, and have the added benefit of being useful for sleep. However, as this class of antidepressant is often associated with anticholinergic side effects, they are sometimes poorly tolerated. In addition, worsening confusion is often seen with the use of this class of medication, making it a group that is often avoided following TBI of greater severity. The most commonly used medication in this class is amitriptyline.

Monoamine oxidase inhibitors (MAOis) are considered to have excellent efficacy for refractory depression. However, the extensive list of drug and food interactions in this class makes this a category that most clinicians avoid following TBI.

Bupropion is an antidepressant medication in the aminoketone class. Its mechanism of action differs from that of tricyclics, SSRIs, MAOis, and SNRIs. It is theorized that its mechanism of action is both dopaminergic and noradrenergic.[104] This drug differs from other antidepressants in that it has an activating effect, rendering the patient more alert. It is also not associated with the sexual side effects, sedation, and weight gain seen with many other antidepressants, especially the SSRIs. In theory, its mechanism of action and side effect profile would seem to make it an ideal medication for use following brain injury. One case report has suggested improvement in refractory motor restlessness following TBI with this medication.[105] However, caution must be used with this medication, especially in more severely injured patients, because of the associated risk of lowering the seizure threshold. Most clinicians prefer to avoid bupropion for patients with TBI for this reason.

Other medications are often useful as adjunct medications for the treatment of depression. In particular, the traditional neurostimulants such as methylphenidate, are often used as "bridge" medications while starting another antidepressant because of the delayed onset of action of other antidepressants.[106,107] Other dopaminergic medications may also be used in this way, although they are not usually as efficacious (Table 11.4).

TABLE 11.5
Medications for Anxiety

Medication	Dosing (Start/Max)	Common Side Effects	Comments
Buspirone	Start: 5 mg bid Max: 20 mg tid	Dizziness, nervousness, insomnia, lightheadedness, nausea, headache	Avoid in combination with MAOis
Citalopram	Start: 20 mg daily Max: 40 mg daily	QT prolongation, nausea, dizziness, decreased libido	Contraindicated with MAOis, monitor for serotonin syndrome
Escitalopram	Start: 10 mg daily Max: 20 mg daily	Suicide risk, nausea, diarrhea, insomnia, decreased libido	Contraindicated with MAOis, monitor for serotonin syndrome
Paroxetine	Start: 20 mg daily Max: 50 mg daily	Asthenia, sweating, nausea, diarrhea, decreased appetite, somnolence, dizziness, tremor, dry mouth, decreased libido	Contraindicated with MAOis, monitor for serotonin syndrome
Fluoxetine	Start: 20 mg daily Max: 60 mg daily	Unusual dreams, decreased libido, anorexia, tremor	Contraindicated with MAOis, monitor for serotonin syndrome
Sertraline	Start: 25 mg daily Max: 200 mg daily	Nausea, diarrhea, tremor, decreased libido	Not a first-line agent for anxiety, must titrate very slowly; contraindicated with MAOis

MAOis, monoamine oxidase inhibitors.

Anxiety

The second most common mood disorder seen following TBI is anxiety. One meta-analysis found that 37% of subjects with brain injury experienced "clinically relevant anxiety."[108] Anxiety has been associated with poorer outcomes, including poorer return to work rates and community reintegration following TBI.[109] Additionally, recent research has suggested a strong relationship between anxiety and subjective neurocognitive fatigue following TBI.[110] Therefore anxiety remains one of the most significant barriers to successful outcomes following TBI.

Complicating the treatment of anxiety is the fact that most anxiolytic medications are associated with significant cognitive side effects and may have an adverse impact on neuroplasticity and recovery. Benzodiazepines are the primary culprit in this area. Although demonstrably efficacious for many symptoms present following TBI, benzodiazepines are associated with impairment of neurologic recovery mechanisms and are therefore medications traditionally believed to be avoided following TBI.[111] Add to this the fact that benzodiazepines are strongly associated with sedation and disruption of normal sleep architecture, strong consideration should be given to using other medication classes before using a benzodiazepine for the routine treatment of anxiety following TBI.

The class of SSRIs are noted to be good for the treatment of anxiety. Like with treatment of depression, the side effect profile is relatively favorable, and these medications are both efficacious and well tolerated. Paroxetine, citalopram, and escitalopram are probably the most effective medications in this class, although paroxetine is often associated with clinically significant sedation. Citalopram and escitalopram have both been associated with reduction of anxiety symptoms in both rodent and human studies following TBI.[112–114]

Buspirone is a 5-HT1A receptor agonist that is associated with anxiolytic effects. It does not have affinity for GABA receptors. It has mild affinity for D2 dopamine receptors. Although clinical use of busprione has been historically thought to be associated with serotonergic syndrome, more recent research has largely dispelled this notion.[115] It has been found to be an effective anxiolytic with a benign side effect profile[116] for individuals with TBI (Table 11.5).[117]

Emotional Lability/Mania

Emotional lability is often associated with other psychiatric issues following TBI and may exacerbate the expression of these issues. Often, treatment of lability is necessary in association with treatment of other underlying mood conditions. Comorbid treatment of mood issues with a mood-stabilizing medication has often been found to be more effective than treatment with a solitary agent alone. This is particularly true in the case of patients with agitated or explosive behavior.

Historically, emotional lability has been treated in psychiatric populations with lithium salts. Although lithium can be an effective treatment, its narrow therapeutic window and the need for reliable administration make it a difficult medication to use in the TBI population. It additionally may be associated with adverse outcomes.[118-124] However, more recent evidence suggesting potential neuroprotective effects may warrant its reevaluation as a useful treatment following TBI, if conditions for appropriate therapeutic management are present.[125-130]

More commonly, mood-stabilizing antiepileptic drugs (AEDs) are the drugs of choice for emotional lability following TBI.[131,132] Carbamazepine and valproic acid are frequently used. Both work relatively quickly, but both are associated with issues requiring frequent laboratory monitoring. Carbamazepine is associated with bone marrow suppression, which may result in anemia and pancytopenia. It is also associated with development of the syndrome of inappropriate antidiuretic

hormone release. Valproic acid is associated with hepatic enzyme impairment, blood dyscrasias, and considerable sedation and weight gain. Another AED often used for emotional lability, which may have a superior side effect profile, is lamotrigine.[133-135] Lamotrigine is associated with a life-threatening rash in a small percentage of patients and must be titrated slowly to avoid this effect. This makes it difficult to effectively use this drug in the inpatient setting. Of these three medications, valproic acid tends to have the strongest mood-stabilizing effect.

SSRIs have also been frequently used for mood stabilization, but traditionally with those with more of a depressed affect.[114,136,137] Caution should be exercised for individuals with bipolar-type presentation, as monotherapy with SSRIs may result in mania (Table 11.6).

Involuntary Emotional Expressive Disorder

A mood disorder that has received considerable attention recently is the involuntary emotional expressive disorder (IEED). This syndrome is also known by many different names, such as pseudobulbar affect disorder, emotional incontinence, and involuntary laughing and crying. The hallmark of this disorder is outbursts

TABLE 11.6
Medications for Emotional Lability/Mania

Medication	Dosing (Start)	Common Side Effects	Comments
Valproic acid	125 mg bid	Hepatic impairment, sedation, weight gain, rash	Monitor for hepatic impairment
Carbamazepine	100 mg bid	Blood dyscrasias, SIADH, hepatic impairment, rash	May cause SIADH, blood dyscrasias including pancytopenia
Lamotrigine	25 mg daily/400 mg daily in divided doses	Suicidal thoughts, dizziness, ataxia, somnolence, headache, diplopia, blurred vision, nausea, vomiting, and rash	May cause life-threatening rash, use extreme caution in patients already taking valproic acid
Citalopram	20 mg/40 mg daily	QT prolongation, nausea, dizziness, decreased libido	Contraindicated with MAOis, monitor for serotonin syndrome
Escitalopram	10 mg/20 mg	Suicide risk, nausea, diarrhea, insomnia, decreased libido	Contraindicated with MAOis, monitor for serotonin syndrome
Paroxetine	20 mg/50 mg	Asthenia, sweating, nausea, diarrhea, decreased appetite, somnolence, dizziness, tremor, dry mouth, decreased libido	Contraindicated with MAOis, monitor for serotonin syndrome
Fluoxetine	20 mg/60 mg	Unusual dreams, decreased libido, anorexia, tremor	Contraindicated with MAOis, monitor for serotonin syndrome
Sertraline	25 mg/200 mg	Nausea, diarrhea, tremor, decreased libido	Not a first-line agent for anxiety, must titrate very slowly; contraindicated with MAOis

TABLE 11.6
Medications for Emotional Lability/Mania—cont'd

Medication	Dosing (Start)	Common Side Effects	Comments
Lithium	300 mg tid/titrate to therapeutic level	Tremor, polyuria, thirst, nausea,	Difficult to use in TBI due to narrow therapeutic window significant toxicity with supratherapeutic levels, may cause renal or hepatic impairment; may cause encephalopathy with concomitant administration of neuroleptics; use caution with diuretics, calcium channel blockers, SSRI's, acetazolamide
Valproic Acid	125 mg bid	Hepatic impairment, sedation, weight gain, rash	Monitor for hepatic impairment
Carbamazepine	100 mg bid	Blood dyscrasias, SIADH, hepatic impairment, rash	May cause SIADH, blood dyscrasias including pan-cytopenia

bid, twice daily; *MAOis*, monoamine oxidase inhibitors; *SSRIs*, selective serotonin reuptake inhibitors; *TBI*, traumatic brain injury; *tid*, thrice daily.

of expressed emotion, particularly laughing or crying, that occur out of proportion to the feeling of the individual. This disorder often results in socially awkward situations wherein the expression of emotion is inappropriate for the setting. For instance, the individual may involuntarily begin laughing uncontrollably at a funeral or in a church. Individuals with IEED will state that the emotion expressed is either inconsistent or out of proportion to how they actually feel internally. In addition, it is characteristic for the emotional expression to start and stop suddenly. The physiologic explanation of this syndrome is theorized to be disruption of pathways that connect the centers of emotional experience to the centers of emotional expression in the brain.

A combination treatment of dextromethorphan and quinidine (DXM-Q, brand name Nuedexta) has been formulated specifically to treat this condition.[138–142] Dextromethorphan has been known to have psychoactive properties for many years, yet its duration of action is quite short because of its rapid metabolism. Quinidine blocks the metabolism of dextromethorphan, increasing the duration of action. Because quinidine may affect the QT interval, it is necessary to perform electrocardiography before and after the initiation of this medication. Additionally, clinicians should be aware of the theoretical risk of seizures with the administration of dextromethorphan, although this has not seemed to be a problem in clinical practice.

Recent literature has suggested that SSRIs and TCAs may be equally effective in the treatment of IEED as DXM-Q.[143–145] Several case reports have suggested a significant improvement in IEED symptoms with sertraline in particular. One open-label trial suggested that the combination of paroxetine and DXM-Q was successful.[146] Another medication with anecdotal reports of benefit in IEED is lamotrigine (Table 11.7).[147]

Neuroses/Perseveration/Paranoia

Frequently, patients with brain injury will experience paranoid ideation, perseveration, or other neurotic behaviors or thought processes during their rehabilitation course. Often, these symptoms interfere with the rehabilitation process as the object of paranoid ideation often is associated with the treating clinicians. This is most likely to occur during the period of posttraumatic amnesia (PTA), although it can persist for longer periods. Typical perseverative thought processes often involve ideas that individuals feel that they need to leave the rehabilitation setting immediately to take care of some sort of business and that the treating therapists and physicians are somehow intending to harm them. Other subjects of perseveration include pain. When pain is the subject of the perseveration, it becomes difficult to engage the patient in any type of therapeutic activity because the patient believes that the pain will be exacerbated.

The treatments for neuroses, paranoia, and perseverative behavior are similar. In most cases, low doses of an atypical neuroleptic works quite well. Risperidone, ziprasidone, olanzapine, and quetiapine are all often useful. With all of these medications, the clinician

TABLE 11.7
Medications for Involuntary Emotional Expressive Disorder

Medication	Dosing (Start/Max)	Common Side Effects	Comments
DXM/q	Tabs contain 20 mg DXM and 10 mg Q Start: 1 tab daily Max: 1 tab bid	Diarrhea, dizziness, cough, vomiting, asthenia, peripheral edema, urinary tract infection, influenza, increased γ-glutamyltransferase, and flatulence	May cause QT prolongation; get EKG before and after starting. Contraindicated with MAOis
Citalopram	Start: 20 mg daily Max: 40 mg daily	QT prolongation, nausea, dizziness, decreased libido	Contraindicated with MAOis, monitor for serotonin syndrome
Escitalopram	Start: 10 mg daily Max: 20 mg daily	Suicide risk, nausea, diarrhea, insomnia, decreased libido	Contraindicated with MAOis, monitor for serotonin syndrome
Paroxetine	Start: 20 mg daily Max: 50 mg daily	Asthenia, sweating, nausea, diarrhea, decreased appetite, somnolence, dizziness, tremor, dry mouth, decreased libido	Contraindicated with MAOis, monitor for serotonin syndrome
Fluoxetine	Start: 20 mg daily Max: 60 mg daily	Unusual dreams, decreased libido, anorexia, tremor	Contraindicated with MAOis, monitor for serotonin syndrome
Sertraline	Start: 25 mg daily Max: 200 mg daily	Nausea, diarrhea, tremor, decreased libido	Not a first-line agent for anxiety, must titrate very slowly; contraindicated with MAOis

DXM, dextromethorphan; *MAOis*, monoamine oxidase inhibitors; *Q*, quinidine.

must monitor sedation, akathisia, metabolic function including glucose metabolism, and extrapyramidal side effects. The newer neuroleptic aripiprazole has outstanding potential for use in this area because it seems to be less associated with the typical extrapyramidal side effects and sedation than the other medications. However, this medication takes longer to reach steady state and therefore may not be as useful in the inpatient setting, where rapid efficacy is necessary. If monotherapy with a neuroleptic is ineffective, often the addition of a mood-stabilizing agent will result in success. Carbamazepine and valproic acid are both effective in this situation.

Use of neurostimulant medications in patients exhibiting these symptoms should be avoided. Often, neurostimulants will aggravate these symptoms. If a patient is on a neurostimulant medication and is exhibiting these symptoms, the first step is to stop those medications to see if the symptoms resolve (Table 11.8).

Psychosis/Hallucinations

Some patients with brain injury may exhibit florid hallucinations and psychotic behavior. In many cases, the psychotic behavior is associated with overtreatment with neurostimulant medications. Amantadine, which is becoming more commonly used following brain injury, is the most common culprit. However, all dopaminergic medications can be associated with psychosis. When this occurs, the first step is to discontinue the potentially offending medications.

If discontinuation of other medications does not result in resolution of the psychotic behavior, the treatment of choice is atypical neuroleptic medications. For patients with brain injury, risperidone, ziprasidone, olanzapine, and quetiapine have all been used with success. In a meta-analysis on evidence to support treatment of neurobehavioral consequences in 2006, olanzapine was reported to have the best objective evidence for the treatment of psychotic symptoms following TBI.[148] Treatment with typical neuroleptics, particularly haloperidol, is considered to be contraindicated following brain injury. Several studies have demonstrated worse functional outcomes in both animal and human studies for individuals given haloperidol following brain injury.[149-156] Additionally there are several case reports of individuals with brain injury developing neuroleptic malignant syndrome (NMS) following administration of haloperidol.[157-160] Patients with TBI appear to be more at risk for developing NMS than the general population. The explanation for this phenomenon is that individuals with TBI are dopamine-depleted or dopamine-insufficient as a result of their injury. Placing these patients on a high-potency neuroleptic may tip the balance and result in NMS (Table 11.9).

TABLE 11.8
Medications for Neuroses/Perseveration/Paranoia

Medication	Starting Dose	Common Side Effects	Comments
Risperidone	0.5 mg prn	Sedation, akathisia, metabolic impairment	
Quetiapine	25 mg prn	Sedation, anticholinergic side effects	May result in confusion in elderly patients
Olanzapine	2.5 mg prn	Sedation, rash, metabolic impairment, weight gain, hypotension, dizziness	Available as injection; may have a paradoxical arousal effect at low doses
Ziprasidone	Oral 20 mg prn IM 10 mg prn	QT prolongation, hypotension, dizziness, electrolyte disturbance, metabolic changes, akathisia	Available as injection
Valproic acid	125 mg bid	Hepatic impairment, sedation, weight gain, rash	Not for monotherapy
Carbamazepine	100 mg bid	Blood dyscrasias, SIADH, hepatic impairment, rash	Not for monotherapy

IM, intramuscular; *SIADH*, syndrome of inappropriate antidiuretic hormone release.

TABLE 11.9
Medications for Psychosis/Hallucinations

Medication	Starting Dose	Common Side Effects	Comments
Risperidone	0.5 mg prn	Sedation, akathisia, metabolic impairment	
Quetiapine	25 mg prn	Sedation, anticholinergic side effects	May result in confusion in elderly patients
Olanzapine	2.5 mg prn	Sedation, rash, metabolic impairment, weight gain, hypotension, dizziness	Available as injection; may have a paradoxical arousal effect at low doses
Ziprasidone	Oral 20 mg prn IM 10 mg prn	QT prolongation, hypotension, dizziness, electrolyte disturbance, metabolic changes, akathisia	Available as injection

IM, intramuscular.

Aggression/Explosive Behavior

Aggressive behavior often needs to be differentiated from "agitation" following TBI. Classically, individuals exhibiting agitated behavior are still in a state of PTA, and are beginning to emerge into the ability to perform purposeful behavior, whereas individuals with TBI may exhibit aggressive behavior at any point in their recovery. The aggressive behavior is usually in response to an external stimuli, and is not internally driven as in the classically agitated, confused patient. These individuals often have injury to the limbic system, particularly the amygdalae, resulting in dysregulation of emotional responses.

Treatment for aggressive outbursts and explosive behavior is often refractory to treatment typically utilized in agitated patients. The most efficacious treatment is often β-blockade, particularly with propranolol.[161] Careful monitoring of cardiac function is necessary, as bradycardia and hypotension may limit the use of this class of medications. Also, the clinician must monitor the patient for development of depression, which is strongly associated with β-blockade.

Other treatments utilized for aggressive/explosive behavior have included mood-stabilizing agents, atypical neuroleptics, and SSRIs.[114,137,148,161] Recently, studies have suggested that amantadine may have a role in this situation.[162] Theoretically, amantadine improves cognitive processing speed, which may improve irritability that is associated with aggression and explosive behavior. However, clinicians must closely monitor the frequency of the outbursts and abandon this course of treatment if the patient's condition worsens (Table 11.10).

NEUROLOGIC ISSUES
Posttraumatic Seizures

Posttraumatic seizures (PTSs) are classified as immediate, early, or late PTSs. Immediate seizures occur within 24 h of the inciting event. Early seizures occur after 24 h

TABLE 11.10
Medications for Aggression/Explosive Behavior

Medication	Starting Dose	Common Side Effects	Comments
Propranolol	10 mg bid	Diarrhea, vomiting, dizziness, fatigue	Hypotension, bradycardia, bronchial asthma, decompensated heart failure, pheochromocytoma, second- or third-degree heart block
Valproic acid	125 mg bid	Hepatic impairment, sedation, weight gain, rash	Not for monotherapy
Carbamazepine	100 mg bid	Blood dyscrasias, SIADH, hepatic impairment, rash	Not for monotherapy
Risperidone	0.5 mg prn	Sedation, akathisia, metabolic impairment	Do not use with paliperidone
Quetiapine	25 mg prn	Sedation, anticholinergic side effects	May result in confusion in elderly patients
Olanzapine	2.5 mg prn	Sedation, rash, metabolic impairment, weight gain, hypotension, dizziness	Available as injection; may have a paradoxical arousal effect at low doses
Ziprasidone	Oral 20 mg prn IM 10 mg prn	QT prolongation, hypotension, dizziness, electrolyte disturbance, metabolic changes, akathisia	Available as injection
Citalopram	Start: 20 mg daily Max: 40 mg daily	QT prolongation, nausea, dizziness, decreased libido	Contraindicated with MAOis, monitor for serotonin syndrome
Escitalopram	Start: 10 mg daily Max: 20 mg daily	Suicide risk, nausea, diarrhea, insomnia, decreased libido	Contraindicated with MAOis, monitor for serotonin syndrome
Paroxetine	Start: 20 mg daily Max: 50 mg daily	Asthenia, sweating, nausea, diarrhea, decreased appetite, somnolence, dizziness, tremor, dry mouth, decreased libido	Contraindicated with MAOis, monitor for serotonin syndrome
Fluoxetine	Start: 20 mg daily Max: 60 mg daily	Unusual dreams, decreased libido, anorexia, tremor	Contraindicated with MAOis, monitor for serotonin syndrome
Amantadine	Start: 100 mg bid Max: 200 mg bid Dose in morning and at noon	Dizziness, insomnia, nausea	Contraindicated in pregnancy, breastfeeding; likely is epileptogenic

bid, twice daily; *IM*, intramuscular; *MAOis*, monoamine oxidase inhibitors; *SIADH*, syndrome of inappropriate antidiuretic hormone release.

but within 7 days of the inciting event. Late seizures occur more than 7 days after the trauma. Posttraumatic epilepsy (PTE) is defined as recurrent and unprovoked seizures.[163] Immediate and early PTSs are considered provoked, whereas late PTSs are considered unprovoked. Therefore two late seizures must occur before diagnosing one with PTE.

Several clinical trials have shown that AEDs are effective in reducing early PTS but do not appear to alter the natural history of late PTSs.[164] According to the latest guidelines issued by the Brain Trauma Foundation in 2007, PTS prophylaxis is recommended for the

first 7 days following TBI.[165] A number of AEDs have been studied for prophylaxis of PTSs following TBI. Phenytoin has been the most well-studied AED for PTS prophylaxis. The first double-blind placebo-controlled trial involving the use of phenytoin for PTS prophylaxis was published in 1990.[166] Subjects received either phenytoin or placebo for 12 months. The percentage of early seizures in the phenytoin group was 3.6% versus 14.2% for the placebo group. At 1 year, the percentage of subjects in the phenytoin group who had experienced at least one seizure was 26.5% versus only 15.7% in the placebo group. These findings demonstrated the

TABLE 11.11
Common Medications for Seizures Following Traumatic Brain Injury

Medication	Dosing (Start/Max)	Common Side Effects	Contraindications
Phenytoin	Prophylaxis: 100 mg tid Max: 625 mg/day	Rash, gingival enlargement, ataxia, nystagmus, constipation, nausea/vomiting, confusion	Concomitant use with delavirdine, concomitant use with rilpivirine
Valproate	Prophylaxis: 250 mg tid Max: 60 mg/kg/day	Peripheral edema, alopecia, weight gain **Serious:** Thrombocytopenia, hepatotoxicity, hyperammonemia encephalopathy	Hepatic disease, urea cycle disorders, mitochondrial disorders
Levetiracetam	Prophylaxis: 500 mg bid Max: 3000 mg/day	Loss of appetite, decreased bone mineral density, dizziness, irritability	
Carbamazepine	Prophylaxis: 200 mg bid Max: 1200 mg/day	Hypotension, constipation, nausea, vomiting, diplopia, nystagmus **Serious:** Agranulocytosis, aplastic anemia	Bone marrow depression, concomitant use of monoamine oxidase inhibitors or nonnucleoside reverse transcriptase inhibitors
Lamotrigine	25 mg daily/400 mg daily in divided doses	Vomiting, coordination abnormality, dyspepsia, nausea, dizziness, rhinitis, anxiety, insomnia, infection, pain, weight decrease, chest pain, and dysmenorrhea	May cause life-threatening rash, use extreme caution in patients already taking valproic acid

bid, twice daily; *tid*, thrice daily.

benefit of seizure prophylaxis only for the first 7 days following TBI.

Other AEDs have also been studied, although less extensively than phenytoin. One other study evaluated valproic acid for the prophylaxis of late PTS in moderate or severe TBI.[167] Subjects were randomized to phenytoin treatment group for 1 week, valproic acid treatment group for 1 month, or valproic acid treatment group for 6 months. There was no significant difference in early PTS between groups. Although there was no statistical difference in late PTS between the groups, there were more seizures at 6 months in both valproic acid groups when compared with the phenytoin group (15% in phenytoin group treated for 1 week, 16% in valproic acid group treated for 1 month, and 24% in valproic acid group treated for 6 months). This study further highlighted that longer duration of seizure prophylaxis did not decrease the incidence of late PTS.

Levetiracetam is a newer AED that is commonly used for PTS prophylaxis. This has not been as extensively studied as phenytoin or valproic acid. One study compared levetiracetam with phenytoin in 52 subjects with severe TBI.[168] Each group was treated for 7 days with either levetiracetam or phenytoin. There was no significant difference in early PTS between the groups.

The Brain Trauma Foundation recommends the use of phenytoin for early PTS prophylaxis. However, in clinical practice, newer AEDs such as levetiracetam are commonly used because of more favorable pharmacokinetic and side effect profiles. Additionally, there have been some data to suggest that phenytoin may negatively affect cognitive outcomes at 6 months when used for seizure prophylaxis.[169] There was no difference in cognitive outcomes noted at 12 or 24 months when comparing the phenytoin and control groups (Table 11.11).

Disorder of Initiation

Disorders of initiation are likely underappreciated during the early phases of rehabilitation following TBI, even though their incidence has been reported as high as 67% following TBI.[170] Those who have disorders of initiation will typically do well in a structured rehabilitation program. They may struggle, however, in real-world situations with less structure. Disorders of initiation are sometimes referred to as apathy, which is defined as diminished motivation in the presence of normal consciousness, attention, cognitive capacity, and mood.[170] It should be noted, however, that patients with initiation disorders are not "unmotivated" to participate in rehabilitation—in fact, they typically do well participating in rehabilitation when cued to do so. Instead, the neurologic insult has impaired their ability to initiate this behavior on their own.

TABLE 11.12
Medications for Disorder of Initiation

Medication	Dosing (Start/Max)	Common Side Effects	Contraindications
Methylphenidate	Start: 5–10 mg bid Max: 60 mg/day	Nervousness, insomnia, anorexia, tachycardia, palpitations, dizziness	Angina, concomitant use of monoamine oxidase inhibitors, glaucoma, heart failure, hyperthyroidism, severe hypertension
Dextroamphetamine/amphetamine	Start: 5–10 mg bid Max: 60 mg/day	Nervousness, insomnia, anorexia, tachycardia, palpitations, dizziness	Angina, concomitant use of monoamine oxidase inhibitors, glaucoma, heart failure, hyperthyroidism, severe hypertension
Amantadine	Start: 50–100 mg bid Max: 200 mg bid	Nausea, insomnia, hallucinations, agitation, anxiety	Contraindicated in pregnancy, breastfeeding
Bromocriptine	Start: 2.5 mg bid Max: 10 mg bid	Nausea, constipation, diarrhea, dizziness	Breastfeeding, syncopal migraine, uncontrolled hypertension
Pramipexole	Start: 0.125 mg tid Max: 1.5 mg tid	Orthostatic hypotension, constipation, nausea, dizziness, extrapyramidal movements, insomnia	None

bid, twice daily; *tid*, thrice daily.

Before initiating pharmacologic therapy for the treatment of disorders of initiation, other medical conditions that could contribute to the clinical presentation, such as hydrocephalus, neuroendocrine dysfunction, or mood disorder, should be ruled out. If a mood disorder is present, consideration should be given to starting more activating antidepressants, such as fluoxetine, sertraline, desipramine, or venlafaxine.

There has been little systematic research performed studying disorders of initiation following TBI. Pharmacologic treatment of disorders of initiation typically target the dopaminergic and norepinephrine pathways. Typical agents include neurostimulants, such as methylphenidate or dextroamphetamine/amphetamine, which increase both dopamine and norepinephrine. Dopamine receptor agonists, such as bromocriptine or pramipexole, may also be considered. Powell reported on 11 patients with TBI or subarachnoid hemorrhage who all showed improvement in their baseline assessments of participation in therapy after initiating bromocriptine and increasing by 2.5 mg every week up to a dose of 5–10 mg twice a day.[171] Amantadine, which increases the endogenous release of dopamine and also targets the glutamatergic pathway, may also improve initiation.[41]

No single agent has been shown to be superior to another for the treatment of disorders of initiation. Selection of pharmacologic therapy should take into account the presence of other neurobehavioral comorbidities such as depression or attention deficits (Table 11.12).

Movement Disorders

Mechanical head trauma may disrupt deep brain motor nuclei (basal ganglia, thalamus, subthalamus) and cerebellum, as well as the white matter tracts associated with these structures.[172] Retrospective studies have estimated the prevalence of movement disorders following severe TBI at approximately 22%.[173] Tremors, dystonia, parkinsonism, myoclonus, and choreiform movements are the most common movement disorders that manifest following head trauma.

Tremor is the most common movement disorder following TBI.[172] There are four types of tremor: rest, postural, action, and intention tremor. Resting tremor is often associated with parkinsonism. Postural tremor occurs with steady tonic contraction, such as holding a utensil, whereas action tremor occurs with smooth movement. Intentional tremor can be thought of as the terminal exacerbation of an action tremor. Approximately 20% of severe TBI survivors will develop a tremor.[173] Fortunately, this is more often transient than permanent. Systemic illness or medications often may be related to the presence of the tremor. Antipsychotics, including metoclopramide, are often used in the brain injury population and may cause tremors. There have been no controlled trials that have investigated the efficacy of medications for the management of posttraumatic tremors. Before treating posttraumatic tremors, consideration should be given as to whether or not the tremor is interfering with the patient's function.

First-line treatment for action and intentional tremors includes propranolol, a nonselective β-antagonist. Primidone is an antiepileptic that is commonly used to treat action or intentional tremor. Other antiepileptics, such as levetiracetam or topiramate, may also be considered.

Dystonia is excessive contraction of agonist and antagonist muscles. Dystonia may often be overlooked in the TBI population given that hypertonia is often attributed to spasticity. Cogwheeling with passive movement of the extremities may be appreciated on examination when dystonia is present. If the passive resistance to movement is not velocity dependent, it suggests that hypertonia may be attributed to dystonic rigidity. Anticholinergic medications, such as trihexyphenidyl, are often used to treat dystonia. However, in the TBI population this is not the ideal drug of choice for the treatment of dystonia because of sedation and negative impact on cognition. Trial of dopaminergic agents in the TBI population for the treatment of dystonia is a reasonable option, especially in patients who are in need of neurostimulation. Dopaminergic agents have provided contradictory results for the treatment of dystonia. Some studies have reported on improvement of dystonia with carbidopa/levodopa,[174] whereas others have reported worsening dystonia. The varied response is likely due to the heterogeneity in mixed population studies.[175] Botulinum toxin has been shown to be safe and effective in the treatment of dystonia in several open and controlled studies.[176]

Parkinsonism is the occurrence of two or more of the following: rigidity, resting tremor, and bradykinesia.[172] Parkinsonism can occur when the nigrostriatal dopaminergic projections or basal ganglia are damaged as a result of the traumatic injury. Dopaminergic agents typically used in idiopathic Parkinson disease are the most effective treatment for posttraumatic parkinsonism (see Table 11.13).

Myoclonus is described as lighteninglike jerks that can be either focal or multifocal. Any disease process that causes cortical irritability can cause myoclonus. Historically, valproic acid and clonazepam have been used as first-line agents for the treatment of myoclonus. As mentioned earlier, given the known inhibitory effects of benzodiazepines on neural plasticity and the negative influence on cognition, it is preferable to avoid the use of clonazepam in the TBI population. More recently, there has been increasing evidence that levetiracetam is also effective in the treatment of myoclonus.[177] This is especially encouraging given levetiracetam's relatively favorable pharmacokinetic and side effect profile.

Chorea is a hyperkinetic movement disorder that can be seen following TBI. Chorea is typically described as having the appearance of dancing or restless fidgeting. Athetosis may be considered a subtype of chorea and is at the slower end of the spectrum. Ballism is on the other end of the spectrum and may result in violent flinging of the extremity. These hyperkinetic movement disorders are thought to be due to impaired inhibitory basal ganglia output.[172] Neuroleptics are typically the first-line agent for the treatment of chorea (Table 11.13).[178]

Fatigue

Defining fatigue is difficult because it is a multidimensional construct.[179] Physiologic fatigue is functional organ failure generally caused by excessive energy consumption and depletion of essential substrates of physiologic functioning, such as hormones or neurotransmitters. Psychologic fatigue is defined as a state of weariness related to reduced motivation, prolonged mental activity, or boredom that occurs in situations such as chronic stress, anxiety, or depression.[180]

Mental fatigue is among one of the most common symptoms reported following TBI.[181] The prevalence of fatigue varies by study ranging from 30% to 70%.[182] The cause of fatigue following TBI continues to be debated, although it is likely multifactorial in nature. For instance, comorbidities such as depression, insomnia, and neuroendocrine abnormalities are likely to influence one's subjective sense of fatigue. One study found no significant difference in fatigue ratings across the severity spectrum of TBI.[183] Greater time since injury was associated with higher fatigue levels. Similar rates of fatigue between the severe and mild TBI populations highlights the subjective nature of fatigue in that the experience of fatigue is reliant on awareness. The mild TBI population likely has a greater awareness of fatigue compared with the severe TBI population.

The coping hypothesis suggests that individuals with TBI expend greater psychophysiologic costs to maintain stable performance over time. One study evaluated the relationship between subjective fatigue and performance on a vigilance task.[184] Individuals with TBI performed at a stable level throughout the 45-min vigilance task but had higher subjective ratings of fatigue compared with the control population.

When considering pharmacologic options for the treatment of posttraumatic fatigue, consideration should first be given to the treatment of comorbidities that may be influencing one's subjective experience of fatigue. When treating depression, consideration may be given to using more activating antidepressant medications, such as fluoxetine, sertraline, or

TABLE 11.13
Medications for Movement Disorders

Problem	Medication	Dosing (Start/Max)	Common Side Effects	Contraindications
Action/intention tremor	Propranolol	Start: 10 mg tid Max: 160 mg bid	Diarrhea, vomiting, dizziness, fatigue	Hypotension, bradycardia, bronchial asthma, decompensated heart failure, pheochromocytoma, second- or third-degree heart block
Action/intention tremor	Primidone	Start: 12.5 mg qhs Max: 250 mg qhs	Ataxia, vertigo	Porphyria
Dystonia	Trihexyphenidyl	Start: 1 mg daily Max: 15 mg/day divided qid	Nausea, xerostomia, dizziness, blurred vision, nervousness, sedation	Narrow-angle glaucoma
Dystonia/Parkinsonism	Carbidopa/levodopa	Start: 10/100 mg tid–qid Max: 200/2000 mg/day	Nausea, confusion, dizziness, headache	Narrow-angle glaucoma, history of melanoma, concomitant administration of MAOis
Parkinsonism	Amantadine	Start: 50–100 mg bid Max: 200 mg bid	Nausea, insomnia, hallucinations, agitation, anxiety	Pregnancy or breastfeeding
Parkinsonism	Pramipexole	Start: 0.125 mg tid Max: 1.5 mg tid	Orthostatic hypotension, constipation, nausea, dizziness, extrapyramidal movements, insomnia, hallucinations	Malignant melanoma, orthostatic hypotension, psychotic disorders, renal insufficiency
Parkinsonism	Ropinirole	Start: 0.25 mg tid Max: 4 mg tid	Orthostatic hypotension, constipation, nausea, dizziness, fatigue	Orthostatic hypotension, bradycardia, psychotic disorders, dyskinesia, renal failure
Myoclonus	Valproic acid	Start: 125–250 mg bid Max: 60 mg/kg/day	Peripheral edema, alopecia, weight gain **Serious:** Thrombocytopenia, hepatotoxicity, hyperammonemia encephalopathy	Hepatic disease, urea cycle disorders, mitochondrial disorders
Myoclonus	Clonazepam	Start: 0.5 mg bid–tid Max: 4 mg/day	Ataxia, dizziness, fatigue	Acute narrow-angle glaucoma, liver disease
Myoclonus	Levetiracetam	Start: 250 mg bid Max: 1500 mg bid	Vomiting, decreased bone mineral density, dizziness, irritability, fatigue	pancytopenia, blood dyscrasias, renal insufficiency, psychosis
Chorea	Risperidone	Start: 0.5 mg bid Max: 16 mg/day	Sedation, akathisia, metabolic impairment	Do not use with paliperidone
Chorea	Olanzapine	Start: 2.5–5 mg daily Max: 20 mg/day	Sedation, rash, metabolic impairment, weight gain, hypotension, dizziness	Breast cancer, diabetes, hypercholesterolemia, neutropenia, parkinsonism, QT prolongation, orthostatic hypotension

bid, twice daily; *tid,* thrice daily.

TABLE 11.14
Medications for Fatigue

Medication	Dosing (Start/Max)	Common Side Effects	Contraindications
Fluoxetine	Start: 20 mg daily Max: 80 mg/day	Diarrhea, nausea, insomnia, anxiety	Concomitant use of monoamine oxidase inhibitors, concomitant use of pimozide or thioridazine
Sertraline	Start: 25–50 mg daily Max: 200 mg/day	Diarrhea, nausea, dizziness, abnormal ejaculation, reduced libido	Concomitant use of monoamine oxidase inhibitors, concomitant use of disulfiram, pimozide
Modafinil	Start: 100 mg bid Max: 400 mg/day	Nausea, headache, insomnia, anxiety	psychosis, hypertension, angina, severe liver or kidney disease.
Methylphenidate	Start: 5–10 mg bid Max: 60 mg/day	Nervousness, insomnia, anorexia, tachycardia, palpitations, dizziness	Angina, concomitant use of monoamine oxidase inhibitors, glaucoma, heart failure, hyperthyroidism, severe hypertension
Dextroamphetamine/amphetamine	Start: 5 mg bid Max: 60 mg/day	Nervousness, insomnia, anorexia, tachycardia, palpitations, dizziness	Angina, concomitant use of monoamine oxidase inhibitors, glaucoma, heart failure, hyperthyroidism, severe hypertension
Amantadine	Start: 50–100 mg bid Max: 200 mg bid	Nausea, insomnia, hallucinations, agitation, anxiety	Contraindicated in pregnancy, breastfeeding

bid, twice daily.

SNRIs. Neuroendocrine abnormalities should also be corrected because hypothyroidism or hypogonadism could potentially be contributing to fatigue. It is important to treat insomnia because this can certainly contribute to fatigue.

Neurostimulants are the most common form of pharmacologic treatment of posttraumatic fatigue. Modafinil was studied in a randomized placebo-controlled trial in 53 patients with severe TBI.[11] There was no significant difference in Fatigue Severity Scale with a total daily dose of modafinil 400 mg at weeks 4 and 10. There was a significant improvement in the Epworth Sleepiness Scale at weeks 4 and 10. Methylphenidate was found to significantly improve mental fatigue in a dose-dependent manner, as assessed by the Mental Fatigue Scale in a group of 51 subjects with mild TBI.[185] Other neurostimulants such as amantadine and dextroamphetamine/amphetamine could also be considered, but there have not been systematic studies that have investigated their use in posttraumatic fatigue (Table 11.14).

Paroxysmal Sympathetic Hyperactivity

A syndrome of agitation, restlessness, diaphoresis, hyperthermia, hypertension, tachycardia, tachypnea, hypertonia, and extensor posturing is often seen following severe TBI. There have been a number of terms

given to this syndrome over the years including dysautonomia, autonomic (sympathetic) storming, diencephalic seizures, or midbrain dysregulatory syndrome. Paroxysmal sympathetic hyperactivity (PSH) has been proposed as an all-encompassing term for the syndrome.[186]

Activation of the sympathetic nervous system is one of the most common features of PSH syndrome. Propranolol is frequently used in PSH to blunt sympathetic outflow. Propranolol is a nonselective β-antagonist that acts on the β-1 and β-2 receptors. It is highly lipophilic and therefore crosses the blood-brain barrier. Labetalol and clonidine may also be considered for blockade of sympathetic hyperactivity. Labetalol is a nonselective β-receptor antagonist and selective α-blocker (α-1 receptors). Labetalol is considered moderately lipophilic. Clonidine is an α-2 agonist that lowers blood pressure and also can have a behavior-stabilizing effect.

It can be useful to consider other clinical entities that mimic PSH syndrome when selecting other agents to treat clinical features of PSH. NMS has several overlapping clinical features of PSH, including hyperthermia, rigidity, and autonomic instability. NMS is typically seen with long-term use of antipsychotic agents with potent dopamine blockade. There have also been case reports of NMS with the withdrawal

TABLE 11.15
Medications for Paroxysmal Sympathetic Hyperactivity (PSH)

Medication	Dosing (Start/Max)	Common Side Effects	Contraindications
Propranolol	Start: 10 mg tid Max: 320 mg/day	Diarrhea, vomiting, dizziness, fatigue	Hypotension, bradycardia, bronchial asthma, decompensated heart failure, pheochromocytoma, second- or third-degree heart block
Labetalol	Start: 50 mg bid Max: 2400 mg/day	Orthostatic hypotension, nausea, dizziness, nasal congestion, fatigue	Bronchial asthma, cardiogenic shock, second- and third-degree heart block, severe bradycardia
Clonidine	Start: 0.1 mg bid Max: 2.4 mg/day	Xerostomia, headache, somnolence	Hypotension
Bromocriptine	Start: 2.5 mg bid Max: 10 mg bid	Nausea, constipation, diarrhea, dizziness	Breastfeeding, syncopal migraine, uncontrolled hypertension
Dantrolene	Start: 25 mg daily Max: 400 mg qid	Flushing, diarrhea, somnolence hepatotoxicity	Hepatic disease
Morphine	Start: 15 mg q 4 hours Max: Dependent on opioid tolerance	Pruritus, constipation, nausea, light headedness, urinary retention	Concomitant use of MAOis, GI obstruction, hypercarbia, respiratory depression

bid, twice daily.

of dopaminergic agents, such as carbidopa/levodopa or amantadine.[187] This is particularly important to consider given that patients with TBI are often placed on neuroleptic agents, such as haloperidol for "agitation." Use of metoclopramide has also been known to induce NMS.[188] Consideration should be given to initiating dopaminergic agents, such as bromocriptine, a D_2 receptor agonist, in a patient with PSH, particularly those who present with muscle rigidity, hyperthermia, and autonomic instability.

Clinical features that mimic malignant hyperthermia (tachycardia, hyperthermia, and tachypnea) should also be considered when treating PSH. Malignant hyperthermia has been reported to occur in cases of TBI without an inciting event, such as surgery or anesthesia.[189] Dantrolene is commonly used to treat malignant hyperthermia. Dantrolene blocks calcium release from the sarcoplasmic reticulum, resulting in the relaxation of sustained skeletal muscle contraction. This may help decrease hyperthermia and muscle rigidity. Dantrolene should be considered in a patient with PSH who presents with hyperthermia and sustained muscle contraction.

In refractory cases of PSH, consideration can be given to the use of morphine. Morphine is an opiate agonist. Morphine may be an effective agent in treating several features of PSH including hypertension, tachypnea, and tachycardia (Table 11.15).

Spasticity and Rigidity

Hypertonia is commonly seen following severe TBI. Hypertonia is increased resistance to passive movement and can have several causes. It is important to consider the different causes of hypertonia as each will have different treatment strategies.

Spasticity is a form of hypertonia that is defined as velocity-dependent resistance to passive muscle stretch. A positive relationship exists between the velocity with which the muscle is stretched (or joint moved) and resistance to movement. The control of muscle tone involves a feedback loop, which integrates information about muscle activity, position, and velocity.[190] When there is CNS damage following TBI, there may be loss of descending inhibitory influences in the muscle stretch reflex pathway, resulting in spasticity.

There are several pharmacologic agents used to treat spasticity following TBI. Most agents act on the CNS to facilitate the inhibitory influences on the muscle stretch reflex pathway that may be decreased due to CNS damage following TBI. Benzodiazepines were the first class of medications used to treat spasticity. Within the benzodiazepine family, diazepam is the one most commonly used to treat spasticity. Diazepam agonizes the GABA$_A$ receptor, resulting in hyperpolarization and inhibitory outflow from the brainstem reticular formation and spinal cord descending tracts.[191] Benzodiazepines, however, should generally be avoided as first-line agents for the treatment of spasticity because of sedative effects and known inhibition of neuroplasticity.

Baclofen is also a GABA agonist that is commonly used to treat spasticity. Unlike diazepam, which is an agonist of the GABA$_A$ receptor, baclofen is a GABA$_B$ agonist. It causes hyperpolarization of the cell at both the presynaptic and postsynaptic levels, resulting in inhibition of both the monosynaptic and polysynaptic reflex pathways.[190] Much of the research in the use of baclofen for the treatment of spasticity has been performed in the spinal cord injury and multiple sclerosis populations. There has been little systematic research in the brain injury population. The sedative effects of baclofen are expected to be less than those of diazepam; however, sedation should be monitored for and patients cautioned of this potential side effect. Abrupt withdrawal should be avoided because there have been instances of new-onset seizures with abrupt withdrawal.[192] There has been conflicting evidence as to whether or not baclofen lowers the seizure threshold.

Tizanidine is an α-2 agonist that has been relatively well studied for the management of spasticity in TBI. Activation of the α-2 receptor results in inhibition of the release of excitatory neurotransmitters, such as glutamate and aspartate, because of negative feedback. Common side effects include hypotension and dizziness, but most prominently, and of particular concern in the brain injury population, it can also cause sedation. It also has the potential to cause liver damage, so liver function tests should be performed before the initiation of treatment, and again at 1, 3, and 6 months. A randomized placebo-controlled trial studied tizanidine in an acquired brain injury population. The primary outcome measure was change in the Modified Ashworth Scale of the wrist flexors assessed at 6 weeks. Tizanidine was started at twice daily dosing of 2 mg/day and increased to 36 mg/day, as tolerated. There was no statistical difference in the primary outcome at 6 and 18 weeks.[193]

Similar to tizanidine, clonidine is also an α-2 agonist. It acts both on the locus coeruleus and at the spinal cord level, enhancing presynaptic inhibition at the spinal cord level. It has demonstrated some efficacy in the treatment of spasticity, but primarily in the spinal cord injury population.[194] It should be noted that there is concern that clonidine may impair motor recovery following acquired brain injury.[195]

Dantrolene is an intriguing choice for the management of spasticity in the TBI population in that its mechanism of action is peripheral action, therefore it does not cause sedation. It acts by inhibiting the release of calcium from the sarcoplasmic reticulum, therefore inhibiting skeletal muscle contraction. Its most well-known side effect is for hepatotoxicity. Liver function tests should be checked weekly for the first month and then at least every other month for the first year.

Chemical neurolysis is commonly used to treat spasticity that is refractory to oral medications. Chemical neurolysis is particularly effective for the treatment of focal spasticity. There are two main agents for chemical neurolysis—phenol and botulinum toxin. Phenol was the first neurolytic agent used to treat spasticity. It decreases spasticity by denaturing proteins of both the motor and sensory nerves, resulting in decreased skeletal muscle tone. Its duration of effect is typically longer than that of botulinum toxin. Typical duration of action is three to 9 months, but it can also be longer.

Unlike phenol, botulinum toxin does not affect the sensory nerves. Botulinum toxin was approved for use in the United States in 1989. There are currently two botulinum toxin serotypes available for use in the United States—types A and B. Botulinum toxin inhibits the presynaptic release of acetylcholine from the synaptic vesicle. The Soluble NSF Attachment Protein Receptor (SNARE) complex attaches the synaptic vesicle to the cell membrane, thus allowing the release of acetylcholine into the neuromuscular junction. Botulinum toxin serotypes A and B act on different SNARE complex proteins. Type A cleaves Soluble NSF Attachment Protein-25 (SNAP-25), a protein attached to the acetylcholine vesicle, whereas Type B cleaves synaptobrevin, a protein attached to the cell membrane. The efficacy of botulinum toxin for the treatment of spasticity has been demonstrated in multiple sclerosis and TBI populations.[196,197]

Systemic side effects of botulinum toxin are possible. Relatively mild side effects include headache, flulike symptoms, fatigue, and nausea. More serious side effects include respiratory depression, dysphagia, and generalized weakness. Botulinum toxin serotype B seems to have more parasympathetic side effects, such as dry mouth and visual disturbance.[198]

Intrathecal baclofen may also be used for the treatment of generalized spasticity. Intrathecal baclofen was first approved by the Food and Drug Administration for use in the United States in 1996.[190] The advantage of an intrathecal delivery system is that a much lower dose of baclofen may be used to obtain adequate control of spasticity. With an intrathecal pump, baclofen is delivered into the subarachnoid space of the spinal

TABLE 11.16
Medications for Spasticity

Medication	Dosing (Start/Max)	Common Side Effects	Contraindications
Diazepam	Start: 2 mg tid Max: 10 mg qid	Hypotension, muscle weakness, somnolence	Acute narrow-angle glaucoma, myasthenia gravis, severe hepatic insufficiency, severe respiratory insufficiency, sleep apnea
Baclofen	Start: 5 mg tid Max: 80 mg/day	Hypotension, somnolence, urinary retention	None
Tizanidine	Start: 2 mg tid Max: 36 mg/day	Hypotension, xerostomia, asthenia, dizziness, somnolence	Concomitant use of potent CYP1A2 inhibitors
Clonidine	Start: 0.1 mg bid Max: 2.4 mg/day	Xerostomia, headache, somnolence	Hypotension
Dantrolene	Start: 25 mg daily–tid Max: 400 mg/day	Flushing, diarrhea, somnolence **Serious:** hepatotoxicity	Hepatic disease
Phenol	Dosing varies based on targeted muscles and severity of spasticity	Injection site reaction	None
Botulinum toxin	Dosing varies based on targeted muscles and severity of spasticity Max: 600 units	Injection site reaction **Serious:** Dysphagia	None but caution use in neuromuscular diseases

bid, twice daily.

cord. Although intrathecal baclofen may be used to treat spasticity in both the upper and lower extremities, it is typically more effective for the treatment of lower extremity spasticity because of limitations regarding catheter placement high in the cervical spine due to narrowing of the spinal canal. Before implantation of the intrathecal baclofen pump, a trial is first conducted to determine whether or not the patient had an adequate response to intrathecal baclofen. Risks associated with intrathecal baclofen pump implantation include infection, pump failure, catheter dislodgement or kinking, and cerebrospinal fluid leaks. Although rare, failure of the pump or catheter can lead to baclofen withdrawal and associated seizures.

As mentioned at the beginning of this section, care should be taken to differentiate the cause of hypertonia as different causes have varying treatment strategies. Refractory hypertonia despite escalating doses of spasticity medications should raise the suspicion that dystonia may be the cause of hypertonia. This is particularly true if cogwheeling of the extremity with passive range of motion is noted on examination. Resistance to passive range of motion that is not velocity dependent suggests the presence of dystonia or paratonia. It is possible that the presentation of hypertonia may be a mixed picture of spasticity, paratonia, or dystonic rigidity. This must be kept in mind when evaluating patients with hypertonia, as the treatment paradigms are different for these different conditions. (Table 11.16).

CONCLUSION

Medication management following TBI can be very challenging yet rewarding. Astute observation is critical in the practice. The information in this chapter should be considered as guidelines, and is not intended to replace the judgment of the clinician. As always, please refer to detailed prescribing information before the use of any medication.

REFERENCES

1. Sawyer E, Mauro LS, Ohlinger MJ. Amantadine enhancement of arousal and cognition after traumatic brain injury. *Ann Pharmacother.* 2008;42(2):247–252.
2. Giacino JT, Whyte J, Bagiella E, et al. Placebo-controlled trial of amantadine for severe traumatic brain injury. *N Engl J Med.* 2012;366(9):819–826.

3. Meythaler JM, Brunner RC, Johnson A, Novack TA. Amantadine to improve neurorecovery in traumatic brain injury-associated diffuse axonal injury: a pilot double-blind randomized trial. *J Head Trauma Rehabil.* 2002;17(4):300–313.

4. Passler MA, Riggs RV. Positive outcomes in traumatic brain injury-vegetative state: patients treated with bromocriptine. *Arch Phys Med Rehabil.* 2001;82(3):311–315.

5. Haig AJ, Ruess JM. Recovery from vegetative state of six months' duration associated with Sinemet (levodopa/carbidopa). *Arch Phys Med Rehabil.* 1990;71(13):1081–1083.

6. Matsuda W, Komatsu Y, Yanaka K, Matsumura A. Levodopa treatment for patients in persistent vegetative or minimally conscious states. *Neuropsychol Rehabil.* 2005;15(3–4):414–427.

7. Matsuda W, Matsumura A, Komatsu Y, Yanaka K, Nose T. Awakenings from persistent vegetative state: report of three cases with parkinsonism and brain stem lesions on MRI. *J Neurol Neurosurg Psychiatr.* 2003;74(11):1571–1573.

8. Krimchansky BZ, Keren O, Sazbon L, Groswasser Z. Differential time and related appearance of signs, indicating improvement in the state of consciousness in vegetative state traumatic brain injury (VS-TBI) patients after initiation of dopamine treatment. *Brain Inj.* 2004;18(11):1099–1105.

9. Dhamapurkar SK, Wilson BA, Rose A, Watson P, Shiel A. Does modafinil improve the level of consciousness for people with a prolonged disorder of consciousness? a retrospective pilot study. *Disabil Rehabil.* 2016:1–7.

10. Kaiser PR, Valko PO, Werth E, et al. Modafinil ameliorates excessive daytime sleepiness after traumatic brain injury. *Neurology.* 2010;75(20):1780–1785.

11. Jha A, Weintraub A, Allshouse A, et al. A randomized trial of modafinil for the treatment of fatigue and excessive daytime sleepiness in individuals with chronic traumatic brain injury. *J Head Trauma Rehabil.* 2008;23(1):52–63.

12. Bomalaski MN, Claflin ES, Townsend W, Peterson MD. Zolpidem for the treatment of neurologic disorders: a systematic review. *JAMA Neurol.* 2017;74(9).

13. Chatelle C, Thibaut A, Gosseries O, et al. Changes in cerebral metabolism in patients with a minimally conscious state responding to zolpidem. *Front Hum Neurosci.* 2014;8:917.

14. Clauss RP. Neurotransmitters in coma, vegetative and minimally conscious states, pharmacological interventions. *Med Hypotheses.* 2010;75(3):287–290.

15. Gosseries O, Charland-Verville V, Thonnard M, Bodart O, Laureys S, Demertzi A. Amantadine, apomorphine and zolpidem in the treatment of disorders of consciousness. *Curr Pharm Des.* 2014;20(26):4167–4184.

16. Noormandi A, Shahrokhi M, Khalili H. Potential benefits of zolpidem in disorders of consciousness. *Expert Rev Clin Pharmacol.* 2017;10(9).

17. Singh R, McDonald C, Dawson K, et al. Zolpidem in a minimally conscious state. *Brain Inj.* 2008;22(1):103–106.

18. Thonnard M, Gosseries O, Demertzi A, et al. Effect of zolpidem in chronic disorders of consciousness: a prospective open-label study. *Funct Neurol.* 2013;28(4):259–264.

19. Tucker C, Sandhu K. The effectiveness of zolpidem for the treatment of disorders of consciousness. *Neurocrit Care.* 2016;24(3):488–493.

20. Whyte J, Myers R. Incidence of clinically significant responses to zolpidem among patients with disorders of consciousness: a preliminary placebo controlled trial. *Am J Phys Med Rehabil.* 2009;88(5):410–418.

21. Whyte J, Rajan R, Rosenbaum A, et al. Zolpidem and restoration of consciousness. *Am J Phys Med Rehabil.* 2014;93(2):101–113.

22. Martin RT, Whyte J. The effects of methylphenidate on command following and yes/no communication in persons with severe disorders of consciousness: a meta-analysis of n-of-1 studies. *Am J Phys Med Rehabil.* 2007;86(8):613–620.

23. Moein H, Khalili HA, Keramatian K. Effect of methylphenidate on ICU and hospital length of stay in patients with severe and moderate traumatic brain injury. *Clin Neurol Neurosurg.* 2006;108(6):539–542.

24. Patrick PD, Blackman JA, Mabry JL, Buck ML, Gurka MJ, Conaway MR. Dopamine agonist therapy in low-response children following traumatic brain injury. *J Child Neurol.* 2006;21(10):879–885.

25. Fridman EA, Krimchansky BZ, Bonetto M, et al. Continuous subcutaneous apomorphine for severe disorders of consciousness after traumatic brain injury. *Brain Inj.* 2010;24(4):636–641.

26. Margetis K, Korfias SI, Gatzonis S, et al. Intrathecal baclofen associated with improvement of consciousness disorders in spasticity patients. *Neuromodulation.* 2014;17(7):699–704. Discussion 704.

27. Pistoia F, Sacco S, Sara M, Franceschini M, Carolei A. Intrathecal baclofen: effects on spasticity, pain, and consciousness in disorders of consciousness and locked-in syndrome. *Curr Pain Headache Rep.* 2015;19(1):466.

28. Sara M, Pistoia F, Mura E, Onorati P, Govoni S. Intrathecal baclofen in patients with persistent vegetative state: 2 hypotheses. *Arch Phys Med Rehabil.* 2009;90(7):1245–1249.

29. Whyte J, Hart T, Vaccaro M, et al. Effects of methylphenidate on attention deficits after traumatic brain injury: a multidimensional, randomized, controlled trial. *Am J Phys Med Rehabil.* 2004;83(6):401–420.

30. Willmott C, Ponsford J. Efficacy of methylphenidate in the rehabilitation of attention following traumatic brain injury: a randomised, crossover, double blind, placebo controlled inpatient trial. *J Neurol Neurosurg Psychiatr.* 2009;80(5):552–557.

31. Kaelin DL, Cifu DX, Matthies B. Methylphenidate effect on attention deficit in the acutely brain-injured adult. *Arch Phys Med Rehabil.* 1996;77(1):6–9.

32. Plenger PM, Dixon CE, Castillo RM, Frankowski RF, Yablon SA, Levin HS. Subacute methylphenidate treatment for moderate to moderately severe traumatic brain injury: a preliminary double-blind placebo-controlled study. *Arch Phys Med Rehabil.* 1996;77(6):536–540.

33. Bleiberg JGW, Cederquist J, Reeves D, Lux W. Effects of dexedrine on performance consistency following brain injury: a double-blind placebo crossover case study. *Neuropsychiatr Neuropsychol Behav Neurol.* 1993;6(4):245–248.

34. Hornstein A, Lennihan L, Seliger G, Lichtman S, Schroeder K. Amphetamine in recovery from brain injury. *Brain Inj.* 1996;10(2):145–148.

35. Tramontana MG, Cowan RL, Zald D, Prokop JW, Guillamondegui O. Traumatic brain injury-related attention deficits: treatment outcomes with lisdexamfetamine dimesylate (Vyvanse). *Brain Inj.* 2014;28(11):1461–1472.

36. Zhang L, Plotkin RC, Wang G, Sandel ME, Lee S. Cholinergic augmentation with donepezil enhances recovery in short-term memory and sustained attention after traumatic brain injury. *Arch Phys Med Rehabil.* 2004;85(7):1050–1055.

37. Khateb A, Ammann J, Annoni JM, Diserens K. Cognition-enhancing effects of donepezil in traumatic brain injury. *Eur Neurol.* 2005;54(1):39–45.

38. Ripley DL. Atomoxetine for individuals with traumatic brain injury. *J Head Trauma Rehabil.* 2006;21(1):85–88.

39. Ripley DL, Morey CE, Gerber D, et al. Atomoxetine for attention deficits following traumatic brain injury: results from a randomized controlled trial. *Brain Inj.* 2014;28(12):1514–1522.

40. Whyte J, Vaccaro M, Grieb-Neff P, Hart T, Polansky M, Coslett HB. The effects of bromocriptine on attention deficits after traumatic brain injury: a placebo-controlled pilot study. *Am J Phys Med Rehabil.* 2008;87(2):85–99.

41. Kraus MF, Maki PM. Effect of amantadine hydrochloride on symptoms of frontal lobe dysfunction in brain injury: case studies and review. *J Neuropsychiatr Clin Neurosci.* 1997;9(2):222–230.

42. Schneider WN, Drew-Cates J, Wong TM, Dombovy ML. Cognitive and behavioural efficacy of amantadine in acute traumatic brain injury: an initial double-blind placebo-controlled study. *Brain Inj.* 1999;13(11):863–872.

43. Zafonte RD, Bagiella E, Ansel BM, et al. Effect of citicoline on functional and cognitive status among patients with traumatic brain injury: citicoline brain injury treatment trial (COBRIT). *JAMA.* 2012;308(19):1993–2000.

44. Callahan CD, Hinkebein J. Neuropsychological significance of anosmia following traumatic brain injury. *J Head Trauma Rehabil.* 1999;14(6):581–587.

45. Cardenas DD, McLean Jr A, Farrell-Roberts L, Baker L, Brooke M, Haselkorn J. Oral physostigmine and impaired memory in adults with brain injury. *Brain Inj.* 1994;8(7):579–587.

46. Weinberg RM, Auerbach SH, Moore S. Pharmacologic treatment of cognitive deficits: a case study. *Brain Inj.* 1987;1(1):57–59.

47. Morey CE, Cilo M, Berry J, Cusick C. The effect of Aricept in persons with persistent memory disorder following traumatic brain injury: a pilot study. *Brain Inj.* 2003;17(9):809–815.

48. Trovato M, Slomine B, Pidcock F, Christensen J. The efficacy of donepezil hydrochloride on memory functioning in three adolescents with severe traumatic brain injury. *Brain Inj.* 2006;20(3):339–343.

49. Silver JM, Koumaras B, Chen M, et al. Effects of rivastigmine on cognitive function in patients with traumatic brain injury. *Neurology.* 2006;67(5):748–755.

50. Tenovuo O, Alin J, Helenius H. A randomized controlled trial of rivastigmine for chronic sequels of traumatic brain injury-what it showed and taught? *Brain Inj.* 2009;23(6):548–558.

51. de la Tremblaye PB, Bondi CO, Lajud N, Cheng JP, Radabaugh HL, Kline AE. Galantamine and environmental enrichment enhance cognitive recovery after experimental traumatic brain injury but do not confer additional benefits when combined. *J Neurotrauma.* 2017;34(8):1610–1622.

52. Effgen GB, Morrison 3rd B. Memantine reduced cell death, astrogliosis, and functional deficits in an in vitro model of repetitive mild traumatic brain injury. *J Neurotrauma.* 2017;34(4):934–942.

53. Rao VL, Dogan A, Todd KG, Bowen KK, Dempsey RJ. Neuroprotection by memantine, a non-competitive NMDA receptor antagonist after traumatic brain injury in rats. *Brain Res.* 2001;911(1):96–100.

54. Elovic EP, Zafonte RD. Ginkgo biloba: applications in traumatic brain injury. *J Head Trauma Rehabil.* 2001;16(6):603–607.

55. Diamond BJ, Shiflett SC, Feiwel N, et al. Ginkgo biloba extract: mechanisms and clinical indications. *Arch Phys Med Rehabil.* 2000;81(5):668–678.

56. Kim YH, Ko MH, Na SY, Park SH, Kim KW. Effects of single-dose methylphenidate on cognitive performance in patients with traumatic brain injury: a double-blind placebo-controlled study. *Clin Rehabil.* 2006;20(1):24–30.

57. Speech TJ, Rao SM, Osmon DC, Sperry LT. A double-blind controlled study of methylphenidate treatment in closed head injury. *Brain Inj.* 1993;7(4):333–338.

58. Kraus MF, Smith GS, Butters M, et al. Effects of the dopaminergic agent and NMDA receptor antagonist amantadine on cognitive function, cerebral glucose metabolism and D2 receptor availability in chronic traumatic brain injury: a study using positron emission tomography (PET). *Brain Inj.* 2005;19(7):471–479.

59. McDowell S, Whyte J, D'Esposito M. Differential effect of a dopaminergic agonist on prefrontal function in traumatic brain injury patients. *Brain.* 1998;121(pt 6):1155–1164.

60. Berthier ML, Green C, Higueras C, Fernandez I, Hinojosa J, Martin MC. A randomized, placebo-controlled study of donepezil in poststroke aphasia. *Neurology.* 2006;67(9):1687–1689.

61. Berthier ML, Hinojosa J, Martin Mdel C, Fernandez I. Open-label study of donepezil in chronic poststroke aphasia. *Neurology.* 2003;60(7):1218–1219.

62. Hong JM, Shin DH, Lim TS, Lee JS, Huh K. Galantamine administration in chronic post-stroke aphasia. *J Neurol Neurosurg Psychiatr.* 2012;83(7):675–680.

63. Whiting E, Chenery HJ, Chalk J, Copland DA. Dexamphetamine boosts naming treatment effects in chronic aphasia. *J Int Neuropsychol Soc.* 2007;13(6):972–979.

64. Walker-Batson D, Curtis S, Natarajan R, et al. A double-blind, placebo-controlled study of the use of amphetamine in the treatment of aphasia. *Stroke.* 2001;32(9):2093–2098.

65. Berthier ML, Green C, Lara JP, et al. Memantine and constraint-induced aphasia therapy in chronic poststroke aphasia. *Ann Neurol.* 2009;65(5):577–585.

66. Enderby P, Broeckx J, Hospers W, Schildermans F, Deberdt W. Effect of piracetam on recovery and rehabilitation after stroke: a double-blind, placebo-controlled study. *Clin Neuropharmacol.* 1994;17(4):320–331.

67. Kessler J, Thiel A, Karbe H, Heiss WD. Piracetam improves activated blood flow and facilitates rehabilitation of poststroke aphasic patients. *Stroke.* 2000;31(9):2112–2116.

68. Huber W, Willmes K, Poeck K, Van Vleymen B, Deberdt W. Piracetam as an adjuvant to language therapy for aphasia: a randomized double-blind placebo-controlled pilot study. *Arch Phys Med Rehabil.* 1997;78(3):245–250.

69. Bragoni M, Altieri M, Di Piero V, Padovani A, Mostardini C, Lenzi GL. Bromocriptine and speech therapy in non-fluent chronic aphasia after stroke. *Neurol Sci.* 2000;21(1):19–22.

70. Ashtary F, Janghorbani M, Chitsaz A, Reisi M, Bahrami A. A randomized, double-blind trial of bromocriptine efficacy in nonfluent aphasia after stroke. *Neurology.* 2006;66(6):914–916.

71. Leemann B, Laganaro M, Chetelat-Mabillard D, Schnider A. Crossover trial of subacute computerized aphasia therapy for anomia with the addition of either levodopa or placebo. *Neurorehabil Neural Repair.* 2011;25(1):43–47.

72. Seniow J, Litwin M, Litwin T, Lesniak M, Czlonkowska A. New approach to the rehabilitation of post-stroke focal cognitive syndrome: effect of levodopa combined with speech and language therapy on functional recovery from aphasia. *J Neurol Sci.* 2009;283(1–2):214–218.

73. Brooke MM, Questad KA, Patterson DR, Bashak KJ. Agitation and restlessness after closed head injury: a prospective study of 100 consecutive admissions. *Arch Phys Med Rehabil.* 1992;73(4):320–323.

74. Nott MT, Chapparo C, Baguley IJ. Agitation following traumatic brain injury: an Australian sample. *Brain Inj.* 2006;20(11):1175–1182.

75. Fugate LP, Spacek LA, Kresty LA, Levy CE, Johnson JC, Mysiw WJ. Definition of agitation following traumatic brain injury: I. A survey of the brain injury special interest group of the American Academy of Physical Medicine and Rehabilitation. *Arch Phys Med Rehabil.* 1997;78(9):917–923.

76. Sandel ME, Mysiw WJ. The agitated brain injured patient. Part 1: definitions, differential diagnosis, and assessment. *Arch Phys Med Rehabil.* 1996;77(6):617–623.

77. Lombard LA, Zafonte RD. Agitation after traumatic brain injury: considerations and treatment options. *Am J Phys Med Rehabil.* 2005;84(10):797–812.

78. Feeney DM, Gonzalez A, Law WA. Amphetamine, haloperidol, and experience interact to affect rate of recovery after motor cortex injury. *Science (New York, NY).* 1982;217(4562):855–857.

79. Goldstein LB. Neuropharmacology of TBI-induced plasticity. *Brain Inj.* 2003;17(8):685–694.

80. Fleminger S, Greenwood RJ, Oliver DL. Pharmacological management for agitation and aggression in people with acquired brain injury. *Cochrane Database Syst Rev.* 2006;(4):Cd003299.

81. Fugate LP, Spacek LA, Kresty LA, Levy CE, Johnson JC, Mysiw WJ. Measurement and treatment of agitation following traumatic brain injury: II. A survey of the brain injury special interest group of the American Academy of Physical Medicine and Rehabilitation. *Arch Phys Med Rehabil.* 1997;78(9):924–928.

82. Chatham Showalter PE, Kimmel DN. Agitated symptom response to divalproex following acute brain injury. *J Neuropsychiatr Clin Neurosci.* 2000;12(3):395–397.

83. Chatham-Showalter PE. Carbamazepine for combativeness in acute traumatic brain injury. *J Neuropsychiatr Clin Neurosci.* 1996;8(1):96–99.

84. Azouvi P, Jokic C, Attal N, Denys P, Markabi S, Bussel B. Carbamazepine in agitation and aggressive behaviour following severe closed-head injury: results of an open trial. *Brain Inj.* 1999;13(10):797–804.

85. Kant R, Smith-Seemiller L, Zeiler D. Treatment of aggression and irritability after head injury. *Brain Inj.* 1998;12(8):661–666.

86. Ratey JJ, Leveroni CL, Miller AC, Komry V, Gaffar K. Low-dose buspirone to treat agitation and maladaptive behavior in brain-injured patients: two case reports. *J Clin Psychopharmacol.* 1992;12(5):362–364.

87. Rosati DL. Early polyneuropharmacologic intervention in brain injury agitation. *Am J Phys Med Rehabil.* 2002;81(2):90–93.

88. Hammond FM, Bickett AK, Norton JH, Pershad R. Effectiveness of amantadine hydrochloride in the reduction of chronic traumatic brain injury irritability and aggression. *J Head Trauma Rehabil.* 2014;29(5):391–399.

89. Mathias JL, Alvaro PK. Prevalence of sleep disturbances, disorders, and problems following traumatic brain injury: a meta-analysis. *Sleep Med.* 2012;13(7):898–905.

90. Ouellet MC, Beaulieu-Bonneau S, Morin CM. Sleep-wake disturbances after traumatic brain injury. *Lancet Neurol.* 2015;14(7):746–757.

91. American Sleep Disorders Association, Diagnostic Classification Steering Committee. *The International Classification of Sleep Disorders : Diagnostic and Coding Manual.* Rochester, MN, USA: ASDA; 1990.

92. Goldstein LB. Prescribing of potentially harmful drugs to patients admitted to hospital after head injury. *J Neurol Neurosurg Psychiatr.* 1995;58(6):753–755.

93. Schallert T, Hernandez TD, Barth TM. Recovery of function after brain damage: severe and chronic disruption by diazepam. *Brain Res.* 1986;379(1):104–111.

94. Flanagan SR, Greenwald B, Wieber S. Pharmacological treatment of insomnia for individuals with brain injury. *J Head Trauma Rehabil.* 2007;22(1):67–70.

95. Stahl SM. Mechanism of action of trazodone: a multifunctional drug. *CNS Spectr.* 2009;14(10):536–546.

96. Grima NA, Ponsford JL, St Hilaire MA, Mansfield D, Rajaratnam SM. Circadian melatonin rhythm following traumatic brain injury. *Neurorehabil Neural Repair.* 2016;30(10):972–977.

97. Kemp S, Biswas R, Neumann V, Coughlan A. The value of melatonin for sleep disorders occurring post-head injury: a pilot RCT. *Brain Inj.* 2004;18(9):911–919.

98. Lequerica A, Jasey N, Portelli Tremont JN, Chiaravalloti ND. Pilot study on the effect of Ramelteon on sleep disturbance after traumatic brain injury: preliminary evidence from a clinical trial. *Arch Phys Med Rehabil.* 2015;96(10):1802–1809.

99. Hammond FM, Barrett RS, Shea T, et al. Psychotropic medication use during inpatient rehabilitation for traumatic brain injury. *Arch Phys Med Rehabil.* 2015;96 (suppl 8). S256–S253.e214.

100. Seel RT, Macciocchi S, Kreutzer JS. Clinical considerations for the diagnosis of major depression after moderate to severe TBI. *J Head Trauma Rehabil.* 2010;25(2):99–112.

101. Kreutzer JS, Seel RT, Gourley E. The prevalence and symptom rates of depression after traumatic brain injury: a comprehensive examination. *Brain Inj.* 2001;15(7):563–576.

102. Fleminger S, Oliver DL, Williams WH, Evans J. The neuropsychiatry of depression after brain injury. *Neuropsychol Rehabil.* 2003;13(1–2):65–87.

103. Weeks DL, Greer CL, Bray BS, Schwartz CR, White Jr JR. Association of antidepressant medication therapy with inpatient rehabilitation outcomes for stroke, traumatic brain injury, or traumatic spinal cord injury. *Arch Phys Med Rehabil.* 2011;92(5):683–695.

104. Jefferson JW, Pradko JF, Muir KT. Bupropion for major depressive disorder: pharmacokinetic and formulation considerations. *Clin Ther.* 2005;27(11):1685–1695.

105. Teng CJ, Bhalerao S, Lee Z, et al. The use of bupropion in the treatment of restlessness after a traumatic brain injury. *Brain Inj.* 2001;15(5):463–467.

106. Zhang WT, Wang YF. Efficacy of methylphenidate for the treatment of mental sequelae after traumatic brain injury. *Medicine.* 2017;96(25):e6960.

107. McIntyre RS, Lee Y, Zhou AJ, et al. The efficacy of psychostimulants in major depressive episodes: a systematic review and meta-analysis. *J Clin Psychopharmacol.* 2017;37(4):412–418.

108. Osborn AJ, Mathias JL, Fairweather-Schmidt AK. Prevalence of anxiety following adult traumatic brain injury: a meta-analysis comparing measures, samples and postinjury intervals. *Neuropsychology.* 2016;30(2):247–261.

109. Dahm J, Ponsford J. Comparison of long-term outcomes following traumatic injury: what is the unique experience for those with brain injury compared with orthopaedic injury? *Injury.* 2015;46(1):142–149.

110. Schiehser DM, Delano-Wood L, Jak AJ, et al. Predictors of cognitive and physical fatigue in post-acute mild-moderate traumatic brain injury. *Neuropsychol Rehabil.* 2016:1–16.

111. Larson EB, Zollman FS. The effect of sleep medications on cognitive recovery from traumatic brain injury. *J Head Trauma Rehabil.* 2010;25(1):61–67.

112. Mahesh R, Pandey DK, Katiyar S, Kukade G, Viyogi S, Rudra A. Effect of anti-depressants on neuro-behavioural consequences following impact accelerated traumatic brain injury in rats. *Indian J Exp Biol.* 2010;48(5):466–473.

113. Pandey DK, Yadav SK, Mahesh R, Rajkumar R. Depression-like and anxiety-like behavioural aftermaths of impact accelerated traumatic brain injury in rats: a model of comorbid depression and anxiety? *Behav Brain Res.* 2009;205(2):436–442.

114. Perino C, Rago R, Cicolini A, Torta R, Monaco F. Mood and behavioural disorders following traumatic brain injury: clinical evaluation and pharmacological management. *Brain Inj.* 2001;15(2):139–148.

115. Gillman PK. Triptans, serotonin agonists, and serotonin syndrome (serotonin toxicity): a review. *Headache.* 2010;50(2):264–272.

116. Cheng JP, Leary JB, Sembhi A, Edwards CM, Bondi CO, Kline AE. 5-hydroxytryptamine1A (5-HT1A) receptor agonists: a decade of empirical evidence supports their use as an efficacious therapeutic strategy for brain trauma. *Brain Res.* 2016;1640(pt A):5–14.

117. Kline AE, Olsen AS, Sozda CN, Hoffman AN, Cheng JP. Evaluation of a combined treatment paradigm consisting of environmental enrichment and the 5-HT1A receptor agonist buspirone after experimental traumatic brain injury. *J Neurotrauma.* 2012;29(10):1960–1969.

118. Deb S, Crownshaw T. The role of pharmacotherapy in the management of behaviour disorders in traumatic brain injury patients. *Brain Inj.* 2004;18(1):1–31.

119. Forlenza OV, Coutinho AM, Aprahamian I, et al. Long-term lithium treatment reduces glucose metabolism in the cerebellum and hippocampus of nondemented older adults: an [(1)(8)F]FDG-PET study. *ACS Chem Neurosci.* 2014;5(6):484–489.

120. Hirvonen MR, Paljarvi L, Naukkarinen A, Komulainen H, Savolainen KM. Potentiation of malaoxon-induced convulsions by lithium: early neuronal injury, phosphoinositide signaling, and calcium. *Toxicol Appl Pharmacol.* 1990;104(2):276–289.

121. Megna J, O'Dell M. Ataxia from lithium toxicity successfully treated with high-dose buspirone: a single-case experimental design. *Arch Phys Med Rehabil.* 2001;82(8):1145–1148.

122. Milutinovic A. Lithium chloride could aggravate brain injury caused by 3-nitropropionic acid. *Bosn J Basic Med Sci.* 2016;16(4):261–267.

123. Parmelee DX, O'Shanick GJ. Carbamazepine-lithium toxicity in brain-damaged adolescents. *Brain Inj.* 1988;2(4):305–308.

124. Unger J, Decaux G, L'Hermite M. Rhabdomyolysis, acute renal failure endocrine alterations and neurological sequelae in a case of lithium selfpoisoning. *Acta Clin Belg.* 1982;37(4):216–223.

125. Cruz C, Jetter KM, Stewart JT. Lithium treatment for posthead injury volatility. *Psychosomatics.* 2015;56(5):576–579.

126. Dell'Osso L, Del Grande C, Gesi C, Carmassi C, Musetti L. A new look at an old drug: neuroprotective effects and therapeutic potentials of lithium salts. *Neuropsychiatr Dis Treat.* 2016;12:1687–1703.

127. Leeds PR, Yu F, Wang Z, et al. A new avenue for lithium: intervention in traumatic brain injury. *ACS Chem Neurosci.* 2014;5(6):422–433.

128. Noguchi KK, Johnson SA, Kristich LE, et al. Lithium protects against anaesthesia neurotoxicity in the infant primate brain. *Sci Rep.* 2016;6:22427.

129. Nonaka S, Chuang DM. Neuroprotective effects of chronic lithium on focal cerebral ischemia in rats. *Neuroreport.* 1998;9(9):2081–2084.

130. Zhou K, Xie C, Wickstrom M, et al. Lithium protects hippocampal progenitors, cognitive performance and hypothalamus-pituitary function after irradiation to the juvenile rat brain. *Oncotarget.* 2017;8(21):34111–34127.

131. Beresford TP, Arciniegas D, Clapp L, Martin B, Alfers J. Reduction of affective lability and alcohol use following traumatic brain injury: a clinical pilot study of anticonvulsant medications. *Brain Inj.* 2005;19(4):309–313.

132. Dikmen SS, Machamer JE, Winn HR, Anderson GD, Temkin NR. Neuropsychological effects of valproate in traumatic brain injury: a randomized trial. *Neurology.* 2000;54(4):895–902.

133. Naguy A, Al-Enezi N. Lamotrigine uses in psychiatric practice-beyond bipolar prophylaxis a hope or hype? *Am J Ther.* 2017. https://doi.org/10.1097/MJT.0000000000000535.

134. Pachet A, Friesen S, Winkelaar D, Gray S. Beneficial behavioural effects of lamotrigine in traumatic brain injury. *Brain Inj.* 2003;17(8):715–722.

135. Whiting WL, Sullivan GA, Stewart JT. Lamotrigine treatment for agitation following traumatic brain injury. *Psychosomatics.* 2016;57(3):330–333.

136. Ashman TA, Cantor JB, Gordon WA, et al. A randomized controlled trial of sertraline for the treatment of depression in persons with traumatic brain injury. *Arch Phys Med Rehabil.* 2009;90(5):733–740.

137. Lee HB, Lyketsos CG, Rao V. Pharmacological management of the psychiatric aspects of traumatic brain injury. *Int Rev Psychiatr (Abingdon, England).* 2003;15(4):359–370.

138. Doody RS, D'Amico S, Cutler AJ, et al. An open-label study to assess safety, tolerability, and effectiveness of dextromethorphan/quinidine for pseudobulbar affect in dementia: PRISM II results. *CNS Spectr.* 2016;21(6):450–459.

139. Hammond FM, Alexander DN, Cutler AJ, et al. PRISM II: an open-label study to assess effectiveness of dextromethorphan/quinidine for pseudobulbar affect in patients with dementia, stroke or traumatic brain injury. *BMC Neurol.* 2016;16:89.

140. Nguyen L, Thomas KL, Lucke-Wold BP, Cavendish JZ, Crowe MS, Matsumoto RR. Dextromethorphan: an update on its utility for neurological and neuropsychiatric disorders. *Pharmacol Ther.* 2016;159:1–22.

141. Roman MW. NueDexta: a treatment for pseudobulbar affect. *Issues Ment Health Nurs.* 2015;36(12):1019–1021.

142. Stahl SM. Dextromethorphan-quinidine-responsive pseudobulbar affect (PBA): psychopharmacological model for wide-ranging disorders of emotional expression? *CNS Spectr.* 2016;21(6):419–423.

143. Balakrishnan P, Rosen H. The causes and treatment of pseudobulbar affect in ischemic stroke. *Curr Treat Options Cardiovasc Med.* 2008;10(3):216–222.

144. Okun MS, Riestra AR, Nadeau SE. Treatment of ballism and pseudobulbar affect with sertraline. *Arch Neurol.* 2001;58(10):1682–1684.

145. Takeuchi H, Iwamoto K, Mukai M, Fujita T, Tsujino H, Iwamoto Y. Effective use of sertraline for pathological laughing after severe vasospasm due to aneurysmal subarachnoid hemorrhage: case report. *Neurol Med Chir.* 2014;54(3):231–235.

146. Schoedel KA, Pope LE, Sellers EM. Randomized open-label drug-drug interaction trial of dextromethorphan/quinidine and paroxetine in healthy volunteers. *Clin Drug Investig.* 2012;32(3):157–169.

147. Chahine LM, Chemali Z. Du rire aux larmes: pathological laughing and crying in patients with traumatic brain injury and treatment with lamotrigine. *Epilepsy Behav.* 2006;8(3):610–615.

148. Warden DL, Gordon B, McAllister TW, et al. Guidelines for the pharmacologic treatment of neurobehavioral sequelae of traumatic brain injury. *J Neurotrauma.* 2006;23(10):1468–1501.

149. Hoffman AN, Cheng JP, Zafonte RD, Kline AE. Administration of haloperidol and risperidone after neurobehavioral testing hinders the recovery of traumatic brain injury-induced deficits. *Life Sci.* 2008;83(17–18):602–607.

150. Ukai W, Ozawa H, Tateno M, Hashimoto E, Saito T. Neurotoxic potential of haloperidol in comparison with risperidone: implication of Akt-mediated signal changes by haloperidol. *J Neural Transm (Vienna, Austria: 1996).* 2004;111(6):667–681.

151. Wilson MS, Gibson CJ, Hamm RJ. Haloperidol, but not olanzapine, impairs cognitive performance after traumatic brain injury in rats. *Am J Phys Med Rehabil.* 2003;82(11):871–879.

152. Goldstein LB. Basic and clinical studies of pharmacologic effects on recovery from brain injury. *J Neural Transplant Plast.* 1993;4(3):175–192.

153. Hynes MD, Anderson CD, Gianutsos G, Lal H. Effects of haloperidol, methyltyrosine and morphine on recovery from lesions of lateral hypothalamus. *Pharmacol Biochem Behav.* 1975;3(5):755–759.

154. Kline AE, Hoffman AN, Cheng JP, Zafonte RD, Massucci JL. Chronic administration of antipsychotics impede behavioral recovery after experimental traumatic brain injury. *Neurosci Lett.* 2008;448(3):263–267.

155. Kline AE, Massucci JL, Zafonte RD, Dixon CE, DeFeo JR, Rogers EH. Differential effects of single versus multiple administrations of haloperidol and risperidone on functional outcome after experimental brain trauma. *Crit Care Med.* 2007;35(3):919–924.

156. Phelps TI, Bondi CO, Ahmed RH, Olugbade YT, Kline AE. Divergent long-term consequences of chronic treatment with haloperidol, risperidone, and bromocriptine on traumatic brain injury-induced cognitive deficits. *J Neurotrauma.* 2015;32(8):590–597.

157. Bellamy CJ, Kane-Gill SL, Falcione BA, Seybert AL. Neuroleptic malignant syndrome in traumatic brain injury patients treated with haloperidol. *J Trauma.* 2009;66(3):954–958.

158. Shaikh N, Al-Sulaiti G, Nasser A, Rahman MA. Neuroleptic malignant syndrome and closed head injury: a case report and review. *Asian J Neurosurg.* 2011;6(2):101–105.

159. Vincent FM, Zimmerman JE, Van Haren J. Neuroleptic malignant syndrome complicating closed head injury. *Neurosurgery.* 1986;18(2):190–193.

160. Wilkinson R, Meythaler JM, Guin-Renfroe S. Neuroleptic malignant syndrome induced by haloperidol following traumatic brain injury. *Brain Inj.* 1999;13(12):1025–1031.

161. Fava M. Psychopharmacologic treatment of pathologic aggression. *Psychiatr Clin North Am.* 1997;20(2):427–451.

162. McGrane IR, Loveland JG, Zaluski HJ. Adjunctive amantadine treatment for aggressive behavior in children: a series of eight cases. *J Child Adolesc Psychopharmacol.* 2016;26(10):935–938.

163. Verellen RM, Cavazos JE. Post-traumatic epilepsy: an overview. *Therapy.* 2010;7(5):527–531.

164. Fisher RS, van Emde Boas W, Blume W, et al. Epileptic seizures and epilepsy: definitions proposed by the International League Against Epilepsy (ILAE) and the International Bureau for Epilepsy (IBE). *Epilepsia.* 2005;46:470–472.

165. Brain Trauma Foundation. Guidelines for the management of severe traumatic brain injury. *J Neurotrauma.* 2007;24(s1):S1–S106.

166. Temkin N, Dimken S, Wilensky J. A randomized, double-blind study of phenytoin for the prevention of post-traumatic seizures. *N Engl J Med.* 1990;323(8):497–502.

167. Temkin N, Dimken S, Anderson G. Valproate therapy for prevention of posttraumatic seizures: a randomized trial. *J Neurosurg.* 1999;91:593–600.

168. Szaflarski J, Sangha K, Lindsell C. Prospective, randomized, single blind comparative trial of intravenous levetiracetam versus phenytoin for seizure prophylaxis. *Neurocrit Care.* 2010;12:165–172.

169. Dikmen S, Temkin N, Miller B. Neurobehavioral effects of phenytoin prophylaxis of posttraumatic seizures. *JAMA.* 1991;265:1271–1277.

170. Marin R, Wilkosz P. Disorders of diminished motivation. *J Head Trauma Rehabil.* 2005;20(4):377–388.

171. Powell J, Al-Adawi S, Morgan J. Motivational deficits after brain injury: effects of bromocriptine in 11 patients. *J Neurol Neurosurg Psychiatr.* 1996;60:416–421.

172. O'Suilleabbain P, Dewey R. Movement disorders after head injury. *J Head Trauma Rehabil.* 2004;19(4):305–313.

173. Krauss J, Trankle R, Kopp K. Post-traumatic movement disorders in survivors of severe head injury. *Neurology.* 1996;47(6):1488–1492.

174. Fletcher N, Thompson P, Scadding J. Successful treatment of childhood onset symptomatic dystonia with levodopa. *J Neurol Neurosurg Psychiatr.* 1993;56(8):865–870.

175. Cloud L, Jinnah H. Treatment strategies for dystonia. *Expert Opin Pharmacother.* 2010;11(1):5–15.

176. Hallett M, Benecke R, Blitzer A, Comella C. Treatment of focal dystonias with botulinum toxin. *Toxicon.* 2009;54(5):628–633.

177. Frucht S, Louis E, Chuang C. A pilot tolerability and efficacy study o flevetiracetam in patients with chronic myoclonus. *Neurology.* 2001;57:1112–1114.

178. Kant R, Zeiler D. Hemiballismus following closed head injury. *Brain Inj.* 1996;10(2):155–158.

179. Ponsford J, Zeiler D, Parcell D. Fatigue and sleep disturbance following traumatic brain injury: their nature, causes, and potential treatments. *J Head Trauma Rehabil.* 2012;27(3):224–233.

180. Lee K, Hicks G, Nino-Murcia G. Validity and reliability of a scale to assess fatigue. *Psychiatr Res.* 1991;36:291–298.

181. Belmont A, Agar N, Azouvi P. Subjective fatigue, mental effort, and attention deficits after severe traumatic brain injury. *Neurorehabil Neural Repair.* 2009;23(9):939–944.

182. Dijkers M, Bushnik T. Assessing fatigue after traumatic brain injury: an evaluation of the Barroso Fatigue Scale. *J Head Trauma Rehabil.* 2008;23:3–16.

183. Ponsford J, Ziino C. Measurement and prediction of subjective fatigue following traumatic brain injury. *J Int Neuropsychol Soc.* 2005;11:416–425.

184. Ziino C, Ponsford J. Vigilance and fatigue following traumatic brain injury. *J Int Neuropsychol Soc.* 2006;12(1):100–110.

185. Johansson B, Wentzel A, Andrell P. Methylphenidate reduces mental fatigue and improves processing speed in persons suffered a traumatic brain injury. *Brain Inj.* 2015;29(6):758–765.

186. Blackman J, Patrick P, Buck M. Paroxysmal autonomic instability with dystonia after brain injury. *Neurol Rev.* 2004;61:321–328.

187. Friedman J, Feinberg S, Feldman R. A neuroleptic malignant like syndrome due to levodopa therapy withdrawal. *JAMA.* 1985;254:2792–2795.

188. Friedman L, Weinrauch L, D'Elia J. Metoclopramide-induced neuroleptic malignant syndrome. *Arch Intern Med.* 1987;147:1495–1497.

189. Feuerman T, Gade G, Reynolds R. Stress-induced malignant hyperthermia in a head-injured patient: case report. *J Neurosurg.* 1988;68:297–299.

190. Eisenberg M, Jasey N. Spasticity and muscle overactivity as components of the upper motor neuron syndrome. In: Fontera W, ed. *Delisa's Physical Medicine & Rehabilitation.* Vol. 5. Philadelphia: Lippincott Williams & Wilkins; 2010:1319–1410.

191. Tseng T, Wang S. Locus of action of centrally acting muscle relaxants, diazepam and tybamate. *J Pharmacol Exp Ther.* 1971;178(2):350–360.

192. Kofler M, Kofter M, Leis A. Prolonged seizure activity after baclofen withdrawal. *Neurology.* 1992;42(3):697–698.

193. Simpson D, Gracies J, Yablon S. Botulinum neurotoxin versus tizanidine in upper limb spasticity: a placebo controlled study. *J Neurol Neurosurg Psychiatr.* 2009;80:380–385.

194. Yablon S, Sipski M. Effect of transdermal clonidine on spinal spasticity: a case series. *Am J Phys Med Rehabil.* 1993;72(3):154–157.

195. Goldstein L. The Sygen in Acute Stroke Study Investigators. Common drugs may influence motor recovery after stroke. *Neurology.* 1995;45(5):865–871.

196. Snow B, Tsui J, Bhatt M. Treatment of spasticity with botulinum toxin: a double-blind study. *Ann Neurol.* 1990;28(4):512–515.

197. Yablon S, Agana B, Ivanhoe C. Botulinum toxin in severe upper extremity spasticity among patients with traumatic brain injury: an open-labeled trial. *Neurology.* 1996;47(4):512–515.

198. Dubow J, Kim A, Leikin J. Visual system side effects caused by parasympathetic dysfunction after botulinum toxin type B injections. *Mov Disord.* 2005;20(7):877–880.

CHAPTER 12

Posttraumatic Pain Management

MICHAEL H. MARINO, MD • THOMAS K. WATANABE, MD

EPIDEMIOLOGY

Given the fact that trauma is the precipitating event for a traumatic brain injury (TBI), it is not surprising that pain is one of the most common complaints after TBI. Many patients with TBI's sustain injuries to other parts of their body as well as the head. Although the term "polytrauma" has gained greater recognition in the military setting, this concept is important when considering painful conditions that arise in the general TBI population as well. Studies on the prevalence of pain acutely are complicated by the difficulty that some patients may have in reporting pain because of their clinical and/or cognitive status. Some studies have examined the prevalence of pain more chronically. Nampiaparampil performed a systematic review on the prevalence of chronic pain after TBI and noted headaches in 58% of all patients and chronic pain in 75% of patients with mild TBI and 32% of patients with moderate or severe TBI.[1] This somewhat surprising finding regarding the relationship between TBI severity and pain complaints has also been reported in some studies that have evaluated the prevalence of posttraumatic headaches (PTH),[2] but not others.[3]

Another systematic review was performed by Dobscha and colleagues to better understand the relationship between polytrauma with TBI and pain. Although the results were limited because of a lack of high-quality studies, an association between pain and psychologic factors was noted.[4] This underscores the multidimensional nature of pain in this context. They also attempted to identify reliable assessment tools of pain and functional limitations related to pain but were not able to do so. Using serial interviews at 3, 6, and 12 months postinjury, the incidence of PTH in the first year after TBI in a moderate to severe TBI population was reported as 71%, although for individuals the complaints did not always persist throughout the period studied.[3]

PATHOPHYSIOLOGY

The sensation of pain and its intensity begins with the peripheral receptors (nociceptors) that are activated by thermal, mechanical, and chemical stimuli. Nociceptors are found in the skin, muscle and viscera. They are connected to primary afferent neurons, which represent the first-order neurons in the pain system. These primary afferents consist of A-δ-fibers and C-fibers. A-δ-fibers are myelinated, thin neurons that are 1–5 μm in diameter with small receptive fields that have conduction velocities of 5–30 m/s. Pain from A-δ-fibers comes from thermoreceptors and mechanoreceptors. It is perceived as fast, sharp, well localized, and well defined. C-fibers are small unmyelinated fibers 0.25–1.5 μm in diameter with conduction velocities of 0.5–2 m/s. Pain from C-fibers comes from thermoreceptors, mechanoreceptors, and chemoreceptors. It is perceived as slow, diffuse, poorly localized, burning, or throbbing.[5]

These peripheral first-order afferents have cell bodies in the dorsal root ganglia and enter the spinal cord via the dorsal horn. From here, two distinct and conceptually important pain pathways diverge into the direct and indirect pathways. The direct pathway is also called the lateral pathway or neospinothalamic tract. The direct pathway is of critical importance in acute pain, as it conveys information detailing the type of pain and its location from the nociceptors.[6] In the direct pathway, the first-order neurons entering the spinal cord via the dorsal horn form their first synapse in the nucleus proprius. From the nucleus proprius, these second-order neurons ascend between 1 and 3 levels and then cross via the anterior white commissure to the contralateral side of the spinal cord and become the spinothalamic tract. The spinothalamic tract ascends and synapses at the ventroposterolateral (VPL) nucleus of the thalamus. From the VPL, third-order neurons project to the primary somatosensory cortex of parietal lobe.[7]

The indirect pathway is also called the medial pathway. The paleospinothalamic, spinomesencephalic, and spinoreticular tracts make up the indirect pathway. The indirect pathway is of critical importance in chronic pain and in the mediation of the autonomic, endocrine, arousal, and affective response to pain. The indirect pain pathway also begins centrally at the level of the second-order neurons in the dorsal horn.[6] The paleospinothalamic tract ascends from the dorsal horn bilaterally in the ventrolateral spinal cord to its synapses in reticular formation and the intralaminar and midline nuclei of the thalamus. It then projects throughout the limbic system, including the anterior cingulate gyrus. The spinomesencephalic tract projects to the midbrain periaqueductal gray. Like the paleospinothalamic tract, it also synapses on the midline and intralaminar nuclei of the thalamus. Its projections are then distributed broadly to the limbic system and throughout the cortex. The spinoreticular tract travels in the anterior white matter of the spinal cord and terminates in the medullary pontine reticular formation and then onto the midline and intralaminar nuclei of the thalamus. It also projects broadly into the cortex and limbic system.[6,7] Projections of the indirect pathway to the reticular formation are responsible for the arousal aspects of pain. The widespread projections to the limbic system and anterior cingulate gyrus are responsible for the affective and motivational aspects of pain. The periaqueductal gray plays an important role as an antinociceptive center. It stimulates the surrounding brainstem structures to decrease pain via descending inhibitory signals to the dorsal horn cells.[8]

Pain pathways for the head and face are anatomically separate from those for the rest of the body. The trigeminal sensory system provides sensation for the face and the front of the scalp. The upper three cervical dorsal roots carry sensory afferents from the upper neck and posterior scalp. The primary nociceptive afferents from the meninges are carried via the ophthalmic division of cranial nerve V. The brain parenchyma itself has no nociceptive afferents. The ear and external auditory canal have sensory afferents carried by cranial nerves IX and X. Primary nociceptive afferents from cranial nerves V, IX, and X travel to the spinal tract and the trigeminal nerve nucleus.[9]

Peripheral and central pain pathways can become sensitized to painful stimuli, which results in hyperresponsiveness to stimuli or spontaneous discharges in the absence of stimuli.[10] Peripheral sensitization can occur by local inflammatory processes and mediators released during injury that can lower the activation threshold for primary nociceptive afferents. Mediators of the inflammatory response such as cytokines, prostaglandins, and leukotrienes also increase the sensitivity of the nociceptors. Substances such as bradykinin, substance P, serotonin, and histamine are released directly from the nociceptors and also increase their sensitivity.[11] Peripheral sensitization can also occur via the process of windup. In windup, sensitization occurs as the activated C-fiber-evoked responses in the dorsal horn become progressively larger in magnitude. This process

stops in the absence of a painful stimulus. Central sensitization involves increased excitability of dorsal horn neurons due to lowered activation thresholds and increased spontaneous activity. Additionally, the receptive field for dorsal horn neurons can expand, further contributing to central sensitization. These processes result in hyperalgesia and allodynia.[12]

ASSESSMENT OF PAIN

Assessment of pain in the patient with brain injury can represent a unique challenge. Altered levels of arousal and memory can interfere with patients' ability to reliably report their subjective experience of pain. For patients who are accurate and reliable historians, standard pain interview questions are appropriate. Assessment of the time of onset, location, intensity, duration, frequency, character, and exacerbating and alleviating factors is advised. It is also useful to inquire about how significantly the pain interferes with day to day activity. Objective rating scales that can be used by reliable patients include the visual analog scale (VAS), the verbal analog scale, the numeric rating scale (NRS), and the picture or faces pain scale. All these scales are easily administered in the clinical setting. The VAS is a 10-cm line with one end representing no pain and the other end representing extreme pain. Patients are asked to place a mark along the line representing the level of their pain. The VAS has shown good validity and reliability in acute[13] and chronic pain.[14] It is useful for measuring change in pain levels in the same patient across different points of time and after specific interventions. The verbal analog scale or verbal rating scale uses a list of adjectives to describe the level of pain intensity. Verbal rating scales have been found to be valid measures of pain and are also sensitive to pain treatments.[15,16] Patients must be literate and familiar with the adjectives used on the scale. Some patients may become frustrated if the best word to describe their pain is not included in the list of adjectives on the scale. The NRS uses a range of digits (for example, 0–10 or 0–100) to rate pain intensity. These tests are quick and easy to administer and do not require literacy or familiarity with particular adjectives. They have been found to be valid for measuring pain and also show sensitivity to treatments.[17,18] The faces pain scale uses a series of photographs or drawings of faces displaying varying levels of pain and discomfort. Patients choose which face best represents their level of pain. The faces pain scale has been demonstrated to be a valid measure of pain and is also sensitive to treatments. The faces pain scale is particularly useful in children, who tend to prefer it, but it is also valid in adults.[19–21] It should be noted that all these scales primarily assess the intensity of pain but do not assess the pain location, affective and behavioral components of pain, or its impact on daily functioning. Pain drawings are effective to measure pain location. The VAS and verbal analog scale can be modified to measure the affective components of pain, and these can be used quickly in the clinical setting. However, they have not been proven to be reliable in truly differentiating the affective component from the pain intensity.[22]

For patients with chronic pain or significant affective or behavioral pain components, longer and more in-depth formal assessments are advised. Referral to specialty pain clinics should be strongly considered for patients with chronic pain and with significant affective symptoms, behavioral changes, and functional deficits related to their pain. A multidisciplinary approach and evaluation should be performed and can include neuropsychologic evaluation. Commonly used assessments such as the McGill Pain Questionnaire, Multidisciplinary Pain Inventory, Short Form-36 Health Survey, Sickness Impact Profile, Beck Depression Inventory, Beck Anxiety Inventory, and Minnesota Multiphasic Personality Inventory are frequently incorporated in a neuropsychologic assessment of pain and aid the clinician in developing a comprehensive picture and treatment plan.[5]

For patients who are unable to accurately respond due to cognitive or communication deficits, there are other options to objectively assess pain. A variety of observational pain scales exist, such as the Faces, Legs, Activity, Cry, Consolability (FLACC) Scale. Like other observational pain scales, the FLACC was designed to objectively measure nonverbal behaviors to assess pain. FLACC was originally developed for infants and preverbal children, but it has been validated for use in adults with cognitive impairment.[5] Measuring pain in patients with disorders of consciousness (DOC) is even more challenging and controversial. One of the central questions in patients with DOC is whether or not they can perceive the subjective experience of pain. To answer this question, one must differentiate between nociception and pain. Nociception involves the basic processing of noxious stimuli. In nociception, peripheral receptors detect tissue damage/injury and carry sensory information via the lateral/direct pain pathway to the primary somatosensory cortex (S1) and secondary somatosensory cortices (S2).[23] Activation of the lateral network is responsible for the sensory discriminative aspects of pain.[24] To experience the subjective sensation of pain, the medial/indirect pathway must be activated. The medial pain pathway involves the cingulate, anterior insula, and prefrontal cortices. The medial pathway is involved in the motivational-affective and cognitive-evaluative aspects of pain processing.[25,26]

Several studies have shown differences in the activation of the medial pathway in patients in the vegetative state compared with patients in the minimally conscious state. Laureys et al. used positron emission tomography (PET) imaging to study brain metabolism in patients with DOC in response to electrical stimulation of the median nerve. Patients in the vegetative state showed severely impaired functional connectivity in the corticocortical pathways connecting the primary somatosensory cortex and the secondary somatosensory cortex compared with healthy controls. They concluded that the impaired connectivity between S1 and higher order associative cortices reduced the likelihood that pain is experienced in an integrated manner in patients in the vegetative state.[27] Conversely, Boly et al. also used PET imaging to evaluate brain activation in patients in the minimally conscious state compared with healthy controls in response to noxious stimuli. They found similar patterns of activation of the medial network in minimal consciousness compared to controls, including activity in the S2, insular cortex, posterior parietal cortex, and anterior cingulate cortex. They concluded that it was likely that minimally conscious patients perceive unpleasant aspects of pain.[28] However, Markl et al. evaluated functional magnetic resonance imaging (MRI) activation triggered by noxious stimuli in 15 patients in the vegetative state due to nontraumatic injury, compared with 15 healthy controls. In their sample, 30% had some degree of activation of the medial pain pathway, including the anterior cingulate cortex and the anterior insular cortex. Although activation and connectivity was reduced in the vegetative group, there still exists the possibility of processing the affective-emotional components of pain to some level.[29]

The Nociceptive Coma Scale (NCS) is an observational pain assessment tool developed with the specific purpose of assessing nociception in patients with DOC. The initial version was composed of four subscales assessing motor, verbal, and visual responses to noxious stimuli.[30] In a study of 40 patients with DOC, the NCS was found to be have good interrater reliability and good concurrent validity compared with the FLACC scale, Neonatal Infant Pain Scale, the Pain Assessment in Advanced Dementia Scale, and the Checklist of Nonverbal Pain Indicators. Additionally, it had greater sensitivity and broader score range than those measures, with lower scores for patients in the vegetative state compared with those who were minimally conscious.[31] The NCS was revised into the NCS Revised (which no longer included a visual response subscore) after a follow-up study of 64 patients with DOC showed no differences in the visual subscale score between noxious and nonnoxious stimulation.[32]

PAINFUL CONDITIONS

Painful Orthopedic and Musculoskeletal Conditions

Extremity fractures are common in TBI and are frequently a source of pain. Extremity injuries occur in as many as 60% of patients with head injury.[33] Although most bony injuries are diagnosed on an initial skeletal survey when a patient presents emergently for care, sometimes complete orthopedic evaluation is delayed due to the need to treat life-threatening injuries. Additionally, comatose or confused patients are unable to accurately communicate regarding areas of pain or tenderness, which require further evaluation.[34] It is estimated that up to 10% of orthopedic injuries will be missed initially.[35] For these reasons, clinicians working with patients with TBI need to have a high index of suspicion for missed fractures and orthopedic injuries. Extremity fractures are sources of pain in themselves, but they also increase the risk of developing several other painful conditions. Internal rotation contractures and adhesive capsulitis are common complications following shoulder girdle fracture. The bones of the shoulder girdle are the most commonly injured upper limb bones in patients with TBI. Injuries commonly occur to the acromioclavicular joint, clavicle or sternoclavicular joint. Therapeutic range of motion exercises should be started as soon as medically possible following shoulder girdle fractures. Brachial plexus injuries are also potentially painful conditions and are common after shoulder girdle fractures. Radial nerve injury should be suspected in all cases of humeral fracture. Elbow fractures are associated with ulnar nerve injury and heterotopic ossification (HO).[34] HO is seen in greater than 60% of operatively managed acetabular fractures.[36]

Once a fracture is identified, it is critical for the treating rehabilitation team to be confident that proper orthopedic care has been instituted to minimize the pain and risk for further fracture-related complications such as hardware failure, displacement, or nonunion. Kushwaha and Garland advocate for early surgical treatment of patients with extremity fractures once intracranial edema has reached the peak level and has begun to subside at approximately 7–10 days postinjury.[34] Proper orthopedic care also involves

clear guidelines on the weight-bearing status, range of motion restrictions, and the method of application of long braces and splints. Modalities should be strongly considered to reduce pain from fractures. The authors suggest cryotherapy in particular because of its role in reducing inflammation and pain. We also advocate for the use of a stepwise approach of pharmacologic treatment of fracture pain starting with nonnarcotic medications. Acetaminophen is a good first-line choice given its favorable side effect profile and analgesic properties. Nonsteroidal antiinflammatory medications (NSAIDs) can be added if acetaminophen is ineffective. If pain remains problematic and is interfering with progress in rehabilitation or causing significant distress, then opiate narcotics should be considered. Adjunctive pain control can be attempted with medications such as gabapentin and pregabalin, both of which have been shown to improve pain control while decreasing opiate requirements.[37] The use of topical lidocaine patches is of questionable value in terms of analgesic effect and decreasing opiate requirements.[38]

Painful contractures are another potential pain generator for patients with TBI. Painful contractures can come from a variety of different mechanisms. They may arise from severe spasticity with progressive loss of range of motion, reduced mobility due to pain, progressive bone formation from HO, or prolonged positioning due to weakness. The reader is referred to the chapter on spasticity for treatment of contractures related to spasticity and treatment of painful muscle spasms. Commonly used spasmolytic medications are listed in Table 12.1. The best approach for painful contractures is to prevent them from occurring. Mobilization and rehabilitation efforts should start as soon as possible and continue through the full course of recovery. Early mobilization in the neurologic intensive care setting has been shown to be safe and effective at improving mobility.[39]

Hemiplegic shoulder pain is common in patients with TBI and stroke. Prevalence of shoulder pain in TBI is estimated to range between 4% and 24%.[40] One series of patients with TBI admitted to an acute inpatient rehabilitation unit found the prevalence of hemiplegic shoulder pain to be 62%.[41] The differential diagnosis of the painful hemiplegic shoulder is broad and includes fractures, spasticity, deep vein thrombosis, peripheral nerve injury (including plexopathy), complex regional pain syndrome (CRPS), rotator cuff injury, painful subluxation, central pain syndrome, and HO. The most important step in treating the painful hemiplegic shoulder is finding the correct diagnosis. In a patient with a painful hemiplegic shoulder, it is suggested that

TABLE 12.1
Common Medications Used to Address Painful Conditions for Patients After Traumatic Brain Injury

Medication	Primary Mechanisms of Action	Common Side Effects	Metabolism
Acetaminophen	Inhibits prostaglandin synthesis	Nausea, symptoms related to liver toxicity	Liver (multiple CYP isozymes)
NSAIDs	Block release of cyclooxygenase:	Dizziness, nausea, diarrhea, constipation	Liver
Cox-1 (multiple)	Cox-1	Increased risk of GI side effects vs. Cox-2	Multiple CYP isozymes
Cox-2 (celecoxib)	Cox-2	Increased risk of CV side effects versus Cox-1	CYP2C9
Tricyclic antidepressants	Inhibit norepinephrine and serotonin reuptake	Cardiac conduction abnormalities, sedation, anticholinergic (especially tertiary amines), lower seizure threshold	Liver (CYP2D6)
Serotonin norepinephrine reuptake inhibitors	Inhibit serotonin and norepinephrine reuptake	Nausea, somnolence, headache (all); dry mouth and fatigue (duloxetine); insomnia, dizziness, nervousness (venlafaxine)	Liver (CYP2D6, CYP1A2)
ANTICONVULSANTS			
Carbamazepine	Stabilizes neuronal sodium channels	Ataxia, dizziness, nausea, vomiting, SIADH	Liver (CYP3A4)
Gabapentin	Not well defined	Fatigue, somnolence, dizziness	Renal
Pregabalin	Not well defined	Dizziness, somnolence, visual changes, fatigue	Renal
Opioids	Via opiate receptors	Somnolence, constipation, mood disturbances, respiratory depression, abuse risk	Liver (CYP3A)
Triptans	5-HT$_{1B}$ and 5-HT$_{1D}$ receptor agonist leads to intracranial arterial vasoconstriction (some controversy), inhibition of release of substance P, and calcitonin gene–related peptide	Paresthesias, neck tightness, nausea, somnolence, fatigue (relative frequency varies among different triptans)	Liver (MAO-A and CYP1A2)
β-Blockers (propranolol)	β$_1$ and β$_2$ receptor blocker	Bradycardia, hypotension, lethargy, fatigue, respiratory distress	Liver (CYP2D6 and CYP1A2)
ANTISPASMODICS			
Dantrolene	Blocks calcium release from sarcoplasmic reticulum	Dizziness, weakness, fatigue, drowsiness, diarrhea, hepatotoxicity	Liver (various microzymes)
Tizanidine	α$_2$-Agonist	Dizziness, dry mouth, hypotension, somnolence, hepatotoxicity	Liver (CYP1A2)
Baclofen	GABA$_B$ agonist to increase inhibitory signals to dampen spinal reflex arc	Somnolence, dizziness, nausea, cognitive deficits	Liver, with the majority excreted unchanged by kidney

5-HT, 5-hydroxytryptamine; *Cox-1*, cyclooxygenase-1; *Cox-2*, cyclooxygenase-2; *CV*, cardiovascular; *CYP*, cytochrome P450; *GABA*, γ-aminobutyric acid; *GI*, gastrointestinal; *MAO*, monoamine oxidase; *NSAIDs*, nonsteroidal antiinflammatory drugs; *SIADH*, syndrome of inappropriate antidiuretic hormone.

one start by generating a differential diagnosis based on knowledge of the mechanism of injury (i.e., TBI vs. non-TBI vs. stroke). For instance, fractures, peripheral nerve injuries, brachial plexopathies, and rotator cuff tears are much more likely in traumatic injuries than in nontraumatic injuries. Taking a careful pain history will help to narrow down the differential further, provided the patient is able to communicate effectively. Next, observation and visual inspection is important to look for signs of swelling, warmth, discoloration, skin changes, obvious bony deformity, or subluxation. This can be followed by physical examination looking for the presence of allodynia or hyperpathia. Examination of active and passive range of motion should ensue, with careful attention being paid to the degree of spasticity and loss of range of motion with external rotation and abduction. Further imaging with x-ray, venous Doppler ultrasound, MRI, electromyography/nerve conduction studies. or triple phase bone scan may be required for diagnosis of fractures, deep vein thrombosis, rotator cuff injury, peripheral nerve injury, or CRPS, respectively.

Heterotopic Ossification

HO is the formation of abnormal, ectopic bone containing bone marrow inside soft tissues. It can be seen following peripheral trauma (fractures, dislocations, burns, and postsurgery) and central nervous system (CNS) injury, such as stroke, TBI, or cerebral anoxia. When HO follows CNS injury, it is referred to as neurologic heterotopic ossification (NHO).[42] Although estimates of the incidence of HO can vary widely, from as low as 11% to as high as 76%, the incidence of symptomatic HO is approximately 10% in patients with TBI.[43,44] NHO develops from concomitant injury to the CNS and to peripheral tissues surrounding joints.[45] These injuries stimulate an inflammatory cascade that releases growth factors and cytokines that cause proliferation of fibroblasts and collagen deposition at the peripheral injury site. Sites of peripheral injuries tend to be significantly hypoxic, and this hypoxic environment stimulates the congregation of mesenchymal cells and osteoprogenitor cells, which further differentiate into chondrocytes. The chondrocytes deposit cartilage, and remodeling of the cartilage matrix stimulates angiogenesis. Newly formed blood vessels bring a blood supply, which alters the hypoxic environment and leads to the differentiation of osteoprogenitor cells into osteoblasts. Osteoblasts deposit osteoid on the previous cartilage sites. Mineralization and remodeling of the heterotopic bone into mature lamellar bone with Haversion canals occurs slowly over time.[46] The presence of Haversion canals, blood vessels, and a marrow cavity make HO unique from other conditions causing ectopic bone formation, such as dystrophic calcification.[47]

NHO is considered a painful condition, largely due to the high levels of inflammation found surrounding the affected joints. Clinically, areas of HO are associated with warmth, swelling, erythema, and soft tissue breakdown. Additionally, as more bone is laid down, joint mobility is compromised and can ultimately lead to ankyloses in painful or uncomfortable positions. Overall, 20% of patients with NHO develop painful nerve impingement or entrapment and contractures. The only established treatment for HO is surgical excision.[48] Indications for surgery include nerve or blood vessel entrapment, limited active function (such as actively moving a limb), limited passive function (such as being seated properly or impaired access for hygiene), and pain. Up until recently, HO excision surgery was delayed until the HO matured and was fully formed because of the risk of recurrence. However, new evidence suggests that the rate of HO recurrence is not affected by HO maturity. A survey of 570 patients with NHO who underwent surgical excision was published in 2011.[43] The researchers found that recurrence of NHO postexcision was not associated with the cause of CNS injury (traumatic injury, stroke, or cerebral anoxia), sex, age at the time of injury, presence of multisite NHO, or time from the CNS injury to the time of surgery. In this series, 181 surgeries were performed within the first year without any recurrence of HO through the 6 months follow-up period. Conversely, in 1999, Lazarus et al. studied 24 patients with NHO about the elbow who underwent surgical excision. They found that a long delay before surgery had a negative effect on recovery of range of motion postsurgery.[49] Other concerns with prolonged delay before surgery for an ankylosed joint include bone loss of the articular structure (i.e., femoral head) and increased risk of perioperative fracture.[50] Surgery can be considered once there is clear indication and the patient is medically stable and appropriate for surgery.

No pharmacologic treatment is available to reverse the process of NHO by decreasing the burden of cartilage and bone matrix once it has been laid down. Instead, pharmacologic treatment of NHO is aimed at slowing down the process of laying down new bone. Etidronate is a bisphosphonate that has been shown to prevent HO formation by inhibiting the mineral phase of hydroxyapatite crystals. Etidronate has a role in decreasing inflammation if given intravenously early in the course of HO in patients with spinal cord injury.[51] It may provide some pain relief by blocking the inflammation in HO but otherwise is not thought to have significant analgesic effects. The NSAIDs indomethacin and rofecoxib have been used successfully to prevent HO formation following hip surgery and TBI,[52,53] although rofecoxib has been withdrawn from the market because of safety concerns. Unfortunately, there is a paucity of evidence supporting their efficacy in slowing down or halting the process of NHO following TBI once the process has already started. Given the large amount of inflammation described in NHO, NSAIDs are still considered useful agents in treating pain and inflammation. Indomethacin can be prescribed in short-acting formulation at a dose of 25 mg three times per day or in its long-acting formulation at a dose of 75 mg once daily.[52] Potential treatment effects of NSAIDs need to be considered against side effects including increased risk of bleeding, gastritis, impaired bone healing, and renal injury. Impaired bone healing is an important consideration given how commonly fractures co-occur in patients with TBI.

NEUROPATHIC PAIN

Patients with TBI may develop posttraumatic neuropathic pain as a consequence of the underlying primary traumatic injury. Neuropathic pain may result from a number of different lesions and have multiple underlying pathophysiologic mechanisms. Although a comprehensive discussion of this condition is beyond the scope of this chapter, when treating patients with traumatic brain injuries and associated painful conditions it is helpful to have a general understanding of some of the more common neuropathic pain conditions as a starting point for the diagnosis and management of these conditions. For this discussion, neuropathic pain is categorized as peripheral pain, central pain, and CRPS.

Peripheral Neuropathic Pain

Patients who sustain a TBI may also have a number of other associated injuries. Among them are injuries to the peripheral nerves. One study in a general trauma population identified an overall incidence of peripheral nerve injuries of 2.8%. Almost half of these injuries were in patients who were involved in motor vehicle crashes. The radial nerve was the most common upper extremity nerve injury, and the peroneal nerve, the most common lower extremity nerve injury.[54] Although damage to the afferent neuronal pathways is an important component, other mechanisms are also involved, including spontaneous ectopic activity of primary afferent neurons, peripheral sensitization,

and central sensitization.[55] Although diagnosis can be challenging when evaluating a patient with cognitive and/or language deficits, characterization of the pain can be helpful. This type of pain is often described as tingling, burning, or shooting. Hypoesthesia, hypoalgesia, hyperalgesia, and allodynia may be present on examination.

Most of the larger randomized controlled trials regarding the pharmacologic treatment of peripheral neuropathic pain have focused on more common conditions such as diabetic neuropathy or postherpetic neuralgia. For these conditions, level A evidence supports the use of tricyclic antidepressants (TCAs), some serotonin-norepinephrine reuptake inhibitors (SNRIs), gabapentin, and pregabalin.[56] There is much less evidence regarding neuropathic pain secondary to traumatic nerve injuries, although some evidence exists suggesting that the cause may not be an important factor with regard to pharmacologic efficacy.[57] Gordh and colleagues reported efficacy in some secondary outcome measures of pain in a randomized, double-blind, placebo-controlled study using gabapentin.[58] Ranoux and colleagues demonstrated the efficacy of botulinum toxin A compared with placebo using a numerical pain rating scale as the primary outcome measure.[59]

The evidence supporting nonpharmacologic management of peripheral traumatic neuropathic pain is also limited. In part due to the relatively low risk, transcutaneous electrical nerve stimulation has been employed. Similarly, repetitive transcutaneous magnetic stimulation has also been employed with some weak evidence of efficacy, although results are often short lived. More invasive surgical intervention such as spinal cord stimulation, deep brain stimulation, and motor cortex stimulation, as well as intrathecal drug delivery systems, are also available.

Central Pain

Central pain is pain that is related to a lesion of the CNS. This pain has been studied most closely in patients with stroke and is often referred to as central poststroke pain (CPSP). Some of the other most frequent conditions in which central pain has been studied are spinal cord injury and multiple sclerosis. Another term often encountered is "thalamic syndrome," which highlights the presumed pathophysiologic role of the spinothalamic tract. Lesions involving the spinothalamocortical system result in sensory deficits that may lead to the disinhibition of thalamic nuclei and the evolution of spontaneous pain and/or allodynia.[60] It is likely that central sensitization, as described previously, plays a role in this process. Central pain is often characterized as burning, throbbing, tingling, or shooting. It can be spontaneous or evoked. Allodynia and hyperalgesia are often considered to be key components in the diagnosis of CPSP. Information regarding central pain after TBI is limited. Ofek and colleagues performed a study comparing patients with TBI who had chronic pain with a group of patients with TBI who did not report chronic pain and with a group of pain-free volunteers. The group that complained of chronic pain had findings consistent with the characteristics of central pain including allodynia and dysesthesias. This group also had an increase in dysregulation of pain and temperature sensations, with a significant decrease in thermal sensation in the painful regions rather than the pain-free regions. These findings, as well as the described symptoms, support the conclusion that these patients were experiencing central pain.[61]

Information regarding pharmacologic management of central pain is limited to causes other than TBI. A recent systematic review using the Grading of Recommendations Assessment, Development and Evaluation (GRADE) classification system gave strong support for the use of TCAs, SNRIs, pregabalin, and gabapentin.[57] Jungehulsing and colleagues published a double-blind placebo-controlled study of patients with CPSP using levetiracetam, demonstrating that this drug was not effective.[62] Mixed results have been reported using lamotrigine in double-blind, placebo-controlled, crossover studies.[63,64] As will be discussed, the side effect profiles of drugs must be taken into account when choosing an intervention.

Several nonpharmacologic approaches have been studied regarding the management of central pain. Repetitive transcranial magnetic stimulation has been studied with mixed results. Hosomi and colleagues demonstrated a reduction in pain scores for patients with CPSP and demonstrated alterations and cortical excitability for those patients who did respond.[65] A double-blind, placebo-controlled trial by de Oliveira et al. failed to demonstrate improvement in CPSP.[66] More invasive procedures such as motor cortex stimulation have also been utilized with some positive results.

Complex Regional Pain Syndrome

CRPS is a painful condition that may be seen after TBI. One study of 100 consecutive patients who were evaluated upon admission to an inpatient brain injury rehabilitation unit reported a 12% incidence of CRPS diagnosed by triple-phase bone scan. Compared with patients who did not have CRPS, risk factors included associated upper extremity injuries and lower Glasgow Coma Score.[67] Classically, CRPS is divided into two types,

with type 1 being defined as having no evidence of nerve damage, whereas type 2 having associated nerve damage. There are several different diagnostic criteria that have been employed, and a number of different diagnostic tests have been proposed. In part, this is likely because the pathophysiology has not been fully characterized. Clinically, in addition to pain the affected limb is often warm, erythematous, and swollen. Over time, the presentation may change to the limb appearing cooler with atrophic skin. Diagnostic testing may include a triple-phase bone scan, with increased uptake in all three phases being considered diagnostic.[68]

Given the lack of a unifying pathophysiologic process, it is not surprising that a number of different interventions have been employed with varying degrees of success. Pharmacologic interventions may include the use of NSAIDs, although there is greater evidence for the use of oral corticosteroids among the antiinflammatory medications. A recent Cochrane review identified weak evidence supporting the use of bisphosphonates and calcitonin, with minimal evidence available to support the use of other oral medications. There was weak evidence that blocking sympathetic nerves with local anesthetics was not effective and that intravenous blockade with guanethidine was not affected by and associated with complications. Daily intravenous ketamine had some support, although complications were also noted with this intervention.[69]

Among nonpharmacologic interventions, there is some evidence that physical and occupational therapy may decrease pain. Management of edema, desensitization, and maintenance of movement and range of motion are also important elements in maintaining function.[70] Mirror therapy has also been demonstrated to be effective in a randomized, sham controlled study of 24 patients with poststroke CRPS 1.[71] Behavioral interventions have also been employed with varying degrees of success.

POSTTRAUMATIC HEADACHES

PTH are defined by the International Classification of Headache Disorders criteria as those that develop within 1 week after head trauma.[72] This is the most common complaint after TBI, with incidence reported as high as 90%. There is some debate as to whether the severity of injury is related to the incidence of PTH.[73] Female gender and a history of headaches before TBI are also risk factors. The pathophysiology of PTH is multifactorial, as is the clinical presentation. Based on the clinical presentation, clinicians often attempt to classify headaches as a way of guiding treatment.

It should be noted that PTH may present with mixed headache types.

Posttraumatic Migraine Headaches

Migraine headaches have been identified as the most common type of PTH for both mild and more severe injuries. It is typically intense, unilateral, and may be accompanied by complaints of nausea/emesis, visual changes, photophobia, and phonophobia. Patients do not need to have a history of migraines to develop this type of PTH. Pharmacologic management is usually divided into abortive agents (medications that are taken when a headache develops) and prophylactic agents (medications taken to decrease the incidence of headaches). Options for abortive medications include NSAIDs, acetaminophen, opioids, and vasoactive medications such as triptans and ergotamine. Triptans are considered first-line medications for migraine headaches in the general population assuming that there are no medical contraindications. They are effective, and because they are specific to the management of migraines, their efficacy can also be helpful regarding the diagnosis of the type of headache. Use of ergots and acetaminophen also are supported by more than one Class 1 study.[74]

Prophylactic or preventative medications for migraine headache should be considered when there are six or more migraine headache days per month, or a lesser number if the migraine headaches are causing more severe impairment. Increased use of abortive medications may lead to the development of medication overuse headaches or chronic migraines. There are a number of medications that can be used for migraine prophylaxis, including TCAs, calcium channel blockers, β-blockers, and anticonvulsants such as valproic acid and topiramate.[75] When choosing a medication, side effects including, but not limited to, cognitive effects must be considered in the TBI population. When appropriate, nonpharmacologic interventions such as relaxation and behavioral therapy should also be employed. Botulinum toxin is also an effective prophylactic intervention.

Tension-Type Headaches

Tension-type headache is the second most common type of PTH. There is no specific pathophysiologic cause for this headache type. It is often grouped with cervicogenic headaches (headaches with a confirmed cervical source, usually related to cervical vertebral joints and spinal nerves) and myofascial headaches under the category of musculoskeletal PTH. Tension-type headaches are described as mild to moderate in severity, usually bilateral and involving the forehead or temples, and can be described as pressure or bandlike. Nausea and vomiting are not typically seen, and these headaches are often not aggravated by routine physical activity. On examination, trigger points may be identified. These are areas where palpation leads to referred pain in other areas and may reproduce the patient's headache pain. Tenderness in the neck area may indicate increased muscle tension but by itself would not be useful for differentiating tension-type headache from the more narrowly defined cervicogenic headaches.

Tension-type headaches are subdivided as episodic and chronic by the International Headache Society criteria, with chronic being defined as occurring greater than 15 days per month on an average for greater than 3 months while meeting other criteria for tension-type headache.[72] Underlying pathophysiologic processes including chronic peripheral nociceptive sensitivity and stimulation leading to central sensitization likely play a role. Chronic release of pain-related peptides such as bradykinin, prostaglandins, and histamine has also been implicated. Accordingly, initial management aims to decrease pain and inflammation. Antiinflammatory medications and acetaminophen are appropriate initial interventions, and for headaches associated with cervical pain, modalities and physical therapy should be considered unless contraindicated, for example, with neck instability. Studies also support the efficacy of behavioral interventions, which may not be appropriate for a subset of patients with TBI. A multimodal approach based on the management of tension-type headache in the general population should be considered, especially for more chronic cases.[76]

Other Types of Posttraumatic Headaches

Temporomandibular joint dysfunction may be seen after trauma to the head, or may be a preexisting condition exacerbated by trauma. This headache type is typically located in the temporal region and may be exacerbated by chewing. On examination, there is often evidence of an excessive lateral shift, or even clicking or locking when the patient is asked to open and close the mouth. Management may include NSAIDs, changing to softer diets, and the use of oral appliances. Physical therapy may play a role in restoring normal motion, and behavioral and psychologic interventions may also be appropriate as emotional disturbances may worsen the symptoms.[77]

Injury to the head may lead to peripheral nerve injuries. This may be from direct trauma or surgical interventions. This pain is usually described as sharp, shooting or burning. Palpation may lead to identification of the area of injury with reproduction of the headache pain. The greater occipital nerve is one of the nerves most commonly injured. The pain is often described as radiating from the back of the head to the periorbital area. This nerve is often injured due to a blow to the back of the head or with whiplash injuries. This headache can be diagnosed by performing a local anesthetic block to the site where pain is reproduced by palpation.[78] This injection may lead to long-term improvement. Medications used for neuropathic pain such as TCAs, SNRIs, and anticonvulsants may also be considered. Other invasive interventions such as radiofrequency ablation have also been employed.

An acute headache, often associated with deterioration in mental status and nausea and vomiting, may be related to increased intracranial pressure. This may be related to a new hemorrhage or acute hydrocephalus. Papilledema is a sign of increased intracranial pressure, and there also may be accompanying focal neurologic changes. Emergent evaluation and management is warranted. Patients may also develop headaches related to low cerebrospinal fluid (CSF) pressure. Patients who have had craniectomies, shunt procedures, or are at risk of CSF leaks may develop these types of headaches. CSF leaks related to head trauma may be identified by clear rhinorrhea or otorrhea. If the patient has had a lumbar puncture, that site should be evaluated for a leak. Treatment is related to identifying the site of the leak. Headache related to craniectomy, that is, the "sunken flap syndrome," often worsens when the patient is upright. Headache may be accompanied by complaints of dizziness or a frank decline in functional status.[79] This condition is managed by cranioplasty unless surgically contraindicated. In cases in which headache is accompanied by fever, nuchal rigidity, and perhaps purulent drainage from a wound site, meningitis or other intracranial infectious process should be immediately ruled out.

Visual deficits are common after TBI, regardless of the severity of injury. These visual deficits may lead to complaints of headache, especially related to visual activities or at times exposure to bright light. A study of combat-injured service members with TBI revealed that almost 50% of participants had convergence insufficiency and accommodative insufficiency. Pursuit and saccadic dysfunctions were noted in 23%, and 87% reported difficulties with reading.[80] Strain with visual activities often leads to headaches described as temporal or "behind the eyes." Management involves identification and treatment of the underlying pathology, and often involves collaboration with specialists in optometry or ophthalmology.

PHARMACOLOGIC CONSIDERATIONS TO TREAT PAIN FOR PATIENTS WITH TRAUMATIC BRAIN INJURY

A number of different pain conditions common in patients with TBI have been described. As part of this discussion, various medications have been identified as being potentially efficacious. However, in the context of rehabilitation of TBI, specific side effects need to be taken into account when making decisions regarding the pharmacologic management of pain. Information regarding specific drugs including their mechanisms of action, metabolism, and relevant side effects are listed in Table 12.1. Many patients are prescribed a number of medications, therefore drug interactions need to be considered, including the effects on metabolism of concomitant medications. General principles regarding pharmacologic management of patients with TBI include minimization of medications and choosing medications that are less likely to interfere with the rehabilitation process. As part of minimizing the overall number of medications, it may be possible to choose a medication that addresses more than one problem. For instance, if pain and depression coexist, it may be possible to prescribe one medication to address both problems.

It is worth highlighting some of the more relevant side effects regarding the TBI population. As noted in Table 12.1, many of the medications discussed have sedation or lethargy listed as side effects. These are common findings or complaints after TBI, and are often the limiting factor when balancing pain management with overall function. Note also that the majority of the medications listed are hepatically metabolized. Patients are often on a number of different medications that are metabolized by the liver, so care must be taken to not overburden the hepatic system. Additionally, some drugs may enhance systems that break down medications (e.g., cytochrome P450), resulting in decreased drug activity at a given dosage.

SUMMARY

Painful conditions are a common component of the clinical presentation of patients with TBI. Clinicians need to be aware of the potential pain generators, especially in patients who may not be able to communicate their distress effectively or accurately. Pain may be a means of identifying previously undiagnosed medical problems. Undertreatment of pain can lead to physical and emotional distress, negatively affecting the outcome. However, pain management must be judicious because inappropriate treatment may also lead to unnecessary complications or poorer patient outcomes.

REFERENCES

1. Nampiaparampil DE. Prevalence of chronic pain after traumatic brain injury: a systematic review. *JAMA.* 2008;300(6):711–719.
2. Uomoto JM, Esselman PC. TBI and chronic pain: differential types and rates by head injury severity. *Arch Phys Med Rehabil.* 1993;74(1):61–64.
3. Hoffman JM, Lucas S, Dikmen S, et al. Natural history of headache after traumatic brain injury. *J Neurotrauma.* 2011;28(9):1719–1725.
4. Dobscha SK, Clark ME, Morasco BJ, et al. Systematic review of the literature on pain in patients with polytrauma including traumatic brain injury. *Pain Med.* 2009;10(7):1200–1217.
5. Zasler N, Martelli M, Nicholson K. Chronic pain. In: Silver J, McAllister T, Yudofsky S, eds. *Textbook of Traumatic Brain Injury.* 2nd ed. Washington DC: American Psychiatric; 2011:375–393.
6. Zasler N, Horn J, Martelli M, Nicholson K. Post-traumatic pain disorders: medical assessment and management. In: Zasler N, Katz D, Zafonte R, eds. *Brain Injury Medicine: Principles and Practice.* New York: Demos; 2007:697–721.
7. Blumenfeld H. Somatosensory pathways. In: Blumenfeld H, ed. *Neuroanatomy through Clinical Cases.* 2nd ed. Sunderland, MA: Sinauer Associates; 2011:275–316.
8. Bolay H, Moskowitz M. Mechanisms of pain modulations in chronic syndromes. *Neurology.* 2002;59(5):82–87.
9. Bartsch T, Goadsby P. Increased responses in trigeminocervical nociceptive neurons to cervical input after stimulation of the dura mater. *Brain.* 2003;126(8):1801–1813.
10. Nicholson K. Pain associated with lesion, disorder or dysfunction of the central nervous system. *Neurorehabilitation.* 2000;14(1):3–14.
11. McMahon S, David L, Bevan S. Inflammatory mediators and modulators of pain. In: McMahon S, Koltzenburg M, eds. *Wall and Melzack's Textbook of Pain.* 5th ed. Philadelphia: Elsevier/Churchill Livingstone; 2006:49–72.
12. Li J, Simone D, Larson A. Windup leads to characteristics of central sensitization. *Pain.* 1999;79(1):75–82.
13. Bijur P, Silver W, Gallagher J. Reliability of the visual analog scale for reliability of acute pain. *Acad Emerg Med.* 2001;8(12):1153–1157.
14. McCormack H, Horne D, Sheather S. Clinical applications of visual analogue scales: a critical review. *Psychol Med.* 1988;18(4):1007–1019.
15. Ohnhaus E, Adler R. Methodological problems in the measurement of pain: a comparison between the verbal rating scale and the visual analogue scale. *Pain.* 1975;1(4):379–384.
16. Fox E, Melzack R. Transcutaneous electrical stimulation and acupuncture: comparison of treatment for low-back pain. *Pain.* 1976;2(2):141–148.
17. Jensen M, Karoly P, Braver S. The measurement of clinical pain intensity: a comparison of six methods. *Pain.* 1986;27(1):117–126.
18. Paice J, Cohen F. Validity of a verbally administered numeric rating scale to measure cancer pain intensity. *Cancer Nurs.* 1997;20(2):88–93.
19. Bieri D, Reeve R, Champion G, Addicoat L, Ziegler J. The Faces Pain Scale for the self-assessment of the severity of pain experienced by children: development, initial validation, and preliminary investigation for ratio scale properties. *Pain.* 1990;41(2):139–150.
20. Wong D, Baker C. Pain in children: comparison of assessment scales. *Pediatr Nurs.* 1988;14(1):9–17.
21. Stuppy D. The Faces Pain Scale: reliability and validity with mature adults. *Appl Nurs Res.* 1988;11(2):84–89.
22. Haefeli M, Elfering A. Pain assessment. *Eur Spine J.* 2006;15(1):S17–S24.
23. Chatelle C, Thibaut A, Whyte J, De Val M, Laureys S, Schnakers C. Pain issues in disorders of consciousness. *Brain Inj.* 2014;28(9):1202–1208.
24. Ploner M, Schmitz F, Freund HJ, Schnitzler A. Parallel activation of primary and secondary somatosensory cortices in human pain processing. *J Neurophysiol.* 1999;81(6):3100–3104.
25. Vogt B. Pain and emotion interactions in subregions of the cingulate gyrus. *Nat Rev Neurosci.* 2005;6(1):533–544.
26. Shackman A, Salomons T, Slagter H, Fox A, Winter J, Davidson R. The integration of negative affect, pain and cognitive control in the cingulate cortex. *Nat Rev Neurosci.* 2011;12(1):154–167.
27. Laureys S, Faymonville M, Peigneux P, et al. Cortical processing of noxious somatosensory stimuli in the persistent vegetative state. *Neuroimage.* 2002;17(2):732–741.
28. Boly M, Faymonville M, Schnackers C, et al. Perception of pain in the minimally conscious state with PET activation: an observational study. *Lancet Neurol.* 2008;7(11):1013–1020.
29. Markl A, Yu T, Vogel D, Muller F, Kotchoubey B, Lang S. Brain processing of pain in patients with unresponsive wakefulness syndrome. *Brain Behav.* 2013;3(2):95–103.
30. Schnakers C, Chatelle C, Vanhaudenhuyse A, et al. The Nociception Coma Scale: a new tool to assess nociception in disorders of consciousness. *Pain.* 2010;148(2):215–219.
31. Schnakers C, Chatelle C, Majerus S, Gosseries O, De Val M, Laureys S. Assessment and detection of pain in noncommunicative severely brain-injured patients. *Expert Rev Neurother.* 2010;10(11):1725–1731.
32. Chatelle C, Majerus S, Whyte J, Laureys S, Schnakers C. A sensitive scale to assess nociceptive pain in patients with disorders of consciousness. *J Neurol Neurosurg Psychiatry.* 2012;83(12):1233–1237.
33. Groswasser Z, Cohen M, Blankstein E. Polytrauma associated with traumatic brain injury: incidence, nature and impact on rehabilitation outcome. *Brain Inj.* 1990;4(2):161–166.
34. Kushwaha V, Garland D. Extremity fractures in the patient with a traumatic brain injury. *J Am Acad Orthop Surg.* 1998;6(5):298–307.
35. Garland D, Bailey S. Undetected injuries in head-injured adults. *Clin Orthop.* 1981;155(2):162–165.

36. Webb L, Bosse M, Mayo K, Lange R, Miller M, Swiont-kowski M. Results in patients with craniocerebral trauma and operatively managed acetabular fractures. *J Orthop Trauma*. 1990;4(4):376–382.

37. Dauri M, Faria S, Gatti A, Celidonio L, Carpenedo R, Sabato AF. Gabapentin and pregabalin for the acute post-operative pain management. A systematic-narrative review of the recent clinical evidences. *Curr Drug Targets*. 2009;10(8):716–733.

38. Bai Y, Miller T, Tan M, Law L, Gan T. Lidocaine patch for acute pain management: a meta-analysis of prospective controlled trials. *Curr Med Res Opin*. 2015;31(3):575–581.

39. Klein K, Mulkey M, Bena J, Albert N. Clinical and psychological effects of early mobilization in patients treated in a neurologic ICU: a comparative study. *Crit Care Med*. 2015;43(4):865–873.

40. Lahz S, Bryant R. Incidence of chronic pain following traumatic brain injury. *Arch Phys Med Rehabil*. 1993;77(9):889–891.

41. Leung J, Moseley A, Fereday S, Jones T, Fairbairn T, Wyndham S. The prevalence and characteristics of shoulder pain after traumatic brain injury. *Clin Rehabil*. 2007;21(2):171–181.

42. Balboni T, Gobezie R, Mamon H. Heterotopic ossification: pathophysiology, clinical features, and the role of radiotherapy for prophylaxis. *Int J Radiat Oncol Biol Phys*. 2006;65(5):1289–1299.

43. Genet F, Jourdan C, Schnitzler A, et al. Troublesome heterotopic ossification after central nervous system damage: a survey of 570 surgeries. *PLoS One*. 2011;6(1):e16632.

44. Garland D, Blum C, Waters R. Periarticular heterotopic ossification in head-injured adults. Incidence and location. *J Bone Joint Surg Am*. 1980;62(7):1143–1146.

45. Genêt F, Kulina I, Vaquette C, et al. Neurological heterotopic ossification following spinal cord injury is triggered by macrophage-mediated inflammation in muscle. *J Pathol*. 2015;236(2):229–240.

46. Brady R, Shultz S, McDonald S, Obrien T. Neurological heterotopic ossification: current understandings and future directions. *Bone*. 2017. https://doi.org/10.1016/j.bone.2017.05.015.

47. Atzeni F, Sarzi-Puttini P, Bevilacqua M. Calcium deposition and associated chronic diseases (atherosclerosis, diffuse idiopathic skeletal hyperostosis, and others). *Rheum Dis Clin North Am*. 2006;32(2):413–426.

48. Sullivan M, Torres S, Mehta S, Ahn J. Heterotopic ossification after central nervous system trauma: a current review. *Bone Joint Res*. 2013;2(3):51–57.

49. Lazarus M, Guttmann D, Rich C, Keenan M. Heterotopic ossification resection about the elbow. *Neurorehabilitation*. 1999;12(2):145–153.

50. Genet F, Marmorat J, Lautridou C, Schnitzler A, Mailhan L, Denormandie P. Impact of late surgical intervention on heterotopic ossification of the hip after traumatic neurological injury. *J Bone Joint Surg Br*. 2009;91(11):1493–1498.

51. Banovac K. The effect of etidronate on late development of heterotopic ossification after spinal cord injury. *J Spinal Cord Med*. 2000;23(1):40–44.

52. Banovac K, Williams JM, Patrick LD, Haniff YM. Prevention of heterotopic ossification in spinal cord injury with indomethacin. *Spinal Cord*. 2001;39(7):370–374.

53. Banovac K, Williams J, Patrick L, Levi A. Prevention of heterotopic ossification in spinal cord injury with COX-2 selective inhibitor (rofecoxib). *Spinal Cord*. 2004;42(12):707–710.

54. Noble J, Munro CA, Prasad VS, Midha R. Analysis of upper and lower extremity peripheral nerve injuries in a population of patients with multiple injuries. *J Trauma Acute Care Surg*. 1998;45(1):116–122.

55. Baron R, Binder A, Wasner G. Neuropathic pain: diagnosis, pathophysiological mechanisms, and treatment. *Lancet Neurol*. 2010;9(8):807–819.

56. Attal N, Cruccu G, Baron RA, et al. EFNS guidelines on the pharmacological treatment of neuropathic pain: 2010 revision. *Eur J Neurol*. 2010;17(9):1113–e88.

57. Finnerup NB, Attal N, Haroutounian S, et al. Pharmacotherapy for neuropathic pain in adults: a systematic review and meta-analysis. *Lancet Neurol*. 2015;14(2):162–173.

58. Gordh TE, Stubhaug A, Jensen TS, et al. Gabapentin in traumatic nerve injury pain: a randomized, double-blind, placebo-controlled, cross-over, multi-center study. *Pain*. 2008;138(2):255–266.

59. Ranoux D, Attal N, Morain F, Bouhassira D. Botulinum toxin type A induces direct analgesic effects in chronic neuropathic pain. *Ann Neurol*. 2008;64(3):274–283.

60. Kumar B, Kalita J, Kumar G, Misra UK. Central post-stroke pain: a review of pathophysiology and treatment. *Anesth Analg*. 2009;108(5):1645–1657.

61. Ofek H, Defrin R. The characteristics of chronic central pain after traumatic brain injury. *Pain*. 2007;131(3):330–340.

62. Jungehulsing GJ, Israel H, Safar N, et al. Levetiracetam in patients with central neuropathic post-stroke pain–a randomized, double-blind, placebo-controlled trial. *Eur J Neurol*. 2013;20(2):331–337.

63. Vestergaard K, Andersen G, Gottrup H, Kristensen BT, Jensen TS. Lamotrigine for central poststroke pain a randomized controlled trial. *Neurology*. 2001;56(2):184–190.

64. Breuer B, Pappagallo M, Knotkova H, Guleyupoglu N, Wallenstein S, Portenoy RK. A randomized, double-blind, placebo-controlled, two-period, crossover, pilot trial of lamotrigine in patients with central pain due to multiple sclerosis. *Clin Ther*. 2007;29(9):2022–2030.

65. Hosomi K, Kishima H, Oshino S, et al. Cortical excitability changes after high-frequency repetitive transcranial magnetic stimulation for central poststroke pain. *Pain*. 2013;154(8):1352–1357.

66. de Oliveira RA, de Andrade DC, Mendonça M, et al. Repetitive transcranial magnetic stimulation of the left premotor/dorsolateral prefrontal cortex does not have analgesic effect on central poststroke pain. *J Pain*. 2014;15(12):1271–1281.

67. Gellman H, Keenan MA, Stone L, Hardy SE, Waters RL, Stewart C. Reflex sympathetic dystrophy in brain-injured patients. *Pain*. 1992;51(3):307–311.

68. Borchers AT, Gershwin ME. Complex regional pain syndrome: a comprehensive and critical review. *Autoimmun Rev.* 2014;13(3):242–265.

69. O'Connell NE, Wand BM, McAuley J, Marston L, Moseley GL. Interventions for treating pain and disability in adults with complex regional pain syndrome- an overview of systematic reviews. *Cochrane Database Syst Rev.* 2013;4:CD009416.

70. Harden RN, Oaklander AL, Burton AW, et al. Complex regional pain syndrome: practical diagnostic and treatment guidelines. *Pain Med.* 2013;14(2):180–229.

71. Caccio A, De Blasis E, Necozione S, Santilla V. Mirror feedback therapy for complex regional pain syndrome. *N Engl J Med.* 2009;361(6):634–636.

72. Headache Classification Committee of the International Headache Society (IHS). The international classification of headache disorders, (beta version). *Cephalalgia.* 2013;33(9):629–808.

73. Watanabe TK, Bell KR, Walker WC, Schomer K. Systematic review of interventions for post-traumatic headache. *PM R.* 2012;4(2):129–140.

74. Marmura MJ, Silberstein SD, Schwedt TJ. The acute treatment of migraine in adults: the American Headache Society evidence assessment of migraine pharmacotherapies. *Headache.* 2015;55(1):3–20.

75. Estemalik E, Tepper S. Preventive treatment in migraine and the new US guidelines. *Neuropsychiatr Dis Treat.* 2013;9(1):709–720.

76. Bendtsen L, Evers S, Linde M, Mitsikostas DD, Sandrini G, Schoenen J. EFNS guideline on the treatment of tension-type headache–report of an EFNS task force. *Eur J Neurol.* 2010;17(11):1318–1325.

77. Murphy MK, MacBarb RF, Wong ME, Athanasiou KA. Temporomandibular joint disorders: a review of etiology, clinical management, and tissue engineering strategies. *Int J Oral Maxillofac Surg.* 2013;28(6):e393–e414.

78. Blumenfeld A, Ashkenazi A, Napchan U, et al. Expert consensus recommendations for the performance of peripheral nerve blocks for headaches–a narrative review. *Headache.* 2013;53(3):437–446.

79. Ashayeri K, Jackson EM, Huang J, Brem H, Gordon CR. Syndrome of the trephined: a systematic review. *Neurosurgery.* 2016;79(4):525–534.

80. Brahm KD, Wilgenburg HM, Kirby J, Ingalla S, Chang CY, Goodrich GL. Visual impairment and dysfunction in combat-injured service members with traumatic brain injury. *Optom Vis Sci.* 2009;86(7):817–825.

CHAPTER 13

Neuroimaging in Traumatic Brain Injury

DAVID F. TATE, PHD • ELISABETH A. WILDE, PHD • GERRY E. YORK, MD •
ERIN D. BIGLER, PHD, ABPP

INTRODUCTION

Our ability to visualize the brain in vivo after traumatic brain injury (TBI) has seen dramatic improvements in acquisition and analyses since the advent of computed tomography (CT) and magnetic resonance imaging (MRI) more than 40 years ago. The ability to visualize the integrity of tissue, to localize abnormalities, and to track the evolution and progression of posttraumatic change continues to shape our clinical, biological, and functional understanding of brain injury in ways that are only beginning to be applied to rehabilitation. The purpose of this chapter is to briefly describe common imaging findings in patient populations with TBI, discuss the implication of these findings for rehabilitation, review recent studies that have used imaging to track rehabilitation in patients with TBI, and to describe methods that might improve our ability to utilize imaging to guide therapeutic efforts in the individual patient. Given the multiple ways in which brain imaging can extract both structural and functional aspects of both intact and damaged neural systems, the rehabilitation clinician and team has more objective information about neural system involvement and rehabilitation planning.[1]

COMMON COMPUTED TOMOGRAPHY AND MAGNETIC RESONANCE IMAGING FINDINGS IN TRAUMATIC BRAIN INJURY

CT and MRI have long been the primary methods for examining the integrity of the brain after a traumatic event. Imaging in TBI is described in detail in several reviews,[2-5] and typically the findings are summarized by modality (i.e., CT, MRI, structural, functional) and/or metric (volume, shape, diffusion scalar metrics). The following is a brief overview of common postinjury findings and their potential usefulness in understanding rehabilitation outcomes.

Computed Tomography Imaging Findings

In the emergency department, CT imaging is the primary method for assessing acute (within 7 days)

injury following head trauma. CT has several significant advantages over MRI in this setting, including its rapid acquisition, wide clinical accessibility in most medical centers (24/7), relative cost, and few contraindications (particularly in situations in which certain kinds of medical devices are being used and medical history may not be readily available). CT is also sensitive and specific in the evaluation of hemorrhage location, mass effect, abnormal changes in the size of ventricles (particularly helpful in assessing midline shift), and any bone injuries. The ability to identify the location, size, and any secondary brain parenchymal effects of hemorrhages and edema is clinically critical, as it allows for immediate neurosurgical guidance. However, because it involves ionizing radiation, CT is usually only clinically indicated when there are certain neurologic indications (i.e., initial low Glasgow Coma Scale [GCS] score, worsening symptom presentation, declining level of consciousness, pupillary asymmetry, repeated vomiting, focal neurologic signs) as outlined in one or more sets of consensus guidelines.[6] Importantly, CT is limited in its ability to detect nonhemorrhagic injuries, such as cortical contusion, diffuse axonal injury (DAI), and early cerebral edema associated with increased intracranial pressure.

Lesion location and gross findings

Qualitatively, the evaluation of CT findings in the clinical setting is typically used to identify the extent of lesions, the impact these lesions have on adjacent brain tissue (i.e., mass effect, compressed ventricle), and the location of lesions. This information is often communicated to the clinical staff via a brief descriptive report and combined with clinical presentation to guide any necessary surgical intervention.

Quantitative studies utilizing CT imaging in TBI are inherently limited. However, lesion volume counts and measures of midline shift from day of injury (DOI) have been used in research studies for some time. For example, the evaluation of CT data was reported in a large study of patients with TBI and revealed promising implementation of computer-aided diagnosis technology in measuring lesions.[7] Importantly, the quantification of midline shift and hemorrhage volume correlate significantly with morbidity and mortality in severe TBI and may also hold predictive value in less severe TBI when there are positive findings on DOI CT.[8] Positive CT findings have also been associated with several clinical indicators, such as general length of hospital stay, length of intensive care unit stay, neurosurgical intervention, and depth of coma.[9,10] Specific to rehabilitation, volumetric analysis of DOI CT has also been associated with cognitive Functional Independence Measure (FIM) scores at rehabilitation admission and discharge and inversely associated with discharge to home following rehabilitation.[11] Similarly, presence of CT-identified brainstem pathology is associated with poor outcome and low FIM scores at the time of discharge (Bigler et al. PMID: 16998426) However, predicting a specific functional outcome, such as cognitive performance, often results in mixed significant and nonsignificant associations when the entire spectrum of TBI severity is considered.[9,12] On the other hand, broader measures of quality of life have shown more consistent associations across the spectrum of TBI severity when positive CT findings at the DOI are present, possibly owing to the global nature of these measures and their relative insensitivity to specific localized effects or injury profiles. As described, these studies demonstrate a significant relation between positive imaging findings on CT and several functional outcomes. However, there is still a large amount of variability at the individual level that is missed by these group analyses and epidemiologic methods.

Prognostic accuracy and temporal changes
Clinical guidelines generally recommend the use of CT within the first 7 days (acute stage) post injury. Once the patient is beyond the acute stage of injury, CT is typically used only when there are MRI contraindications (i.e., pacemaker or ferromagnetic metal in the body). Regardless, CT imaging can and has been used to predict and follow changes in the brain over periods of time following brain injury. In fact, several studies have demonstrated the value of DOI CT imaging for predicting significant imaging and clinical abnormalities months and even years post injury. More specifically, positive findings on DOI CT imaging can be used to predict gray matter atrophy in the frontal and temporal lobes (see Fig. 13.1).[13,14] Quantitative structural features gleaned from CT imaging (lesion volume, lesion location) show improved prognostic capabilities over qualitative features (Marshall CT classification) when predicting 6-month mortality in patients with TBI.

In addition to these group-level descriptive studies, case studies or clinical cases have been followed using CT imaging. This prospective approach can reveal the progressive nature of injuries and even discern between subtle pathologic aspects of brain injury (see Fig. 13.2). However, the paucity of prospective research using CT imaging makes it difficult to determine what rehabilitation or treatment planning implications these changes might have beyond the individual patient.

Computed tomography summary
CT will continue to be the primary clinical tool in the evaluation of acute head injury severity, as it provides rapid determination of injury that might require surgical intervention. In addition, it has also been shown to provide important prognostic information, and with improvements in quantitative evaluation, it may provide additional insights into the management and rehabilitation of symptoms post TBI.

Magnetic Resonance Imaging Findings
Despite the utility of CT, especially its speed in acquisition, MRI has several advantages over CT that have benefited both clinical and imaging research of TBI. First, the tissue contrast and the resolution are superior to CT, making it possible to visualize gray and white matter anatomy more clearly. Second, the multiple-parameter settings make it possible to emphasize different tissue types using the same imaging equipment (see Fig. 13.3). Consequently, MRI can detect more subtle abnormalities that may go unnoticed when using CT imaging only. In fact, direct comparison of CT and MRI findings in TBI demonstrates that as many as 30% of the patients with mild TBI with a negative CT scan have hemorrhagic and nonhemorrhagic diffuse axonal abnormalities on MRI.[8,15] Third, MRI allows visualization in sagittal and coronal planes as well as the axial plane, which may improve visibility of certain structures of interest. Fourth, because MRI does not use ionizing radiation, it can be used in prospective studies more safely than CT. Fifth, there are a growing number of automated methods for quantifying anatomic and functional features (i.e., see Fig. 13.4). Combined, these advantages have led to the widespread use of MRI in TBI research. This has, in turn, contributed to important clinical insights that improve our understanding of the diagnosis, prognosis, and treatment planning.

Structural imaging findings
The primary clinical and research applications of MRI are to assess the structural integrity of tissue and to quantify the size and shape of lesions, gray/white

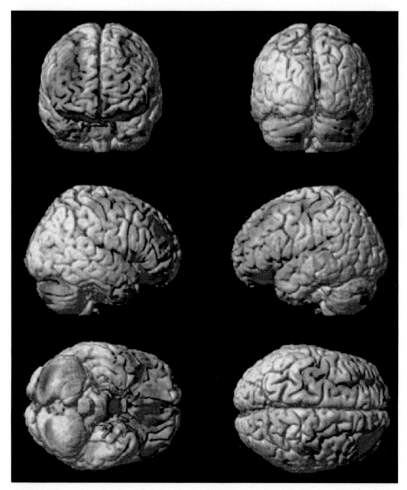

FIG. 13.1 Composite image showing the areas of the brain most vulnerable to brain injury. The *red areas* in the frontal and temporal lobe and the cerebellum are common areas of atrophy that can be predicted when positive day of injury computed tomography findings are observed. (Image used with permission from American Psychological Association.)

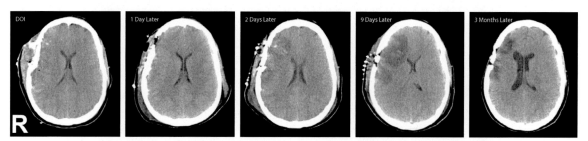

FIG. 13.2 Computed tomography scan from acute traumatic brain injury, with initial scan demonstrating multiple foci of subarachnoid hemorrhage, cortical contusion, and early edema in the right frontal and parietal lobes laterally. One day later, there is more diffuse edema in the left frontal lobe and corona radiata, which continues to worsen by 2 days post injury. At 9 days post injury, most of the acute hemorrhage has resolved with residual edema in the frontal and parietal lobes. By 3 months post injury, there is encephalomalacia in these regions and obvious ex vacuo enlargement of the right lateral ventricle. *DOI*, day of injury.

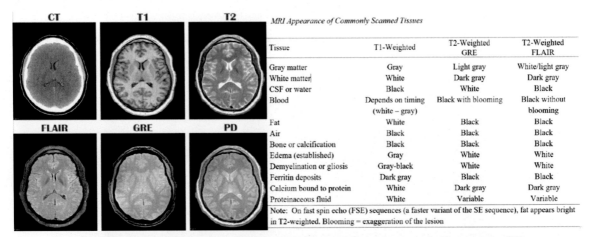

CT	T1	T2
FLAIR	GRE	PD

MRI Appearance of Commonly Scanned Tissues

Tissue	T1-Weighted	T2-Weighted GRE	T2-Weighted FLAIR
Gray matter	Gray	Light gray	White/light gray
White matter	White	Dark gray	Dark gray
CSF or water	Black	White	Black
Blood	Depends on timing (white – gray)	Black with blooming	Black without blooming
Fat	White	Black	Black
Air	Black	Black	Black
Bone or calcification	Black	Black	Black
Edema (established)	Gray	White	White
Demyelination or gliosis	Gray-black	White	White
Ferritin deposits	Dark gray	Black	Black
Calcium bound to protein	White	Dark gray	Dark gray
Proteinaceous fluid	White	Variable	Variable

Note: On fast spin echo (FSE) sequences (a faster variant of the SE sequence), fat appears bright in T2-weighted. Blooming = exaggeration of the lesion

FIG. 13.3 Illustration and table showing the contrast differences between computed tomography (CT) and several magnetic resonance imaging (MRI) sequences commonly used to assess traumatic brain injury. There is a significant improvement in the contrast between CT and MRI, whereby cerebrospinal fluid (CSF), gray matter, and white matter become more visible. The table outlines various tissue types and the expected appearance in the MRI sequence. *FLAIR*, fluid-attenuated inversion recovery; *GRE*, gradient echo; *PD*, proton density.

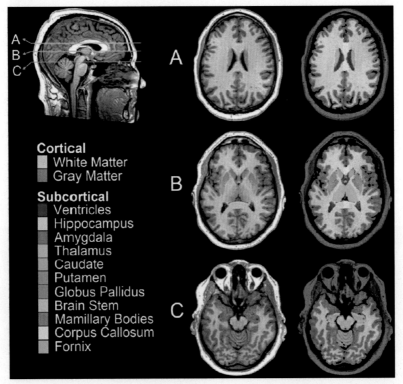

Cortical
White Matter
Gray Matter

Subcortical
Ventricles
Hippocampus
Amygdala
Thalamus
Caudate
Putamen
Globus Pallidus
Brain Stem
Mamillary Bodies
Corpus Callosum
Fornix

FIG. 13.4 Image showing the automated label mapping capabilities of FreeSurfer, which is a commonly used automated volumetric tool. Each segmented image (axial colored maps) shows the different cortical and subcortical labels visible at the different levels of the brain. (Image used with permission from Oxford University Press, Inc.)

matter structures, and cortical thickness. Across the spectrum of TBI severity, MRI consistently demonstrates global and regional atrophy of gray and white matter volumes. Closer inspection of these data clearly shows that the frontal and temporal lobes are particularly vulnerable because of the bony features of the skull in the frontal and temporal regions as well as the meningeal attachments that act as rigid restraints. However, these global imaging abnormalities are not always related to functional change, especially in patients with mild TBI.[16] To date, most quantitative structural MRI studies in TBI have included mixed samples of patients across the range of TBI severity, vary in chronicity of injury, are cross-sectional in nature, and have limited evidence of relationships between imaging and functional outcomes.

However, there are a few important conclusions that can be gleaned from structural MRI studies to date. First, it is clear from studies that include the full range of severity that several regions of the brain tend to be more vulnerable to the effects of TBI, including the frontal and temporal poles, medial temporal lobe structures (including the hippocampus), inferior frontal gyri, and deep white matter.[17,18] In addition, overall brain volume loss seems to be a common finding in patients with TBI, with the patients with moderate and severe TBI experiencing the most volume loss.[19,20] However, patients with mild TBI also demonstrate volume loss compared with healthy controls that may become evident only when examined in a prospective manner.[21,22] More sophisticated postprocessing methods of structural MRI (e.g., cortical thickness, hippocampal shape) demonstrate diffuse abnormalities in TBI, including white matter loss.[19,23,24] Importantly, only a few studies demonstrate relationships between structural imaging abnormalities and cognitive outcomes.[25–27] Thus the clinical utility of structural imaging studies has been limited when trying to understand the clinical significance of any abnormalities that might be observed in patients with mild TBI.

Another more recent focus in TBI research is the quantification of the volume and shape of subcortical structures. Volumetric findings have been noted in the thalamus, hippocampus, putamen, and pallidum.[28–32] In one manuscript by our group, significant differences were noted for several subcortical gray matter structures, including the thalamus, amygdala, and nucleus accumbens. These findings combined with research findings from animal models of TBI that have shown negative pathologic influence involving the nucleus accumbens on outcome suggest a connection between imaging findings and rehabilitation that

requires further study.[33] The commonness of post-TBI symptoms that relate to mood regulation, drive, fatigability, and motivation, which are often major hindrances to rehabilitation, may relate to subcortical pathology at the level of the basal ganglia.

Susceptibility-weighted imaging findings

The multimodal capabilities of MRI are particularly useful when examining TBI. Simple adjustments to the sequence parameters allow the clinician and researcher to emphasize different tissue and pathologic characteristics. Susceptibility-weighted imaging (SWI) has demonstrated additional sensitivity to injury in patients with mild TBI, which is not available in conventional MRI techniques. In fact, one of the main clinical applications of SWI to date is the detection of microhemorrhages, shearing, and DAI in TBI.[34,35] SWI is up to six times more sensitive to injury after TBI, detecting subtle lesions (i.e., small punctate lesions typically located at the gray/white matter boundaries) and venous changes (i.e., venous undulations/bulbs) previously unobserved in conventional MRI sequences. In one study, SWI detected previously unobserved lesions in 22% of patients with mild TBI with persistent cognitive symptoms.[36] Importantly, similar rates have also been reported by others.[37] In addition, several studies have also delineated a clear relationship between the number/volume of SWI lesions and functional outcomes of patients with TBI,[38–40] including significant relationships between clinical measures such as GCS score, length of hospital stay, and intellectual function.[40] With additional analyses, additional predictive value could be derived from SWI findings.

Diffusion magnetic resonance imaging findings

Diffusion magnetic resonance imaging (dMRI) has been touted by many as an imaging method that could provide unique pathologic and functional insight into the changes associated with mild TBI. dMRI differs from conventional structural MRI in that it is sensitive to the microstructural changes in white matter that may be at the primary locus of injury in mild TBI.[41,42] Because this sequence is tuned to the orientation and degree of water movement in living tissue, the local changes in these measurements can provide important quantifiable information regarding the microstructure of the underlying tissue. Typically, four scalar metrics are derived from the tissue, including fractional anisotropy (FA), mean diffusivity, axial diffusivity, and radial diffusivity. In healthy brain parenchyma, white matter is highly organized (e.g., higher FA values), making

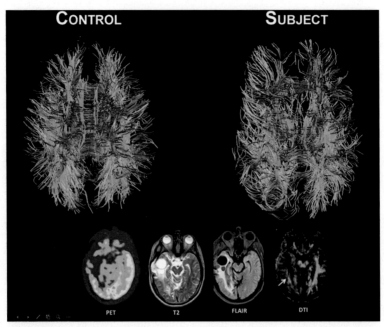

FIG. 13.5 Illustration of whole brain tractography generated from diffusion magnetic resonance imaging data showing the difference between a healthy age- and gender-matched control and a patient with traumatic brain injury. Of the two images, the control tractography results in more organized appearance of white matter fiber tracks that are visibly noted. *DTI*, diffusion tensor imaging; *FLAIR*, fluid-attenuated inversion recovery; *PET*, positron emission tomography.

tracking of white matter pathways easier and improving the sensitivity of this measure to white matter injury across a variety of neurologic disorders (see Fig. 13.5).

Given the sensitivity of dMRI in imaging white matter, it has garnered much interest in investigating TBI. This has led to numerous studies that have been reviewed extensively elsewhere,[2,43,44] and as a group this literature is difficult to accurately summarize without acknowledging the significant methodological (i.e., dMRI processing methods) and sample (i.e., TBI severity, military, civilian, age, time since injury, sample size) differences between the studies. However, the following few representative studies that focus on the connection between significant dMRI findings and outcomes (cognitive, mood, or symptoms) highlight findings that improved our diagnostic and prognostic understanding and perhaps even may be used to inform rehabilitation.

Using simple region of interests (ROIs) and/or voxel-based methods across TBI severity and patient populations (i.e., sports, military/veterans, civilian), studies have demonstrated significant differences in various scalar metrics (predominately FA) for several ROIs, including the corpus callosum, cingulate gyrus, cerebellar peduncles, superior longitudinal fasciculus,

and orbitofrontal white matter.[45-49] Significant findings were consistently worse with increasing TBI severity,[50] with multiple TBI exposures,[51] and with the presence of additional common comorbid conditions (i.e., posttraumatic stress disorder [PTSD][52,53]; major depressive disorder [MDD][47,54]; alcohol use disorder).[55] In addition, significant relationships have been shown between many of these scalar metrics and poorer outcomes, including worse symptom reporting and mood problems, including suicidality.[48,49] Worsening cognitive performance across several domains, including processing speed, executive function, and memory, is also commonly associated with worse dMRI measures.

Prospective studies have improved our understanding of the evolution and progression of the dMRI metrics following TBI. In the Ljungqvist et al. study, dMRI measures in the corpus callosum continued to show change 6 and 12 months post injury when compared with controls (continued reductions in FA).[56] In the Edlow et al. study, changes (reductions in FA) over time were correlated with outcomes, including dementia rating scale scores.[57] In the Dennis et al. study, differences in dMRI measures were not noted until in the chronic phase in patients with TBI having reduced FA that is related to

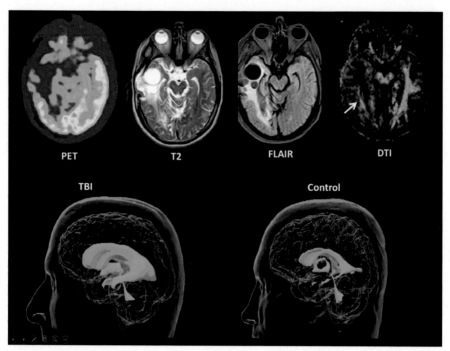

FIG. 13.6 This illustration shows a comparison of the kind of clinically relevant information that comes from integrating the information gathered from multiple methods to image the damaged brain. Because the brain is a symmetric organ, when a radiotracer is administered to the brain, the uptake of that tracer also should be symmetric, but as shown in the upper left positron emission tomography (PET) image, there is no tracer uptake. Although the magnetic resonance imaging sequences show a large posttraumatic cystic formation and clearly abnormal signal findings throughout the temporal lobe, the PET findings straightforwardly demonstrate there is no functional activity in the regions surrounding the cystic formation. *DTI*, diffusion tensor imaging; *FLAIR*, fluid-attenuated inversion recovery; *TBI*, traumatic brain injury.

cognitive performance, including memory and executive function.[58] In a study examining dMRI-derived metrics as predictors of functional outcome following rehabilitation in children with TBI, FA in the ipsilesional corticospinal tract provided relatively high predictive accuracy (sensitivity = 95%, specificity = 78%), which exceeded the predictive ability of lesion volume or other clinical variables. Mean FA of the ipsilesional corticospinal tract also correlated positively with the pediatric functional independence measure (WeeFIM) discharge motor scores.[59,60]

Thus it is our opinion that dMRI will have a significant impact on rehabilitation efforts as future studies continue to delineate the important relationships between the dMRI metrics and clinical outcomes. Future studies that focus on rehabilitation more specifically will help clinicians identify the structural connectivity patterns most likely to result in successful response to treatment or at the very least identify patterns that may more accurately predict the heterogeneous outcomes common in patient populations with TBI.

Magnetic resonance imaging summary

Conventional MRI is better able to identify abnormalities after TBI than CT alone. Global, regional, and more specific MRI abnormalities are related to TBI severity, making structural MRI a powerful diagnostic, prognostic, and scientific tool. Importantly, it is possible that MRI sensitivity and specificity could be dramatically improved by finding ways to combine the pathologic features from various imaging sequences (see Fig. 13.6). For example, it is clear from the illustration that unique information from each of the MRI sequences provides distinctive information about the extent and distribution of injury pathology in the individual patient. One might reasonably conclude that, together this information might improve the ability of the clinician to predict outcome or recovery. For example, everything observable in the images presented in Fig. 13.7 is potentially quantifiable. Application of the automated structural image analysis method, Free-Surfer (https://surfer.nmr.mgh.harvard.edu/), allows

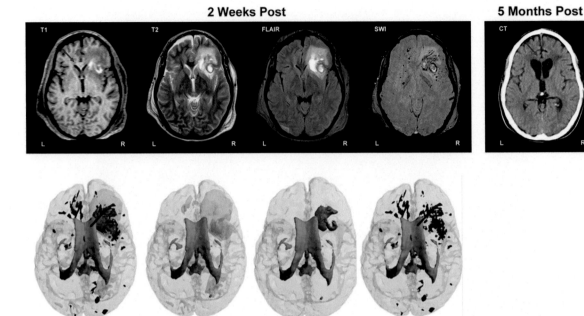

FIG. 13.7 This illustration shows the contrast differences from four magnetic resonance imaging (MRI) sequences (top row) 2 weeks post TBI. Each sequence emphasizes different tissue and pathologic characteristics (i.e., edema [FLAIR], hemosiderin deposits [SWI]) associated with injury. The 5-month follow-up computed tomography (CT) scan shows the dramatic increase in ventricular size (*red arrows*) and frontal atrophy compared with the more acute MRI scans. The images in the second row are the 3-dimensional renderings of the injured tissue types captured by each of the sequences (*darker red blobs*). These combined images show that the value of information from multiple sources may provide a better characterization of the extent and nature of injury following TBI. *FLAIR*, fluid-attenuated inversion recovery; *SWI*, susceptibility-weighted imaging; *TBI*, traumatic brain injury.

the computation of the volume of any ROI. In severe brain injury, generalized atrophy is commonplace, and even though the MRI was obtained approximately 2 weeks post injury, a significant decrease in brain volume was emerging and already quantifiable, with an approximate 50-cc reduction from estimates of preinjury volume. However, as can be seen in the follow-up CT scan at 5 months post injury, the volume loss is clearly visible in terms of the prominent ventricular dilation (hydrocephalus ex vacuo) and prominence of cortical sulci and excess cerebrospinal fluid (CSF) that replaces the lost parenchymal volume. By 5 months, estimates of brain parenchymal volume loss were over 150 cc. Such global losses associated with brain structural integrity are associated with greater neuropsychological impairment, in particular memory and processing speed.[61] Furthermore, corpus callosum volume loss was evident at 2 weeks post injury, indicating loss of interhemispheric integrity, which can be visualized when the 5-month comparison is viewed, by

comparing the size (width, see red arrow in Fig. 13.7) of the corpus callosum just above the anterior horn of the lateral ventricles. For the rehabilitation clinician, recognition of these types of quantitative image analysis findings may allow prediction of impaired processing speed, provide objective information to help guide therapies, and track improvement over time.

DIRECT EXAMINATION OF IMAGING FINDINGS TRACKING REHABILITATION OUTCOMES

The current literature includes a growing number of articles that examine the effects of treatment on the brain after a TBI.[62] These studies show many changes in imaging findings associated with treatment effects and cognitive improvement and suggest significant neuroplastic capacity, even in the chronic phase post injury.[63]

Functional MRI (fMRI) and resting state fMRI (rsfMRI) have been particularly useful in documenting pretreatment to posttreatment changes. These imaging sequences measure subtle changes in the cerebral blood flow over time using the blood oxygen level–dependent (BOLD) contrast. These changes in blood flow are thought to be linked to neuronal activity, and as such, functional maps of connectivity can be quantified and visualized during an active task or during rest in the scanner. Studies utilizing these methods have grown rapidly, making this literature somewhat difficult to summarize (like dMRI findings), and findings from these studies are reviewed extensively elsewhere.[64]

For example, Han and colleagues[65] examined both structural (cortical thickness) and functional imaging changes after 8 weeks (12 sessions) of either strategy or knowledge-based training in a large (n = 60) sample of participants with mild to moderate TBI. These results demonstrate a difference in change patterns between the two therapies, with the strategy therapy showing complex structural and functional connectivity patterns between pretreatment and posttreatment time points. Furthermore, the changes where shown to be associated with improvements in cognitive performance on a test of simple attention and processing speed (i.e., Trails A). In a study of story memory rehabilitation techniques in TBI, Chiaravalloti and colleagues demonstrated significant changes between baseline and posttreatment functional imaging.[66] More specifically, there was an interaction between groups (treatment vs. control) for BOLD signal changes within the anterior cingulate, posterior insula, and cerebellum, with the treatment group demonstrating significant relative improvements compared with controls. In the Chen et al.[67] study of attention training following TBI, improvements in behavioral measures of attention and executive control were demonstrated after 5 weeks of intensive training (ten 2-h group trainings, three 1-h individual trainings, and 20 h at home practice). Additional improvements in the extrastriate cortex were significant independent of baseline fMRI. Improvements of prefrontal functional signal were shown to be dependent on baseline functional signal and preintervention scores on attention measures. In another manuscript directly examining the effects of rehabilitation,[68] the authors demonstrated significant improvement in functional imaging measures (i.e., amygdala, subcallosal gyrus, anterior cingulate gyrus, and lateral prefrontal gyrus) following virtual exposure therapy to treat PTSD symptoms in service members with TBI. Although additional research is needed to fully appreciate the effects of rehabilitation following TBI, these studies seem to validate the principle of using imaging in the understanding of the biological effects and general efficacy of traditional cognitive rehabilitation in TBI.[62]

In addition to measurement of cognitive rehabilitation interventions, the potential benefits of other therapeutic treatments have also been examined. In a small pilot randomized clinical trial, Yuan and colleagues[69] demonstrated imaging-detectable treatment effects in structural connectivity measures in a group of adolescents with mild TBI and persistent postconcussion symptoms undergoing aerobic training as compared with a comparison group participating in a stretching intervention; these imaging changes were also related to improvement in symptom report.

Finally, neuroimaging has been applied in persons with chronic TBI to guide and tailor rehabilitation strategies, as well as to select patients who may benefit most from therapies. Strangman and colleagues collected fMRI measures while participants performed a verbal memory task.[70] The magnitude of the activation of the fMRI predicted rehabilitation success following a 12-week cognitive rehabilitation intervention; extreme underactivation or overactivation of the ventrolateral prefrontal cortex was associated with less successful learning after rehabilitation.

In other experimental approaches in TBI rehabilitation, transcranial direct current stimulation has begun to garner some important interest and MRI evidence to augment more traditional therapeutic approaches. In this rehabilitation paradigm, traditional cognitive therapies are combined with electrical stimulation. This electrical stimulation seems to create a preparatory brain state that allows the patient to benefit more directly or efficiently from the traditional cognitive rehabilitation. For example, in adult[71] patient populations with TBI (across the spectrum of TBI severity), improvements in attention and communicative abilities were demonstrated. In addition, rfMRI results showed improvements in the BOLD response in the middle temporal gyrus, superior temporal gyrus, cingulate gyrus, and precentral gyrus that were associated with improvements in cognitive measures. In addition, 3-month follow-up testing also demonstrated stable cognitive performance and improved electroencephalography measures (amplitude of low-frequency fluctuation). This augmentation approach to rehabilitation in TBI may yet prove to be a required feature of future rehabilitation efforts that can be used to supplement and improve rehabilitation outcomes regardless of treatment choice. As summarized in the review by Galetto and Sacco,[62] there are just a handful of functional neuroimaging studies that have monitored changes over time. Nonetheless, the approach of using a multimodal method to assess both the functional and structural integrity of neural systems and ROIs in response to rehabilitation therapies holds great promise.

FUTURE DIRECTIONS AND CONCLUSIONS

One criticism and potential limitation of imaging research in TBI is that studies often rely on group analyses. The group approach can be misleading, as the spatial distribution and functional outcomes in patients with TBI are often heterogeneous.[72] This heterogeneity limits the usefulness of imaging when one attempts to use the findings to inform a more personalized approach to the rehabilitation process. For imaging to inform rehabilitation, new patient-centric or individualized medicine methods will need to be applied.

Another limitation to this literature is that many of our assumptions about what imaging variables are associated with important clinical outcomes are dependent on cross-sectional analyses. This is quickly changing, but any significant findings are or should be limited to associations and should not be considered causal. Debate persists regarding the optimal time to acquire imaging for use in prognostication, as the expected pattern of quantitative results may change from the acute to subacute to chronic phases of injury[57]; this may be particularly true of diffusion imaging. An additional criticism is that many studies rely on sample sizes that are insufficient. The studies that examined treatment outcomes directly relied on sample sizes between 8 and 31 participants. In fact, most studies include only less than 10 participants in the treatment arm. Conclusions from these smaller sample sizes require additional validation, although important hypotheses can be derived from the findings as they stand currently.

REFERENCES

1. Konigs M, Pouwels PJ, Ernest van Heurn LW, et al. Relevance of neuroimaging for neurocognitive and behavioral outcome after pediatric traumatic brain injury. *Brain Imaging Behav*. 2017. https://doi.org/10.1007/s11682-017-9673-3.
2. Asken BM, DeKosky ST, Clugston JR, Jaffee MS, Bauer RM. Diffusion tensor imaging (DTI) findings in adult civilian, military, and sport-related mild traumatic brain injury (mTBI): a systematic critical review. *Brain Imaging Behav*. 2017. https://doi.org/10.1007/s11682-017-9708-9.
3. Bigler ED. Systems biology, neuroimaging, neuropsychology, neuroconnectivity and traumatic brain injury. *Front Syst Neurosci*. 2016;10:55.
4. Blennow K, Brody DL, Kochanek PM, et al. Traumatic brain injuries. *Nat Rev Dis Primers*. 2016;2:16084.
5. Shin SS, Bales JW, Edward Dixon C, Hwang M. Structural imaging of mild traumatic brain injury may not be enough: overview of functional and metabolic imaging of mild traumatic brain injury. *Brain Imaging Behav*. 2017;11(2):591–610.
6. Shetty VS, Reis MN, Aulino JM, et al. ACR appropriateness criteria head trauma. *J Am Coll Radiol*. 2016;13(6):668–679.
7. Maas AI, Hukkelhoven CW, Marshall LF, Steyerberg EW. Prediction of outcome in traumatic brain injury with computed tomographic characteristics: a comparison between the computed tomographic classification and combinations of computed tomographic predictors. *Neurosurgery*. 2005;57(6):1173–1182. Discussion 1173–1182.
8. Yuh EL, Cooper SR, Ferguson AR, Manley GT. Quantitative CT improves outcome prediction in acute traumatic brain injury. *J Neurotrauma*. 2012;29(5):735–746.
9. Prieto-Palomino MA, Curiel-Balsera E, Arias-Verdu MD, et al. Relationship between quality-of-life after 1-year follow-up and severity of traumatic brain injury assessed by computerized tomography. *Brain Inj*. 2016;30(4):441–451.
10. Stawicki SP, Wojda TR, Nuschke JD, et al. Prognostication of traumatic brain injury outcomes in older trauma patients: a novel risk assessment tool based on initial cranial CT findings. *Int J Crit Illn Inj Sci*. 2017;7(1):23–31.
11. Majercik S, Bledsoe J, Ryser D, et al. Volumetric analysis of day of injury computed tomography is associated with rehabilitation outcomes after traumatic brain injury. *J Trauma Acute Care Surg*. 2017;82(1):80–92.
12. Lee H, Wintermark M, Gean AD, Ghajar J, Manley GT, Mukherjee P. Focal lesions in acute mild traumatic brain injury and neurocognitive outcome: CT versus 3T MRI. *J Neurotrauma*. 2008;25(9):1049–1056.
13. Bigler ED, Burr R, Gale S, et al. Day of injury CT scan as an index to pre-injury brain morphology. *Brain Inj*. 1994;8(3):231–238.
14. Bigler ED, Ryser DK, Gandhi P, Kimball J, Wilde EA. Day-of-injury computerized tomography, rehabilitation status, and development of cerebral atrophy in persons with traumatic brain injury. *Am J Phys Med Rehabil*. 2006;85(10):793–806.
15. Mittl Jr RL, Yousem DM. Frequency of unexplained meningeal enhancement in the brain after lumbar puncture. *AJNR Am J Neuroradiol*. 1994;15(4):633–638.
16. Slobounov S, Gay M, Johnson B, Zhang K. Concussion in athletics: ongoing clinical and brain imaging research controversies. *Brain Imaging Behav*. 2012;6(2):224–243.
17. Bigler ED, Tate DF. Brain volume, intracranial volume, and dementia. *Invest Radiol*. 2001;36(9):539–546.
18. Levin HS, Zhang L, Dennis M, et al. Psychosocial outcome of TBI in children with unilateral frontal lesions. *J Int Neuropsychol Soc*. 2004;10(3):305–316.
19. Bigler ED, Abildskov TJ, Petrie J, et al. Heterogeneity of brain lesions in pediatric traumatic brain injury. *Neuropsychology*. 2013;27(4):438–451.
20. Gale SD, Baxter L, Roundy N, Johnson SC. Traumatic brain injury and grey matter concentration: a preliminary voxel based morphometry study. *J Neurol Neurosurg Psychiatr*. 2005;76(7):984–988.

21. Levine B, Kovacevic N, Nica EI, et al. The Toronto traumatic brain injury study: injury severity and quantified MRI. *Neurology.* 2008;70(10):771–778.
22. MacKenzie JD, Siddiqi F, Babb JS, et al. Brain atrophy in mild or moderate traumatic brain injury: a longitudinal quantitative analysis. *AJNR Am J Neuroradiol.* 2002;23(9):1509–1515.
23. Merkley TL, Bigler ED, Wilde EA, McCauley SR, Hunter JV, Levin HS. Diffuse changes in cortical thickness in pediatric moderate-to-severe traumatic brain injury. *J Neurotrauma.* 2008;25(11):1343–1345.
24. Tate DF, York GE, Reid MW, et al. Preliminary findings of cortical thickness abnormalities in blast injured service members and their relationship to clinical findings. *Brain Imaging Behav.* 2014;8(1):102–109.
25. Bergeson AG, Lundin R, Parkinson RB, et al. Clinical rating of cortical atrophy and cognitive correlates following traumatic brain injury. *Clin Neuropsychol.* 2004;18(4):509–520.
26. Monti JM, Voss MW, Pence A, McAuley E, Kramer AF, Cohen NJ. History of mild traumatic brain injury is associated with deficits in relational memory, reduced hippocampal volume, and less neural activity later in life. *Front Aging Neurosci.* 2013;5:41.
27. Wilde EA, Newsome MR, Bigler ED, et al. Brain imaging correlates of verbal working memory in children following traumatic brain injury. *Int J Psychophysiol.* 2011;82(1):86–96.
28. Beauchamp MH, Ditchfield M, Maller JJ, et al. Hippocampus, amygdala and global brain changes 10 years after childhood traumatic brain injury. *Int J Dev Neurosci.* 2011;29(2):137–143.
29. Gooijers J, Chalavi S, Beeckmans K, et al. Subcortical volume loss in the thalamus, putamen, and pallidum, induced by traumatic brain injury, is associated with motor performance deficits. *Neurorehabil Neural Repair.* 2016;30(7):603–614.
30. Isoniemi H, Kurki T, Tenovuo O, Kairisto V, Portin R. Hippocampal volume, brain atrophy, and APOE genotype after traumatic brain injury. *Neurology.* 2006;67(5):756–760.
31. Spanos GK, Wilde EA, Bigler ED, et al. Cerebellar atrophy after moderate-to-severe pediatric traumatic brain injury. *AJNR Am J Neuroradiol.* 2007;28(3):537–542.
32. Takayanagi Y, Gerner G, Takayanagi M, et al. Hippocampal volume reduction correlates with apathy in traumatic brain injury, but not schizophrenia. *J Neuropsychiatr Clin Neurosci.* 2013;25(4):292–301.
33. Wang L, Conner JM, Nagahara AH, Tuszynski MH. Rehabilitation drives enhancement of neuronal structure in functionally relevant neuronal subsets. *Proc Natl Acad Sci USA.* 2016;113(10):2750–2755.
34. Haacke EM, Tang J, Neelavalli J, Cheng YC. Susceptibility mapping as a means to visualize veins and quantify oxygen saturation. *J Magn Reson Imaging.* 2010;32(3):663–676.
35. Lawrence TP, Pretorius PM, Ezra M, Cadoux-Hudson T, Voets NL. Early detection of cerebral microbleeds following traumatic brain injury using MRI in the hyper-acute phase. *Neurosci Lett.* 2017;655:143–150.
36. Tate DF, Gusman M, Kini J, et al. Susceptibility weighted imaging and white matter abnormality findings in service members with persistent cognitive symptoms following mild traumatic brain injury. *Mil Med.* 2017;182(3):e1651–e1658.
37. Riedy G, Senseney JS, Liu W, et al. Findings from structural MR imaging in military traumatic brain injury. *Radiology.* 2016;279(1):207–215.
38. Beauchamp MH, Beare R, Ditchfield M, et al. Susceptibility weighted imaging and its relationship to outcome after pediatric traumatic brain injury. *Cortex.* 2013;49(2):591–598.
39. Spitz G, Bigler ED, Abildskov T, Maller JJ, O'Sullivan R, Ponsford JL. Regional cortical volume and cognitive functioning following traumatic brain injury. *Brain Cogn.* 2013;83(1):34–44.
40. Tong KA, Ashwal S, Holshouser BA, et al. Diffuse axonal injury in children: clinical correlation with hemorrhagic lesions. *Ann Neurol.* 2004;56(1):36–50.
41. Basser PJ, Mattiello J, LeBihan D. MR diffusion tensor spectroscopy and imaging. *Biophys J.* 1994;66(1):259–267.
42. Pierpaoli C, Basser PJ. Toward a quantitative assessment of diffusion anisotropy. *Magn Reson Med.* 1996;36(6):893–906.
43. Koerte IK, Lin AP, Willems A, et al. A review of neuroimaging findings in repetitive brain trauma. *Brain Pathol.* 2015;25(3):318–349.
44. Wilde EA, Bouix S, Tate DF, et al. Advanced neuroimaging applied to veterans and service personnel with traumatic brain injury: state of the art and potential benefits. *Brain Imaging Behav.* 2015;9(3):367–402.
45. Little DM, Kraus MF, Joseph J, et al. Thalamic integrity underlies executive dysfunction in traumatic brain injury. *Neurology.* 2010;74(7):558–564.
46. Matsushita M, Hosoda K, Naitoh Y, Yamashita H, Kohmura E. Utility of diffusion tensor imaging in the acute stage of mild to moderate traumatic brain injury for detecting white matter lesions and predicting long-term cognitive function in adults. *J Neurosurg.* 2011;115(1):130–139.
47. Matthews SC, Strigo IA, Simmons AN, O'Connell RM, Reinhardt LE, Moseley SA. A multimodal imaging study in U.S. veterans of Operations Iraqi and Enduring Freedom with and without major depression after blast-related concussion. *Neuroimage.* 2011;54(suppl 1):S69–S75.
48. Messe A, Caplain S, Paradot G, et al. Diffusion tensor imaging and white matter lesions at the subacute stage in mild traumatic brain injury with persistent neurobehavioral impairment. *Hum Brain Mapp.* 2011;32(6):999–1011.
49. Yurgelun-Todd DA, Bueler CE, McGlade EC, Churchwell JC, Brenner LA, Lopez-Larson MP. Neuroimaging correlates of traumatic brain injury and suicidal behavior. *J Head Trauma Rehabil.* 2011;26(4):276–289.
50. Kraus MF, Susmaras T, Caughlin BP, Walker CJ, Sweeney JA, Little DM. White matter integrity and cognition in chronic traumatic brain injury: a diffusion tensor imaging study. *Brain.* 2007;130(Pt 10):2508–2519.

51. Davenport ND, Lim KO, Armstrong MT, Sponheim SR. Diffuse and spatially variable white matter disruptions are associated with blast-related mild traumatic brain injury. *Neuroimage.* 2012;59(3):2017–2024.

52. Davenport ND, Lamberty GJ, Nelson NW, Lim KO, Armstrong MT, Sponheim SR. PTSD confounds detection of compromised cerebral white matter integrity in military veterans reporting a history of mild traumatic brain injury. *Brain Inj.* 2016;30(12):1491–1500.

53. Waltzman D, Soman S, Hantke NC, et al. Altered microstructural caudate integrity in posttraumatic stress disorder but not traumatic brain injury. *PLoS One.* 2017;12(1):e0170564.

54. Spitz G, Alway Y, Gould KR, Ponsford JL. Disrupted white matter microstructure and mood disorders after traumatic brain injury. *J Neurotrauma.* 2017;34(4):807–815.

55. Lange RT, Shewchuk JR, Rauscher A, et al. A prospective study of the influence of acute alcohol intoxication versus chronic alcohol consumption on outcome following traumatic brain injury. *Arch Clin Neuropsychol.* 2014;29(5):478–495.

56. Ljungqvist J, Nilsson D, Ljungberg M, Esbjornsson E, Eriksson-Ritzen C, Skoglund T. Longitudinal changes in diffusion tensor imaging parameters of the corpus callosum between 6 and 12 months after diffuse axonal injury. *Brain Inj.* 2017;31(3):344–350.

57. Edlow BL, Copen WA, Izzy S, et al. Diffusion tensor imaging in acute-to-subacute traumatic brain injury: a longitudinal analysis. *BMC Neurol.* 2016;16:2.

58. Dennis EL, Jin Y, Villalon-Reina JE, et al. White matter disruption in moderate/severe pediatric traumatic brain injury: advanced tract-based analyses. *Neuroimage Clin.* 2015;7:493–505.

59. Ressel V, O'Gorman Tuura R, Scheer I, van Hedel HJ. Diffusion tensor imaging predicts motor outcome in children with acquired brain injury. *Brain Imaging Behav.* 2016;11(5):1373–1384.

60. Strauss S, Hulkower M, Gulko E, et al. Current clinical applications and future potential of diffusion tensor imaging in traumatic brain injury. *Top Magn Reson Imaging.* 2015;24(6):353–362.

61. Tate DF, Khedraki R, Neeley ES, Ryser DK, Bigler ED. Cerebral volume loss, cognitive deficit, and neuropsychological performance: comparative measures of brain atrophy: II. Traumatic brain injury. *J Int Neuropsychol Soc.* 2011;17(2):308–316.

62. Galetto V, Sacco K. Neuroplastic changes induced by cognitive rehabilitation in traumatic brain injury: a review. *Neurorehabil Neural Repair.* 2017;31(9):800–813. https://doi.org/10.1177/1545968317723748.

63. Caeyenberghs K, Verhelst H, Clemente A, Wilson PH. Mapping the functional connectome in traumatic brain injury: what can graph metrics tell us? *Neuroimage.* 2016.

64. McDonald BC, Saykin AJ, McAllister TW. Functional MRI of mild traumatic brain injury (mTBI): progress and perspectives from the first decade of studies. *Brain Imaging Behav.* 2012;6(2):193–207.

65. Han K, Davis RA, Chapman SB, Krawczyk DC. Strategy-based reasoning training modulates cortical thickness and resting-state functional connectivity in adults with chronic traumatic brain injury. *Brain Behav.* 2017;7(5):e00687.

66. Chiaravalloti ND, Dobryakova E, Wylie GR, DeLuca J. Examining the efficacy of the modified story memory technique (mSMT) in persons with TBI using functional magnetic resonance imaging (fMRI): the TBI-MEM trial. *J Head Trauma Rehabil.* 2015;30(4):261–269.

67. Chen AJ, Novakovic-Agopian T, Nycum TJ, et al. Training of goal-directed attention regulation enhances control over neural processing for individuals with brain injury. *Brain.* 2011;134(Pt 5):1541–1554.

68. Roy MJ, Francis J, Friedlander J, et al. Improvement in cerebral function with treatment of posttraumatic stress disorder. *Ann N Y Acad Sci.* 2010;1208:142–149.

69. Yuan W, Wade SL, Quatman-Yates C, Hugentobler JA, Gubanich PJ, Kurowski BG. Structural connectivity related to persistent symptoms after mild TBI in adolescents and response to aerobic training: preliminary investigation. *J Head Trauma Rehabil.* 2017;32(6).

70. Strangman GE, O'Neil-Pirozzi TM, Goldstein R, et al. Prediction of memory rehabilitation outcomes in traumatic brain injury by using functional magnetic resonance imaging. *Arch Phys Med Rehabil.* 2008;89(5):974–981.

71. Sacco K, Galetto V, Dimitri D, et al. Concomitant use of transcranial direct current stimulation and computer-assisted training for the rehabilitation of attention in traumatic brain injured patients: behavioral and neuroimaging results. *Front Behav Neurosci.* 2016;10:57.

72. Ware JB, Hart T, Whyte J, Rabinowitz A, Detre JA, Kim J. Inter-subject variability of axonal injury in diffuse traumatic brain injury. *J Neurotrauma.* 2017;34(14):2243–2253.

CHAPTER 14

Disorders of Consciousness

SUNIL KOTHARI, MD • EKUA GILBERT-BAFFOE, MD •
KATHERINE A. O'BRIEN, PHD

Some survivors of traumatic brain injury (TBI) experience a prolonged disorder of consciousness (DoC). Although the rehabilitation needs of these patients significantly overlap with those of other subpopulations of TBI, there are issues specific to the care of patients with DoC (Fig. 14.1); these are the focus of this chapter.

TAXONOMY AND NOMENCLATURE

An understanding of the nomenclature and taxonomy of the various DoCs is essential in caring for these patients. Broadly speaking, DoCs can be divided into two categories: states of unconsciousness (*coma* and *vegetative state* [VS]) and states of consciousness (*minimally conscious state* [MCS]) (Box 14.1). To understand the differences between these conditions, it is important to first distinguish between the concepts of *arousal* and *awareness*. Arousal refers to the overall level of wakefulness. However, by itself, wakefulness is not sufficient for consciousness. That is because consciousness also requires awareness, in particular, of one's self or one's environment. In fact, in clinical practice, consciousness has been *defined* as the state of awareness of one's self and/or environment. Although other conceptions of consciousness exist,[1] the understanding of consciousness as a state of awareness is currently universally assumed in clinical practice.

Differing degrees of arousal and awareness distinguish the three primary DoCs from each other (Table 14.1). Specifically, coma is defined as the complete absence of spontaneous or stimulus-induced arousal, as evidenced by the lack of any eye opening. Because there is no arousal, awareness is not present either. In the VS, arousal has returned (although it may fluctuate); this is heralded by the return of eye opening. However, the patient continues to lack awareness. For this reason, the VS has sometimes been referred to as a state of "wakeful unconsciousness." The MCS is characterized by the return of awareness of self and/or environment, although the degree of awareness can be minimal and variable. Finally, patients are considered to have emerged from the MCS if they have regained the capacity for functional object use and/or functional communication (Box 14.1).

It is important to note that coma is a self-limited state, rarely lasting more than 4 weeks. After that period, patients will have either died or emerged into a VS (although there has been a recent case report of a prolonged coma[2]). The transition from coma to VS is usually obvious, heralded as it is by eye-opening and the return of apparent sleep-wake cycles. However, differentiating between the VS and the MCS can be more challenging. The diagnosis of MCS is contingent on detecting behaviors that constitute definite evidence of awareness of the self and/or environment. The presence of actions such as command following, communication, or object manipulation represents clear evidence of consciousness, whereas other behaviors may be more ambiguous in their interpretation (Table 14.2).

For example, it is important to recognize that certain behaviors that may *appear* to indicate consciousness can be present in the VS, including yawning, chewing, tearing, smiling, and vocalization. In and of themselves, these behaviors do not indicate consciousness. However, if some of them (for example, affective behaviors such as tearing or smiling) reproducibly occur in the setting of an appropriate environmental stimulus, they may indicate consciousness. For example, a patient would likely be considered aware if she tears up only at the mention of her daughter's name, but not in response to other words or names. Similarly, vocalization can only be considered a sign of consciousness if it is contingently related to an appropriate environmental stimulus. Otherwise, only intelligible verbalization (i.e., of words) would constitute evidence of consciousness. With regard to the response to painful stimuli, it is important to distinguish between posturing and true localization. Likewise, although spontaneous movement may be present in the VS, it is typically only reflexive or patterned in character. Finally, it is possible to have visual startle in a VS; therefore only sustained

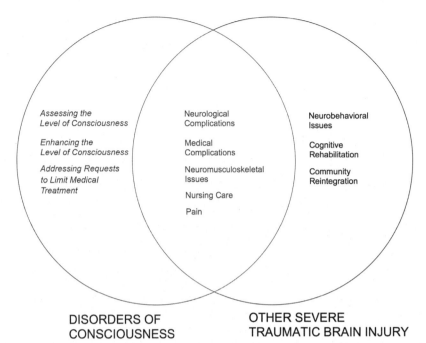

FIG. 14.1 Major issues in DoC rehabilitation (within the spectrum of TBI rehabilitation). *DoC,* disorder of consciousness; *TBI,* traumatic brain injury.

BOX 14.1
Spectrum of Disorders of Consciousness

UNCONSCIOUS CONDITIONS:
Coma: complete loss of spontaneous and stimulus-induced arousal
Vegetative state: return of basic arousal; state of wakeful unawareness

CONSCIOUS CONDITIONS:
MCS: return of awareness; but awareness may be minimal in degree and inconsistent in manifestation
    MCS minus: presence of nonlinguistically mediated behavior only (e.g., *nonreflexive movement, visual pursuit*)
    MCS plus: presence of linguistically mediated behavior (e.g., *command following, verbalization, communication*)
Emerged from MCS: return of functional object use and/or functional communication.

MCS, minimally conscious state.

TABLE 14.1
Arousal and Awareness in Disorders of Consciousness

	Arousal	**Awareness**
Coma	–	–
Vegetative state	+/++	–
MCS	+/++	+
Emerged from MCS	++	++

MCS, minimally conscious state.

---

fixation and/or pursuit is considered unequivocal evidence of consciousness.

There is some evidence that there is a general sequence of recovery of behaviors from the VS through the MCS and beyond.[3,4] Specifically, it appears that nonreflexive movement and visual fixation/pursuit are frequently the first behaviors to emerge. This is often followed by the ability to indicate "yes/no" responses and follow commands. The latest behaviors to emerge in many patients are object manipulation and verbalization.[3,4] Of course, these are general patterns and may not reflect the trajectory of recovery for any individual patient. Within the category of MCS, a distinction is sometimes made between *MCS plus* and *MCS minus*. *MCS plus* is characterized by the presence of any linguistically mediated behaviors, such as intelligible

TABLE 14.2
Repertoire of Behaviors in the Vegetative and Minimally Conscious States

	Vegetative State	**Minimally Conscious State**
Response to Pain	Posturing	Localization
Movement	Reflexive/patterned/involuntary	Nonreflexive
Visual	Startle	Fixation/pursuit
Affective	Random	Contingent
Vocal	Vocalization only	Intelligible verbalization
Response to commands	–	Inconsistent
Communication	–	Unreliable yes/no[a]
Object use	–	Object manipulation[a]

[a]Functional communication and/or functional object use indicate emergence from the minimally conscious state.

verbalization, command following, or communication.[5,6] A patient in the MCS who lacks any evidence of linguistically mediated behavior is considered to be in an *MCS minus* state, such as a patient who demonstrates only nonreflexive movement and visual pursuit. Finally, it is again emphasized that, with regard to the MCS, the behaviors being discussed are often subtle and variable in manifestation.

As mentioned previously, patients are considered to have emerged from the MCS if they demonstrate evidence of functional communication and/or functional object use. These behaviors were chosen as the "exit criteria" from the MCS because of their relationship to personal autonomy and meaningful social interaction.[7] In the MCS, yes/no responses, although present, are often unreliable and inaccurate. Functional communication, by contrast, requires the ability to provide *accurate* yes/no responses to basic questions. Likewise, although patients in the MCS can *manipulate* objects, functional object use involves the knowledge of the appropriate *use* of common objects.[7]

It is important to note that the term *vegetative state* has, over the years, accrued many negative connotations amongst the public (and even among many healthcare professionals). The label often has the unfortunate implication that the patient is a "vegetable," although the original use of this term was simply meant to convey the preservation of vegetative functions in these patients (such as respiration, cardiac function, digestion, elimination, etc.).[8] For this reason, there have been calls to replace the term vegetative state with an alternate, such as "wakeful unconsciousness" or "unresponsive wakefulness syndrome." Of the substitutes suggested, the one that seems to have the most support

in the field is *unresponsive wakefulness syndrome* (UWS); this term is already widely used in Europe.[9] Although this chapter will use the term *vegetative state* in deference to clinical usage in the United States, clinicians are encouraged to consider introducing one of the alternate terms in discussions with family members. Another set of terms that had been widely used in the past are the temporal markers, *persistent* or *permanent*. Although patients can remain in a VS or an MCS indefinitely, the use of temporal adjectives such as *persistent* or *permanent* is now discouraged; instead, the patient's condition should be described as well as the duration of time that the patient has remained in that condition (e.g., "VS for 8 months").[7]

Finally, although the categorization of DoCs into coma, VS, and MCS is currently normative for the field, there have been challenges to the validity of the conceptualization of consciousness underlying such distinctions. These challenges have been accompanied by calls for more complex, nuanced models of consciousness.[10] However, although theoretically compelling, these changes have not yet affected clinical practice, therefore the traditional approach and terminology is employed for this chapter.

EPIDEMIOLOGY

Accurate figures for the incidence and prevalence of DoC in the United States are not available, for a variety of reasons.[11] Because there is no widely used diagnostic code (such as the International Classification of Diseases or ICD-10) for the MCS, large registries and datasets are not able to capture these patients. The problem is compounded by the fact that the term *minimally conscious state* has not been widely adopted outside of specialized circles, so that even qualitative review of diagnoses listed in medical records would tend to miss these patients. In addition, these patients are located in a variety of different venues (long-term acute care facilities, skilled nursing facilities, rehabilitation centers, nursing homes, residences, etc.), making locating and tracking them quite challenging. Finally, because of neurologic recovery, patients who might have a DoC at one point in time, may not at a later time (or they might evolve from, for example, the VS into the MCS). In the face of all these challenges, the best estimate we have is that there are approximately 35,000 people in the United States in the VS and another 280,000 in the MCS.[12] For the reasons outlined, however, it is likely that these figures underestimate the true prevalence of DoC in the United States.

NEURAL SUBSTRATE OF CONSCIOUSNESS

There has been extensive research on the neural substrate of consciousness over the last two decades.[13-23] Although there is not space to review the specific results of this research, a general finding is of relevance to rehabilitation clinicians, namely that although certain structures, especially the thalamus, are frequently damaged in patients with a DoC,[24-26] consciousness itself is not localized to any single area of the brain. Rather, consciousness seems to be subserved by large-scale, integrated corticothalamic networks; patients with higher levels of consciousness demonstrate more widespread activation and a greater degree of integration of these networks.[15,16,27] There have been several proposed models of these networks; a well-known one, the "mesocircuit model," is shown in Fig. 14.2.[28] This model illustrates the extensive interconnections between different cortical regions, subcortical nuclei, and the thalamus. It is also noted that the connections can be either excitatory or inhibitory; it is the relative balance between total excitation and inhibition that determines the overall level of activation of the network and thus, presumably, the level of consciousness. The figure also illustrates putative mechanisms of action of various treatment modalities; this will be discussed further later. One further consequence of the fact that consciousness seems to be a function of large-scale integrated networks is that, with a few exceptions, it is difficult to rely on the results of structural imaging (such as magnetic resonance imaging [MRI]) to determine the current or expected level of consciousness. Indeed, the identity, location, and activity of these networks have been clarified almost exclusively through the use of functional imaging.[13-23]

ASSESSMENT AND DIAGNOSIS: GENERAL PRINCIPLES

Numerous studies have documented high rates of misdiagnosis of patients with a DoC; in particular, patients who are conscious are frequently diagnosed as being in a VS.[29-31] The most recent study to date[31] found that over 40% of patients diagnosed as being in a VS (based on qualitative bedside evaluations by multidisciplinary teams) were discovered to be conscious when assessed with a standardized behavioral measure (the Coma Recovery Scale-Revised [CRS-R]). Moreover,

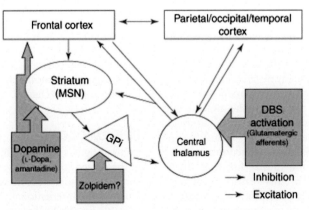

FIG. 14.2 Hypothesized "mesocircuit" model of the neural substrate of consciousness. *DBS*, deep brain stimulation; *GPi*, Globus Pallidus Interna; *MSN*, Medium Spiny Neurons.

10% of patients diagnosed as being in an MCS had in fact already emerged from the MCS. These figures are consistent with the earlier studies and underscore the systemic underestimation of consciousness in severely brain injured individuals.

The high rates of misdiagnosis are likely related to numerous factors. These factors can helpfully be categorized into those related to the examiner and those related to the patient.[32] With regard to examiners, a significant issue is simply the lack of knowledge about DoC amongst many providers, especially in terms of the distinction between the VS and the MCS. This increases the likelihood of misidentifying or misinterpreting behaviors. Another factor is the sole reliance on bedside qualitative neurologic examinations, to the exclusion of incorporating standardized assessments. The study mentioned earlier illustrates the relative insensitivity of unstructured, qualitative examinations relative to standardized instruments. Finally, there are often only a limited number of evaluations performed. The lack of serial examinations runs the risk of "undersampling" behavior, thereby missing evidence of awareness, which is often subtle and inconsistent.

In addition to examiner-related factors, the very nature of DoC poses significant challenges to assessment. For example, superimposed sensory, motor, and cognitive impairments may confound the assessment. These may include sensory deficits (such as impaired hearing or vision), unrecognized paresis or paralysis, or unidentified cognitive issues (such as aphasia or apraxia). Additionally, patients with DoC often have their level of consciousness impaired by other issues (concurrent medical problems, sedating medications, etc.) that may cause them to appear less aware than they really are. Finally, as previously mentioned, the behavioral variability that is the hallmark of the MCS often leads to diagnostic inaccuracy.

The consequences of misdiagnosis are high,[33] often having profound implications for prognosis, access to care, and treatment. In particular, questions about limiting or withdrawing treatment arise much more frequently for patients who are thought to be in a VS. Even if medical care is pursued, access to specialized rehabilitation services are much more limited for someone thought to be in a VS than for someone in an MCS. Finally, even the goals of treatment are affected by the perceived level of consciousness; for example, attempts to establish communication systems are understandably only likely to be pursued in those patients thought to be conscious.

Given the importance of correctly determining the level of consciousness as well as the known high rate of misdiagnosis, the accurate assessment of the level of consciousness should be a foundational goal for any rehabilitation program that cares for patients with DoC. The *goal* of this assessment is to elicit and correctly identify signs of awareness (in particular, by distinguishing behaviors that might be automatic or reflexive from those that represent awareness or intention). The *process* of evaluation should include (1) multiple evaluations over time, (2) be done utilizing different modes of assessment, (3) be administered by multiple examiners, (4) be performed under optimal environmental conditions, (5) and should be done at various times of day. This approach ensures a large and varied "data sample," which is often required to detect subtle and inconsistent evidence of consciousness. In addition, it is important that patients be examined under conditions of appropriate stimulation to ensure that impaired arousal does not prevent the manifestation of signs of consciousness. Specific methods of evaluation are discussed in the following sections.

However, before initiating the formal assessment process, it is important that clinicians first evaluate for the presence of conditions that can mimic or overlap with a DoC (Box 14.2). For example, a patient with locked-in syndrome may have limited ability to demonstrate relevant behaviors, but this is due to profound paralysis rather than a deficit in consciousness. Nonetheless, because these patients can appear behaviorally similar to patients with DoC, they can be mistakenly diagnosed with a DoC with adverse or even catastrophic consequences. Another condition that can be mistaken for a DoC is akinetic mutism. In this

---

BOX 14.2
Conditions and Deficits That Can Confound the Assessment of Consciousness

- Akinetic mutism
- Catatonia
- Locked-in state
- Widespread paresis or paralysis (e.g., critical illness polyneuropathy/myopathy)
- Bilateral cranial nerve III palsies
- Profound primary sensory deficits (e.g., *blindness, deafness*)
- Higher order sensory, motor, or cognitive deficits (e.g., *aphasia, apraxia*)

condition, the deficit is one of *drive* rather than consciousness. As with the locked-in syndrome, patients with akinetic mutism often have minimal motor output despite having relatively intact awareness. However, it is the deficit in initiation rather than motor paralysis that is the underlying cause. Finally, clinicians should be familiar with catatonia, because its manifestation also mimics that of DoC and because it often responds very well to treatment.[34]

In addition to the general conditions that can mimic or overlap with a DoC, clinicians should assess for the presence of specific deficits that can confound the assessment of consciousness (Box 14.2). These include motor deficits such as widespread paralysis or even focal weakness, as seen, for example, in bilateral cranial nerve III palsies (which, by precluding eye opening, may result in an inaccurate diagnosis of persistent coma). Sensory deficits, in particular profound deficits in hearing or vision, can undermine assessments of consciousness because many of the stimuli or instructions provided occur through either the visual or the auditory system. Finally, the presence of higher order cognitive deficits such as aphasia or apraxia can suggest a falsely lower level of consciousness, either by interfering with the comprehension of instructions or by preventing motor behaviors that would indicate the true level of awareness.[35,36] For example, a recent study identified that globally aphasic patients without a DoC could be misidentified as being in an MCS.[36]

The evaluation for the conditions and deficits described earlier would likely involve both physical examination and ancillary testing. In particular, structural imaging (such as an MRI) should be reviewed to assess for the presence of lesions that can be correlated with the conditions or deficits described. Electrophysiologic studies can also be useful. For example, an electromyography can be used to evaluate for critical illness polyneuropathy, or myopathy in patients with minimal or no motor output. Likewise, visual and auditory evoked potentials may be useful in assessing the structural integrity of auditory or visual pathways.

ASSESSMENT AND DIAGNOSIS: BEHAVIORAL ASSESSMENTS

Although there has recently been a great deal of investigation into technologically based diagnostic tests, behavioral assessment remains the "gold standard" for determining the level of consciousness of patients with DoC. There are three major forms that these behavioral

---

> **BOX 14.3**
> **Assessments of Consciousness**
>
> **BEHAVIORAL**
> Qualitative evaluation
> Formal assessments
> - Standardized scale (e.g., CRS-R)
> - IQBA
>
> **NONBEHAVIORAL[a]**
> - Pupillometry
> - EMG (e.g., surface EMG)
> - Neurophysiologic (e.g., ERPs, TMS-EEG)
> - Functional neuroimaging (e.g., fMRI)

CRS-R, Coma Recovery Scale-Revised; *EEG*, electroencephalography; *EMG*, electromyography; *ERP*, event-related potential; *fMRI*, functional magnetic resonance imaging; *IQBA*, individualized quantitative behavioral assessment; *TMS*, transcranial magnetic stimulation.
[a]Not yet routinely utilized in clinical practice.

---

evaluations can take (Box 14.3): qualitative evaluation, standardized scales, and individualized quantitative behavioral assessment (IQBA). Although qualitative assessments by themselves have significant disadvantages, as evidenced by the high rate of misdiagnosis when they are the primary form of evaluation, they may still yield valuable information. In particular, the greater the complexity and frequency of the behavior, especially if appropriately related to environmental stimuli, the more weight a qualitative observation carries in terms of evidence of awareness. For example, even a single verbalization may be sufficient to establish that a patient is conscious. On the other hand, a simple behavior, such as moving a finger, is insufficient to establish consciousness. Even with these less complex or frequent behaviors, however, qualitative observations can be useful for suggesting areas of further investigation. For example, a family may believe that the patient can move his fingers late in the evening when he seems to be at his most alert. Although the team may not have directly witnessed this behavior, the qualitative observation may trigger more focused attention on this behavior as a potential sign of consciousness and/or mode of communication. A template for a bedside qualitative examination of a patient with a DoC is summarized in (Box 14.4); this is modified from a recent excellent discussion of these issues.[38]

However, because behaviors in patients with DoC are, when present, inconsistent and ambiguous, qualitative evaluations usually need to be supplemented (or even supplanted by) more formal assessments.

> **BOX 14.4**
> **Bedside Evaluation of a Patient With A Disorder of Consciousness**
>
> - Observation of spontaneous activity
>   - Movements (purposeful/complex vs. posturing vs. reflex/patterned)
>   - Vocalizations or verbalizations
>   - Eye movements (pursuit/tracking vs. nonspecific roving vs. no movement)
> - Observation of response to environment
>   - Observe for changes in facial expression contingent on relevant environmental stimuli (e.g., familiar voices, particular conversation, music, pictures)
>   - Observe for intentional reach for or manipulation of objects on or around the patient (e.g., pulling at tubes, clothing, items placed in hands)
>   - Observe for gestural behaviors indicating communicative intent (e.g., yes/no signals)
> - Responses to targeted stimulation
>   - Noxious stimulation (localization vs. reflexive/generalized movements)
>   - Visual fixation or tracking to stimuli (e.g., with salient stimuli such as a mirror or familiar picture)
>   - Verbal stimulation
>   - Generic stimulation (e.g., social greeting; patient's name)
>   - Simple commands: choose commands favoring areas of potentially preserved movement; avoid responses that may represent reflexive behaviors (e.g., squeeze hand); allow adequate time for response
>   - Eye (e.g., "look up" or "blink twice")
>   - Limb (e.g., "show two fingers" or "make a fist" or "raise your arm")
>   - Oral (e.g., "open your mouth" or "stick out your tongue")
>   - Axial (e.g., "lean forward" or "lean your head")
>   - "Stop moving" or "hold still"

The primary formal evaluation tool used is a scale that standardizes both administration and scoring. An expert panel conducted a review of available scales and determined that six of them were appropriate for use in patients with DoC.[39] Of these six, one, the CRS-R[40] was recommended for use with "minor reservations" (the remainder were recommended with "moderate reservations"). Although these other scales have their advantages, in what follows the focus will be on the CRS-R, both because of the recommendation it received by the expert panel and because it appears to be the most widely used scale in the United States.

The CRS-R is a 23-item scale composed of six subscales that assess function in the domains of arousal, auditory function, visual function, oromotor/verbal function, motor function, and communication. Within each subscale, items are organized hierarchically, based on the neurologic complexity of the behavior of interest. Scores can range from a low of 0 to a high of 23. As alluded to earlier, the CRS-R has reasonably strong psychometric properties.[39,41] It is important to note that the presence or absence of consciousness is not determined by the total score on the CRS-R. Rather, the presence of specific behaviors within each subscale indicates whether a patient is in a VS, in an MCS, or has emerged from MCS. Thus the total score is more helpful in following overall trends over time rather than providing specific diagnostic information.

The CRS-R takes approximately 15–30 min to administer. It has been recommended that the instrument be administered at least five times within a 2-week period to reduce the risk of misdiagnosis.[42] As with all assessments, the CRS-R should ideally be administered during periods of maximal arousal (and the administration of the instrument includes an "arousal facilitation protocol" to address hypoarousal during the assessment). As with most scales, the initial training and experience in use affect the quality of data obtained. Of interest, a recent study found that in almost half of the sample, the scoring improved when the CRS-R was administered with a family member or caregiver and that, moreover, in 16% of the sample, the improvement in score resulted in a change in the defined level of consciousness (e.g., from VS to MCS or from MCS to emerged from MCS).[43] In summary, the administration of a standardized scale is now considered the standard of care in DoC rehabilitation programs and the CRS-R is likely the best choice of scale at the present time.

Although a standardized scale such as the CRS-R forms the core of the behavioral assessment of the

TABLE 14.3 Example of an Individualized Quantitative Behavioral Assessment		
	Right Hand Moves	**No Response**
Command: "Move your right hand"	24	76
Contracommand: "Hold still"	12	88
Observation	9	91

patients with DoC, there is another formal method of evaluation that can supplement it: the individualized quantitative behavioral assessment or IQBA.[44,45] An IQBA is a method of using a single-subject experimental design to assist in answering specific clinical questions about residual cognitive and behavioral capacities. It is especially useful if the behavioral responses are infrequent or ambiguous. An example of a situation in which an IQBA might be utilized is if there is uncertainty as to whether a patient is following a command or not. This might be because the frequency with which the patient seems to follow the command is fairly low or because the patient seems to perform the movement of interest spontaneously at times. In this situation, a behavior to be performed ("commanded") is identified, based both on the patient's neuromuscular status and any qualitative observation of spontaneous movement. Then, both the stimuli (command) and response are operationally defined ahead of time. The patient is observed under three conditions: *rest* (no command), *command*, and *contracommand* ("hold still"), and the frequency of the behavior of interest is tabulated and analyzed statistically to determine if it occurs at a rate greater than predicted by chance.

For example (Table 14.3), the team or the family may observe that the patient moves her right hand spontaneously. However, when asked to do so on command, the response rate is too infrequent to confirm that she is following the command. Moreover, the patient is noted to move her right hand at other times, unrelated to any commands. In this situation, the team would define what type and degree of hand movement would constitute following the command. Then each examiner would, after a set period of observation, give the patient both the command ("move your right hand") as well as the "contracommand" ("hold still"). The frequency of hand movement (as operationalized ahead of time) is counted after each condition

(observation, command, contracommand). The data can then be entered into a table (Table 14.3). In this example, if one were to simply look at the frequency of hand movement after the command "move your right hand," it would be difficult to know for certain whether or not the patient was following the command. However, when the command condition is compared to a contracommand and an observation period, it can be seen that although the patient's response rate is low in the command condition, it is statistically significantly higher than the other two conditions, suggesting the ability to follow the command. In most cases of IQBA administration, the IQBA is administered by multiple team members daily for a period of 1 to 2 weeks after which time the aggregate data are analyzed.

In addition to command following, IQBAs have been used to assess visual function, communication ability, and emotional responses.[44,45] On occasion, an IQBA can detect signs of consciousness earlier than the CRS-R.[46] This is not because of a flaw in the CRS-R. Rather, the attention to methodological consistency that is required of standardized measures such as the CRS-R precludes the ability to adjust for clinically meaningful individual variation. For example, if a scale requires a response within 10 seconds to be considered positive but the patient always responds at 11 seconds (due to slowed processing), the patient will not receive credit for what may be genuine responses, especially if they are consistent. The IQBA allows for the probing and investigation of behaviors that might not be identified by a standardized scale. Therefore the standardized scale (such as the CRS-R) and the IQBA should be considered as complementary because they serve different purposes.

ASSESSMENT AND DIAGNOSIS: NONBEHAVIORAL ASSESSMENTS

It is now recognized that a subset of patients who appear to be in a VS based on behavioral assessments are actually conscious, when assessed through nonbehavioral modalities such as functional neuroimaging or electrophysiologic measures. In one well-known report, a patient who was determined to be in a VS (based on extensive behavioral assessments) was found to be able to both follow commands and answer simple yes/no questions when assessed by functional MRI (fMRI).[48] Specifically, when asked to perform a motor imagery task (imagining the swinging of a tennis racket) or a spatial imagery task (walking through their home, while "looking" around), the same areas of the patient's brain were activated as in healthy controls (indicating that the patient was able to follow mental-imagery commands). Next, the patient was asked a series of basic questions and was instructed to, for example, imagine swinging a tennis racket if the answer was "yes" or walking through their home if the answer was "no." In this manner, the patient was able to accurately answer a brief series of very basic questions when assessed through fMRI.[47]

What this report (and others) have demonstrated is that, even with extensive and appropriate behavioral assessments, the cognitive capacities of a subset of patients is likely being underestimated, even to the point that patients are being diagnosed as being in a VS when they are, to varying degrees, conscious. This state has been characterized in various ways, namely, "complete cognitive-motor dissociation,"[49] "functional locked-in syndrome,"[5] etc. Regardless of what this state is called, the point is that there are a subset of patients with DoC who are known to be conscious only via technologically based assessments. A recent meta-analysis of 37 studies (which included over a 1000 patients) estimated that roughly 15% of patients with a clinical diagnosis of VS are able to follow commands by modifying their brain activity.[50] Although not utilized in routine clinical practice currently, it is likely that these technologically based modalities will, in the near future, supplement routine behavioral assessments. Therefore it is important that rehabilitation clinicians understand the basic principles and issues involved with the use of these techniques.

All these modalities (Box 14.3), which are meant to detect evidence of consciousness that is not behaviorally discernible, fall into two general categories: those that reveal behavioral output (such as subclinical muscle activation) that cannot be detected on bedside evaluation and those that assess brain activity directly (for example, in the form of cerebral electrical activity). An example of the former category is pupillometry. This involves the use of a device to detect and quantify subtle changes in pupillary diameter.[51] Because it is well-established that pupillary diameter reliably and consistently changes in response to mental activity (such as visual attention, mental imagery, and semantic expectations), the presence of these changes in an appropriate setting can indicate the presence of mental processing and, thus, consciousness.[52,53] A recent report demonstrated that this phenomenon could be exploited to establish communication with locked-in patients (and also detect pupillary evidence of consciousness in an MCS patient).[54]

Another example of a modality that detects subclinical behavioral responses is surface electromyography (sEMG). sEMG can be used to detect muscle activation

that does not result in visible muscle contraction, either because the activation itself is subthreshold or because extrinsic factors, such as spasticity or contractures, prevent the muscle from visibly contracting. When paired with structured command-following protocols (such as used in an IQBA), sEMG has been shown to detect command-following in patients who were otherwise determined to be in a VS.[55,56] It is important to note that there were some patients who were clearly in an MCS, based on behavioral assessment, who were not able to activate the sEMG reliably to command. In other words, there is a risk of false-negative findings, especially if only one assessment is performed.[57] However, as long as this caveat is kept in mind and, furthermore, as long as the strict methodological protocols of a command-following IQBA are followed, sEMG offers an easily accessible modality for supplementing the bedside assessment of patients with DoC.

Pupillometry and sEMG are designed to identify behavioral responses that are not detectable on bedside evaluations, whereas other ancillary modalities directly assess for cerebral activity that might represent conscious activity.[50,58-64] The two most common modalities in this category are functional neuroimaging (e.g., fMRI) and electrophysiologic measures. Examples of electrophysiologic measures include global EEG measures (such as complexity or reactivity),[65,66] EEG paired with transcranial magnetic stimulation (TMS),[67] and cognitive event-related potentials (ERPs).[59] Regardless of whether they involve imaging or electrophysiology, these modalities all attempt to identify brain activity that is thought to represent consciousness. Utilizing these modalities, there are three different approaches to test for consciousness in patients. The first is to utilize an *active paradigm*, in which the patient must execute a cognitive task and the cerebral correlates of task execution are identified. An example of this is the fMRI study discussed earlier,[47,48] wherein patients were asked to perform a mental imagery task and the execution of the task was confirmed if the appropriate areas of the brain were activated. Active paradigms represent the strongest evidence of consciousness because they are premised on the patient *willfully* modulating their brain activity.

Passive paradigms, by contrast, rely on detecting changes in brain activity in response to an external stimulus. These paradigms do not require the intentional participation of the patient. An example of a passive paradigm would be the presence of a specific electrophysiologic waveform on hearing one's own name (but not when hearing other names). Positive results on passive paradigms do not serve as strong evidence for the presence of consciousness because, as will be discussed shortly, it is known that there can be a significant amount of unconscious cognitive processing in the brain. Finally, there are *resting state paradigms*, in which assumptions are made about the patient's level of consciousness by extrapolating from known patterns of resting brain activity.[68] This paradigm likely provides the weakest evidence of the presence of consciousness.

These modalities, which directly assess brain activity to detect evidence of consciousness, have been extensively reviewed elsewhere.[50,58–64] Because these techniques are not yet routinely used in clinical practice, the remainder of the discussion will focus on several important points that should be kept in mind as these modalities begin to be more widely used. First, as mentioned previously, it is important to distinguish *cognition* from *consciousness*. Although it may seem counterintuitive, the brain engages in a great deal of cognitive processing that we are not consciously aware of.[69] This is especially true of basic sensory processing (e.g., auditory or visual), but even fairly high-level cognitive processing (e.g., semantic or affective) may occur without there being a corresponding subjective perception or experience.[58] Thus the presence of covert cognitive processing in a patient with a DoC does not automatically imply the presence of consciousness. This is especially true of the passive paradigms described previuosly. As a result, positive findings with passive paradigms need to be interpreted cautiously and, if possible, active paradigms should be utilized whenever possible.

A second point is that the majority of these studies demonstrated that negative findings were not uncommon in patients who were clearly known to be conscious on behavioral assessment. In other words, almost all these modalities had false-negatives, with patients known to be conscious failing to show a response on imaging or electrophysiologic measures. Thus lack of a response on these modalities *cannot* be used to exclude the possibility of consciousness. Finally, beside the issue of accessibility of many of these modalities (such as fMRI), there are concerns regarding the degree of technical expertise required to administer these techniques and the corresponding risk of technical errors, which may falsely suggest the presence or absence of consciousness in any given patient. All the foregoing issues will need to be addressed before these modalities are ready for routine clinical use; however, as they do become more widely used, clinicians will be able to supplement their behavioral assessments with these techniques. This "multimodal" approach to assessment will likely significantly enhance diagnostic accuracy.[31,70,71]

A final point should be made about these modalities. Although the focus has been on their role in detecting evidence of "covert consciousness," these techniques have other potential roles as well. For example, there is growing evidence that the presence of covert cognitive processing in patients with DoC portends a better prognosis and that these techniques have a role to play in prognostication.[5,63,72–79] Also, the presence of covert cognition likely implies that the neural networks that subserve consciousness are intact, if not fully activated. If so, these techniques may help identify those patients for whom treatment and rehabilitative efforts are especially indicated. This hypothesis of underactivated neural networks as a target for treatment will be further discussed later. Finally, it is noted that the willful modulation of brain activity that is the focus of the active paradigms also form the basis of brain-computer interfaces for communication and environmental control, which will also be further discussed further later.

TREATMENT: GENERAL APPROACH

Treatment of patients with a DoC has several different objectives. First, basic bodily functions such as respiration, nutrition, elimination, and skin integrity need to be optimized. Moreover, concurrent medical and neurologic issues need to be managed and the risk of further medical and neurologic complications minimized. Finally, neuromusculoskeletal issues, such as spasticity and contractures, need to be aggressively managed. The approach to these objectives is similar to that for other TBI populations and is briefly discussed in the Medical, Neurologic, and Neuromuscular Issues section and more extensively elsewhere in this textbook.

Another goal of treatment that overlaps considerably with treatment approaches to other patients with TBI is the attempt to magnify and leverage residual abilities (motor and cognitive) to increase functional abilities. For example, this could involve targeting the spasticity and contractures in a limb that appears to be under some degree of volitional control so that it can be used to communicate or physically interact with the environment. Assistive technology can have a significant role to play in these situations; these neuroprosthetic devices are also treated in more depth elsewhere in this textbook. Of note is the possibility that brain-computer interfaces might further augment the functional capacities of these patients.[80–82] However, because these devices often rely on a fairly

BOX 14.5
Potentially Reversible Causes of Impaired
Consciousness

- Understimulation/undermobilization
- Disrupted sleep-wake cycles
- Sedating medications
- Concurrent medical conditions (e.g., infection, hypoxemia, metabolic abnormalities, etc.)
- Neuroendocrine abnormalities
- Intracranial abnormalities (e.g., hydrocephalus, large subdural hygromas)
- Seizures (e.g., nonconvulsive status epilepticus)

BOX 14.6
Interventions to Enhance the Level of
Consciousness

GENERAL REHABILITATION INTERVENTIONS
- Sensory stimulation
- Mobilization (sitting, standing)
- Interpersonal interaction

PHARMACOLOGIC AGENTS
- Neurostimulants
- GABA agonists
- Other

ENERGY MODALITIES[a]
Electrical
- DBS
- tDCS
- rTMS
- VNS
Ultrasound
- LIFU

BIOLOGICAL THERAPIES[a]
- Stem cell therapy

DBS, deep brain stimulation; *GABA*, γ-aminobutyric acid; *LIFU*, low-intensity focused ultrasound; *rTMS*, repetitive transcranial magnetic stimulation; *tDCS*, transcranial direct current stimulation; *VNS*, vagus nerve stimulation;
[a]Not yet routinely utilized in clinical practice.

high level of cognitive function to be successful, there are challenges to adapting their use for patients in an MCS.[80–82]

As with other areas of TBI rehabilitation, it is important for clinicians to address potentially reversible causes of impaired mentation (Box 14.5). The clinician should attempt to screen for all these issues through a combination of the history, physical examination, and ancillary testing. In particular, close monitoring of sleep-wake cycles is warranted, as the lack of sufficient rest can significantly affect arousal and therefore neurofunctional capacities. Also, a thorough review of medications should be made with the aim of eliminating or substituting for any medications that may potentially adversely affect arousal or other cognitive abilities. Screening for and treating all general medical conditions (e.g., infection, metabolic abnormalities, etc.) is indicated given the vulnerability of the injured brain to what would otherwise be minor medical issues. At least some form of neuroendocrine screening is also warranted. Finally, both structural imaging (e.g., CT or MRI) and electrophysiologic evaluation (e.g., EEG) should be routinely obtained, to help identify any possible neurologic causes that may be impairing consciousness. Clinicians should not underestimate the degree to which identifying and treating these secondary causes of impaired mentation can improve the patient's level of consciousness.

INTERVENTIONS TO ENHANCE THE LEVEL OF CONSCIOUSNESS

In addition to the goals and interventions described earlier, the one therapeutic objective that is unique to the DoC population is the attempt to modulate (and ideally enhance) the degree or level of awareness by directly targeting the neurophysiologic substrate responsible for mediating consciousness. Although several treatments are known to be efficacious (or show promise) (Box 14.6), the exact target or mechanism of action of these interventions is not clear. One hypothesis[15–17,28] is that, at least in some patients, the neural networks subserving consciousness (or awareness) are at least partially intact, although underactivated. If these networks can be activated, the patient's degree or level of consciousness should correspondingly improve. There are several points to be made about this hypothesis (Fig. 14.3). First, two patients may appear clinically similar (for example, in a VS) but for very different reasons. In one case, the neural networks subserving awareness are no longer intact. This would imply that there is no target for intervention to enhance the patient's level of consciousness. Another patient in a VS may have at least partially intact neural networks, which, however, are underactivated. In this

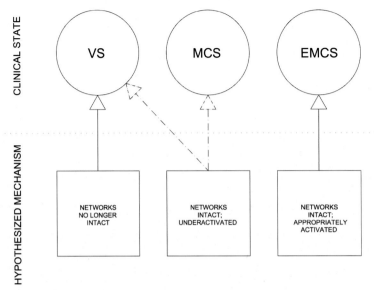

FIG. 14.3 Level of consciousness as determined by the degree of activation of neural networks subserving consciousness. *MCS*, minimally conscious state; *VS*, vegetative state.

case, increasing the activation of these networks could theoretically enhance a patient's level of consciousness, even to the point that they shift from VS to the MCS (or from the MCS to having emerged from the MCS).

If this hypothesis is correct, it would provide at least a partial explanation of the efficacy of some of these treatments. It would also suggest that it might be possible to distinguish between patients who have the potential to respond to treatment (because the relevant neural networks are at least partially intact) and those who do not (because their neural networks are no longer intact), thereby allowing for resources to be more efficiently and appropriately targeted. For example, one could look for functional neuroimaging or electrophysiologic evidence of intact network function (even if there is no apparent behavioral correlate) and target these patients for treatment.[83]

Although we have been discussing neural networks underlying *awareness*, it is also possible that there are additional or alternative targets for some of the interventions used in the field. For example, it is likely that some interventions work because they improve *arousal*. Although they have no direct effect on awareness networks, they may improve the patient's level of consciousness as a consequence of enhancing arousal. Alternatively, if the patient has a significant deficit in *drive* (analogous to abulic or akinetic mute patients), it is theoretically possible to activate those networks, thereby leading to an improvement in behavioral

output. Regardless of whether the target is arousal, drive, or awareness itself (or some other neurobehavioral domain), the idea underlying the hypothesis remains that the interventions should be aimed at activating preserved neural networks.

Standard rehabilitation interventions are thought to play a role in enhancing the level of consciousness (Box 14.6). These include sensorimotor stimulation as well as interpersonal interaction. Patients with DoC frequently have significant improvements within the first 24–48 h of beginning a rehabilitation program, before any medical interventions have been initiated, supporting the idea that the sensory stimulation, mobilization, and interpersonal interaction that they experience upon admission are having a benefit. With regard to sensory stimulation, it is important to note that what may be most important is the generic sensory stimulation patients experience in a typical rehabilitation program rather than a formal program of structured (unimodal or multimodal) targeted sensory stimulation. There is little evidence to support the efficacy of the latter,[84] although recent reviews suggest that this is partly due to the methodological limitations of the studies themselves rather than lack of efficacy of the interventions.[85,86] This is an area that requires further investigation. Another potential form of sensory stimulation that might enhance consciousness is vestibular stimulation,[87,88] although this is still an underexplored modality in this context.

In contrast to the situation with sensory stimulation, there is empirical evidence that mobilization can enhance the level of consciousness of patients with DoC.[89,90] In particular, a recent randomized controlled trial[90] found that the addition of verticalization (achieved through a tilt table) to a standard DoC rehabilitation program increased the rate of recovery (as measured by the CRS-R). This would suggest that the intensive mobilization that occurs in rehabilitation programs (e.g., sitting program, standing program, functional electrical stimulation cycling, body-weight-supported gait therapy, etc.) can have an effect on consciousness. As in the case of sensory stimulation, it is unclear if the apparent effect is mediated by direct activation of networks subserving awareness or activation of more basic arousal mechanisms (or both).

Finally, it is likely that interpersonal interaction itself can positively affect the level or degree of consciousness. Extrapolation from other fields (for example, child development) would seem to support this possibility. Moreover, there is functional neuroimaging evidence that patients with DoC often have strong cerebral activation in response to voices, especially of those with whom they have an emotional bond[91-93] Also, a recent report suggests that increased interaction with family members seems to accelerate the recovery of consciousness.[94] All these interventions—sensory stimulation, motor mobilization, and interpersonal interaction—might be helpfully conceptualized as forms of environmental enrichment.[95] There can be other components to this type of enrichment, for example, the potential benefit of being outdoors on a regular basis (or possibly interacting with domestic animals). It is also possible that the documented benefit of music therapy in patients with DoC is at least partially (although not wholly) attributable to its complex ability to stimulate the sensory, motor, and emotional systems simultaneously.[96-99]

In addition to the rehabilitation interventions just discussed, there are medical treatments that are likely to be of benefit (Box 14.6). The majority of these can be thought of as falling into two large categories, based on the mechanism of action: pharmacologic manipulation and targeted energetic therapy (primarily electrical). A third category of treatments, biological therapies, such as stem cell therapy,[100] has been much less studied than the other interventions. Pharmacologic interventions have long been used in these settings, although the evidence for their specific efficacy in DoC is still limited. In general, many of the same agents that are used in other areas of TBI

rehabilitation can be used with patients with DoC; these are discussed in more detail elsewhere in this textbook. What follows are a few remarks specifically addressing their use in DoC; this topic is treated more extensively in several recent reviews.[101-103]

The agents most often used are considered central nervous system (CNS) stimulants and specifically target catecholaminergic pathways. Of these, amantadine has the strongest evidence base supporting its use, primarily due to the results of a randomized controlled trial investigating its role in posttraumatic DoC.[104] This study, discussed in more detail in the chapter on pharmacotherapy, found that administration of amantadine in the subacute period (4–16 weeks after injury) accelerated the recovery of consciousness in patients with posttraumatic DoC. Based on this evidence, it is reasonable to recommend that all patients with a posttraumatic DoC within this time frame should receive amantadine unless otherwise contraindicated. Fig. 14.2 illustrates a potential mechanism of action of amantadine according to the mesocircuit hypothesis discussed previously. Of the other stimulant medications, levodopa, bromocriptine, methylphenidate, amphetamine, and modafinil are possible options, although the evidence base in the DoC population is both limited (in terms of quantity and methodological quality) and inconsistent[105]; thus specific recommendations are not possible.

In addition to stimulants, γ-aminobutyric acid (GABA) agonists, which have often been considered CNS depressants, have been shown to have a role to play in enhancing the level of consciousness of some patients with DoC.[107] In particular, zolpidem has been shown in a placebo-controlled, double-blind single-dose crossover study to improve the consistency and complexity of behavioral responses in approximately 5% of patients.[108] An open-label study found a slightly higher response rate of approximately 20%.[109] Although the response rate is not high, it seems reasonable to consider a zolpidem trial in all patients with DoC (for whom it is not contraindicated) given the relatively low risk associated with the medication. A hypothesized mechanism of action for the ability of GABA agonists to enhance the level of consciousness is illustrated in Fig. 14.2. According to this "mesocircuit hypothesis",[28] zolpidem inhibits a structure (the globus pallidus interna) that itself is inappropriately inhibiting a circuit involved with consciousness. Thus by "inhibiting the inhibitor," zolpidem facilitates a more normal level of activation of the circuit. Finally, it is noted that there is some suggestive evidence that another GABA agonist, intrathecal baclofen (ITB), may also enhance the level of consciousness in some patients with DoC, although whether the improvement is due solely to improved motor output (resulting from treatment of spasticity) or whether there is a direct effect on consciousness itself still needs to be clarified.[110–112,131]

Other than the medications already discussed, there is some evidence to support the possible role of other pharmacologic agents such as selective seratonin reuptake inhibitors, lamotrigine, and donepezil.[101–103] As with all the other medications discussed (with the exception of amantadine and zolpidem), there is not enough evidence to make specific recommendations. However, this does not mean that trials of agents other than amantadine and zolpidem are not warranted. In fact, given the relatively low risks of most of these medications, empirical trials with these agents would be justified. However, as with medication trials with other TBI populations, treatment goals should be identified and operationally defined, objective measures administered regularly to track response, and the medication itself be given at an adequate dose for an appropriate amount of time. This approach is described in more detail elsewhere in the textbook.

Pharmacotherapy is currently the mainstay of medical interventions for DoC. However, there has also been significant work in the area of "applied energy therapy" in DoC, almost exclusively in the form of electrical stimulation.[103,113] These electrical therapies include noninvasive treatments such as repetitive TMS[114–116] and transcranial direct current stimulation (tDCS)[117–119] as well as invasive treatments such as vagus nerve stimulation[120] and deep brain stimulation (DBS).[83,121,122] Of these modalities, DBS currently has the strongest evidence of efficacy because of the methodological rigor of the most recent study (even though the investigation involved only one patient).[83] In this patient, the stimulation electrodes were placed in the central thalamus; Fig. 14.2 illustrates a potential mechanism of action based on the mesocircuit hypothesis. Unfortunately, due to fiscal and regulatory barriers, DBS is not currently available for clinical use for patients with DoC in the United States.[123,124] The remainder of the therapies require further study before their routine use in clinical practice can be recommended. However, it is noted that, given the apparent relatively low risk profile of tDCS, some clinicians and centers may already be offering this modality of treatment to selected patients. Finally, note is made of early work on low-intensity focused ultrasound as a mode of treatment.[125]

MEDICAL, NEUROLOGIC, AND NEUROMUSCULAR ISSUES

The medical, neurologic, and neuromusculoskeletal issues faced by patients with DoC are similar to those faced by other patients with significant TBI (Fig. 14.1) and are treated more extensively elsewhere in this textbook. However, although the issues faced by patients with DoC are similar, they are often more severe in their manifestation. Recent studies have found a high burden of medical complications in patients with DoC as well as a higher rate of acute care transfers than other patients with TBI in rehabilitation facilities.[126,128,129] Common medical and neurologic issues identified in these studies included infections, paroxysmal sympathetic hyperactivity, hydrocephalus, metabolic disturbances, and seizures.[128–130] One study found that the rate of new complications seems to diminish as a function of time in an inpatient rehabilitation program and not as a function of time since injury,[128] suggesting that the close medical and neurologic monitoring and management in rehabilitation units can reduce the rate of these complications.

As with the medical and neurologic issues, neuromuscular issues such as weakness, spasticity, and contractures are often much more severe in patients with DoC than in other patients with TBI. They carry added significance in this population because, as previously discussed, motor output is an important means for these patients to indicate their true level of consciousness. In addition, adequate management of these issues will allow for reduced pain, improved positioning/mobilization, and possibly the increased capacity and efficacy of voluntary movement. Thus the comprehensive and effective management of these neuromuscular issues is a priority for these patients. Frequent utilization of treatments such as nerve and muscle blocks and ITB pumps[110–112,131] and neuro-orthopedic procedures such as tendon lengthenings[132] are warranted. In addition to obvious spasticity and contractures, clinicians should routinely screen patients for potentially occult neuromusculoskeletal conditions such as occult fractures, heterotopic ossification, peripheral nerve injuries, and the presence of critical illness polyneuropathy/myopathy.

Finally, it is important to monitor for and address pain.[37,106,133–135] Patients with a DoC are at high risk for painful conditions. The neuromusculokeletal issues that these patients face are often painful, and there are frequently other potential sources of noxious stimuli (e.g., skin breakdown, constipation, instrumentation). Also, recent functional neuroimaging studies seem to confirm clinical experience, namely that patients in

MCS are capable of feeling pain.[37,106,133–135] Although it is currently not thought that patients in a true VS are capable of feeling pain, the high rate of misdiagnosis of VS as well as the phenomenon of covert awareness would suggest that adequate analgesic control be the goal for all patients, regardless of the presumed level of consciousness. A recently devised scale, the Nociception Coma Scale-Revised, may be a useful tool for identifying pain and monitoring response to treatment in ambiguous cases.[37] Finally, although adequate analgesic control is both a clinical and ethical imperative in these patients, it is recognized that it may sometimes require medications that adversely affect arousal. In these cases, clinicians and caregivers should have discussions about the benefits of improved arousal relative to optimal pain control. The balance between these two goals may shift over time. For example, it may be appropriate to minimize potentially sedating analgesic medications during the early phases of assessment of the level of consciousness and then introduce them again at a later time.

OUTCOMES IN DISORDER OF CONSCIOUSNESS

Prognosis and outcome are key questions in DoC, for both clinicians and families. Unfortunately, older studies in this area are limited by both diagnostic inaccuracy and a lack of conceptual clarity. In particular, most of these studies did not make distinctions between the various DoCs. This is a significant issue because recent evidence suggests that outcome is directly tied to diagnosis, with patients in MCS having much better outcomes than those in VS.[136] More recent studies, although few in number, have provided more helpful information regarding outcomes in DoC. When reviewing these studies, it is important to be clear about what the outcome of interest is; these outcomes can include mortality, recovery of consciousness, and functional recovery. This section will focus primarily on the latter two outcomes because these tend to be of most relevance to rehabilitation clinicians. However, it is noted that most studies have suggested a relatively high mortality rate after DoC, especially for those with chronic DoC.[137–139]

The most comprehensive review on *recovery of consciousness* in the VS is several decades old[137] and thus prone to the limitations of the older studies described earlier. However, although potentially affecting the actual percentages reported, these conceptual and methodological limitations likely do not affect the general patterns and correlations observed. Specifically, this review found that outcome in VS was directly related both to the etiology and the time since onset. Patients with traumatic VS had much better outcomes than patients with nontraumatic VS. Also, regardless of the etiology, the longer one remained in a VS, the lower the chances of recovery of consciousness. Thus over half (52%) of the adults in a posttraumatic VS at 1 month had recovered consciousness at 1 year. However, the number recovering consciousness drops to 35% for those in a posttraumatic VS at 3 months and to just 16% for those who remain in a posttraumatic VS at 6 months.[137] For those who remained in a VS at 12 months, the prognosis for recovery of consciousness was found to be very low. However, late recovery of consciousness is possible and has been reported multiple times,[137,140,141] suggesting that the prospects for late recovery are better than previously thought. For those who do recover consciousness after posttraumatic VS, *functional outcome* can vary and is again directly related to the time that the patient was in a VS.[137] Specifically, for those who were in VS at 1 month, approximately half of those recovering consciousness in a year will be *severely disabled* according to the Glasgow Outcome Scale (GOS). The other half will show *moderate disability* or *good recovery* by GOS criteria. However, for those who regain consciousness after being in a posttraumatic VS for at least 6 months, the likelihood of severe disability (according to GOS criteria) is three times higher than the likelihood of having a moderate disability or good recovery.[137]

As stated earlier, the prognosis for the MCS is much better than that for the VS. One study found that the probability of a favorable outcome was much greater for patients in a posttraumatic MCS (38%) than in a posttraumatic VS (2%).[136] Several recent studies have examined the outcomes in patient who were admitted to an inpatient rehabilitation setting with DoC. One study[142] of patients with DoC admitted approximately 35 days after injury found that, at 1 year, nearly half of the patients had achieved recovery to daytime independence at home and 22% had returned to work or school. Another study[143] of patients with posttraumatic DoC admitted to an inpatient rehabilitation program (approximately 1 month postinjury) found that almost 20% of patients were found capable of living without in-house supervision at follow-up ranging from 1 to 5 years. In addition, almost 20% demonstrated employment potential in either a sheltered or a competitive employment setting. Many of the patients in the studies just mentioned had emerged from a DoC during their stay in inpatient rehabilitation. Another study examined outcomes in more severely affected patients, namely those who remained in DoC at the time of *discharge* from inpatient rehabilitation. In this study of patients with posttraumatic DoC, close to 20% of patients performed independently on basic motor and cognitive subscales of the Functional Independence Measure at 2 years.[127] These studies suggest that outcomes from posttraumatic DoC are much better than commonly believed.

Although there is accumulating knowledge about outcomes after DoC in *general*, the ability to prognosticate in individual cases is still limited. As has been discussed, there are several clinical "rules of thumb" (based on the studies discussed earlier, as well as others[144]): patients with a traumatic DoC have a much better prognosis than those with a nontraumatic (especially anoxic) DoC, patients in an MCS have a better prognosis than patients in a VS at equivalent points in time, and the rate of recovery is positively correlated with outcome. There is also evidence that structural neuroimaging may be mildly helpful in prognosticating after posttraumatic DoC; in particular, deeper lesions on MRI (e.g., at the level of the brainstem) are associated with poorer outcomes.[145] However, our ability to translate these general findings to accurate prognoses for individual patients is still very limited.

There are several promising ancillary techniques that may improve our ability to prognosticate in the future. In particular, several of the modalities discussed previously (e.g., functional neuroimaging, ERP) may allow for the identification of a subset of patients with DoC who have a better prognosis. Specifically, those patients who show evidence of covert cognitive abilities appear to recover more quickly and have better outcomes than patients who have similar clinical (behavioral) examinations but lack evidence of covert cognitive capacities.[5,63,72–79] This is unsurprising in so far as the presence of residual cognitive abilities, whether they are detected behaviorally or through ancillary measures, are likely a marker of preserved (although underactivated) neural networks. There are also other electrophysiologic techniques, which are not designed to detect covert cognitive capacities, which may, nonetheless, be useful in predicting outcome.[146] It is anticipated that, in the years to come, at least some of these ancillary modalities will play a larger and more frequent role in prognostication in DoC.

FAMILIES AND CAREGIVERS

As is the case with all severe brain injuries, attention to the needs of families and caregivers is a crucial part of the rehabilitation process. However, families and caregivers of patients with a DoC have certain needs and experiences that are unique to this population. This often begins in acute care, even before a patient with DoC is admitted to a rehabilitation program, when families are often confronted with questions and decisions regarding the continuation or cessation of life-sustaining medical treatment. They are frequently approached early on with recommendations for palliative treatment or organ donation, often within just a few hours of their loved one's injury.[147,148] As a result, families can feel pressured and resentful, and as a result, they frequently adopt a defensive position, feeling the need to fight for their loved one's life in opposition to the healthcare system. A lack of trust in the healthcare system, especially acute care physicians, can develop, and, if it does, it often colors the family's interactions with the rehabilitation clinicians whom they subsequently encounter.[147] However, even though these families have often made the explicit and intentional decision to keep the patient alive, they frequently have doubts and feel guilt about the decision(s) they made, especially later, when they see that the patient is not recovering as expected and instead remains in a DoC.[148]

During the rehabilitation stay, this perceived lack of improvement (at least relative to the families' initial expectations as well as in comparison to other patients whom they may encounter) is a central experience. For families, DoC often represents a condition of *ambiguous loss*, which is a situation without resolution in which their loved one is experienced as "physically present but psychologically absent."[149] Traditional approaches to grief may not be entirely appropriate in these settings, given the lack of finality and the ambiguity of the patient's status as "present" or "absent." Rehabilitation clinicians should be aware of the phenomena just described—the possible mistrust of the healthcare system that was advocating for early withdrawal of treatment, the doubt and guilt that might be experienced regarding decisions made in the acute care setting, and the experience of ambiguous loss—so as to better appreciate and engage with the family's psychologic experience.

Compounding these psychologic difficulties are the cognitive challenges families face in understanding consciousness and its operationalization by the clinical team. Consciousness itself is a very abstract concept, and there is not even agreement in clinical or philosophical circles as to how to best conceptualize it.[1] Even the various clinical categories of DoC can be difficult to comprehend. This is especially true of the VS, given our everyday (and intuitive) experience of the deep relationship between arousal and awareness. Families may struggle to understand how their loved one could have their eyes open and yet be unconscious. It is imperative that the rehabilitation team do their best to educate the family, in understandable terms, about the different categories of DoC as well as the various methods of assessment of consciousness to be utilized. In fact, properly informed, there is reason to believe that families can play an integral role in the assessment process.

The observations of family and caregivers are often quite valuable and provide an important supplement to the assessments performed by the clinical team. Part of the value of the families' observations is simply a function of the significant amount of time they spend with the patient, often at times (e.g., evenings, nights) when the clinical team is not present. Thus they have a large number of "data points," increasing the chances that they will observe behavior that less frequent observation might miss. Moreover, knowing the patient well, family members may be able to detect subtle changes that might not be apparent to the treating professionals. Finally, it has been shown that patients with DoC are often more likely to respond to the voice of a family member than a treating clinician.[91-93] This suggests that families may actually be better positioned to elicit behavior from the patient, thereby enhancing the likelihood that behavior relevant to the assessment of consciousness is detected.

Thus despite the general suspicion that families and caregivers may "overperceive" and overinterpret behaviors, it is more likely that, on balance, the advantages of incorporating their observations outweighs the potential drawbacks. Recent evidence seems to support this position. One study found a 76% match rate in families' beliefs about the patient's level of consciousness and the diagnostic assessment performed by the clinical team. Interestingly, 17% of families thought their loved one had a lower level of consciousness (than the clinical team) and only 7% cases believed their loved one was better.[150] In another study, discussed previously, almost half of the CRS-R scores were higher when the family actively participated in the administration of the measure. Moreover, in 16% of these instances, the improvement in score resulted in a patient being reclassified as in an MCS rather than a VS.[43]

In addition to the issues unique to DoC discussed previously, family members of patients with DoC have the same needs for information, training, and support as do caregivers of patients with less severe brain injuries. The needs for training and support are even more intensive for families who decide to take their loved one home after discharge. Clinicians should prepare for ongoing material and psychologic support to continue well after discharge, given the evidence for the potentially high levels of burden (and often distress) that caregivers of patients with DoC often face.[149,151-155]

ETHICAL ISSUES

A number of ethical issues arise in the context of the care of patients with DoC. These include the ethical implications of diagnostic and prognostic uncertainty,[156] the conduct of research with these patients,[157,158] responding to requests for novel diagnostic or therapeutic interventions,[159] and the ethical implications of covert awareness.[160,161] However, some of the most challenging situations—clinically, psychologically, and ethically—are requests to limit or withdraw medical treatment, especially for patients who might be in an MCS.[162] There is both legal and ethical consensus that it is permissible to withdraw treatment for someone in a chronic VS (if there is sufficient evidence of their wishes to that effect),[163,164] whereas there is no consensus—either legally or ethically—should a similar request arise in the context of a patient in an MCS.[165-168] In these situations, an ethics consultation or the involvement of an ethics committee should be sought.

DoC PROGRAMS AND SYSTEMS OF CARE

Much of the content of this chapter can be summarized in the form of goals of a DoC rehabilitation program (Box 14.7). As can be seen, although some of the goals are specific to patients with DoC, the majority represents goals of any program that treats patients with moderate to severe TBI. Still, having these goals in mind may help the clinical team maintain focus by anchoring interventions to specific aims. It can also be helpful in orienting families and caregivers to the expected objectives of the patient's stay. Two recently published accounts provide excellent examples of actual programs that are centered on these goals.[95,169] Unfortunately, despite the apparent benefits of a DoC rehabilitation program, the majority of patients with DoC lack access to such services.

This is partly due to a clinical mindset that still persists about these patients, namely, one of "therapeutic nihilism."[147] At a clinical level, it is assumed

---

BOX 14.7
Goals of a Disorders of Consciousness Program

- Assess current level of consciousness
- Address reversible causes of impaired consciousness
- Initiate interventions to enhance consciousness
- Establish a system of communication
- Identify and magnify residual voluntary movement
- Address restrictions in range of motion
- Intensive mobilization and environmental enrichment
- Prevent and manage secondary medical complications
- Optimize respiration/nutrition/elimination/integument
- Provide family education/training/support
- Establish a plan for aftercare

---

that the prognosis for these patients is uniformly poor and that there are no treatments available to alter that trajectory. At the level of values, it is often assumed by clinicians that living with a DoC precludes "quality of life"; this assumption can color, consciously or unconsciously, decisions about the nature and extent of treatment (and even whether to withhold treatment). Thus especially in the acute care setting, DoC is often viewed through the prism of end-of-life care[147] and discussions with families often revolve around Do Not Resuscitate orders and palliative care.[148] The option of referring a patient to a specialized DoC rehabilitation program is less likely to arise; rather, if the patient survives, the plans more often center around long-term placement, either at a nursing home or with family.

However, even if clinicians wanted to refer patients to DoC programs, there are systemic barriers to accessing these services. Most notably, many patients with DoC do not meet eligibility requirements, set by the payer, for rehabilitation services. This is true for many providers of health insurance, whether public or private.[170] Also, even if patients with DoC are admitted to a rehabilitation facility, their length of stay is often significantly limited. Unfortunately, lack of access to specialized rehabilitation services is likely leading to a higher rate of complications and less progression of the level of consciousness.[12] There are several efforts underway to attempt to remedy this situation, from the development of clinical practice recommendations to efforts at advocacy.

At a policy level, a compelling case has been made by an expert panel to "front-load" the specialized services offered to these patients.[12] That is, rather than have patients start at a lower level of care until they are "ready" for rehabilitation, it has been proposed that these patients, after medical and neurologic stabilization, be transferred to a specialized DoC program, with goals as outlined earlier (Box 14.7). After an initial stay in such a program, those patients who have improved sufficiently can be transitioned to standard brain injury rehabilitation, whereas those who have not can be transferred to a less intensive level of care, with systems in place for close monitoring and transition back to a specialized DoC program if indicated. A program with some similarities to this proposal is currently in place in the VA system; if it proves successful, it might serve as a model for programs in the civilian sector.[95]

A forceful case has been made to view access to quality care for patients with DoC as an ethical and political imperative.[147,171] Our systems of care have not kept pace with our improved understanding of these conditions, including the knowledge that prognosis is better than once thought and that treatment can further alter the trajectory towards improvement, both in neurologic status and quality of life. Not only do people with a DoC lack access to care, they are also segregated from the rest of the population, often housed in long-term facilities with no meaningful attempt made at improving their status or integrating them into the community. For these reasons, it has been argued that the right to care for patients with DoC is one of the premier civil rights issues of our time.[147]

REFERENCES

1. Schneider S, Velmans M, eds. *The Blackwell Companion to Consciousness.* 2nd ed. Malden, MA: Wiley-Blackwell; 2017.
2. Bagnato S, Boccagni C, Sant'Angelo A, et al. Long-lasting coma. *Funct Neurol.* 2014;29(3):201–205.
3. Lannin NA, Cusick A, McLachlan R, Allaous J. Observed recovery sequence in neurobehavioral function after severe traumatic brain injury. *Am J Occup Ther.* 2013;67(5):543–549.
4. Taylor CM, Aird VH, Tate RL, Lammi MH. Sequence of recovery during the course of emergence from the minimally conscious state. *Arch Phys Med Rehabil.* 2007;88(4):521–525.
5. Bruno M-A, Vanhaudenhuyse A, Thibaut A, Moonen G, Laureys S. From unresponsive wakefulness to minimally conscious PLUS and functional locked-in syndromes: recent advances in our understanding of disorders of consciousness. *J Neurol.* 2011;258(7):1373–1384.

6. Bruno M-A, Majerus S, Boly M, et al. Functional neuroanatomy underlying the clinical subcategorization of minimally conscious state patients. *J Neurol.* 2012;259(6):1087–1098.

7. Giacino JT, Kalmar K. Diagnostic and prognostic guidelines for the vegetative and minimally conscious states. *Neuropsychol Rehabil.* 2005;15(3–4):166–174.

8. Jennett B, Plum F. Persistent vegetative state after brain damage. A syndrome in search of a name. *Lancet (London, England).* 1972;1(7753):734–737.

9. Laureys S, Celesia GG, Cohadon F, et al. Unresponsive wakefulness syndrome: a new name for the vegetative state or apallic syndrome. *BMC Med.* 2010;8(1):68.

10. Bayne T, Hohwy J, Owen AM. Are there levels of consciousness? *Trends Cogn Sci.* 2016;20(6):405–413.

11. Fins JJ, Master MG, Gerber LM, Giacino JT. The minimally conscious state. *Arch Neurol.* 2007;64(10):1400.

12. Berube J, Fins JJ, Giacino JT, et al. *The Mohonk Report: A Report to Congress on Disorders of Consciousness: Assessment, Treatment, and Research Needs.* Charlottesville, VA: National Brain Injury Research, Treatment, and Training Foundation; 2006.

13. Koch C, Massimini M, Boly M, Tononi G. Neural correlates of consciousness: progress and problems. *Nat Rev Neurosci.* 2016;17(5):307–321.

14. Bachmann T, Hudetz AG. It is time to combine the two main traditions in the research on the neural correlates of consciousness: C = L × D. *Front Psychol.* 2014;5:940.

15. Rodriguez Moreno D, Schiff ND, Giacino J, Kalmar K, Hirsch J. A network approach to assessing cognition in disorders of consciousness. *Neurology.* 2010;75(21):1871–1878.

16. Schiff ND, Rodriguez-Moreno D, Kamal A, et al. fMRI reveals large-scale network activation in minimally conscious patients. *Neurology.* 2005;64(3):514–523.

17. Chennu S, Annen J, Wannez S, et al. Brain networks predict metabolism, diagnosis and prognosis at the bedside in disorders of consciousness. *Brain.* 2017;140(8):2120–2132.

18. Demertzi A, Soddu A, Laureys S. Consciousness supporting networks. *Curr Opin Neurobiol.* 2013;23(2):239–244.

19. Di Perri C, Stender J, Laureys S, Gosseries O. Functional neuroanatomy of disorders of consciousness. *Epilepsy Behav.* 2014;30:28–32.

20. Vanhaudenhuyse A, Demertzi A, Schabus M, et al. Two distinct neuronal networks mediate the awareness of environment and of self. *J Cogn Neurosci.* 2011;23(3):570–578.

21. Di Perri C, Bahri MA, Amico E, et al. Neural correlates of consciousness in patients who have emerged from a minimally conscious state: a cross-sectional multimodal imaging study. *Lancet Neurol.* 2016;15(8):830–842.

22. Lant ND, Gonzalez-Lara LE, Owen AM, Fernández-Espejo D. Relationship between the anterior forebrain mesocircuit and the default mode network in the structural bases of disorders of consciousness. *Neuroimage Clin.* 2016;10:27–35.

23. Boly M, Seth AK. Modes and models in disorders of consciousness science. *Arch Ital Biol.* 2012;150(2–3):172–184.

24. Adams JH, Jennett B, McLellan DR, Murray LS, Graham DI. The neuropathology of the vegetative state after head injury. *J Clin Pathol.* 1999;52(11):804–806.

25. Graham DI, Adams JH, Murray LS, Jennett B. Neuropathology of the vegetative state after head injury. *Neuropsychol Rehabil.* 2005;15(3–4):198–213.

26. Lutkenhoff ES, Chiang J, Tshibanda L, et al. Thalamic and extrathalamic mechanisms of consciousness after severe brain injury. *Ann Neurol.* 2015;78(1):68–76.

27. Schiff ND, Ribary U, Moreno DR, et al. Residual cerebral activity and behavioural fragments can remain in the persistently vegetative brain. *Brain.* 2002;125(Pt 6):1210–1234.

28. Schiff ND. Recovery of consciousness after brain injury: a mesocircuit hypothesis. *Trends Neurosci.* 2010;33(1):1–9.

29. Andrews K, Murphy L, Munday R, Littlewood C. Misdiagnosis of the vegetative state: retrospective study in a rehabilitation unit. *BMJ.* 1996;313(7048):13–16.

30. Childs NL, Mercer WN, Childs HW. Accuracy of diagnosis of persistent vegetative state. *Neurology.* 1993;43(8):1465–1467.

31. Schnakers C, Vanhaudenhuyse A, Giacino J, et al. Diagnostic accuracy of the vegetative and minimally conscious state: clinical consensus versus standardized neurobehavioral assessment. *BMC Neurol.* 2009;9(1):35.

32. Giacino JT, Schnakers C, Rodriguez-Moreno D, Kalmar K, Schiff N, Hirsch J. Behavioral assessment in patients with disorders of consciousness: gold standard or fool's gold? *Prog Brain Res.* 2009;177:33–48.

33. Farisco M, Petrini C. Misdiagnosis as an ethical and scientific challenge. *Ann Ist Super Sanita.* 2014;50(3):229–233.

34. Saddawi-Konefka D, Berg SM, Nejad SH, Bittner EA. Catatonia in the ICU. *Crit Care Med.* 2014;42(3):e234–e241.

35. Majerus S, Bruno M-A, Schnakers C, Giacino JT, Laureys S. The problem of aphasia in the assessment of consciousness in brain-damaged patients. *Prog Brain Res.* 2009;177:49–61.

36. Schnakers C, Bessou H, Rubi-Fessen I, et al. Impact of aphasia on consciousness assessment. *Neurorehabil Neural Repair.* 2015;29(1):41–47.

37. Schnakers C, Zasler N. Assessment and management of pain in patients with disorders of consciousness. *PM R.* 2015;7(11):S270–S277.

38. Giacino J, Katz D, Garber K, Schiff N. Assessment and rehabilitative management of individuals with disorders of consciousness. In: Zasler N, Katz D, Zafonte R, Arciniegas D, Bullock M, Kreutzer J, eds. *Brain Injury Medicine: Principles and Practice.* 2nd ed. New York: Demos Medical Publishing; 2012:522.

39. Seel RT, Sherer M, Whyte J, et al. Assessment scales for disorders of consciousness: evidence-based recommendations for clinical practice and research. *Arch Phys Med Rehabil.* 2010;91(12):1795–1813.

40. Giacino JT, Kalmar K. *CRS-R Coma Recovery Scale-Revised Administration and Scoring Guidelines.* Johnson Rehabilitation Institution Affiliated with JFK Medical Center. http://www.tbims.org/combi/crs/CRS Syllabus.pdf.

41. La Porta F, Caselli S, Ianes AB, et al. Can we scientifically and reliably measure the level of consciousness in vegetative and minimally conscious states? Rasch analysis of the coma recovery scale-revised. *Arch Phys Med Rehabil.* 2013;94(3):527–535.e1.

42. Wannez S, Heine L, Thonnard M, Gosseries O, Laureys S. The repetition of behavioral assessments in diagnosis of disorders of consciousness. *Ann Neurol.* 2017;81(6):883–889.

43. Sattin D, Giovannetti AM, Ciaraffa F, et al. Assessment of patients with disorder of consciousness: do different coma recovery scale scoring correlate with different settings? *J Neurol.* 2014;261(12):2378–2386.

44. Whyte J, DiPasquale MC. Assessment of vision and visual attention in minimally responsive brain injured patients. *Arch Phys Med Rehabil.* 1995;76(9):804–810.

45. Whyte J, DiPasquale MC, Vaccaro M. Assessment of command-following in minimally conscious brain injured patients. *Arch Phys Med Rehabil.* 1999;80(6):653–660.

46. Block C, Rosenblatt A, O'Brien K, Kothari S. Use of an individualized quantitative behavioral assessment (IQBA) for the early detection of signs of consciousness following brain injury. *J Int Neuropsychol Soc.* 2016; 22(suppl 1).

47. Monti MM, Owen AM. Behavior in the brain: using functional neuroimaging to assess residual cognition and awareness after severe brain injury. *J Psychophysiol.* 2010;24(2):76–82.

48. Monti MM, Vanhaudenhuyse A, Coleman MR, et al. Willful modulation of brain activity in disorders of consciousness. *N Engl J Med.* 2010;362(7):579–589.

49. Schiff ND. Cognitive motor dissociation following severe brain injuries. *JAMA Neurol.* 2015;72(12):1413.

50. Kondziella D, Friberg CK, Frokjaer VG, Fabricius M, Møller K. Preserved consciousness in vegetative and minimal conscious states: systematic review and meta-analysis. *J Neurol Neurosurg Psychiatr.* 2016;87(5):485–492.

51. Larson MD, Behrends M. Portable infrared pupillometry. *Anesth Anal.* 2015;120(6):1242–1253.

52. Laeng B, Sirois S, Gredebäck G. Pupillometry. *Perspect Psychol Sci.* 2012;7(1):18–27.

53. Hartmann M, Fischer MH. Pupillometry: the eyes shed fresh light on the mind. *Curr Biol.* 2014;24(7): R281–R282.

54. Stoll J, Chatelle C, Carter O, Koch C, Laureys S, Einhäuser W. Pupil responses allow communication in locked-in syndrome patients. *Curr Biol.* 2013;23(15):R647–R648.

55. Bekinschtein TA, Coleman MR, Niklison J, Pickard JD, Manes FF. Can electromyography objectively detect voluntary movement in disorders of consciousness? *J Neurol Neurosurg Psychiatr.* 2008;79(7):826–828.

56. Habbal D, Gosseries O, Noirhomme Q, et al. Volitional electromyographic responses in disorders of consciousness. *Brain Inj.* 2014;28(9):1171–1179.

57. Lesenfants D, Habbal D, Chatelle C, Schnakers C, Laureys S, Noirhomme Q. Electromyographic decoding of response to command in disorders of consciousness. *Neurology.* 2016;87(20):2099–2107.

58. Monti MM. Cognition in the vegetative state. *Annu Rev Clin Psychol.* 2012;8(1):431–454.

59. Hauger SL, Schanke A-K, Andersson S, Chatelle C, Schnakers C, Løvstad M. The clinical diagnostic utility of electrophysiological techniques in assessment of patients with disorders of consciousness following acquired brain injury. *J Head Trauma Rehabil.* 2017;32(3): 185–196.

60. Owen AM. Using functional magnetic resonance imaging and electroencephalography to detect consciousness after severe brain injury. *Handb Clin Neurol.* 2015;127:277–293.

61. Harrison AH, Connolly JF. Finding a way in: a review and practical evaluation of fMRI and EEG for detection and assessment in disorders of consciousness. *Neurosci Biobehav Rev.* 2013;37(8):1403–1419.

62. Guldenmund P, Stender J, Heine L, Laureys S. Mindsight: diagnostics in disorders of consciousness. *Crit Care Res Pract.* 2012;2012:624724.

63. Morlet D, Fischer C. MMN and novelty P3 in coma and other altered states of consciousness: a review. *Brain Topogr.* 2014;27(4):467–479.

64. Kirschner A, Cruse D, Chennu S, Owen AM, Hampshire A. A P300-based cognitive assessment battery. *Brain Behav.* 2015;5(6).

65. Casali AG, Gosseries O, Rosanova M, et al. A theoretically based index of consciousness independent of sensory processing and behavior. *Sci Transl Med.* 2013;5(198).

66. Casarotto S, Comanducci A, Rosanova M, et al. Stratification of unresponsive patients by an independently validated index of brain complexity. *Ann Neurol.* 2016;80(5):718–729.

67. Napolitani M, Bodart O, Canali P, et al. Transcranial magnetic stimulation combined with high-density EEG in altered states of consciousness. *Brain Inj.* 2014;28(9):1180–1189.

68. Marino S, Bonanno L, Giorgio A. Functional connectivity in disorders of consciousness: methodological aspects and clinical relevance. *Brain Imaging Behav.* 2016;10(2):604–608.

69. van Gaal S, Lamme VAF. Unconscious high-level information processing. *Neuroscientist.* 2012;18(3):287–301.

70. Coleman MR, Bekinschtein T, Monti MM, Owen AM, Pickard JD. A multimodal approach to the assessment of patients with disorders of consciousness. *Prog Brain Res.* 2009;177:231–248.

71. Schiff ND. Multimodal neuroimaging approaches to disorders of consciousness. *J Head Trauma Rehabil.* 2006;21(5):388–397.

72. Vogel D, Markl A, Yu T, Kotchoubey B, Lang S, Müller F. Can mental imagery functional magnetic resonance imaging predict recovery in patients with disorders of consciousness? *Arch Phys Med Rehabil.* 2013;94(10):1891–1898.

73. Wijnen VJM, Eilander HJ, de Gelder B, van Boxtel GJM. Repeated measurements of the auditory oddball paradigm is related to recovery from the vegetative state. *J Clin Neurophysiol.* 2014;31(1):65–80.

74. Steppacher I, Eickhoff S, Jordanov T, Kaps M, Witzke W, Kissler J. N400 predicts recovery from disorders of consciousness. *Ann Neurol.* 2013;73(5):594–602.

75. Xu W, Jiang G, Chen Y, Wang X, Jiang X. Prediction of minimally conscious state with somatosensory evoked potentials in long-term unconscious patients after traumatic brain injury. *J Trauma Inj Infect Crit Care.* 2012;72(4):1024–1030.

76. Cavinato M, Freo U, Ori C, et al. Post-acute P300 predicts recovery of consciousness from traumatic vegetative state. *Brain Inj.* 2009;23(12):973–980.

77. Qin P, Di H, Yan X, et al. Mismatch negativity to the patient's own name in chronic disorders of consciousness. *Neurosci Lett.* 2008;448(1):24–28.

78. Wijnen VJM, van Boxtel GJM, Eilander HJ, de Gelder B. Mismatch negativity predicts recovery from the vegetative state. *Clin Neurophysiol.* 2007;118(3):597–605.

79. Daltrozzo J, Wioland N, Mutschler V, Kotchoubey B. Predicting coma and other low responsive patients outcome using event-related brain potentials: a meta-analysis. *Clin Neurophysiol.* 2007;118(3):606–614.

80. Chatelle C, Chennu S, Noirhomme Q, Cruse D, Owen AM, Laureys S. Brain–computer interfacing in disorders of consciousness. *Brain Inj.* 2012;26(12):1510–1522.

81. Gibson RM, Owen AM, Cruse D. Brain–computer interfaces for patients with disorders of consciousness. *Prog Brain Res.* 2016;228:241–291.

82. Naci L, Monti MM, Cruse D, et al. Brain-computer interfaces for communication with nonresponsive patients. *Ann Neurol.* 2012;72(3):312–323.

83. Schiff ND, Giacino JT, Kalmar K, et al. Behavioural improvements with thalamic stimulation after severe traumatic brain injury. *Nature.* 2007;448(7153):600–603.

84. Lombardi F, Taricco M, De Tanti A, Telaro E, Liberati A. Sensory stimulation of brain-injured individuals in coma or vegetative state: results of a cochrane systematic review. *Clin Rehabil.* 2002;16(5):464–472.

85. Padilla R, Domina A. Effectiveness of sensory stimulation to improve arousal and alertness of people in a coma or persistent vegetative state after traumatic brain injury: a systematic review. *Am J Occup Ther.* 2016;70(3): 7003180030p.1.

86. Abbate C, Trimarchi PD, Basile I, Mazzucchi A, Devalle G. Sensory stimulation for patients with disorders of consciousness: from stimulation to rehabilitation. *Front Hum Neurosci.* 2014;8:616.

87. Schiff ND, Pulver M. Does vestibular stimulation activate thalamocortical mechanisms that reintegrate impaired cortical regions? *Proc Biol Sci.* February 22, 1999;266(1417):421–423.

88. Vanzan S, Wilkinson D, Ferguson H, Pullicino P, Sakel M. Behavioural improvement in a minimally conscious state after caloric vestibular stimulation: evidence from two single case studies. *Clin Rehabil.* 2017;31(4):500–507.

89. Elliott L, Coleman M, Shiel A, et al. Effect of posture on levels of arousal and awareness in vegetative and minimally conscious state patients: a preliminary investigation. *J Neurol Neurosurg Psychiatr.* 2005;76(2): 298–299.

90. Krewer C, Luther M, Koenig E, Müller F. Tilt table therapies for patients with severe disorders of consciousness: a randomized, controlled trial. Glasauer S, ed. *PLoS One.* 2015;10(12):e0143180.

91. Perrin F, Castro M, Tillmann B, Luauté J. Promoting the use of personally relevant stimuli for investigating patients with disorders of consciousness. *Front Psychol.* 2015;6:1102.

92. Bekinschtein T, Leiguarda R, Armony J, et al. Emotion processing in the minimally conscious state. *J Neurol Neurosurg Psychiatr.* 2004;75(5):788.

93. Machado C, Korein J, Aubert E, et al. Recognizing a mother's voice in the persistent vegetative state. *Clin EEG Neurosci.* 2007;38(3):124–126.

94. Abbasi M, Mohammadi E, Sheaykh Rezayi A. Effect of a regular family visiting program as an affective, auditory, and tactile stimulation on the consciousness level of comatose patients with a head injury. *Jpn J Nurs Sci.* 2009;6(1):21–26.

95. McNamee S, Howe L, Nakase-Richardson R, Peterson M. Treatment of disorders of consciousness in the Veterans Health Administration Polytrauma Centers. *J Head Trauma Rehabil.* 2012;27(4):244–252.

96. Rollnik JD, Altenmüller E. Music in disorders of consciousness. *Front Neurosci.* 2014;8:190.

97. Magee WL, O'Kelly J. Music therapy with disorders of consciousness: current evidence and emergent evidence-based practice. *Ann N Y Acad Sci.* 2015;1337(1): 256–262.

98. O'Kelly J, James L, Palaniappan R, Taborin J, Fachner J, Magee WL. Neurophysiological and behavioral responses to music therapy in vegetative and minimally conscious states. *Front Hum Neurosci.* 2013;7:884.

99. O'Kelly J, Magee WL. Music therapy with disorders of consciousness and neuroscience: the need for dialogue. *Nord J Music Ther.* 2013;22(2):93–106.

100. Hazell AS. The vegetative state and stem cells: therapeutic considerations. *Front Neurol.* 2016;7:118.

101. Ciurleo R, Bramanti P, Calabrò RS. Pharmacotherapy for disorders of consciousness: are "awakening" drugs really a possibility? *Drugs.* 2013;73(17):1849–1862.

102. Mura E, Pistoia F, Sara M, Sacco S, Carolei A, Govoni S. Pharmacological modulation of the state of awareness in patients with disorders of consciousness: an overview. *Curr Pharm Des.* 2013;999(999):5–6.

103. Oliveira L, Fregni F. Pharmacological and electrical stimulation in chronic disorders of consciousness: new insights and future directions. *Brain Inj.* 2011;25(4): 315–327.

104. Giacino JT, Whyte J, Bagiella E, et al. Placebo-controlled trial of amantadine for severe traumatic brain injury. *N Engl J Med.* 2012;366(9):819–826.

105. Martin RT, Whyte J. The effects of methylphenidate on command following and yes/no communication in persons with severe disorders of consciousness. *Am J Phys Med Rehabil.* 2007;86(8):613–620.

106. Pistoia F, Sacco S, Sarà M, Carolei A. The perception of pain and its management in disorders of consciousness. *Curr Pain Headache Rep.* 2013;17(11):374.

107. Pistoia F, Sara M, Sacco S, Franceschini M, Carolei A. Silencing the brain may be better than stimulating it. The GABA effect. *Curr Pharm Des.* 2013;999(999):23–24.

108. Whyte J, Rajan R, Rosenbaum A, et al. Zolpidem and restoration of consciousness. *Am J Phys Med Rehabil.* 2014;93(2):101–113.

109. Thonnard M, Gosseries O, Demertzi A, et al. Effect of zolpidem in chronic disorders of consciousness: a prospective open-label study. *Funct Neurol.* 2013;28(4):259–264.

110. Sarà M, Pistoia F, Mura E, Onorati P, Govoni S. Intrathecal baclofen in patients with persistent vegetative state: 2 hypotheses. *Arch Phys Med Rehabil.* 2009;90(7):1245–1249.

111. Pistoia F, Sacco S, Sarà M, Franceschini M, Carolei A. Intrathecal baclofen: effects on spasticity, pain, and consciousness in disorders of consciousness and locked-in syndrome. *Curr Pain Headache Rep.* 2015;19(1):466.

112. Oyama H, Kito A, Maki H, Hattori K, Tanahashi K. Consciousness recovery induced by intrathecal baclofen administration after subarachnoid hemorrhage -two case reports-. *Neurol Med Chir (Tokyo).* 2010;50(5):386–390.

113. Ragazzoni A, Cincotta M, Giovannelli F, et al. Clinical neurophysiology of prolonged disorders of consciousness: from diagnostic stimulation to therapeutic neuromodulation. *Clin Neurophysiol.* 2017;128(9):1629–1646.

114. Pistoia F, Sacco S, Carolei A, Sarà M. Coticomotor facilitation in vegetative state: results of a pilot study. *Arch Phys Med Rehabil.* August 2013;94(8):1599–1606.

115. Pape TL-B, Rosenow J, Lewis G. Transcranial magnetic stimulation: a possible treatment for TBI. *J Head Trauma Rehabil.* 2006;21(5):437–451.

116. Piccione F, Cavinato M, Manganotti P, et al. Behavioral and neurophysiological effects of repetitive transcranial magnetic stimulation on the minimally conscious state: a case study. *Neurorehabil Neural Repair.* 2011;25(1):98–102.

117. Estraneo A, Pascarella A, Moretta P, et al. Repeated transcranial direct current stimulation in prolonged disorders of consciousness: a double-blind cross-over study. *J Neurol Sci.* 2017;375:464–470.

118. Thibaut A, Bruno M-A, Ledoux D, Demertzi A, Laureys S. tDCS in patients with disorders of consciousness: sham-controlled randomized double-blind study. *Neurology.* 2014;82(13):1112–1118.

119. Angelakis E, Liouta E, Andreadis N, et al. Transcranial direct current stimulation effects in disorders of consciousness. *Arch Phys Med Rehabil.* 2014;95(2):283–289.

120. Corazzol M, Lio G, Lefevre A, et al. Restoring consciousness with vagus nerve stimulation. *Curr Biol.* 2017;27(18):R994–R996.

121. Schiff ND. Moving toward a generalizable application of central thalamic deep brain stimulation for support of forebrain arousal regulation in the severely injured brain. *Ann N Y Acad Sci.* 2012;1265(1):56–68.

122. Shah SA, Schiff ND. Central thalamic deep brain stimulation for cognitive neuromodulation – a review of proposed mechanisms and investigational studies. *Eur J Neurosci.* 2010;32(7):1135–1144.

123. Giacino JT, Fins JJ, Machado A, Schiff ND. Central thalamic deep brain stimulation to promote recovery from chronic posttraumatic minimally conscious state: challenges and opportunities. *Neuromodul Technol Neural Interf.* 2012;15(4):339–349.

124. Fins JJ, Dorfman GS, Pancrazio JJ. Challenges to deep brain stimulation: a pragmatic response to ethical, fiscal, and regulatory concerns. *Ann N Y Acad Sci.* 2012;1265:80–90.

125. Monti MM, Schnakers C, Korb AS, Bystritsky A, Vespa PM. Non-invasive ultrasonic thalamic stimulation in disorders of consciousness after severe brain injury: a first-in-man report. *Brain Stimul.* 2016;9(6):940–941.

126. Nakase-Richardson R, Tran J, Cifu D, et al. Do rehospitalization rates differ among injury severity levels in the NIDRR traumatic brain injury model systems program? *Arch Phys Med Rehabil.* 2013;94(10):1884–1890.

127. Whyte J, Nakase-Richardson R, Hammond FM, et al. Functional outcomes in traumatic disorders of consciousness: 5-year outcomes from the National Institute on disability and rehabilitation research traumatic brain injury model systems. *Arch Phys Med Rehabil.* 2013;94(10):1855–1860.

128. Whyte J, Nordenbo AM, Kalmar K, et al. Medical complications during inpatient rehabilitation among patients with traumatic disorders of consciousness. *Arch Phys Med Rehabil.* 2013;94(10):1877–1883.

129. Ganesh S, Guernon A, Chalcraft L, Harton B, Smith B, Louise-Bender Pape T. Medical comorbidities in disorders of consciousness patients and their association with functional outcomes. *Arch Phys Med Rehabil.* 2013;94(10):1899–1907.

130. Bagnato S, Boccagni C, Sant'Angelo A, Prestandrea C, Virgilio V, Galardi G. EEG epileptiform abnormalities at admission to a rehabilitation department predict the risk of seizures in disorders of consciousness following a coma. *Epilepsy Behav.* 2016;56:83–87.

131. Margetis K, Korfias SI, Gatzonis S, et al. Intrathecal baclofen associated with improvement of consciousness disorders in spasticity patients. *Neuromodul Technol Neural Interf.* 2014;17(7):699–704.

132. Keenan MA, Esquenazi A, Mayer NH. Surgical treatment of common patterns of lower limb deformities resulting from upper motoneuron syndrome. *Adv Neurol.* 2001;87:333–346.

133. Schnakers C, Chatelle C, Demertzi A, Majerus S, Laureys S. What about pain in disorders of consciousness? *AAPS J.* 2012;14(3):437–444.

134. Chatelle C, Thibaut A, Whyte J, De Val MD, Laureys S, Schnakers C. Pain issues in disorders of consciousness. *Brain Inj.* 2014;28(9):1202–1208.

135. Pistoia F, Sacco S, Stewart J, Sarà M, Carolei A. Disorders of consciousness: painless or painful conditions?-Evidence from neuroimaging studies. *Brain Sci.* 2016;6(4).

136. Giacino JT, Kalmar K. The vegetative and minimally conscious states: a comparison of clinical features and functional outcome. *J Head Trauma Rehabil.* 1997;12(4): 36–51.

137. The Multi-Society Task Force on PVS. Medical aspects of the persistent vegetative state. *N Engl J Med.* 1994;330(21):1572–1579.

138. Estraneo A, Moretta P, Loreto V, Lanzillo B, Santoro L, Trojano L. Late recovery after traumatic, anoxic, or hemorrhagic long-lasting vegetative state. *Neurology.* 2010;75(3):239–245.

139. Luaute J, Maucort-Boulch D, Tell L, et al. Long-term outcomes of chronic minimally conscious and vegetative states. *Neurology.* 2010;75(3):246–252.

140. Childs NL, Mercer WN. Late improvement in consciousness after post-traumatic vegetative state. *N Engl J Med.* 1996;334(1):24–25.

141. Voss HU, Uluğ AM, Dyke JP, et al. Possible axonal regrowth in late recovery from the minimally conscious state. *J Clin Invest.* 2006;116(7):2005–2011.

142. Katz DI, Polyak M, Coughlan D, Nichols M, Roche A. Natural history of recovery from brain injury after prolonged disorders of consciousness: outcome of patients admitted to inpatient rehabilitation with 1–4 year follow-up. *Prog Brain Res.* 2009;177:73–88.

143. Nakase-Richardson R, Whyte J, Giacino JT, et al. Longitudinal outcome of patients with disordered consciousness in the NIDRR TBI model systems programs. *J Neurotrauma.* 2012;29(1):59–65.

144. Whyte J, Gosseries O, Chervoneva I, et al. Predictors of short-term outcome in brain-injured patients with disorders of consciousness. *Prog Brain Res.* 2009;177: 63–72.

145. Kothari S, DiTommaso C. Prognosis after severe traumatic brain injury: a practical, evidence-based approach. In: Zasler N, Katz D, Zafonte R, Arciniegas D, Bullock M, Kreutzer J, eds. *Brain Injury Medicine: Principles and Practice.* 2nd ed. New York: Demos Medical Publishing; 2012:248–278.

146. Sarà M, Pistoia F, Pasqualetti P, Sebastiano F, Onorati P, Rossini PM. Functional isolation within the cerebral cortex in the vegetative state. *Neurorehabil Neural Repair.* 2011;25(1):35–42.

147. Fins JJ. *Rights Come to Mind : Brain Injury, Ethics, and the Struggle for Consciousness.* New York: Cambridge University Press; 2015.

148. Kitzinger J, Kitzinger C. The "window of opportunity" for death after severe brain injury: family experiences. *Sociol Health Illn.* 2013;35(7):1095–1112.

149. Giovannetti AM, Covelli V, Sattin D, Leonardi M. Caregivers of patients with disorder of consciousness: burden, quality of life and social support. *Acta Neurol Scand.* 2015;132(4):259–269.

150. Jox RJ, Kuehlmeyer K, Klein A-M, et al. Diagnosis and decision making for patients with disorders of consciousness: a survey among family members. *Arch Phys Med Rehabil.* 2015;96(2):323–330.

151. Soeterik SM, Connolly S, Playford ED, Duport S, Riazi A. The psychological impact of prolonged disorders of consciousness on caregivers: a systematic review of quantitative studies. *Clin Rehabil.* 2017;31(10): 1374–1385.

152. Covelli V, Sattin D, Giovannetti AM, Scaratti C, Willems M, Leonardi M. Caregiver's burden in disorders of consciousness: a longitudinal study. *Acta Neurol Scand.* 2016;134(5):352–359.

153. Pagani M, Giovannetti AM, Covelli V, Sattin D, Raggi A, Leonardi M. Physical and mental health, anxiety and depressive symptoms in caregivers of patients in vegetative state and minimally conscious state. *Clin Psychol Psychother.* 2014;21(5):420–426.

154. Cruzado JA, Elvira de la Morena MJ. Coping and distress in caregivers of patients with disorders of consciousness. *Brain Inj.* 2013;27(7–8):793–798.

155. Leonardi M, Giovannetti AM, Pagani M, Raggi A, Sattin D, on behalf of the National Consortium. Burden and needs of 487 caregivers of patients in vegetative state and in minimally conscious state: results from a national study. *Brain Inj.* 2012;26(10):1201–1210.

156. Johnson LSM. Inference and inductive risk in disorders of consciousness. *AJOB Neurosci.* 2016;7(1):35–43.

157. Fins JJ. Neuroethics and disorders of consciousness: discerning brain states in clinical practice and research. *AMA J Ethics.* 2016;18(12):1182–1191.

158. Graham M, Weijer C, Peterson A, et al. Acknowledging awareness: informing families of individual research results for patients in the vegetative state. *J Med Ethics.* 2015;41(7):534–538.

159. Jox RJ, Bernat JL, Laureys S, Racine E. Disorders of consciousness: responding to requests for novel diagnostic and therapeutic interventions. *Lancet Neurol.* 2012;11(8):732–738.

160. Graham M, Weijer C, Cruse D, et al. An ethics of welfare for patients diagnosed as vegetative with covert awareness. *AJOB Neurosci.* 2015;6(2):31–41.

161. Friedrich O. Knowledge of partial awareness in disorders of consciousness: implications for ethical evaluations? *Neuroethics.* 2013;6(1):13–23.

162. Fins JJ. Affirming the right to care, preserving the right to die: disorders of consciousness and neuroethics after Schiavo. *Palliat Support Care.* 2006;4(2):169–178.

163. Shepherd L. *If that Ever Happens to Me: Making Life and Death Decisions after Terri Schiavo.* 1st ed. Chapel Hill, NC: University of North Carolina Press; 2009.

164. Buckley T, Crippen D, DeWitt AL, et al. Ethics roundtable debate: withdrawal of tube feeding in a patient with persistent vegetative state where the patients wishes are unclear and there is family dissension. *Crit Care*. 2004;8(2):79–84.

165. Huxtable R. "In a twilight world"? Judging the value of life for the minimally conscious patient. *J Med Ethics*. 2013;39(9):565–569.

166. Jackson E. The minimally conscious state and treatment withdrawal: W v M. *J Med Ethics*. 2013;39(9):559–561.

167. Lo B, Dornbrand L, Wolf LE, Groman M. The Wendland case — withdrawing life support from incompetent patients who are not terminally ill. *N Engl J Med*. 2002;346(19):1489–1493.

168. Johnson LSM. The right to die in the minimally conscious state. *J Med Ethics*. 2011;37(3):175–178.

169. Seel RT, Douglas J, Dennison AC, Heaner S, Farris K, Rogers C. Specialized early treatment for persons with disorders of consciousness: program components and outcomes. *Arch Phys Med Rehabil*. 2013;94(10):1908–1923.

170. Fins JJ, Wright MS, Kraft C, et al. Whither the "improvement standard"? Coverage for severe brain injury after Jimmo v. Sebelius. *J L Med Ethics*. 2016;44(1):182–193.

171. Martone M. What does society owe those who are minimally conscious? *J Soc Christ Ethics*. 2006;26:201–217.

CHAPTER 15

Assessment and Cognitive/Behavioral Interventions in Moderate to Severe Traumatic Brain Injury Along the Healthcare Continuum

OCTAVIO A. SANTOS, PHD • JUSTIN J.F. O'ROURKE, PHD, ABPP-CN •
EDAN A. CRITCHFIELD, PSYD, ABPP-CN • JASON R. SOBLE, PHD, ABPP-CN

INTRODUCTION

Providing care for patients with moderate to severe traumatic brain injury (TBI) along the continuum of recovery can be challenging, as patients move from one level of care to another and present with a variety of cognitive impairments that require treatment.[1,2] Cognitive impairment can significantly interfere with day-to-day functioning, including basic activities of daily living (e.g., eating, toileting, bathing, dressing) and/or instrumental activities of daily living (IADLs) (e.g., cleaning, cooking, laundering, shopping), relationships, employment, community participation, and recreation.[3] To minimize the impact of cognitive impairment on daily functioning, treatment usually involves evidence-based interventions that fall into two broad categories: pharmacotherapy (see Chapter 11 for a review of pharmacotherapy) and cognitive rehabilitation. The aim of this chapter is to briefly summarize evidence-based practices in cognitive rehabilitation to improve social functioning, communication, behavior, and academic/vocational performance,[4] with the ultimate goal of enhancing quality of life,[3,5] maximizing cognitive recovery, and reducing functional disability after TBI.[3,6–8]

Treatment plans almost universally include cognitive rehabilitation immediately following moderate to severe TBI given the ubiquitous nature of cognitive impairment from primary and secondary brain injuries following trauma. Ideally, an interdisciplinary treatment team provides cognitive rehabilitation by integrating rehabilitation techniques across multiple disciplines to form a treatment milieu.[9,10] In this context, clinical neuropsychologists are particularly well suited to assist with (1) cognitive rehabilitation across the continuum of recovery by determining the presence, cause, and extent of cognitive impairment after TBI; (2) elucidating and managing emotional/behavioral symptoms; and (3) making treatment recommendations based on objective findings.[5,9,11,12] For these reasons, the remainder of this chapter is written from the perspective of a neuropsychologist; however, it is important to note that the success of cognitive rehabilitation depends on the contributions of multiple disciplines (i.e., physiatrist, neuropsychology, occupational therapy, speech pathology, rehabilitation psychology, recreational therapy, physical therapy). As patients progress through the acute, postacute, and chronic phases of recovery, cognitive rehabilitation assessment and treatment approaches are modified accordingly to meet the unique needs of each patient.

ACUTE TRAUMATIC BRAIN INJURY REHABILITATION: DISORDERS OF CONSCIOUSNESS AND BEHAVIORAL MANAGEMENT

Acute TBI involves the actual injury to the brain and any ensuing secondary neurochemical processes or complications (e.g., increased intracranial pressure, ischemia/hypoxia, disrupted glucose utilization, excitotoxicity, inflammation), resulting in additional cellular/tissue dysfunction or death, which adversely affects functional outcomes.[13,14] Following initial medical stabilization, individuals with greater TBI severity are prone to disorders of consciousness classified as coma, unresponsive wakefulness (formerly "vegetative state"), or minimally conscious state (MCS; see Chapter 14 for detailed explanation of these disorders).[15] Posttraumatic amnesia (PTA; i.e., inability to store consistent day-to-day memories) is also a common confusional state following moderate to severe TBI.[16,17]

Several prognostic indicators in acute TBI have been identified,[18-23] such as injury type/severity, neuroimaging findings, Glasgow Coma Scale[24] scores, length of loss of consciousness, and length/severity of PTA. Neuropsychologic assessment in acute TBI is often limited by patients' presenting medical problems and may not be clinically indicated or even possible.[25] In cases in which a patient is experiencing a disorder of consciousness or PTA, evaluation may initially consist of ongoing, serial bedside assessment of orientation and mental status. The Coma Recovery Scale-Revised[26] and the Orientation Log[27] (O-Log) are commonly used measures to evaluate the level of consciousness, assist with differential diagnosis (e.g., unresponsive wakefulness vs. MCS), track patient status, monitor for resolution of PTA, elucidate eventual prognosis, and carry out early treatment planning.[28]

Using the results of assessment data, cognitive rehabilitation plans can be developed to engage in specific interventions with patients and families,[29] and these cognitive interventions may range from specific techniques, such as errorless learning and spaced retrieval, to simple reorientation to time, place, and situation. Interventions can also be behavioral in nature. Disorientation, agitation, and aggression are common neuropsychiatric disturbances following TBI that can be addressed through nonpharmacologic management, such as behavioral modification techniques, reduced environmental stimulation,[10,30,31] and serial monitoring of behavioral agitation (e.g., Agitated Behavior Scale[32]). Concurrent with patient-focused interventions, neuropsychologists frequently provide ongoing education to families on common cognitive/behavioral symptoms following TBI and typical recovery trajectories for long-term planning purposes.[25]

POSTACUTE TRAUMATIC BRAIN INJURY: FROM A DISORDER OF CONSCIOUSNESS TO A DISORDER OF COGNITION

Patients with moderate to severe TBI begin to exhibit specific cognitive impairment beyond confusion and amnesia after the resolution of PTA. Persisting neurocognitive deficits often include impairments in executive functioning, attention, self-awareness, and declarative memory.[33,34] Symptom presentation and course of cognitive recovery vary widely across patients because of injury characteristics and premorbid individual differences. The effects of primary injury on the brain (e.g., acceleration-deceleration and rotational forces, lesion location), secondary injuries and conditions (e.g., increased intracranial pressure, hypoxia,

hydrocephalus), premorbid characteristics (e.g., prior head injury, educational attainment, substance use, psychiatric conditions, personality), and the availability of acute interventions all affect symptom presentation and recovery course.[35]

Neuropsychologic Assessment of Neurocognitive Disorders

In a rehabilitation setting, within the limitations of the patient, performing elements of the neuropsychologic evaluation allows providers to objectively quantify neurocognitive deficits after TBI, assist with identification of the cause and differential diagnosis, and develop individualized cognitive rehabilitation plans. Compared with other disciplines, the neuropsychologic evaluation takes into account medical, psychiatric, neurologic, and psychosocial factors that affect functioning.[36-43] A typical neuropsychologic assessment consists of a comprehensive clinical interview, examinations of basic sensory and motor functioning, and administration of psychometric test developed to measure specific cognitive domains (i.e., processing speed, attention/concentration, memory/learning, and executive functions) and psychologic functioning (i.e., mood, personality).[44,45]

Interdisciplinary teams use neuropsychologic assessment to differentiate the effects of neurologic damage from TBI and of secondary conditions (e.g., chronic pain, disrupted sleep, substance abuse, current or premorbid psychiatric disorders).[25] Assessment allows rehabilitation professionals to tailor effective treatments to each patient's unique symptom presentation, by characterizing specific cognitive/behavioral impairments and attributing deficits to their proper causes. In addition to assisting rehabilitation professionals, neuropsychologic assessment directly benefits the patient and their family by (1) providing a basis for developing deficit awareness, (2) determining if there has been a true cognitive change, (3) identifying areas of cognitive strength that can be relied upon in treatment, (4) reducing ambiguity about their condition, and (5) providing guidance for the next steps in treatment.[46] Although there are no guidelines for when to conduct full neuropsychologic evaluation, it is typical to conduct neuropsychologic evaluations soon after the resolution of PTA and again approximately 1 year after injury. However, it is common to have several evaluations completed within the year after injury if there are specific questions that need to be addressed. For example, toward the end of acute rehabilitation, neuropsychologic assessment is useful for determining patients' decision-making capacity, ability to return to work, and required levels of supervision upon discharge.[45]

Repeat neuropsychologic evaluation can then be used to monitor recovery and determine the efficacy of interventions.[4,11,47]

Interventions for Neurocognitive Disorders in Postacute Care

As previously indicated, individualized cognitive rehabilitation plans can be developed once specific cognitive/behavioral deficits have been identified via neuropsychologic assessment (or other clinical methods) for intervention. In this context, rehabilitation methods fall on a continuum between deficit-focused approaches and holistic methods.[48] Professionals who lean toward deficit-focused methods engage in treatment by identifying well-defined, quantifiable behaviors without attending to factors that are not directly related to the specific behavior in question (e.g., correcting impulsive behaviors through behavioral modification without attempting to foster insight into the behaviors themselves). Holistic approaches exist on the opposite end of the continuum and focus on the therapeutic milieu (e.g., a supportive and integrated multidisciplinary environment).[9] In holistic rehabilitation, the therapeutic milieu provides a protected environment for patients to reengage in daily activities and social interaction, where failures can be controlled and targets for further intervention can be observed. Interventions in holistic approaches usually include cognitive rehabilitation, individual or group psychologic services, protected work trials, community outings, physical and occupational therapy, and medical management.[36,49,50]

Within each approach to cognitive rehabilitation (i.e., deficit-focused vs. holistic), specific interventions tend to fall into one of three categories: restorative, compensatory, or metacognitive techniques.[51] Of these, restorative and metacognitive strategies are used most frequently in postacute rehabilitation. Compensatory strategies are discussed later (in Late Traumatic Brain Injury Rehabilitation: Outcomes, Interventions, and Extended Care section). Restorative interventions are those that attempt to reestablish functioning within a cognitive domain through the use of drills and exercises for specific deficits.[52,53] Although research has indicated that many restorative interventions have limited benefits,[6] the following have been shown to promote recovery: errorless learning,[54] spaced retrieval,[55] constraint-induced therapy for aphasia,[56] visuospatial training for patients with neglect,[6] and attention process training (APT).[57] Metacognitive training consists of teaching behaviors that facilitate information processing (i.e., "think about their thinking") through the use of specific strategies, such as self-monitoring/self-instruction, strategy training, goal attainment/management, time-pressure management, and problem solving.[52] Common metacognitive training strategies include self-pacing and frequently checking work for errors, working on one task at a time, taking regular breaks to refocus attention, and working in a quiet environment with minimal noise/interruptions.[7,12,36,37,49,58-61] Regardless of the clinician's emphasis on restorative or metacognitive techniques, research has supported the use of cognitive rehabilitation for maximizing overall cognitive functioning following TBI[6-8] and has indicated that involvement from the entire rehabilitation team leads to improved outcomes.[3,9,50]

Assessment and Intervention of Impaired Self-Awareness

As patients enter the postacute recovery phase, many will have difficulty accurately recognizing and appreciating changes in their level of functioning,[42] particularly for more subtle cognitive or emotional impairments compared with deficit(s)-producing physical limitations (e.g., hemiparesis).[62] Deficits in awareness (i.e., anosognosia) may be global or specific (i.e., affecting aspects of cognitive, physical, social, and/or emotional functioning) and are conceptualized in three levels: (1) *intellectual awareness* involves basic understanding that a function is impaired (e.g., patient parrots having "memory problems" and is unable to provide examples or show appreciation of deficit[s]); (2) *emergent awareness* requires not only the ability to understand and appreciate specific deficit(s) (i.e., intellectual awareness) but also to identify in the moment when this problem is occurring; and (3) *anticipatory awareness* requires both intellectual and emergent awareness as well as the anticipation that a problem will occur in certain situations given the presence of specific deficit(s).[63]

A method for assessing self-awareness includes a formal comparison between a patient's self-reported level of functioning and objective test data or report from others (e.g., family members, caregivers, rehabilitation professionals) who can provide a more accurate assessment of functioning. Another approach to measuring awareness includes comparing a patient's predicted performance on a task (e.g., climbing a flight of stairs, grocery shopping, setting up a pillbox) to their actual level of performance. From a rehabilitation perspective, increasing self-awareness is important, as patients who are able to more accurately perceive their deficits have demonstrated better participation in rehabilitation; increased utilization of compensatory strategies and functional ability postdischarge; and higher rates of employment.[64,65] However, improved self-awareness can also bring about an increase in psychiatric symptoms (e.g., adjustment, depression, anxiety, anger, and interpersonal/relationship problems).[66]

Interventions for impaired self-awareness can be developed parallel to Crosson and colleagues'[63] conceptualization of intellectual, emergent, and anticipatory levels of awareness discussed earlier. For example, intellectual awareness can be addressed through education on common sequelae of moderate to severe TBI and the patient's specific deficits. The effectiveness of this intervention often can be increased by presenting the patients with discrepancies between their perceived level of functioning and those reported by others in frequent contact with the patients.[67] Emergent awareness can be improved by providing feedback when patients struggle performing a task given their deficits and/or by using videotaped sessions of such performance difficulties to support others' feedback.[68] Finally, predictive awareness can be addressed through rehabilitation exercises that utilize a "goal, plan, do, review" format in which patients establish a goal and then plan out the steps needed to reach it, while keeping in mind how their strengths and weaknesses will impact performance. Patients then complete the planned steps to reach their goal and review how their performance matched their expectations. Ideally, as the anticipatory awareness improves, patients will incorporate "lessons learned" into their plans in subsequent sessions.[69]

LATE TRAUMATIC BRAIN INJURY REHABILITATION: OUTCOMES, INTERVENTIONS, AND EXTENDED CARE

Patients generally show most rapid improvement in the first 6–12 months after moderate to severe TBI once medically stabilized, although additional recovery can occur for up to 36 months or longer, often with persistent functional limitations. Many factors predict the likelihood of ongoing cognitive and functional deficits, including length of coma, length of PTA, lesion depth on imaging, TBI severity, and age.[70–74] Cognitive impairment that persists for more than 3 months is linked to greater likelihood of disability.[75] Even though a patient may have a number of risk factors for persisting cognitive deficits, cognitive rehabilitation may still be beneficial. For example, despite slower recovery rates and longer hospital stays, most older adult patients undergoing rehabilitation are found to achieve functional improvement and community reintegration.[76] In addition to residual cognitive deficits from trauma,

moderate to severe TBI has been shown to increase the risk for neurodegenerative diseases in later life.[77–79]

Cognitive and Behavioral Interventions in Late Traumatic Brain Injury Rehabilitation

After the post-acute TBI phase, comprehensive interdisciplinary outpatient rehabilitation services provide individualized, coordinated, and outcome-focused interventions designed for patients who are able to reside in the community, but still need treatment to meet their ultimate goals.[4,49,80–84] The care plan should be developed in collaboration with the patient and caregivers to establish goals for improving physical, cognitive, and vocational functioning to maximize independence and community reintegration.[4,49,59] Regular follow-up for patients with ongoing rehabilitation needs is also frequently necessary.[4,36,38,49]

Cognitive rehabilitation interventions in outpatient rehabilitation services may include modeling, guided practice, distributed practice, direct instruction with feedback, paper-and-pencil tasks, communication skills, computer-assisted retraining programs, and use of memory aids.[6,7,38,49,58,60,61,85,86] Effective compensatory strategies need to be (1) individualized to the patient and his or her work setting; (2) well defined, goal directed, practiced repeatedly, and adjusted by professionals/caregivers for maximal effectiveness as the patient improves; and, (3) measurable in a way that can be monitored by the patient.[6,36,38,49,61,85] Cognitive rehabilitation interventions can be provided on a one-on-one basis or in a small group setting,[36,39,49,58,61] and, in most cases, the goal of remediation should not be limited to training a task-specific performance, but rather the training and internalization of regulatory cognitive processes.[36,58,80,81,85,87]

Similar to the postacute phase of recovery, practice standards in cognitive rehabilitation in late recovery include direct attention training (DAT) and metacognitive training,[8,88,89] as well as specific strategies and compensatory techniques for deficits in memory,[8,89] executive functions,[8,90] and pragmatic communication/conversational skills.[89,91] Rooted in the concept of neuroplasticity, DAT involves repeated stimulation of attention to strengthen the underlying neural processes. In DAT, exercises are organized hierarchically according to theoretically grounded models of attention and require sufficient repetition to ensure generalization of gains achieved in cognitive rehabilitation.[6,7,49,85,88,92] An example of DAT is APT in which five attentional components (i.e., focused, sustained, selective, alternating, and divided attentions) are targeted,[11] showing significant improvements in complex attention in patients with TBI[57,93] (metacognitive training is discussed in Postacute Traumatic Brain Injury: From a Disorder of Consciousness to a Disorder of Cognition section).

Strategy training in memory rehabilitation targets (sequences of) behaviors that facilitate information processing, retention, and retrieval (e.g., rehearsal, self-questioning, mnemonics), by providing alternative ways of learning.[11,36,39,49,58,61,89] Such memory strategies require adaptation to the patient's needs, systematic training, and evaluation/modification based on the patient's level of success and acceptance. Compensatory techniques may include training in the use of memory aids (e.g., timers, pocket computers, personal organizers, digital recorders) with direct application to functional activities.[8,11,53,89,90] Importantly, devices should be prescribed based on an individualized needs assessment followed by identification of a device(s) that matches the patient's deficits, along with provision of necessary training to ensure their success and consistent use.[4] Demonstrated benefits of memory aids include support for completion of functional activities, flexibility of treatment options, and high consumer acceptance.[6,7,58]

Considered a major contributor to social isolation after TBI, impairment in social communication co-occurs with cognitive/personality changes and is affected by premorbid/environmental factors, such as prior mental health history, education, prior occupation, patterns of relating, and personality characteristics. Therefore effective treatments for social communication address new deficits and problematic interpersonal patterns that existed before injury. Interventions directed at improving pragmatic communication/conversational skills may include active listening skills, group therapy, family therapy, videotaped interactions, modeling and rehearsal, and training of self-monitoring strategies.[7,36,58–61,85,86,94]

Caregiver's Role in Cognitive/Behavioral Interventions

Since family members often assume care and support intervention applications as patients transition through TBI recovery phases, patients' successful reintegration into the family structure is essential to maximize the quality of life and independence.[95] Given that behavioral/personality changes following TBI (e.g., forgetfulness, poor organization/planning, sleep disturbance, irritability) can persist and be especially distressing for families, it is necessary to provide families/caregivers with recommendations on environmental/routine modifications and implementation of compensatory strategies to improve daily functioning, foster independence, and

alleviate caregiver stress.[3,8,96,97] For example, reducing distractions/clutter at home helps the patient's focus on relevant information. Caregivers can also play an instrumental role in encouraging patients to use a memory notebook to keep track of daily activities and adhere to a sleep hygiene plan. Although irritability may be a symptom of TBI (e.g., lowered frustration tolerance, disturbed sleep, confusion), caregivers should set boundaries with patients, ignore inappropriate/disruptive behaviors, and avoid escalating stressful situations.[4,61,98] Severe and persistent behavioral/personality problems may require admission to a specialized neurobehavioral program involving behavior modification, medication management, social skills training, substance abuse treatment, family therapy, and physical management.[36,61,81,82,99] The ability of families to meet patients' needs is determined by several factors, including social support, investment in providing support, financial resources, and competing family responsibilities (e.g., child rearing, careers).[4,12] Due to the impact of TBI on family members and the significant variability in their ability to cope and accept new roles,[45,82,100–102] rehabilitation professionals should be aware of the common sequelae of TBI; address family concerns about recovery/prognosis; encourage caregivers to get adequate rest, nutrition, exercise, and relaxation; and provide relevant psychologic intervention as described later.[4,36,103,104]

Community Reintegration and Extended Care

Community participation has been shown to promote patients' continued gains in functional recovery and quality of life as well as to reduce caregiver stress[39,49,105–107]; however, patients may fail to reintegrate into their communities without interventions to facilitate skills development. Therefore referral to a specialty team may be needed for evaluation and recommendations regarding community access (i.e., driving, transportation), vocational/recreational activities, safety, independent living skills, social networks, health/wellness, and individual/caregiver supports[4,81,83,104,108] (see Chapter 18 for further information on community reintegration).

Assessment of driving ability is vital for every patients with moderate to severe TBI, because physical, cognitive, and neurobehavioral changes after TBI often affect the ability to drive safely.[6,49,105] A driver rehabilitation program consists of a multifaceted approach that involves an assessment of the cognitive abilities necessary to drive (e.g., processing speed, complex divided attention), vision examination, predriving/behind-the-wheel assessment, education, and training considering the patient's characteristics. A road test conducted by a professional driving instructor or other certified occupational therapist is considered the gold standard for determining driving safety.[109,110]

Vocational rehabilitation helps patients to achieve greater living independence and integration within their workplace, family/relationships, and community through work evaluation, job counseling, education, and training.[36,39,61,83,103,105,111] Similarly, recreation therapy uses activity-based interventions requiring development, strengthening, and maintenance of physical and cognitive skills transferable to "real-world" experiences. Such interventions aim to promote community participation, life satisfaction, and overall health/well-being, especially for patients unable to resume work. Recreation therapy also has the added benefit of identifying useful rewards to use for reinforcing desired behaviors.[4,59,81]

Extended care services aim to maintain patients' maximum level of independence in the least restrictive setting and are sometimes recommended depending on patients'/caregivers' needs.[4,87] Among these services, home-based primary care provides interdisciplinary services for patients with complex chronic disabling conditions to addresses their medical, functional, social, and behavioral needs, including facilitation of structural home adaptations and training to patients and caregivers.[49,83,87,104,112] Homemaker/home health aide services are provided to assist patients with basic activities of daily living and/or IADLs.[4,83] Respite care provides temporary relief from routine caregiving tasks, whereas adult day healthcare is an individualized day program to help patients and caregivers develop the necessary knowledge/skills to manage home care requirements.[4,36,38,83] Community Residential Care (CRC) provides healthcare supervision for patients without families with significant medical, psychiatric, and psychosocial limitations to living independently. Examples of CRC include medical foster homes, assisted/group living homes, family care homes, and some psychiatric homes.[4] Additionally, patients and caregivers may require assistance with nonmedical issues (e.g., guardianship, fiduciary, representative payee, and advanced directives) and may benefit from further assistance from applicable local community agencies (e.g., adult protective services, department of family services).[4,36,59,83,103]

Cultural Diversity Considerations in Traumatic Brain Injury Rehabilitation

Culture influences not only the patient's symptom presentation, perception of illness and disability, expect

ation for recovery, use of rehabilitation services, and potential for improvement but also the clinician's response to the patient/caregiver.[113,114] Community reintegration is also affected by the cultural environment to which the patient wishes to return. Use of a culturally appropriate clinical approach tailored to the patient's needs is necessary for optimal engagement in rehabilitation to maximize outcomes and reduce health disparities.[106] Gaining a sense of trust is important in developing a relationship with patients,[115] and an awareness of patients' worldview and cultural differences in family dynamics facilitates a strong therapeutic alliance. Assessment of cognitive deficits and cognitive rehabilitation in culturally and linguistically diverse individuals should also consider the patient's socioeconomic status, quality of education, and acculturation on test data and interpretation to avoid mischaracterizing cultural differences as cognitive impairment.[116,117] In clinical practice, there is great potential for the development of culturally and linguistically adapted education programs, and future research is greatly needed to better understand cultural factors and their interaction with the patient, clinician, and environment to affect outcomes in rehabilitation from TBI.[106]

CONCLUSIONS

Patients with moderate to severe TBI and their caregivers often face challenges as they transition through the continuum of care, presenting with various complaints related to cognitive impairment requiring treatment. Evidence-based cognitive rehabilitation has been shown to be effective in managing neurocognitive deficits affecting psychosocial functioning. This chapter summarized cognitive rehabilitation practices in moderate to severe TBI, considering acute, postacute, and late rehabilitation phases as well as highlighting neuropsychologic assessment as a comprehensive method to (1) characterize cognitive impairment after resolution of PTA; (2) assist with the differential diagnosis, treatment planning, and monitoring recovery; and (3) determine the efficacy of interventions. Conceptual approaches to cognitive rehabilitation, such as restorative, compensatory, or metacognitive interventions, are often used during the postacute and late TBI rehabilitation phases, some of which have consistently proven increased cognitive outcomes. Assessing and treating self-awareness deficits becomes important for experiencing further gains from cognitive rehabilitation. Family members and caregivers play an instrumental role in the patient's rehabilitation, and require support from healthcare professionals to implement cognitive rehabilitation recommendations and avoid burnout. Thoughtful considerations to diversity variables are necessary to engage both patients and caregivers in rehabilitation to maximize outcomes, facilitate community reintegration, and reduce health disparities. Finally, given the fact that patients may experience persistent neurobehavioral and/or physical problems, extended care services are likely necessary for assuring maximum level of independence and adequate treatment.

REFERENCES

1. Katz DI, Zasler ND, Zafonte RD. Clinical continuum of care and natural history. In: *Brain Injury Medicine: Principles and Practice*. New York, NY: Demos Medical Publishing; 2007:3–13.
2. Murphy MP, Carmine H. Long-term health implications of individuals with TBI: a rehabilitation perspective. *Neurorehabilitation*. 2012;31(1):85–94. https://doi.org/10.3233/NRE-2012-0777.
3. Barman A, Chatterjee A, Bhide R. Cognitive impairment and rehabilitation strategies after traumatic brain injury. *Indian J Psychol Med*. 2016;38(3):172–181. https://doi.org/10.4103/0253-7176.183086.
4. Benedict SM, Belanger HG, Ceperich SD, et al. Veterans health initiative. In: Vanderploeg RD, Cornis-Pop M, eds. *Traumatic Brain Injury: Independent Study Course*. Washington, DC: Department of Veterans Affairs Employee Education System; 2010.
5. Dawson DR, Marcotte TD. Special issue on ecological validity and cognitive assessment. *Neuropsychol Rehabil*. 2017;27(5):599–602. https://doi.org/10.1080/09602011.2017.1313379.
6. Rohling ML, Faust ME, Beverly B, Demakis G. Effectiveness of cognitive rehabilitation following acquired brain injury: a meta- analytic re-examination of Cicerone et al.'s (2000, 2005) systematic reviews. *Neuropsychology*. 2009;23(1):20–39. https://doi.org/10.1037/a0013659.
7. Cicerone KD, Langenbahn DM, Braden C, et al. Evidence-based cognitive rehabilitation: updated review of the literature from 2003 through 2008. *Arch Phys Med Rehabil*. 2011;92(4):519–530. https://doi.org/10.1016/j.apmr.2010.11.015.
8. Cicerone KD, Dahlberg C, Malec JF, et al. Evidence-based cognitive rehabilitation: updated review of the literature from 1998 through 2002. *Arch Phys Med Rehabil*. 2005;86(8):1681–1692. https://doi.org/10.1016/j.apmr.2005.03.024.
9. Prigatano GP. *Principles of Neuropsychological Rehabilitation*. New York, NY: Oxford University Press; 1999.
10. Prigatano GP, Borgaro S, Caples H. Non-pharmacological management of psychiatric disturbances after traumatic brain injury. *Int Rev Psychiatr*. 2003;15:371–379. https://doi.org/10.1080/09540260310001606755.
11. Tsaousides T, Gordon WA. Cognitive rehabilitation following traumatic brain injury: assessment to treatment. *Mt Sinai J Med*. 2009;76(2):173–181. https://doi.org/10.1002/msj.20099.
12. D'Amato RC, Hartlage LCLC. Essentials of neuropsychological assessment: treatment planning for rehabilitation. *Neuropsychol Rehabil*. 2008:3-5.
13. Algattas H, Huang JH. Traumatic brain injury pathophysiology and treatments: early, intermediate, and late phases post-injury. *Int J Mol Sci*. 2013;15(1):309–341. https://doi.org/10.3390/ijms15010309.
14. Stocchetti N, Taccone FS, Citerio G, et al. Neuroprotection in acute brain injury: an up-to-date review. *Crit Care*. 2015;19(1):186. https://doi.org/10.1186/s13054-015-0887-8.
15. Giacino J, Whyte J, Zafonte RD, et al. The minimally conscious state definition and diagnostic criteria. *Neurology*. 2002;58(3):349–353. https://doi.org/10.1212/WNL.58.3.349.
16. Russell WR. Cerebral involvement in head injury: a study based on the examination of two hundred cases. *Brain*. 1932;55(4):549–603. https://doi.org/10.1093/brain/55.4.549.
17. Russell WR, Nathan PW. Traumatic amnesia. *Brain*. 1946;69(4):280–300. https://doi.org/10.1093/brain/69.4.280.
18. Dikmen SS, Corrigan JD, Levin HS, Machamer J, Stiers W, Weisskopf MG. Cognitive outcome following traumatic brain injury. *J Head Trauma Rehabil*. 2009;24(6):430–438. https://doi.org/10.1097/HTR.0b013e3181c133e9.
19. Lingsma HF, Roozenbeek B, Steyerberg EW, Murray GD, Maas AI. Early prognosis in traumatic brain injury: from prophecies to predictions. *Lancet Neurol*. 2010;9(5):543–554. https://doi.org/10.1016/S1474-4422(10)70065-X.
20. Maas AIR, Steyerberg EW, Butcher I, et al. Prognostic value of computerized tomography scan characteristics in traumatic brain injury: results from the IMPACT study. *J Neurotrauma*. 2007;24(2):303–314. https://doi.org/10.1089/neu.2006.0033.
21. Nakase-Richardson R, Sherer M, Seel RT, et al. Utility of post-traumatic amnesia in predicting 1-year productivity following traumatic brain injury: comparison of the Russell and Mississippi PTA classification intervals. *J Neurol Neurosurg Psychiatr*. 2011;82(5):494–499. https://doi.org/10.1136/jnnp.2010.222489.
22. Nakase-Richardson R, Yablon SA, Sherer M. Prospective comparison of acute confusion severity with duration of post-traumatic amnesia in predicting employment outcome after traumatic brain injury. *J Neurol Neurosurg Psychiatr*. 2007;78(8):872–876. https://doi.org/10.1136/jnnp.2006.104190.
23. Nakase-Richardson R, Sepehri A, Sherer M, Yablon SA, Evans C, Mani T. Classification schema of posttraumatic amnesia duration-based injury severity relative to 1-year outcome: analysis of individuals with moderate and severe traumatic brain injury. *Arch Phys Med Rehabil*. 2009;90(1):17–19. https://doi.org/10.1016/j.apmr.2008.06.030.

24. Teasdale G, Jennett B. Assessment of coma and impaired consciousness. A practical scale. *Lancet (London, England)*. 1974;2(7872):81–84.

25. Soble JR, Critchfield EA, O'Rourke JJF. Neuropsychological evaluation in traumatic brain injury. [Special issue] *Phys Med Rehabil Clin North Am*. 2017;28:339–350. https://doi.org/10.1016/j.pmr.2016.12.009.

26. Giacino JT, Kalmar K, Whyte J. The JFK coma recovery scale-revised: measurement characteristics and diagnostic utility. *Arch Phys Med Rehabil*. 2004;85(12):2020–2029. https://doi.org/10.1016/j.apmr.2004.02.033.

27. The Center for Outcome Measurement in Brain Injury. *The Orientation Log*. http://www.tbims.org/combi/olog/.

28. Arciniegas DB, McAllister TW. Neurobehavioral management of traumatic brain injury in the critical care setting. *Crit Care Clin*. 2008;24(4):737–765. https://doi.org/10.1016/j.ccc.2008.06.001.

29. Wilson B, Mateer SO. *Cognitive Rehabilitation, an Integrative Neuropsychological Approach*. vol. 72. 2002. https://doi.org/10.1136/jnnp.72.3.421-a.

30. Lombard LA, Zafonte RD. Agitation after traumatic brain injury. *Am J Phys Med Rehabil*. 2005;84(10):797–812. https://doi.org/10.1097/01.phm.0000179438.22235.08.

31. McAllister TW. Neurobehavioral sequelae of traumatic brain injury: evaluation and management. *World Psychiatr*. 2008;76(2):163–172. https://doi.org/10.1002/msj.20097.

32. Bogner JA, Corrigan JD, Stange M, Rabold D. Reliability of the agitated behavior scale. *J Head Trauma Rehabil*. 1999;14(1):91–96.

33. Roebuck-Spencer T, Sherer M. Moderate and severe traumatic brain injury. In: *Textbook of Clinical Neuropsychology*. New York, NY: Psychology Press; 2008:411–436.

34. Arciniegas DBD, Held K, Wagner P. Cognitive impairment following traumatic brain injury. *Curr Treat Options Neurol*. 2002;4(1):43–57. https://doi.org/10.1007/s11940-002-0004-6.

35. Larrabee GJ. *Forensic Neuropsychology: A Scientific Approach*. 2nd ed. New York, NY: Oxford University Press; 2011.

36. Wilson B, Gracey F, Evans JJ, Bateman A. *Neuropsychological Rehabilitation: Theory, Models, Therapy and Outcome*; 2010.

37. Armstrong CL, Morrow L. *Handbook of Medical Neuropsychology: Applications of Cognitive Neuroscience*; 2010:1–564. https://doi.org/10.1007/978-1-4419-1364-7.

38. Wilson BA. Theoretical approaches to cognitive rehabilitation. In: *Clinical Neuropsychology: A Practical Guide to Assessment and Management for Clinicians*. 2004:345–365.

39. Champion AJ. *Neuropsychological Rehabilitation: A Resource for Group-Based Education and Intervention*; 2006.

40. Bennett TL, Raymond MJ. The neuropsychology of traumatic brain injury. In: *Neuropsychol Handb*. 2008:533–570.

41. Richards PM, Kirk JW. Traumatic brain injury across the lifespan: a neuropsychological tutorial for attorneys. *Psychol Inj L*. 2010;3(1):3–24. https://doi.org/10.1007/s12207-010-9065-0.

42. Rabinowitz AR, Levin HS. Cognitive sequelae of traumatic brain injury. *Psychiatr Clin North Am*. 2014;37(1):1–11. https://doi.org/10.1016/j.psc.2013.11.004.

43. Webbe FM. Sports neuropsychology. In: *Neuropsychol Handb*. 3rd ed. 2008:771–800.

44. Scott JG. Components of the neuropsychological evaluation. In: *The Little Black Book of Neuropsychology*. Boston, MA: Springer US; 2011:127–137. https://doi.org/10.1007/978-0-387-76978-3_4.

45. Lezak MD, Howieson D, Bigler ED, Tranel D. *Neuropsychological Assessment*. 5th ed. New York, NY: Oxford University Press; 2012.

46. Gorske TT, Smith SR. *Collaborative Therapeutic Neuropsychological Assessment*. New York, NY: Springer; 2009. https://doi.org/10.1007/978-0-387-75426-0.

47. Perumparaichallai RK, Husk KL, Myles SM, Klonoff PS. The relationship of neuropsychological variables to driving status following holistic neurorehabilitation. *Front Neurol*. 2014;5. https://doi.org/10.3389/fneur.2014.00056.

48. Wilson B. *Case Studies in Neuropsychological Rehabilitation*; 1999.

49. Sherer M, Sander A. *Handbook on the Neuropsychology of Traumatic Brain Injury*; 2014. https://doi.org/10.1007/978-1-4939-0784-7.

50. Cicerone KD, Mott T, Azulay J, et al. A randomized controlled trial of holistic neuropsychologic rehabilitation after traumatic brain injury. *Arch Phys Med Rehabil*. 2008;89(12):2239–2249. https://doi.org/10.1016/j.apmr.2008.06.017.

51. Eapen B, Allred D, O'Rourke J, Cifu D. Rehabilitation of moderate-to-severe traumatic brain injury. *Semin Neurol*. 2015;35(1):e1–e13. https://doi.org/10.1055/s-0035-1549094.

52. Sohlberg M, Turkstra L. *Optimizing Cognitive Rehabilitation: Effective Instructional Methods*. New York, NY: The Guilford Press; 2011.

53. Koehler R, Wilhelm EE, Shoulson I, Institute of Medicine (U.S.). Committee on Cognitive Rehabilitation Therapy for Traumatic Brain Injury. *Cognitive Rehabilitation Therapy for Traumatic Brain Injury: Evaluating the Evidence*. New York, NY: National Academies Press; 2012.

54. Wilson BA, Baddeley A, Evans J, Shiel A. Errorless learning in the rehabilitation of memory impaired people. *Neuropsychol Rehabil*. 1994;4(3):307–326. https://doi.org/10.1080/09602019408401463.

55. Schacter DL, Rich SA, Stampp MS. Remediation of memory disorders: experimental evaluation of the spaced-retrieval technique. *J Clin Exp Neuropsychol*. 1985;7(1):79–96. https://doi.org/10.1080/01688638508401243.

56. Meinzer M, Djundja D, Barthel G, Elbert T, Rockstroh B. Long-term stability of improved language functions in chronic aphasia after constraint-induced aphasia therapy. *Stroke*. 2005;36(7):1462–1466. https://doi.org/10.1161/01.STR.0000169941.29831.2a.

57. Moore Sohlberg M, McLaughlin KA, Pavese A, Heidrich A, Posner MI. Evaluation of attention process training and brain injury education in persons with acquired brain injury. *J Clin Exp Neuropsychol.* 2000;22(5):656–676. https://doi.org/10.1076/1380-3395(200010)22:5;1-9; FT656.

58. Pella RD, Kendra K, Hill BD, Gouvier WD. Cognitive rehabilitation with brain-damaged patents. In: *Neuropsychol Handb.* 2008:419–467.

59. Duchnick JJ, Ropacki S, Yutsis M, Petska K, Pawlowski C. Polytrauma transitional rehabilitation programs: comprehensive rehabilitation for community integration after brain injury. *Psychol Serv.* 2015;12(3):313–321. https://doi.org/10.1037/ser0000034.

60. Levin H, Shum D, Chan R. *Understanding Traumatic Brain Injury: Current Research and Future Directions*; 2014.

61. Sohlberg MM, Mateer CA. *Cognitive Rehabilitation: An Integrative Neuropsychological Approach.* New York, NY: The Guilford Press; 2001.

62. Sherer M, Boake C, Levin E, Silver BV, Ringholz G, High WM. Characteristics of impaired self-awareness after traumatic brain injury. *J Int Neuropsychol Soc.* 1998;4:380–387.

63. Crosson B, Barco PP, Velozo CA, et al. Awareness and compensation in postacute head injury rehabilitation. *J Head Trauma Rehabil.* 1989;4(3):46–54. https://doi.org/10.1097/00001199-198909000-00008.

64. Fischer S, Gauggel S, Trexler LE. Awareness of activity limitations, goal setting and rehabilitation out come in patients with brain injuries. *Brain Inj.* 2004;18(6):547–562. https://doi.org/10.1080/0269905031 0001645793.

65. Sherer M, Bergloff P, Levin E, High W, Oden K, Nick TG. Impaired awareness and employment outcome after traumatic brain injury. *J Head Trauma Rehabil.* 1998;13(5):52–61. https://doi.org/10.1097/00001199-199810000-00007.

66. Malec JF, Testa JA, Rush BK, Brown AW, Moessner AM. Self-assessment of impairment, impaired self-awareness, and depression after traumatic brain injury. *J Head Trauma Rehabil.* 2007;22(3):156–166. https://doi.org/10.1097/01.HTR.0000271116.12028.af.

67. Schmidt J, Lannin N, Fleming J, Ownsworth T. Feedback interventions for impaired self-awareness following brain injury: a systematic review. *J Rehabil Med.* 2011;43(8):673–680. https://doi.org/10.2340/16501977-0846.

68. Meeter M, Murre JMJ, Janssen SMJ, Birkenhager T, Van Den Broek WW. Retrograde amnesia after electroconvulsive therapy: a temporary effect? *J Affect Disord.* 2011;132(1–2):216–222. https://doi.org/10.1016/j.jad.2011.02.026.

69. Haskins E, Cicerone K, Dams-O'Connor K, Eberle R, Langenbahn D, Shapiro-Rosenbaum A. *Cognitive Rehabilitation Manual; Translating Evidence-Based Recommendations into Practice.* Reston, VA: American Congress of Rehabilitation Medicine; 2012.

70. Braakman R, Gelpke GJ, Habbema JD, Maas AIR, Minderhoud JM. Systematic selection of prognostic features in patients with severe head injury. *Neurosurgery.* 1980;6(4):362–370.

71. Jennett B, Teasdale GM, Braakman R, Minderhoud J, Heiden J, Kurze T. Prognosis of patients with severe head injury. *Neurosurgery.* 1979;4(4):283–289. https://doi.org/10.1227/00006123-197904000-00001.

72. Stablein DM, Miller JD, Choi SC, Becker DP. Statistical methods for determining prognosis in severe head injury. *Neurosurgery.* 1980;6(3):243–248.

73. Chestnut R, Ghajar J, Maas AI. Management and prognosis of severe traumatic brain injury. Part 2: early indicators of prognosis in severe traumatic brain injury. *J Neurotrauma.* 2000;17:557–627.

74. Raymont V, Greathouse A, Reding K, Lipsky R, Salazar A, Grafman J. Demographic, structural and genetic predictors of late cognitive decline after penetrating head injury. *Brain.* 2008;131(2):543–558. https://doi.org/10.1093/brain/awm300.

75. Skandsen T, Finnanger TG, Andersson S, Lydersen S, Brunner JF, Vik A. Cognitive impairment 3 months after moderate and severe traumatic brain injury: a prospective follow-up study. *Arch Phys Med Rehabil.* 2010;91(12):1904–1913. https://doi.org/10.1016/j.apmr.2010.08.021.

76. Cifu D, Kreutzer JS, Marwitz JH, Rosenthal M, Englander J, High W. Functional outcomes of older adults with traumatic brain injury: a prospective, multicenter analysis. *Arch Phys Med Rehabil.* 1996;77(9):883–888. https://doi.org/10.1016/S0003-9993(96)90274-9.

77. Das M, Mohapatra S, Mohapatra SS. New perspectives on central and peripheral immune responses to acute traumatic brain injury. *J Neuroinflamm.* 2012;9(1):236. https://doi.org/10.1186/1742-2094-9-236.

78. Guo Z, Cupples LA, Kurz A, et al. Head injury and the risk of AD in the MIRAGE study. *Neurology.* 2000;54:1316–1323. https://doi.org/10.1212/WNL.54.6.1316.

79. Nemetz PN, Leibson C, Naessens JM, et al. Traumatic brain injury and time to onset of Alzheimer's disease: a population-based study. *Am J Epidemiol.* 1999;149(1):32–40.

80. Stephens JA, Williamson K-NC, Berryhill ME. Cognitive rehabilitation after traumatic brain injury. *OTJR Occup Particip Heal.* 2015;35(1):5–22. https://doi.org/10.1177/1539449214561765.

81. Pickett TC, Bender MC, Gourley E. Head injury rehabilitation of military members. *Mil Neuropsychol.* 2010:175–198.

82. Collins RC, Kennedy MC. Serving families who have served: providing family therapy and support in interdisciplinary polytrauma rehabilitation. *J Clin Psychol.* 2008;64(8):993–1003. https://doi.org/10.1002/jclp.20515.

83. Zasler ND, Katz DI, Zafonte RD. *Brain Injury Medicine: Principles and Practice.* New York, NY: Demos Medical Publishing; 2013. https://doi.org/10.1097/01.HTR.0000300238.28737.54.

84. Laskowitz D, Grant G. *Translational Research in Traumatic Brain Injury*; 2016:1–11.

85. Cicerone KD, Langenbahn DM, Braden C, et al. Evidence-based cognitive rehabilitation: updated review of the literature from 2003 through 2008. *Arch Phys Med Rehabil*. 2011;92(4):519–530. https://doi.org/10.1016/j.apmr.2010.11.015.

86. Kobeissy FH. *Brain Neurotrauma: Molecular, Neuropsychological, and Rehabilitation Aspects*. New York, NY: CRC Press; 2015. https://doi.org/10.1017/CBO9781107415324.004.

87. Cifu DX, Caruso D, Ebooks C. *Traumatic Brain Injury*; 2010. https://doi.org/10.1097/MCC.0b013e32833190da.

88. Sohlberg MM, Avery J, Kennedy M, et al. Practice guidelines for direct attention training. *J Med Speech Lang Pathol*. 2003;11(3):xix–xxxix. https://doi.org/10.1037/t00741-000.

89. Cicerone KD, Dahlberg C, Kalmar K, et al. Evidence-based cognitive rehabilitation: recommendations for clinical practice. *Arch Phys Med Rehabil*. 2000;81(12):1596–1615. https://doi.org/10.1053/apmr.2000.19240.

90. Sohlberg MM, Kennedy MRT, Avery J, et al. Evidence-based practice for the use of external aids as a memory compensation technique. *J Med Speech Lang Pathol*. 2007;15(1):xv-li.

91. Struchen MA. Social communication interventions. In: High WM, et al., ed. *Rehabilitation for Traumatic Brain Injury*. New York, NY: Oxford Univ. Press; 2005:88–117. https://doi.org/10.1007/978-1-4939-0784-7_11.

92. Greenwald BD, Rigg JL. Neurorehabilitation in traumatic brain injury: does it make a difference? *Mt Sinai J Med*. 2009;76(2):182–189.

93. Sohlberg MM, Mateer CA. Effectiveness of an attention-training program. *J Clin Exp Neuropsychol*. 1987;9(2):117–130. https://doi.org/10.1080/01688638708405352.

94. Vanderploeg RD, Schwab K, Walker WC, et al. Rehabilitation of traumatic brain injury in active duty military personnel and veterans: defense and veterans brain injury center randomized controlled trial of two rehabilitation approaches. *Arch Phys Med Rehabil*. 2008;89(12):2227–2238. https://doi.org/10.1016/j.apmr.2008.06.015.

95. Sander AM, Caroselli JS, High WM, et al. Relationship of family functioning to progress in a post-acute rehabilitation programme following traumatic brain injury. *Brain Inj*. 2002;16:649–657. https://doi.org/10.1080/02699050210128889.

96. Dikmen SS, Machamer JE, Powell JM, Temkin NR. Outcome 3 to 5 years after moderate to severe traumatic brain injury. *Arch Phys Med Rehabil*. 2003;84(3):1449–1457. https://doi.org/10.1053/S0003-9993(03)00287-9.

97. Lew HL, Poole JH, Guillory SB, Salerno RM, Leskin G, Sigford B. Persistent problems after traumatic brain injury: the need for long-term follow-up and coordinated care. *J Rehabil Res Dev*. 2006;43(2):vii–x.

98. Pontón MO, Monguió I. Rehabilitation of brain injury among hispanic patients. In: Pontón MO, León-Carrión J, eds. Neuropsychology and the Hispanic Patient: A Clinical Handbook. Mahwah, NJ: Lawrence Erlbaum; 2001:323-335.

99. Uomoto M, McLean A. Care continuum in traumatic brain injury rehabilitation. *Rehabil Psychol*. 1989;34(2):71–79.

100. Kreutzer JS, Marwitz JH, Kepler K. Traumatic brain injury: family response and outcome. *Arch Phys Med Rehabil*. 1992;73(8):771–778.

101. Sander AM. Predictors of psychological health in caregivers of patients with closed head injury. *Brain Inj*. 1997;11(4):235–249.

102. Kreutzer JS, Gervasio AH, Camplair PS. Patient correlates of caregivers' distress and family functioning after traumatic brain injury. *Brain Inj*. 1994;8(3):211–230. https://doi.org/10.3109/02699059409150974.

103. Newby G, Coetzer R, Daisley A, Weatherhead S. *Practical Neuropsychological Rehabilitation in Acquired Brain Injury: A Guide for Clinicians*. London, UK: Karnac Books Ltd; 2013.

104. Reed J, Byard K, Fine H, eds. *Neuropsychological Rehabilitation of Childhood Brain Injury: A Practical Guide*. London, UK: Palgrave Macmillan; 2015.

105. Lillie RA, Kowalski K, Patry BN, Sira C, Tuokko H, Mateer CA. Everyday impact of traumatic brain injury. In: *Neuropsychology Everyday Functioning*. 2010:302–330.

106. Lequerica A, Krch D. Issues of cultural diversity in acquired brain injury (ABI) rehabilitation. *Neurorehabilitation*. 2014;34(4):645–653. https://doi.org/10.3233/NRE-141079.

107. Inzaghi MG, De Tanti A, Sozzi M. The effects of traumatic brain injury on patients and their families: a follow-up study. *Eura Medicophys*. 2005;41(4):265–273.

108. Murrey GJ, Hale FM, Williams JD. Assessment of anosognosia in persons with frontal lobe damage: clinical utility of the Mayo-Portland Adaptability Inventory (MPAI). *Brain Inj*. 2005;19:599–603. https://doi.org/10.1080/02699050400025257.

109. Schultheis MT, Matheis RJ, Nead R, DeLuca J. Driving behaviors following brain injury: self-report and motor vehicle records. *J Head Trauma Rehabil*. 2002;17(1):38–47. https://doi.org/10.1097/00001199-200202000-00006.

110. Rike P-O, Ulleberg P, Schultheis MT, Lundqvist A, Schanke A-K. Behavioural ratings of self-regulatory mechanisms and driving behaviour after an acquired brain injury. *Brain Inj*. 2014;28:1–13. https://doi.org/10.3109/02699052.2014.947632.

111. Arango-Lasprilla JC. Traumatic brain injury in Spanish-speaking individuals: research findings and clinical implications. *Brain Inj*. 2012;26(6):801–804. https://doi.org/10.3109/02699052.2012.655368.

112. Hoge CW, Goldberg HM, Castro CA. Care of war veterans with mild traumatic brain injury–flawed perspectives. *N Engl J Med*. 2009;360(16):1588–1591. https://doi.org/10.1056/NEJMp0810606.

113. Banja JD. Ethics, values, and world culture: the impact on rehabilitation. *Disabil Rehabil*. 1996;18(6):279–284. https://doi.org/10.3109/09638289609165881.

114. Balcazar FE, Suárez-Balcazar Y, Taylor-Ritzler T, Keys C. *Race, Culture, and Disability Rehabilitation Science and Practice*. Ontario, Canada: Jones and Bartlett Publishers; 2010.

115. Alston RJ. Racial identity and cultural mistrust among African-American recipients of rehabilitation services: an exploratory study. *Int J Rehabil Res.* 2003;26(4):289–295.

116. Kennepohl S, Shore D, Nabors N, Hanks R. African American acculturation and neuropsychological test performance following traumatic brain injury. *J Int Neuropsychol Soc.* 2004;10(4):566–577. https://doi.org/10.1017/S1355617704104128.

117. Gasquoine PG. Race-norming of neuropsychological tests. *Neuropsychol Rev.* 2009;19(2):250–262. https://doi.org/10.1007/s11065-009-9090-5.

CHAPTER 16

Prognosis, Outcome Measures, and Prevention

ANDREW J. GARDNER, PHD • ELIZABETH V. ADAMOVA, DO •
ROSS D. ZAFONTE, DO

PROGNOSIS AND OUTCOME MEASURES

Prognosis is part of the essence of every medical presentation and a fundamental responsibility of all clinicians. It is prognosis, not diagnosis, that provides the legitimate foundation for medical intervention.[1] Predicting a likely recovery from disease or illness, however, remains a common challenge in modern medicine. A complete prognosis is characterized by a number of elements and includes estimations pertaining to the expected duration and the level of function and a description of the course of the illness/disease, such as progressive decline, intermittent crisis or sudden, unpredictable crisis, and partial or full recovery.[2] Therefore a variety of metrics can be applied to the prediction of a prognosis. Developing prognostic guidelines based on research literature is challenging, and healthcare professionals often rely on their own clinical experience in formulating a prognosis.[3,4] A number of studies, however, have demonstrated that a clinician's "subjective" estimation of prognoses is often far less accurate than those derived from well-designed studies.[5-7] Another difficulty is that the clinical approach of applying prognostic group data at an individual level also has limitations.[1]

In traumatic brain injury (TBI), these limitations are especially evident at the mild end of the severity spectrum, where the heterogeneity is considered as one of the most significant barriers to finding effective therapeutic interventions.[8] The TBI literature varies in terms of the quality, study design, and research objectives. Often the focus of the research is not to provide guidelines for application in clinical practice, and therefore TBI healthcare providers may not easily derive practical application from studies that report only general associations (for example, the Glasgow Coma Scale [GCS] score on admission to hospital was correlated with outcome). TBI prognosis may be calculated in the context of survival, functional outcomes, cognitive outcomes, physical outcomes, behavioral outcomes, or return to premorbid activities, such as returning to employment.

The most recent guidelines from the American Association of Neurological Surgeons and The Joint Section on Neurotrauma and Critical Care, pertaining to clinical indicators of outcome in TBI, identify that the five factors that are most frequently used to determine the prognosis of *severe TBI* are the GCS score, age, pupillary responses, presence of hypotension, and abnormalities on computed tomography (CT). Several critical factors affect the prognosis in TBI, and each of these will be discussed briefly in this chapter.

Demographic and Premorbid Characteristics

The absence of bilateral pupillary responses after a severe TBI is also associated with a high mortality rate (91%–100%).[9,10] A weaker predictive factor is the presence of hypotension after a severe TBI. The mortality rates in patients who have periods of hypotension range from 42% to 50% compared with 27% or 28% in normotensive patients.[11,12] In a systematic review of multivariable prognostic models for moderate to severe TBI, the best predictors of outcome were reported to be the GCS, pupil reactivity, and CT.[13] In a systematic review of multivariable prognostic models for mild TBI (mTBI), there was no multivariable prognostic model that adequately predicted individual patient outcomes. However, preinjury mental health and early postinjury neuropsychologic functioning were identified as the most robust prognostic factors in the context of multivariable models. In addition, it was found that women and adults with early postinjury anxiety had worse prognoses.[14]

Although the duration of posttraumatic amnesia (PTA) is used as a measure of TBI severity, it is also a reasonable predictor of longer-term outcomes in children[15] and in moderate to severe TBI in adults.[16] Similarly, *time to follow commands* has also been demonstrated as a clinically useful injury severity rating for predicting the outcome in pediatric TBI.[17,18]

Age: One of the most powerful prognostic factors is age. There is an overrepresentation of emergency department (ED) TBI presentations in elderly adults (aged ≥85 years), which is largely reflective of the peak rates of fall-related TBIs occurring most commonly among these age groups[19-22] and in young children (0–4 years). Several studies show an association between older age and worse outcome.[19-54] However, the nature of this association (i.e., age as a continuous risk factor vs. inflection points of increased risk at specific ages) differed among studies. Although the risk for adults appears continuous, the prognosis worsens significantly after the age of 65 years. Studies have varied in their report of an age cutoff for an unlikely outcome of a good recovery.[34,45,47,48] In an analysis of 5600 adult patients with closed TBI, 74% of patients older than 55 years had poor outcome at 6 months compared with 39% of younger patients. The investigators concluded that for every 10 years of age the odds of a negative outcome increased by 40%–50%.[24] Additionally, younger patients were more likely to achieve independent ambulation.[55]

Education: The literature on the level of education and TBI outcome is mixed. Lower educational attainment was not found to be associated with nonproductivity post-TBI,[56] but higher educational levels (greater than 12 years) have also been reported to have a weak association with better outcome.[26] The age of a patient with a severe TBI at presentation is inversely related to the likelihood of death. Although the age-related mortality rate associated with a severe head injury (GCS < 8) falls on a continuum, the critical threshold appears to be around 50 years. The mortality rate of patients with a severe head injury older than 50 years was 78%–84%, whereas it was 28%–38% for patients younger than 50 years.[9,57]

Employment status: Preinjury unemployment has been reported to be associated with continued disability (activity limitations) and nonproductivity (not returning to work or training) at least 1 year post-TBI.[56] Other studies have reported that a majority of previously employed TBI survivors are unemployed 1–3 years postinjury, with figures in the vicinity of 56%.[58,59]

Socioeconomic status and access to healthcare: Socioeconomic status and access to healthcare may also play a role in outcome. Uninsured African American and uninsured Hispanic patients with TBI were found to have an increased risk of mortality compared with their insured counterparts.[60] In addition, uninsured Asians and uninsured African American patients with TBI have a higher risk of mortality than uninsured white patients.[60]

Race: TBI is one area where ethnic minority groups continue to appear to have higher risk for negative outcomes.[61,62] Minorities are at disproportionate risk for TBI and account for nearly half of all brain injury hospitalizations.[63-65] This disparity is most obvious in African Americans, who have a 35% higher TBI incidence than whites[63] and have a higher death rate from TBI.[66]

Gender: The rate of ED TBI presentations in males is 60%–80% higher than in females, with assaults and motor vehicle accidents (MVAs) demonstrating the greatest discrepancies.[19] In terms of sport-related concussion, gender differences relating to outcome and predictors of outcome have been reported, with females typically found to take longer to recover than their male counterparts.[67-70]

Mental health issues: Depression and personality changes have been described as the most common psychiatric syndromes following TBI. Depression has been reported to range between 9% and 36%,[44,45] and personality changes affect more than one-third of severe TBI survivors.[71,72] Following TBI, a significant increase in the prevalence of major depressive disorder (MDD) and generalized anxiety disorder have been reported. For example, in a sample of 48 patients with severe TBI, the most frequent psychiatric disorders were MDD (30.3%) and personality changes (33.3%).[73] However, the potential association between premorbid mental health problems and outcomes following TBI has been less commonly studied. Screening positive for posttraumatic stress disorder was significantly associated with psychiatric history.[74]

Drug and alcohol abuse: Many studies report a history of alcohol and/or drug abuse as a risk factor for poor outcome following TBI.[75-78]

Genetics: Decades of work on genetics, including multiple meta-analytical analyses, confirm that the presence of ApoE-4 correlates with worse chronic outcome from TBI.[79-81] In a Chinese cohort, investigators speculated that the apolipoprotein E (APOE-) 491AA promoter in ε4 carriers was associated with poor clinical outcome in the first week after TBI, as measured by the decline in GCS score or worsening of CT findings.[82] Prior work has suggested that the APOE allele is likely to affect the outcome among those with more severe injuries.[83,84] Possession of the APOE ε4 has been shown to reduce the prospect of a favorable outcome in children and young adults,[85] with evidence that APOE ε4 carriers are more than twice as likely as noncarriers to have an unfavorable outcome at six months after head injury.[85]

Mechanism of Injury

Cause of injury: The International Mission on Prognosis and Analysis of Clinical Trials in Traumatic Brain Injury

(IMPACT) database, a collection of eight randomized controlled trials, found that the cause of injury was not an independent predictor of long-term outcome following TBI (adjusting for age).

Multitrauma: Patients with TBI with extremity fractures after MVAs have been found to have higher cognitive Functional Independence Measure scores at discharge.[86] In a pediatric study, chest injury was associated with poor outcome.[87] However, in other studies, chest or abdomen trauma was not predictive of long-term functional outcome.[88]

Injury Severity and Related Outcome Measures

Severity of injury: TBI severity and acute and subacute clinical presentations play a large role in prognosis. The initial GCS score is inversely correlated with the likelihood of death. An admission GCS score of 3 was associated with mortality rates between 65% and 100%, although 7% of patients with an initial GCS of 3 have a good outcome (Glasgow Outcome Scale [GOS] score of 4 or 5). An initial GCS score of 7 was associated with mortality rates ranging from 15% to 27%.[9,12]

The duration of PTA: there is a long history supporting PTA as the most powerful prognostic tool at the disposal of the rehabilitation clinician.[89] A strong association has been observed between the duration of PTA and outcome, where the longer the duration of PTA, the worse the outcome.[31,48,50,53,90–93]

The duration of coma: A number of studies have examined the association between duration of loss of consciousness (LOC) and outcome.[31,48,50,52,53,93–95] Various parameters were used to define the duration of LOC, the period until which the patient could reliably follow commands, a GCS score greater than 8, or no specifications were reported. The duration of coma has been shown to be a strong prognostic factor in predicting both functional and occupational long-term outcomes. The majority of reported studies reported an association between the duration of coma and outcome[31,48,50,53,93,94] (i.e., the longer the duration of coma, the worse the outcome).

Outcome measures: One study using the Transforming Research and Clinical Knowledge in Traumatic Brain Injury database revealed that one in every three patients with mTBI was functionally impaired (i.e., had a Glasgow Outcome Scale-Extended [GOSE] score ≤ 6) at 3 months postinjury. In addition, 82% of patients with mTBI reported that they were continuing to experience at least one postconcussive symptom at both 6 and 12 months postinjury.[96] Moderate disability (or a good recovery) has been reported in more than 90% of

moderate TBI survivors.[97–100] Risk factors that are associated with poorer outcome in moderate TBI include lower GCS scores (i.e., 9 or 10), older age, and CT scan abnormalities.[97–100] Research has demonstrated that even in individuals with a good recovery, quite often neurobehavioral problems are present and contribute to the morbidity of moderate TBI.[99,100]

Glasgow Coma Scale

The most commonly used measure of severity is the GCS. The GCS score is considered to be a strong and reliable prognostic indicator for outcome in patients with TBI,[25,27,28,30,86,101–140] such that lower GCS scores are typically associated with worse outcomes. Despite the probability of a good outcome decreasing with lower GCS scores, the initial GCS score could potentially be associated with any outcome. As such, the GCS itself does not yield definitive prognoses, but merely a general idea of the TBI severity. In addition, in considering specific aspects of functional outcome among TBI survivors, a single GCS score may not be an ideal or reliable prognostic guide.[104]

The Glasgow Outcome Scale and the Extended Glasgow Outcome Scale

The GOS and the follow-up edition, the GOSE, were developed as a global scale for functional outcome that rates an individual's status into one of five (GOS),[105,106] or one of eight (GOSE),[107] categories (see Table 16.1). GCS score of 3–5, motor score of 1–3, absent verbal response, absent pupillary reaction, or absent oculocephalic reflex were independently predictive of poor functional outcome as measured by the GOS[108] score.

Abbreviated Injury Score

The Abbreviated Injury Score (AIS) assesses the severity of injury in seven body regions, one of which is the head AIS. The head AIS uses neuroradiologic or operative findings in its assessment. The injury assessment score (Injury Severity Score [ISS]) reflects an assessment of the three most severely injured body regions. These anatomic measures have been useful in prognostic models.[109] Head AIS and ISS scores have been associated with both early and long-term outcomes at 5–7 years after hospital discharge. Head AIS of 1–3 and ISS of < 25 were predictive of good recovery compared with head AIS scores of 4–6 and ISS of ≥ 25. Higher ISS scores were also associated with higher mortality rates.[88,110]

Loss of consciousness and posttraumatic amnesia

Measures of TBI severity have included recording the duration of LOC and PTA. LOC and PTA, however, are

TABLE 16.1				
Glasgow Outcome Scale and the Extended Glasgow Outcome Scale				
GLASGOW OUTCOME SCALE			**EXTENDED GLASGOW OUTCOME SCALE**	
Score	Outcome	Definition	Score	Outcome
1	Dead	Dead	1	Dead (D)
2	Persistent vegetative state	Wakefulness without awareness	2	Vegetative state (VS)
3	Severe disability	Conscious but dependent	3	Lower severe disability (SD–)
4	Moderate disability	Independent but disabled	4	Upper severe disability (SD+)
5	Good recovery	Fully integrated into society (may have nondisabling sequelae)	5	Lower moderate disability (MD–)
			6	Upper moderate disability (MD+)
			7	Lower good recovery (GR–)
			8	Upper good recovery (GR+)

Adapted from Jennett B, Bond M. Assessment of outcome after severe brain damage. *Lancet.* 1975;1(7905):480–484, with permission.

not always present in every case of TBI, and therefore they are of limited value in these instances. When PTA is present, its duration is a good indicator of the extent of cognitive and functional deficits after TBI[111] and is considered to be a good predictor of outcome.[112–114] PTA is essentially defined as the period during which an individual is unable to reliably and consistently follow commands. The "time to follow commands" may take into account early complications, but it can be affected by early sedation and the patient requires monitoring over an extended period.

Galveston Orientation and Amnesia Test
The Galveston Orientation and Amnesia Test (GOAT) was the first measure developed to assess the duration of PTA,[115] by assessing the orientation and memory for events preceding and following a TBI.[116] The GOAT and its Modified Orientation and Amnesia Test (MOAT) and Children's Orientation and Amnesia Test (COAT) versions were developed to evaluate cognition serially during the subacute stage of recovery from closed head injury. The GOAT includes 10 questions that assess orientation, biographical recall, and memory (see Fig. 16.2); a score greater than 75 (out of 100) for three consecutive days is considered the threshold for emergence from PTA.[117]

Orientation Log
The Orientation Log(O-Log) was designed for bedside with rehabilitation inpatients.[118] It is a quantitative tool used to quickly measure the orientation status (place, time, and situational domains). It is designed for serial

administration to document change over time.[119] Each of the 10 items are scored as follows:

3 points = spontaneous free recall (i.e., first response)
2 points = correct upon logical cueing (i.e., "that was yesterday, so today must be…")
1 point = correct upon multiple choice or phonemic cueing
0 points = incorrect response despite cueing, inappropriate response, or no response.

A total score out of 30 is derived from the O-Log, and emergence from PTA is considered to have occurred when a patient has performed well enough to achieve a score greater than 24 over two consecutive administrations.[118]

Westmead Post-traumatic Amnesia Scale and its abbreviated form
The Westmead Post-traumatic Amnesia Scale (WPTAS) and its abbreviated form (the A-WPTAS) are also valid measures for determining the length of PTA.[120–124] The WPTAS was designed to assess the ability of individuals who have sustained a TBI to lay down new memories over a 24-h period.[120] The WPTAS measures the orientation (time, person, place), together with memory for new information from 1 day after the next. In individuals with mild TBI, the A-WPTAS has facilitated the assessment of the orientation and capacity to lay down new information over short periods.[125] An individual is considered to have emerged from PTA on the first of three consecutive days where a recall score of 12 has been achieved (Fig. 16.3).[126]

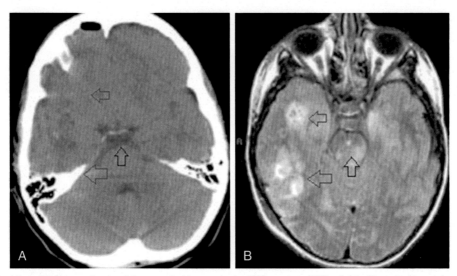

FIG. 16.1 **(A)** Noncontrast axial computed tomography (CT) scan and **(B)** a fluid-attenuated inversion recovery magnetic resonance (MR) image of a 10-year-old boy 48 h after he sustained a severe closed head injury. The region of hyperintense signal in the brain stem (*red arrows*) and the hyperintense signal in the right temporal region (*blue arrows*) are visible on the MR image but cannot be detected on the CT scan.

Question	Error score	Notes
What is your name?	/ 2	Must give both first name and surname.
When were you born?	/ 4	Must give day, month, and year.
Where do you live?	/ 4	Town is sufficient.
Where are you now?		
(a) City	/ 5	Must give actual town.
(b) Building	/ 5	Usually in hospital or rehab center. Actual name necessary.
When were you admitted to this hospital?	/ 5	Date.
How did you get here?	/ 5	Mode of transport.
What is the first event you can remember after the injury?	/ 5	Any plausible event is sufficient (record answer)
Can you give some detail?	/ 5	Must give relevant detail.
Can you describe the last event you can recall before the accident?	/ 5	Any plausible event is sufficient (record answer)
What time is it now?	/ 5	1 for each half-hour error, etc.
What day of the week is it?	/ 3	1 for each day error, etc.
What day of the month is it? (i.e. the date)	/ 5	1 for each day error, etc.
What is the month?	/ 15	5 for each month error, etc.
What is the year?	/ 30	10 for each year error.
Total error		
100 - total error		Can be a negative number.

FIG. 16.2 The Galveston Orientation and Amnesia Test.

Westmead Post Traumatic Amnesia (P.T.A.) Scale

Date of Onset: _____

Initial Examiner: _____   Alternate face cards used in examiners absence: _____

	Date:													
1. How old are you?	A													
	S													
2. What is your date of birth?	A													
	S													
3. What month are we in?	A													
	S													
4. What time of the day is it? (Morning / Afternoon / Night)	A													
	S													
5. What day of the week is it?	A													
	S													
6. What year are we in?	A													
	S													
7. What is the name of this place?	A													
	S													
8. Face	A													
	S													
9. Name	A													
	S													
10. Picture I	A													
	S													
11. Picture II	A													
	S													
12. Picture III	A													
	S													
Orientation:	7													
Recall:	5													
Total:	12													

A = Patient's Answer
S = Patient's Score (1 or 0)
* answers if three options given

FIG. 16.3 Westmead Post-traumatic Amnesia scale. (Adapted from Swan S, Queensland Health Therapy Gold Coast Hospital and Royal Brisbane & Women's Hospital, 2009; from Shores EA, Marosszeky JE, Sandanam J, Batchelor J. Preliminary validation of a clinical scale for measuring the duration of post-traumatic amnesia. *Med J Aust*. 1986;144:569–572, with permission.)

Computed Tomography and Traumatic Brain Injury Outcome

The introduction of CT dramatically improved the ability to detect intracerebral abnormalities. Since its development and subsequent implementation for acute care management, the CT scan has largely become part of routine ED clinical care within the TBI population. The results of CT scans provide important information for TBI prognosis.[27] The presence of subarachnoid hemorrhage,[28,108,127] intraventricular hemorrhage,[127,128] cisternal effacement,[28,127] significant midline shift,[28,127] extradural hemorrhage, or subdural hemorrhage on acute CT scan are all associated with worse outcome, and any one of these findings has been associated with the full range of outcomes. However, evidence of contusions only has a modest effect on the prognosis.[28]

CT classification systems have been developed to associate CT findings with functional outcome, for example, the Marshall CT Classification.[28,127] Data from the large-scale IMPACT study found that the Marshall CT Classification and individual CT characteristics were strong prognostic factors in predicting outcome, as measured by the GOS. Patients with diffuse injuries in class III or IV had worse outcomes. Among patients with mass lesions, the outcome was better for epidural hematomas compared with acute subdural hematomas.[28,127] However, in a 5- to 7-year follow-up of a cohort of pediatric patients with TBI, the presence of subdural or intracerebral hemorrhage was not predictive of outcome.[88]

Magnetic Resonance Imaging and Traumatic Brain Injury Outcome

Structural magnetic resonance imaging (MRI) is more sensitive than CT for detecting abnormalities in the brain after TBI (see Fig. 16.1 for contrast between CT and MRI in the same patient with TBI).[129] More advanced magnetic resonance techniques have demonstrated some promise in improving the sensitivity for detecting subtle TBI-related abnormalities, for example, identifying diffuse axonal injury and nonhemorrhagic contusions.[130,131]

Diffusion tensor imaging (DTI) enables the visualization of white matter tracts.[132] Measures are expressed using various indices such as the fractional anisotropy, which reflects the directionality of water diffusion or the degree of anisotropy. Because axonal injury is common in TBI, DTI is a promising biomarker.

Magnetic resonance spectroscopy allows for measurements of brain metabolites that may be affected by concussion including *N*-acetylaspartate, a marker of neuronal health; glutathione, an antioxidant that is depleted during oxidative stress, which is common after TBI; glutamate, an excitatory neurotransmitter that is altered by TBI; and myoinositol, a marker of glial cell activity.[133,134]

Susceptibility-weighted imaging is a technique that exploits differences in magnetic susceptibility between tissues and is sensitive to microhemorrhages after mild TBI.[134,135]

Resting state functional MRI provides a measurement of the brain's functional connectivity networks.

Arterial spin labeling (ASL) is a method that involves magnetically labeling blood before it enters the brain and is capable of quantifying cerebral blood flow.[136] Because studies report hemodynamic impairment in patients with TBI,[137] ASL represents a strong TBI biomarker candidate.

PREVENTION

To explore relevant preventative TBI strategies, an understanding of the key mechanism of injury is vital. Strategies to minimize and/or neutralize the risks associated with, for example, falls, MVAs, and being stuck against an object, the three mechanisms that accounted for 75% of all TBI-related ED visits, hospitalizations, and deaths in 2013, would be most helpful.[138] Monitoring of epidemiologic patterns of TBI-related ED visits, admissions, and mortality can help identify target populations and mechanisms of injury to inform TBI prevention strategies.

Prevention of Fall-Related Traumatic Brain Injury

Falls are a common cause of injury in the older adult population (those ≥75 years), followed by those aged 0–4 years, followed by those aged 65–74 years.[20,138]

Strategies for older adult fall prevention include the following:

- One of several evidence-based fall prevention initiatives is the Stopping Elderly Accidents, Deaths, and Injuries, created by the Centers for Disease Control and Prevention to guide primary care physicians in the identification of modifiable fall risk factors.[139,140]

- Medical evaluation must incorporate fall risk assessment
  - Identifying those at risk via questionnaires, which may be filled out in the waiting room
    - Reporting any recent falls, near falls, unsteadiness
  - Medication review to decrease iatrogenic causes of hypotension/orthostasis
  - Surgical referral (i.e., cataract surgery, pacemaker)
  - Physical examination (i.e., timed-up-and-go test, sensory and strength testing) to determine the need for appropriate external modification based on strength testing, gait and balance deficits, and visual acuity
    - Mobility aids/proper footwear
    - Vision screening, visual aids
    - Cognitive aids and therapies if cognitive deficits are noted
  - Vitamin D supplementation for patients with low vitamin D levels has been shown to decrease fall risk
- Home safety assessment
  - Alleviation of irregular surfaces/rugs/carpets and clutter
  - Adequate lighting especially near the stairs
  - Coverings to prevent falls on slippery surfaces
  - Safety features in bathrooms and on stairs
- Exercise prescription to improve balance and gait stability and decrease fall risk. Referral may be placed to community balance, gait, and fitness groups. For example, Tai Chi has been shown to reduce the rate of falls and risk of fractures.
- Falls are also a common method of suicide attempts in the older population.
  - Installation of bars on windows
  - Mental health screenings

In the pediatric population, fall prevention is equally important.

- At home, installation of bars on windows and staircases
- Shopping cart safety
- Gym and playground design for children must follow recommendations such as those outlined in the Consumer Product Safety Commission's *Public Playground Safety Handbook*, which includes using age-appropriate equipment, incorporation of shock-absorbing surfaces, and close adult supervision.

Prevention of Transport-Related Traumatic Brain Injury

Preventing motor vehicle crashes through educational programs to enhance driver performance and safety awareness and improving motor vehicle design to increase safety are the strategies being used to reduce the risk of transport-related TBI.

For example, reducing the incident of driving under the influence of alcohol or other drugs, through harsher penalties, greater presence of law enforcement on the roads, and random testing, in addition to advertising and community education and awareness campaigns. Further, public policy and safety laws, including graduated licensing of novice drivers, reduction of speed limits, seat belt and helmet laws, zero tolerance for alcohol/drug intoxication regulations, and road engineering practices.

Multiple studies have reported a decrease in MVA-related deaths and brain injury in response to laws requiring helmet use for bikers, motorcyclists, and other open unrestrained vehicle riders. In California, implementation of a universal helmet use law in 1992 conferred an increase in helmet use to 99% from approximately 50% the year before, and the number of motorcyclist fatalities in that state decreased to approximately 37% during 1991–92.[141] On the other hand, when Florida exempted certain riders from having to wear a helmet in 2000, motorcyclist fatalities per 10,000 motorcycle registrations increased to 21% during the subsequent 2 years. Moreover, death rates have been found to be 20%–40% higher in states with nonexistent or weak laws when compared with states with universal helmet laws. (Car design safety considerations, including airbags, collapsible engine, and electronic stability controls, have had an impact on injury rates.)[142]

Prevention of Work-Related Traumatic Brain Injury

Work-related TBI (WRTBI) constitutes one of the most serious workplace injuries that is more likely than most other work-related injuries to result in hospitalization.[143] For WRTBI, Konda and colleagues[143] identified that males, workers in the youngest (15–24 years of age, followed by 25–34 years of age) and oldest (55 years and older) age groups, and those who work in the primary (e.g., agriculture, forestry, mining or construction) industries were at greater risk of sustaining occupational TBI, with falls constituting the most common mechanism of injury. In addition, there was an increased risk of injury during the first 4 weeks at work, especially in the construction industry, suggesting factors such as the younger workers' poorer risk assessment of occupational hazards, relative lack of work experience, and suboptimal safety training, implicating greater workplace orientation and training as a possible means of preventing and certainly reducing the risks.

Other preventative strategies may target occupations within the construction industry and assess a need for personal protective equipment (netting, guardrails, hole covers, personal arrest systems) and safety training, especially in the youngest workers and during first 4 weeks of employment when injury rates are the highest.[143]

CONCLUSIONS

Prognosis is an important clinical tool for determining medical management. However, predicting recovery in TBI can be especially challenging. One limitation is the variety of metrics that can be applied in studies of prognosis (i.e., survival, functional outcomes, cognitive outcomes, physical outcomes, behavioral outcomes, or return to premorbid activities such as returning to employment). Developing prognostic guidelines based on research literature is challenging, and healthcare professionals may often rely on their own clinical experience in formulating a prognosis.

There are numerous outcome measures that have been developed and validated in TBI populations to assist with this process. Many of these measures have been validated by providing cutoff scores that predict a dichotomous "good versus bad" outcome, and applying these measures across the spectrum of the severity continuum has limitations.

Prevention, implementing strategies to reduce the risk and rates of TBI, is an important societal issue. Efforts focused on legislature regarding sports regulations, veterans' affairs, funding and insurance coverage, as well as safety policies and regulations, education tools and programs, mechanical alterations for a safer environment, fall prevention interventions including effective screening, and community preventative programs will assist in reducing the rates of TBI associated with at-risk activities. Emphasis on specific populations and targeting age groups at greatest risk is important for focused injury prevention and surveillance.

REFERENCES

1. Wiesemann C. The significance of prognosis for a theory of medical practice. *Theor Med Bioeth*. 1998;19(3): 253–261.
2. Vogenberg FR. Predictive and prognostic models: implications for healthcare decision-making in a modern recession. *Am Heal Drug Benefits*. 2009;2(6):218–222.

3. Dawes RM, Faust D, Meehl PE. Clinical versus actuarial judgement. *Science (80-)*. 1989;243(4899):1668–1674.
4. Knaus WA, Wagner DP, Lynn J. Short-term mortality predictions for critically ill hospitalized adults: science and ethics. *Science (80-)*. 1991;254:389–393.
5. Perkins HS, Jonsen AR, Epstein WV. Providers as predictors: using outcome predictors in intensive care. *Crit Care Med*. 1986;14(2):105–110.
6. Chang RW, Lee B, Jacobs S, Lee B. Accuracy of decisions to withdraw therapy in critically ill patients: clinical judgement versus a computer model. *Crit Care Med*. 1989;17(11):1091–1097.
7. Poses RM, Bekes C, Copare FJ, Scott WE. The answer to "What are my chances, doctor?" depends on who is asked: prognostic disagreement and inaccuracy for critically ill patients. *Crit Care Med*. 1989;17(8):827–833.
8. Saatman KE, Duhaime A-C, Bullock R, Maas AIR, Valadka A, Manley GT. Classification of traumatic brain injury for targeted therapies. *J Neurotrauma*. 2008;25(7):719–738.
9. Braakman R, Gelpke GJ, Habbema JD, Maas AI, Minderhoud JM. Systematic selection of prognostic features in patients with severe head injury. *Neurosurgery*. 1980;6(4):362–370.
10. Cordobés F, Lobato RD, Rivas JJ, et al. Observations on 82 patients with extradural hematoma. Comparison of results before and after the advent of computerized tomography. *J Neurosurg*. 1981;54(2):179–186.
11. Chesnut RM, Marshall LF, Klauber MR, et al. The role of secondary brain injury in determining outcome from severe head injury. *J Trauma*. 1993;34(2):216–222.
12. Fearnside MR, Cook RJ, McDougall P, McNeil RJ. The Westmead Head Injury Project outcome in severe head injury. A comparative analysis of pre-hospital, clinical and CT variables. *Br J Neurosurg*. 1993;7(3):267–279.
13. Savola O, Hillbom M. Early predictors of post-concussion symptoms in patients with mild head injury. *Eur J Neurol*. 2003;10(2):175–181.
14. Silverberg ND, Gardner AJ, Brubacher JR, Panenka WJ, Li JJ, Iverson GL. Systematic review of multivariable prognostic models for mild traumatic brain injury. *J Neurotrauma*. 2015;32(8):517–526.
15. Briggs R, Brookes N, Tate R, Lah S. Duration of post-traumatic amnesia as a predictor of functional outcome in school-age children: a systematic review. *Dev Med Child Med*. 2015. https://doi.org/10.1111/dmcn.12674.
16. Walker WC, Ketchum JM, Marwitz JH, et al. A multicentre study on the clinical utility of post-traumatic amnesia duration in predicting global outcome after moderate-sever traumatic brain injury. *J Neurol Neurosurg Psychiatr*. 2010;81(1):87–89.
17. Austin CA, Slomine BS, Dematt EJ, Salorio CF, Suskauer SJ. Time to follow commands remains the most useful injury severity variable for predicting WeeFIM® scores 1 year after paediatric TBI. *Brain Inj*. 2013;27(9):1056–1062.
18. Davis KC, Slomine BS, Salorio CF, Suskauer SJ. Time to follow commands and duration of posttraumatic amnesia predict GOS-E peds scores 1 to 2 years after TBI in children requiring inpatient rehabilitation. *J Head Trauma Rehabil*. 2015.
19. Fu TS, Jing R, Fu WW, Cusimano MD. Epidemiological trends of traumatic brain injury identified in the emergency department in a publicly-insured population, 2002-2010. *PLoS One*. 2016;11(1).
20. Faul M, Xu L, Wald MM, Coronado VG. *Traumatic Brain Injury in the United States: Emergency Department Visits, Hospitalizations, and Deaths*. Atlanta (GA); 2010.
21. Marin JR, Weaver MD, Yealy DM, Mannix RC. Trends in visits for traumatic brain injury to emergency departments in the United States. *JAMA*. 2014;311(18):1917–1919.
22. Fu TS, Jing R, McFaull SR, Cusimano MD. Recent trends in hospitalization and in-hospital mortality associated with traumatic brain injury in Canada: a nationwide, population-based study. *J Trauma Acute Care Surg*. 2015;79(3):449–454.
23. Gray DS, Burnham RS. Preliminary outcome analysis of a long-term rehabilitation program for severe acquired brain injury. *Arch Phys Med Rehabil*. 2000;81(11):1447–1456.
24. Hukkelhoven CW, Steyerberg EW, Rampen AJ, et al. Patient age and outcome following severe traumatic brain injury: an analysis of 5600 patients. *J Neurosurg*. 2003;99(4):666–673.
25. Poon WS, Zhu XL, Ng SC, Wong GK. Predicting one year clinical outcome in traumatic brain injury (TBI) at the beginning of rehabilitation. *Acta Neurochir Suppl*. 2005;93:207–208.
26. Mushkudiani NA, Engel DC, Steyerberg EW, et al. Prognostic value of demographic characteristics in traumatic brain injury: results from the IMPACT study. *J Neurotrauma*. 2007;24(2):259–269.
27. Cremer OL, Moons KGM, van Dijk GW, van Balen P, Kalkman CJ. Prognosis following severe head injury: development and validation of a model for prediction of death, disability, and functional recovery. *J Trauma*. 2006;61(6):1484–1491.
28. Murray GD, Butcher I, McHugh GS, et al. Multivariable prognostic analysis in traumatic brain injury: results from the IMPACT study. *J Neurotrauma*. 2007;24(2):329–337.
29. Livingston DH, Lavery RF, Verhagen AP, et al. Recovery at one year following isolated traumatic brain injury: a Western Trauma Association prospective multicenter trial. *J Trauma*. 2005;59(6):1298–1304.
30. Signorini DF, Andrews PJ, Jones PA, Wardlaw JM, Miller JD. Predicting survival using simple clinical variables: a case study in traumatic brain injury. *J Neurol Neurosurg Psychiatr*. 1999;66(1):20–25.
31. Rao N, Rosenthal M, Cronin-Stubbs D, Lambert R, Barnes P, Swanson B. Return to work after rehabilitation following traumatic brain injury. *Brain Inj*. 1990;4(1):49–56.

32. Kakarieka A, Braakman R, Schakel EH. Clinical significance of the finding of subarachnoid blood on CT scan after head injury. *Acta Neurochir (Wien)*. 1994;129(1–2):1–5.

33. Walder AD, Yeoman PM, Turnball A. The abbreviated injury scale as a predictor of outcome of severe head injury. *Intensive Care Med*. 1995;21(7):606–609.

34. Gomez PA, Lobato RD, Boto GR, De la Lama A, Gonzalez PJ, de la Cruz J. Age and outcome after severe head injury. *Acta Neurochir (Wien)*. 2000;142(4):373–381.

35. Rovlias A, Kotsou S. Classification and regression tree for prediction of outcome after severe head injury using simple clinical and laboratory variables. *J Neurotrauma*. 2004;21(7):886–893.

36. Perel P, Arango M, Clayton T, et al. Predicting outcome after traumatic brain injury: practical prognostic models based on large cohort of international patients. *BMJ*. 2008;336:425–435.

37. Steyerberg EW, Mushkudiani N, Perel P, et al. Predicting outcome after traumatic brain injury: developmental and international validation of prognostic scored based on admission characteristics. *PLoS Med*. 2008;5(8):1251–1261.

38. Nelson DW, Nystron H, MacCuallum R, et al. Extended analysis of early computed tomography scans of traumatic brain injured patients and relations to outcome. *J Neurotrauma*. 2010;27:51–64.

39. Skandsen T, Kvistad KA, Solheim O, Lydersen S, Haavde Strand I, Vik A. Prognostic value of magnetic resonance imaging in moderate and severe head injury: a prospective study of early MRI findings and one-year outcome. *J Neurotrauma*. 2011;28(5):691–699.

40. Skandsen T, Kvistad KA, Solheim O, Lydersen S, Haavde Strand I, Vik A. Prognostic value of magnetic resonance imaging in moderate and severe head injury: a prospective study of early MRI findings and one-year outcome. *J Neurotrauma*. 2011;28:203–215.

41. Yeoman P, Pattani H, Silcocks P, Owen V, Fuller G. Validation of the IMPACT outcome prediction score using the Nottingham head injury dataset. *J Trauma*. 2011;71(2):387–392.

42. Born JD, Albert A, Hans P, Bonnal J. Relative prognostic value of best motor response and brain stem reflexes in patients with severe head injury. *Neurosurgery*. 1985;16:595–600.

43. Choi SC, Muizelaar JP, Barnes TY, Marmarou NA, Brooks DM, Young HF. Prediction tree for severely head-injured patients. *J Neurosurg*. 1991;75(2):251–255.

44. Narayan RK, Enas GG, Choi SC. *Practical Techniques for Predicting Outcome in Severe Head Injury*; 1989.

45. Vollmer DG, Torner JC, Jane JA, et al. Age and outcome following traumatic coma: why do older patients fare worse? *J Neruosurg*. 1991;75(1):S37–S49.

46. Choi SC, Narayan RK, Anderson RL, Ward JD. Enhanced specificity of prognosis in severe head injury. *J Neurosurg*. 1988;69(3):381–385.

47. Pennings JL, Bachulis BL, Simons CT, Slazinski T. Survival after severe brain injury in the aged. *Arch Surg*. 1993;128:787–794.

48. Katz DI, Alexander MP. Traumatic brain injury: predicting course of recovery and outcome for patients admitted to rehabilitation. *Arch Neurol*. 1994;51:661–670.

49. Combes P, Fauvage B, Colonna M, Passagia JG, Chirossel JP, Jacquot C. Severe head injuries: an outcome prediction and survival analysis. *Intensive Care Med*. 1996;22(12):1391–1395.

50. Ellenberg JH, Levin HS, Saydjari C. Posttraumatic amnesia as a predictor of outcome after severe closed head injury. *Arch Neurol*. 1996;53(8):782–791.

51. Hawkins DJ, Lewis FD, Medeiros RS. Impact of length of stay on functional outcomes of TBI patients. *Am Surg*. 2005;71:921–929.

52. Sherer M, Yablon SA, Nakase-Richardson R, Nick TG. Effect of severity of post-traumatic confusion and its constituent symptoms on outcome after traumatic brain injury. *Arch Phys Med Rehabil*. 2008;89:42–47.

53. Tate RL, Lulham JM, Broe GA, Strettles B, Pfaff A. Psychosocial outcome for the survivors of severe blunt head injury: the results from a consecutive series of 100 patients. *J Neurol Psychol*. 1989;52(10):1128–1134.

54. Levin HS, Benton AL, Grossman RG. *Neurobehavioral Consequences of Closed Head Injury*. New York, NY: Oxford University Press; 1982.

55. Katz DI, White DK, Alexander MP, Klein RB. Recovery of ambulation after traumatic brain injury. *Arch Phys Med Rehabil*. 2004;85(6):865–869.

56. Willemse-van Son AH, Ribbers GM, Verhagen AP, Stam HJ. Prognostic factors of long-term functioning and productivity after traumatic brain injury: a systematic review of prospective cohort studies. *Clin Rehabil*. 2007;21(11):1024–1037.

57. Narayan RK, Greenberg RP, Miller JD, et al. Improved confidence of outcome prediction in severe head injury. A comparative analysis of the clinical examination, multimodality evoked potentials, CT scanning, and intracranial pressure. *J Neurotrauma*. 1981;54(6):751–762.

58. Gollaher K, High W, Sherer M, et al. Prediction of employment outcome one to three years following traumatic brain injury (TBI). *Brain Inj*. 1998;12(4):255–263. https://doi.org/10.1080/026990598122557.

59. Ponsford JL, Olver JH, Curran C. A profile of outcome: 2 years after traumatic brain injury. *Brain Inj*. 1995;9(1):1–10. https://doi.org/10.3109/02699059509004565.

60. Berry C, Ley EJ, Mirocha J, Salim A. Race affects mortality after moderate to severe traumatic brain injury. *J Surg Res*. 2010;163(2):303–308. https://doi.org/10.1016/j.jss.2010.03.018.

61. Betancourt JR, Green AR, Carrillo JE, Ananeh-Firempong O. Defining cultural competence: a practical framework for addressing racial/ethnic disparities in health and health care. *Public Health Rep*. 2003;118:293–302.

62. Wong MD, Shapiro MF, Boscardin WJ, Ettner SL. Contribution of major diseases to disparities in mortality. *N Engl J Med.* 2002;347(20):1585–1592.

63. Shafi S, Marquez de la Plata C, Diaz-Arrastia R, et al. Racial disparities in long-term functional outcome after traumatic brain injury. *J Trauma.* 2007;63(6):1263–1270. https://doi.org/10.1097/TA.0b013e31815b8f00.

64. Marquez de la Plata C, Hewlitt M, de Oliveira A, et al. Ethnic differences in rehabilitation placement and outcome after TBI. *J Head Trauma Rehabil.* 2007;22(2):113–121. https://doi.org/10.1097/01.HTR.0000265099.29436.56.

65. Jager TE, Weiss HB, Cohen JH. Traumatic brain injuries evaluated in U.S. emergency departments, 1992-1994. *Acad Emerg Med.* 2000;7:134.

66. Langlois JA, Rutland-Brown W, Thomas KE. *Traumatic Brain Injury in the United States: Emergency Department Visits, Hospitalizations, and Deaths.* Atlanta, GA; 2004.

67. Benedict PA, Baner NV, Harrold GK, et al. Gender and age predict outcomes of cognitive, balance and vision testing in a multidisciplinary concussion center. *J Neurol Sci.* 2015;353(1–2):111–115.

68. Covassin T, Elbin RJ, Harris W, Parker T, Kontos A. The role of age and sex in symptoms, neurocognitive performance, and postural stability in athletes after concussion. *Am J Sports Med.* 2012;40(6):1303–1312.

69. Berz K, Divine J, Foss KB, Heyl R, Ford KR, Myer GD. Sex-specific differences in the severity of symptoms and recovery rate following sports-related concussion in young athletes. *Phys Sport Med.* 2013;41(2):58–63.

70. Brooks BL, Iverson GL, Atkins JE, Zafonte R, Berkner PD. Sex differences and self-reported attention problems during baseline concussion testing. *Appl Neuropsychol Child.* 2015. https://doi.org/10.1080/21622965.2014.1003066.

71. Pelegrin-Valero CA, Gomez-Hernandez R, Munoz-Cespedes JM, Fernandez-Guinea SD, Tirapu-Ustarroz J. Nosologic aspects of personality change due to head trauma. *Rev Neurol.* 2001;32:681–687.

72. Rao V, Spiro JR, Handel S, Onyike CU. Clinical correlates of personality changes associated with traumatic brain injury. *J Neuropsychiatr Clin Neurosci.* 2008;20:118–119.

73. Diaz AP, Schwarzbold ML, Thais ME, et al. Psychiatric disorders and health-related quality of life after severe traumatic brain injury: a prospective study. *J Neurotrauma.* 2012;29(6):1029–1037. https://doi.org/10.1089/neu.2011.2089.

74. Haarbauer-Krupa J, Taylor CA, Yue JK, et al. Screening for post-traumatic stress disorder in a civilian emergency department population with traumatic brain injury. *J Neurotrauma.* 2016.

75. Rutherford W. Postconcussion symptoms: relationship to acute neurological indices, individual differences, and circumstances of injury. In: Levin HS, Eisenberg HM, Benson AL, eds. *Mild Head Injury.* New York, NY: Oxford University Press; 1989:229–245.

76. Dunlop TW, Udvarhelyi GB, Stedem AF, et al. Comparison of patients with and without emotional/behavioral deterioration during the first year after traumatic brain injury. *J Neuropsychiatr.* 1991;3:150–156.

77. Kreutzer JS, Harris JM. Model systems of treatment for alcohol consumption following traumatic brain injury. *Brain Inj.* 1990;4:1–5.

78. Rimel RW, Giordani B, Barth JT, Jane JA. Moderate head injury: completing the clinical spectrum of brain trauma. *Neurosurgery.* 1982;11:344–351.

79. Kassam I, Gagnon F, Cusimano MD. Association of the APOE-epsilon4 allele with outcome of traumatic brain injury in children and youth: a meta-analysis and meta-regression. *J Neurol Neurosurg Psychiatry.* 2016;87(4):433–440.

80. Lawrence DW, Comper P, Hutchison MG, Sharma B. The role of apolipoprotein E episilon (epsilon)-4 allele on outcome following traumatic brain injury: a systematic review. *Brain Inj.* 2015;29(9):1018–1031.

81. Zeng S, Jiang JX, Xu MH, et al. Prognostic value of apolipoprotein E epsilon4 allele in patients with traumatic brain injury: a meta-analysis and meta-regression. *Genet Test Mol Biomark.* 2014;18(3):202–210.

82. Jiang Y, Sun X, Gui L, et al. Correlation between APOE-491AA promoter in epsilon4 carriers and clinical deterioration in early stage of traumatic brain injury. *J Neurotrauma.* 2007;24(24):12.

83. Tierney RT, Mansell JL, Higgins M, et al. Apolipoprotein E genotype and concussion in college athletes. *Clin J Sport Med.* 2010;20(6):464–468.

84. Terrell TR, Bostick RM, Abramson R, et al. APOE, APOE promoter, and Tau genotypes and risk for concussion in college athletes. *Clin J Sport Med.* 2008;18(1).

85. Teasdale GM, Nicoll JAR, Murray G, Fiddes M. Association of apolipoprotein E polymorphism with outcome after head injury. *Lancet.* 1997;350:1069–1071.

86. Cowen TD, Meythaler JM, DeVivo MJ, Ivie CSI, Lebow J, Novack T. Influence of early variables in traumatic brain injury on functional independence measure scores and rehabilitation length of stay and charges. *Arch Phys Med Rehabil.* 1995;76(9):797–803.

87. Chung CY, Chen CL, Cheng PT, See LC, Tang SF, Wong AM. Critical score of Glasgow Coma Scale for pediatric traumatic brain injury. *Pediatr Neurol.* 2006;34(5):379–387.

88. Massagli TL, Michaud LJ, Rivara FP. Association between injury indices and outcome after severe traumatic brain injury in children. *Arch Phys Med Rehabil.* 1996;77(2):125–132.

89. Greenwood R. Value of recording duration of post-traumatic amnesia. *J Neurosurg.* 1997;349:1041–1042.

90. Bishara SN, Partridge FM, Godfrey HPD, Knight G. Post-traumatic amnesia and Glasgow Coma Scale related to outcome in survivors in a consecutive series of patients with severe closed-head injury. *Brain Inj.* 1992;6(4):373–380.

91. Godfrey HPD, Bishara SN, Partridge FM, Knight G. Neuropsychological impairment and return to work following severe closed head injury: implications for clinical management. *N Z Med J.* 1993;106(960):301–303.

92. Nakase-Richardson R, Sepehri A, Sherer M, Yablon SA, Evans C, Mani T. Classification schema of posttraumatic amnesia duration-based injury severity relative to 1-year outcome: analysis of individuals with moderate and severe traumatic brain injury. *Arch Phys Med Rehabil.* 2009;90:17–19.

93. Sidaros A, Engberg AW, Sidaros K, et al. Diffusion tensor imaging during recovery from severe traumatic brain injury and relation to clinical outcome: a longitudinal study. *Brain.* 2008;131:559–572.

94. Formisano R, Voogt RT, Buzzi MG, et al. Time interval of oral feeding recovery as a prognostic factor in severe traumatic brain injury. *Brain Inj.* 2004;18(1):103–109.

95. Facco E, Zuccarello M, Pittoni G, et al. Early outcome prediction in severe head injury: comparison between children and adults. *Childs Nerv Syst.* 1986;2(2):67–71.

96. McMahon P, Hricik A, Yue JK, et al. Symptomatology and functional outcome in mild traumatic brain injury: results from the prospective TRACK-TBI study. *J Neurotrauma.* 2014;31(1):26–33.

97. Compagnone C, D'Avella D, Servadei F, et al. Patients with moderate head injury: a prospective multicenter study of 315 patients. *Neurosurgery.* 2009;64(4):690–697.

98. Fabbi A, Servadei F, Marchesini G, Stein SC, Vandelli A. Early predictors of unfavourable outcomes in subject with moderate head injury in the emergency department. *J Neurol Neurosurg Psychiatr.* 2008;79:567–573.

99. van der Naalt J. Prediction of outcome in mild to moderate head injury: a review. *J Clin Exp Neuropsychol.* 2001;23(6):837–851. https://doi.org/10.1076/jcen.23.6.837.1018.

100. Stein SC. Outcome from moderate head injury. In: Wilberger JE, Povlishock JT, eds. *Neurotrauma.* New York, NY: McGraw-Hill; 1996:755–777.

101. Thakker JC, Splaingard M, Zhu J, Babel K, Bresnahan J, Havens PL. Survival and functional outcome of children requiring endotracheal intubation during therapy for severe traumatic brain injury. *Crit Care Med.* 1997;25(8):1396–1401.

102. White JR, Farukhi Z, Bull C, et al. Predictors of outcome in severely head-injured children. *Crit Care Med.* 2001;29(3):534–540.

103. Asikainen I, Kaste M, Sarna S. Predicting late outcome for patients with traumatic brain injury referred to a rehabilitation programme: a study of 508 Finnish patients 5 years or more after injury. *Brain Inj.* 1998;12(2):95–107.

104. Zafonte RD, Hammond FM, Mann NR, Wood DL, Black KL, Millis SR. Relationship between Glasgow coma scale and functional outcome. *Am J Phys Med Rehabil.* 1996;75(5):364–369.

105. Jennett B, Bond M. Assessment of outcome after severe brain damage. *Lancet.* 1975;1(7905):480–484.

106. Teasdale GM, Pettigrew LE, Wilson JT, Murray G, Jennett B. Analyzing outcome of treatment of severe head injury: a review and update on advancing the use of the Glasgow Outcome Scale. *J Neurotrauma.* 1998;15(8):587–597.

107. Wilson JTL, Pettigrew LEL, Teasdale GM. Structured interviews for the Glasgow outcome scale and the extended Glasgow outcome scale: guidelines for their use. *J Neurotrauma.* 1998;15(8):573–585.

108. Pillai S, Praharaj SS, Mohanty A, Kolluri VR. Prognostic factors in children with severe diffuse brain injuries: a study of 74 patients. *Pediatr Neurosurg.* 2001;34(2):98–103.

109. Foreman BP, Caesar RR, Parks J, et al. Usefulness of the abbreviated injury score and the injury severity score in comparison to the Glasgow Coma Scale in predicting outcome after traumatic brain injury. *J Trauma.* 2007;62(4):946–950.

110. Ducrocq SC, Meyer PG, Orliaguet GA, et al. Epidemiology and early predictive factors of mortality and outcome in children with traumatic severe brain injury: experience of a French pediatric trauma center. *Pediatr Crit Care Med.* 2006;7(5):461–467.

111. Khan F, Baguley IJ, Cameron ID. Rehabilitation after traumatic brain injury. *Med J Aust.* 2003;178(6):290–295.

112. Alexander MP. Mild traumatic brain injury: pathophysiology, natural history, and clinical management. *Neurology.* 1995;45(7):1253–1260.

113. Bowen A, Chamberlain MA, Tennant A, Neumann V, Conner M. The persistence of mood disorders following traumatic brain injury: a 1 year follow-up. *Brain Inj.* 1999;13(7):547–553.

114. Nakase-Richardson R, Sherer M, Seel RT, et al. Utility of post-traumatic amnesia in predicting 1-year productivity following traumatic brain injury: comparison of the Russell and Mississippi PTA classification intervals. *J Neurol Neurosurg Psychiatr.* 2011;82(5):494–499.

115. Zasler ND, Katz DI, Zafonte RD. Clinical continuum of care and natural history. In: *Brain Injury Medicine: Principles and Practice.* New York: Demos Medical Publishing; 2007:3–13.

116. Levin HS, O'Donnell VM, Grossman RG. The Galveston orientation and amnesia test. A practical scale to assess cognition after head injury. *J Nerv Ment Disord.* 1979;167(11):675–684.

117. Cifu DX, Caruso D. *Traumatic Brain Injury.* New York, NY: Demos Medical Publishing; 2010.

118. Jackson WT, Novack TA, Dowler RN. Effective serial measurement of cognitive orientation in rehabilitation: the orientation log. *Arch Phys Med Rehabil.* 1998;79(6):718–720.

119. Novack T. *The Orientation Log.* The Center for Outcome Measurement in Brain Injury; 2000. http://www.tbims.org/combi/olog.

120. Shores EA, Marosszeky JE, Sandanam J, Batchelor J. Preliminary validation of a clinical scale for measuring the duration of post-traumatic amnesia. *Med J Aust.* 1986;144(11):569–572.

121. Shores EA. Comparison of the Westmead PTA Scale and Glasgow Coma Scale as predictors of neuropsychological outcome following extremely severe blunt head injury. *J Neurol Neurosurg Psychiatr.* 1989;52(1):126–127.

122. Meares S, Shores EA, Taylor AJ, Lammél A, Batchelor J. Validation of the Abbreviated Westmead Post-traumatic Amnesia Scale: a brief measure to identify acute cognitive impairment in mild traumatic brain injury. *Brain Inj.* 2011;25(12):1198–1205. https://doi.org/10.3109/02699 052.2011.608213.

123. Shores EA. Further concurrent validity on the Westmead PTA scale. *Appl Neuropsychol.* 1995;2(3–4):167–169.

124. Shores EA, Lammél A, Hullick C, et al. The diagnostic accuracy of the Revised Westmead PTA Scale as an adjunct to the Glasgow Coma Scale in the early identification of cognitive impairment in patients with mild traumatic brain injury. *J Neurol Neurosurg Psychiatr.* 2008;79(10):1100–1106.

125. Ponsford J, Willmott C, Rothwell A, Kelly AM, Nelms R, Ng KT. Use of the Westmead PTA scale to monitor recovery after mild head injury. *Brain Inj.* 2004;18(6):603–614.

126. Tate RL, Pfaff A, Baguley IJ, et al. A multicentre, randomised trial examining the effect of test procedures measuring emergence from post-traumatic amnesia. *J Neurol Neurosurg Psychiatr.* 2006;77(7):841–849.

127. Maas AIR, Steyerberg EW, Butcher I, et al. Prognostic value of computerized tomography scan characteristics in traumatic brain injury: results from the IMPACT study. *J Neurotrauma.* 2007;24(2):303–314.

128. Maas AI, Hukkelhoven CW, Marshall LF, Steyerberg EW. Prediction of outcome in traumatic brain injury with computed tomographic characteristics: a comparison between the computed tomographic classification and combinations of computed tomographic predictors. *Neruosurgery.* 2005;57(6):1173–1182.

129. Orrison WW, Gentry LR, Stimac GK, Tarrel RM, Espinosa MC, Cobb LC. Blinded comparison of cranial CT and MR in closed head injury evaluation. *AJNR Am J Neuroradiol.* 1994;15(2):351–356.

130. Paterakis K, Karantanas AH, Komnos A, Volikas Z. Outcome of patients with diffuse axonal injury: the significance and prognostic value of MRI in the acute phase. *J Trauma.* 2000;49(6):1071–1075.

131. Yokota H, Kurokawa A, Otsuka T, Kobayashi S, Nakazawa S. Significance of magnetic resonance imaging in acute head injury. *J Trauma.* 1991;31(3):351–357.

132. Jeter CB, Hergenroeder GW, Hylin MJ, Redell JB, Moore AN, Dash PK. Biomarkers for the diagnosis and prognosis of mild traumatic brain injury/concussion. *J Neurotrauma.* 2012 121012222107005. https://doi.org/10.1089/neu.2012.2439.

133. Gardner A, Iverson GL, Stanwell P. A systematic review of proton magnetic resonance spectroscopy findings in sport-related concussion. *J Neurotrauma.* 2014;31(1):1–18.

134. Hunter JV, Wilde EA, Tong KA, Holshouser BA. Emerging imaging tools for use with traumatic brain injury research. *J Neurotrauma.* 2012;29(4):654–671.

135. Shenton ME, Hamoda HM, Schneiderman JS, et al. A review of magnetic resonance imaging and diffusion tensor imaging findings in mild traumatic brain injury. *Brain Imaging Behav.* 2012;6(2):137–192. http://www.pu bmedcentral.nih.gov/articlerender.fcgi?artid=3803157& tool=pmcentrez&rendertype=abstract.

136. Kim J, Whyte J, Patel S, et al. Resting cerebral blood flow alterations in chronic traumatic brain injury: an arterial spin labeling perfusion FMRI study. *J Neurotrauma.* 2010;27(8):1399–1411.

137. Maugans TA, Farley C, Altaye M, Leach J, Cecil KM. Pediatric sports-related concussion produces cerebral blood flow alterations. *Pediatrics.* 2012;129(1):28–37.

138. Taylor C, Bell J, Breiding M, Xu L. Traumatic brain injury-related emergency department visits, hospitalizations, and deaths – United States, 2007 and 2013. *MMWR Surveill Summ.* 2017;66(9):1–16.

139. Gillespie LD, Robertson M, Gillespie W, et al. Interventions for preventing falls in older people living in the community (Review). *Cochrane Database Syst Rev.* 2012;(9).

140. Stevens J, Phelan E. Development of STEADI: a fall prevention resource for health care providers. *Health Promot Pract.* 2013;14(5):706–714.

141. Kraus JF, Peek C, McArthur DL, Williams A. The effect of the 1992 California motorcycle helmet use law on motorcycle crash fatalities and injuries. *JAMA.* 1994;272(19):1506–1511.

142. Muller A. Florida's motorcycle helmet law repeal and fatality rates. *Am J Public Health.* 2004;94(4):556–558. https://doi.org/10.2105/AJPH.94.4.556.

143. Konda S, Reichard A, Tiesman H, Hendricks S. Non-fatal work-related traumatic brain injuries treated in US hospital emergency departments, 1998-2007. *Inj Prev J Int Soc Child Adolesc Inj Prev.* 2015;21(2):115–120.

CHAPTER 17

Neuroprosthetics

SHEITAL BAVISHI, DO • JOSEPH ROSENTHAL, MD, MPH •
MARCIA BOCKBRADER, MD, PHD

INTRODUCTION

A neuroprosthetic is any device that can enhance the input or output of a neural system. Although some neuroprosthetics, such as cochlear implants and visual prosthetics, have been around since the 1950s, they are just beginning to emerge as viable interventions in the field of brain injury. Neuroprosthetics encompass a variety of artificial devices or systems that can be used to enhance the motor, sensory, cognitive, visual, auditory, and communicative deficits that arise from acquired brain injuries (ABIs). These include assistive technology (AT), functional electrical stimulation (FES), myoelectric prostheses, robotics, virtual reality (VR) gaming, and brain stimulation. Neuromodulation consists of extracranial stimulation devices such as transcranial direct current stimulation (tDCS) and transcranial magnetic stimulation (TMS) or implanted devices such as brain-computer interfaces (BCIs) and deep brain stimulators. The objective of neuroprosthetics is to allow brain-injured people to participate in everyday life and enhance the quality of life.[1] In this chapter, we will review the different types of neuroprosthetics and their use in brain injury rehabilitation and recovery.

ASSISTIVE TECHNOLOGY, AUGMENTATIVE AND ALTERNATIVE COMMUNICATION, INFORMATION AND COMMUNICATION TECHNOLOGIES

Patients who sustain traumatic brain injuries (TBIs) often will have significant functional limitations due to physical, cognitive, and communication sequelae. These limitations may make it difficult to live independently, interact with their environment, or communicate their needs. They may have trouble turning on lights, answering the phone, using the television, and controlling the thermostat. Electronic devices have been developed to allow persons with such limitations more independence. Other devices can be used to help

those with cognitive deficits remember to take their medicine, be reminded to complete tasks, or take notes and lists.

AT is any item, piece of equipment, or product, which can be acquired commercially, modified, or customized, used to increase, maintain, or improve the functional capabilities of individuals. Augmentative and alternative communication (AAC) includes tools, systems, and strategies that are used specifically to assist or support communication. Information and communications technology (ICT) includes technology such as email, internet, and mobile phones that enable users to access, store, transmit, and manipulate information (Table 17.1).[2]

Switches

Switches are devices that can be connected to other devices to control them. They come in various styles, esthetics, and functionality. Switches can be simple or more complex and can be activated in different ways (push, pull, sip puff, pressing, blinking). Simple versions may use buttons or joysticks. More complex ones involve pressure change devices activated by air movement controlled by the mouth or eye gaze systems. Switches can be generic, connect to various devices with adapter cords, or be designed with a specific functionality for a device. Single switches are less physically demanding, but they are slower when there are more options to scan. On the other hand, multiswitch scanning is more cognitively and physically complicated but allows the options to be organized in such ways that choices can be made faster.

Choosing the most appropriate switch depends on multiple variables. The patient's cognitive and physical abilities, complexity of what is being controlled, cost, and mounting options should be considered. Often, multiple switches will need to be trialed before settling on the best option. Utilizing an AT center or library can allow patients to try different switches before purchasing.

TABLE 17.1 Types of Devices	
Assistive technology	Low tech: Planners/organizers Calendars Journals Switches High tech: Personal digital assistant Digital voice recorders Computers Cameras Smart phones Environmental control devices
Augmentative and alternative communication	Low Tech: Communication boards Yes/No buttons High Tech: Text to talk Eye gaze systems
Information and communication technologies	Tablets Computers Internet Mobile apps Telerehabilitation

Environmental Control

To live independently or to be left alone, a person must be able to interact with his or her environment. Lights need to be turned on and off, electronics need to be activated, and the thermostat needs to be controlled. A person with significant physical and mobility impairments may find it difficult to get to devices or may not have the dexterity to control them. More complicated devices like electronic thermostats may be difficult to operate for patients with cognitive impairments. Therefore to be able to control their environment, patients with TBIs may need devices designed to simplify environmental control.

Multiple commercial products have been developed that allow control over lights and electronics by a single device. Electronic devices are now sold as "smart devices" and are able to be remotely controlled by a single device. Apps have been developed that allow users to use their smartphones, electronic tablets, and computers to remotely control devices throughout their homes, including lights, alarm systems, thermostats, and televisions. Devices that are not designed to be remotely controlled can be plugged into electronic switches that can be controlled remotely, essentially turning them into smart devices.

Voice-activated devices are becoming more commercially available. Products that connect to multiple smart devices throughout a home environment allow people to speak commands to activate them (e.g., Amazon Alexa, Google Home). This allows patients with significant physical impairments to manage their environment around them without the assistance of others.

Not all patients with TBIs will be able to utilize all environmental control products. Patients with physical impairments such as severe ataxia or tetraparesis may be limited in what devices they can physically utilize. Those with severe cognitive deficits may not be able to understand how to access and utilize the centralized remote device. Patients with significant verbal communication impairments, such as aphasia and dysarthria, would be limited in the use of voice activation products. Therefore a thorough assessment of a patient's needs and abilities is crucial to advise and prescribe which devices may increase a patient's independence.

Electronic Memory Aids

Cognitive deficits after TBI are quite common. Problems with memory, attention, and executive function are common and can significantly limit an individual's independence. More and more, technology is being used to compensate. Some devices have been adapted to help, whereas others have been specifically designed to fill a specific need. These devices come in various styles. Some have a single purpose, whereas others, such as smartphones, are more complex and have multiple functions.

Multiple types of devices can be used for reminders. Alarms can be set on watches and mobile phones to remind someone to complete a task. Smartphone and tablet apps allow reminder alarms to be set. Some pill boxes come with alarms to remind patients to take their medications on time.

To help with memory, devices such as smartphones, tablets, and personal digital assistants (PDA) can be used to create lists and take notes. Some can even transcribe, eliminating the need to manually type in the information. There is good evidence that devices such as PDAs and smartphones, when used as cognitive aids, improve independence and confidence for individuals who have had TBIs. Studies have shown that use of devices can achieve higher memory goals and increase completion of tasks.[3,3a] Individuals with TBIs report general satisfaction with use of these devices as compensatory memory aids.[4] Digital recorders allow lectures, meetings, and appointments to be recorded and reviewed later. For individuals with attention, memory, and processing speed difficulties, these devices allow them to focus on the speaker instead of taking notes and review the information multiple times.

Considerations for Assistive Technology, Augmentative and Alternative Communication, and Information and Communications Technologies

Use of AT, AAC, and ICT devices requires evaluation of factors that influence the successful use of these devices. Barriers, facilitators, preferred features, and desirable functions need to be assessed before recommending or using an AT or AAC device. Common barriers to successful use could be physical factors (vision, fine motor skills, etc.), cognitive factors (memory, executive function, etc.), psychosocial factors, access to device and funding, support team, and reliability. Facilitators to successful use could be motivation, training, support team, consumer involvement about choice of device, individualized approach (goals and needs), funding, ongoing assessment and reevaluation, etc. Features that need to be considered are ease of use, capacity for storage, and congruency with needs. Therefore proper assessment with an AAC trained therapist is recommended, and ongoing training, repetition, and visits are recommended for both the brain-injured person and the caregiver/support team.[2]

FUNCTIONAL ELECTRICAL STIMULATION AND NEUROMUSCULAR ELECTRICAL STIMULATION

There are various types of noninvasive neuroprosthetic devices that have been developed to stimulate muscles and nerves to increase strength and improve function. These devices are typically used in individuals with upper motor neuron lesions such as TBI, stroke, cerebral palsy, spinal cord injury, and multiple sclerosis because the peripheral nerves need to be intact. Neuromuscular electrical stimulation (NMES) is used to strengthen muscles weakened from disuse and central nervous system injuries. FES is used to stimulate specific muscles to improve a specific function (i.e., grasp or ambulation) in neurologically impaired individuals.

NMES devices are most often small and portable, although some products combine exercise equipment (i.e., stationary bikes) with the NMES devices to increase efficacy. The electrodes that stimulate the muscles are attached to the device using long wires. These electrodes are placed over the targeted muscle groups and then turned on. Muscles are then strengthened by pulsed stimulations. The intensity and frequency of the pulses can be adjusted based on muscle size and patient tolerance. Various muscle groups throughout the limbs can be exercised. There are two types of NMES devices. Cyclic devices, when turned on, send repetitive stimulation signals. They will continue to activate in a repetitive pattern until turned off, and voluntary activation is not required. Electromyography (EMG)-mediated devices stimulate when the patient attempts to volitionally activate specific muscles, providing full activation of the desired movement.

Commercial devices have even been developed that are used to strengthen and improve the coordination of throat muscles used for swallowing in cases of dysphagia. Devices such as VitalStim (DJO Global) have shown improved outcomes over traditional swallow rehabilitation.[5]

FES devices target specific weaknesses and functional deficits. For example, there are commercial devices that treat foot drop by stimulating the common peroneal nerve to activate dorsiflexion during the step phase of gait. Two such devices are the NESS L300 Foot Drop System made by Bioness Inc. and the WalkAide made by Innovative Neurotronics. These devices have been shown to be at least equivalent to ankle-foot orthoses in terms of gait speed, balance, and mobility scores in patients with ABI.[6] They can reduce falls and can have a positive effect on spasticity.[7,8] There is also evidence that use of FES can actually promote neuroplasticity.[9,10] Although more expensive than AFOs, these devices can be used for long term and can be cost-effective neuroprosthetic devices for the treatment of dropped foot.[11]

Other devices have been developed to improve the grip strength and function by stimulating muscles in the forearm. One example is the NESS H200 Wireless Hand Rehabilitation System made by Bioness Inc. Patients place their hand and forearm in the device, and specially placed sensors measure the electrical activity and stimulate to augment the desired actions of the hand and wrist. Small studies have shown that patients with upper extremity hemiparesis after stroke have improved functional outcomes when incorporating FES into their rehabilitation program.[12,13] There is even evidence that use of FES in upper extremity paresis can induce cortical changes in patients with chronic stroke.[14]

Although generally considered safe, NMES and FES should be used with caution in patients with metal implants and cardiac pacemakers and in those unable to respond to painful stimuli. The use of these devices is contraindicated in patients with implanted defibrillators.

Myoelectric Prostheses

Individuals with weak function may benefit from the use of myoelectric orthotics, such as the MyoPro elbow/wrist/hand orthotic, developed by Myomo. This device supports the upper limb, and when it senses muscle activity, it turns on motors that move the limb in the desired motion. It has been shown to improve upper limb function in patients with chronic stroke, and use of the device showed greater improvement in rehabilitation measures than standard repetitive task-specific therapy.[15,16] Although no studies have been conducted on patients with upper limb paresis after TBI, these patients may benefit from the device to improve function and independence.

PERIPHERAL NERVE STIMULATION FOR PAIN RELIEF

Neurostimulation of sensory nerves is a promising modality to manage difficult-to-treat pain. Although these devices are technically not neuroprosthetics, they are worth mentioning here because of the similarities to motor nerve stimulators. There are multiple pain conditions associated with TBI. Headaches, complex regional pain syndrome, and hemiparetic shoulder pain are commonly seen after TBI. These pain syndromes are often very difficult to treat. Various neuromodulation devices have been developed to nonpharmacologically manage pain. These devices will be discussed in more detail in the Chapter 12 on pain.

ROBOTICS

The use of robotic technology for mobility, movement, and rehabilitation is relatively new, but it is potentially a new frontier for patients with neurologic injury, including TBI. There are devices for both the upper and lower limbs with various functionalities. Some are used strictly as therapy rehabilitation tools to promote recovery, whereas others are used as functional devices to improve function. Most important, the devices can be adjusted to fit the patient's needs. Some of the devices have smart technology that adjust the therapies as the patient progresses. Multiple commercially available upper limb devices have been developed that mobilize or promote recovery in elbows, wrists, and hands. Although evidence does show benefit from these devices, the literature has yet to show superiority in functional recovery to conventional upper limb therapy.[17] Other devices have been developed to help patients with paraplegia from spinal cord injury stand and ambulate.

Robotic devices have been developed that incorporate multiple therapeutic strategies into one device for rehabilitation of patients with various neurologic injuries. The Lokomat consists of multiple components including a computer-controlled, powered gait orthosis with motors at each hip and knee joint, a bodyweight support system (BWSS), and a treadmill. Another option is the G-EO; this device also has a BWSS, but instead of a treadmill and exoskeleton, the feet are placed onto moving platforms that simulate ankle, knee, and hip movements of a normal gait pattern. The device is activated when the patient attempts to move the leg and then augments the movement based on the patient's abilities. A unique feature of this type of device is that unlike treadmill training, it allows simulation of stair climbing. Both these types of devices eliminate the need for therapist manpower to assist in movement of the legs during gait training. The literature for use of robotic devices in ambulation is limited, and some controversy exists regarding its superiority to conventional gait therapy in patients with stroke.[18] However, there is evidence that these devices do improve some functional gait measures in patients with TBI while limiting therapist burden.[19]

VIDEO GAMING

Advanced technology for rehabilitation is emerging to enhance conventional therapy paradigms. Video game therapy is being used for motor and cognitive recovery in ABI rehabilitation. Commercially available products have been the forefront of research for video game therapy and are regularly being used in in- and outpatient rehabilitation settings. Video game therapy not only provides additional modalities for improving recovery but also makes therapy fun and improves participation.[20]

Gaming Systems and Computer-Based Systems

Various gaming systems and computer-based systems are available in the market today. Each has technology that can be used for rehabilitation purposes such as balance, hand-eye coordination, visual perception, endurance, and cognition. Video game therapy has been compared to conventional therapy and noted to have improved outcomes for balance and attention in small sample sizes.[21]

Virtual Reality

As opposed to conventional gaming, VR can enhance rehabilitation techniques in real-world environments.

The traditional rehabilitation model is in a gym or clinic setting and cannot place patients in real-world situations. Increasing studies have been incorporating VR into various interventions to allow for opportunities to practice different skills while in a safe/controlled environment.[22] VR can reliably be used to assess Instrumental Activities of Daily Living (IADL) in patients with TBI in a virtual kitchen.[23] VR can provide an immersive environment in which patients can practice cognitive strategies in everyday situations. Specifically, clinicians have been attempting to utilize VR to replicate various scenarios, including shopping at the supermarket, using an ATM, cooking, and driving, to increase the generalizability of strategies in day-to-day scenarios.

Small studies have proved the efficacy of VR in improving walking abilities in children with ABI.[24] Current studies in VR are focusing on feasibility,[25] knowledge translation,[26] and VR environment assessment and development.[27] Development of VR environments that could be used for cognitive and functional rehabilitation is currently the focus of research.

NEUROMODULATION

Fundamentally, neuromodulatory stimulation affects neural activity and, ultimately, behavior through electromagnetic or mechanical modulation of neuronal membrane potentials of the brain. These changes in membrane potential can suppress or enhance firing in neural circuits, altering brain connections and modulating behaviors. Currently, various techniques in neuromodulation such as tDCS, TMS, deep brain stimulation (DBS), transcranial focused ultrasound stimulation (TFUS), and BCIs are being studied to enhance motor and cognitive function in TBI.

In transcranial electric stimulation, scalp surface electrodes generate electrical fields and associated electrical currents (current density field) in the head. TMS uses Faraday's principle to induce electrical currents within the head from magnetic field pulses produced by a coil at the scalp. TFUS uses a piezoelectric crystal to generate high-frequency sound waves at the scalp that penetrate to deep brain structures and mechanically deform and depolarize neural membranes. Implanted microelectrodes can record local electrical field potentials or apply local electrical currents to monitor or modify brain activity.

Brain stimulation is hypothesized to augment neurorehabilitation after brain injury by enhancing plasticity, leading to use-dependent reorganization of connections between brain regions and improved level of function.[28–30] Other mechanisms associated

TABLE 17.2
Brain Stimulation Definitions

Brain Stimulation	Definition
Transcranial magnetic stimulation	Focal, noninvasive brain stimulation that induces a hyperpolarizing or depolarizing electrical field in the brain through brief magnetic pulse(s) applied at the scalp
Transcranial direct current stimulation	Diffuse, noninvasive brain stimulation that modulates the excitability of underlying brain tissue through weak, constant, electrical current applied at the scalp
Deep brain stimulation	Local electrical stimulation of deep brain structures, e.g., thalamus, with surgically implanted electrodes and pulse generator
Transcranial focused ultrasound stimulation	Focal, noninvasive brain stimulation that induces neural depolarization through mechanical perturbation of membranes with high-frequency, low-intensity sound waves
Vagal nerve stimulation	Local stimulation of the vagus nerve at the neck with surgically implanted electrodes and pulse generator

with brain stimulation that may contribute to recovery of function include downregulation of cortical hyperexcitability and suppression of maladaptive plasticity.[31] In addition to modulating excitability within cortical brain circuits, brain stimulation may also cause widespread changes in cerebral blood flow, altering and potentially normalizing the delivery of oxygen and nutrients.[32] Specific treatment effects depend on both stimulation parameters (e.g., intensity, duration, frequency, anatomic site) and patient factors (e.g., medications, genetics, anatomy, time since injury) (Table 17.2).

Transcranial Magnetic Stimulation

TMS is a promising, but experimental, treatment for sequelae of TBI. Open-label studies in mild TBI suggest that left dorsolateral prefrontal cortex (DLPFC) repetitive TMS (rTMS) may improve postconcussive symptoms and headache.[33,34] In addition, several single case reports indicate transient improvement in alertness and command following for patients with disorders of consciousness (DOC) who receive motor cortex (M1) TMS [35,36] or DLPFC TMS,[37,38] although another reported no significant difference in command following between M1 rTMS and sham.[39] There are also mixed findings for the effect of rTMS on post-TBI mood disturbance. Single case reports suggest that 20–30 sessions of low-frequency, inhibitory rTMS to the right DLPFC (with or without excitatory, high-frequency left DLPFC stimulation) may reduce depressive symptoms in mild[40] and severe TBI.[41] However, treatment of suicidal depression in mild TBI with nine sessions of left-sided, excitatory, prefrontal rTMS was not better than sham in a pilot study.[42] Limited evidence from case reports also exists for improved cognitive function with TMS: posttraumatic neurologic neglect improved in a patient receiving left posterior parietal theta burst stimulation[43] and executive dysfunction improved in a patient with chronic TBI with right and left hemisphere frontotemporal rTMS.[44] Additional case reports have demonstrated resolution of posttraumatic musical hallucinations[45] and tinnitus[46] with 10 sessions of low-frequency rTMS. No randomized clinical trials have yet been completed to establish the effects of TMS on cognition,[47] mood, headache, or DOC after TBI; determine optimal stimulation parameters; or identify relevant patient selection criteria. TMS is usually safe and well tolerated, even among patients with brain injury.[40] However, high-frequency, excitatory rTMS is associated with an increased risk of seizures, and two case reports have described TMS-associated seizure events.[38,48]

Transcranial Direct Current Stimulation

tDCS appears to be safe for patients with TBI, with no associated seizures reported and side effects limited to those seen in healthy individuals, including tingling skin sensations, drowsiness, headache, and dizziness.[49–51] tDCS has been studied for posttraumatic headache, TBI-related cognitive and motor impairments, and posttraumatic DOC. A retrospective, open-label study of 44 adolescents with chronic posttraumatic headache demonstrated improvement in headache duration, intensity, and severity with five to nine sessions of frontal, anodal tDCS (0.6–0.9 mA for 30–45 min).[52] However, improvement in postconcussive symptoms in a randomized controlled trial has not yet been shown.[53] In a case series, anodal M1 tDCS (n = 2, 1.5 mA for 15 min) combined with physical therapy produced clinically significant motor improvement in the upper limb Fugl-Meyer test.[54] Improvements for working memory and attention with DLPFC anodal tDCS have also been shown in randomized, double-blind, sham-controlled trials (n = 26, 20 sessions of 1 mA for 20 min[55]; n = 32, 20 sessions of 2 mA for

20 min[56]) and randomized, sham-controlled crossover studies (n = 4, 1 session of 2 mA for 20 min[57]; n = 9, 1 session of 2 mA for 20 min[58]). However, a randomized, sham-controlled trial of left DLPFC anodal tDCS with low dose and short stimulation duration (n = 21, 1 mA for 10 min for 15 sessions[59]) did not improve memory or attention better than sham. Several studies suggest that anodal tDCS may also improve arousal and command following for some patients with TBI with DOC (n = 2 minimally conscious state [MCS], n = 3 vegetative state [VS][60]; n = 19 MCS, n = 6 VS[61]; n = 5 MCS, n = 5 VS[62]), but large randomized controlled trials in DOC have not yet been completed. Patient characteristics, including degree of sparing of cortical connectivity post-TBI, are thought to underlie the differential response of MCS and VS to tDCS, leading to different rates of emergence to consciousness. Furthermore, individual differences in brain anatomy associated with TBI, e.g., posttraumatic skull defects, lesions that increase cerebrospinal fluid relative to brain volume, and presence of shunt hardware, alter current flow and may necessitate prestimulation current density modeling to optimize stimulation parameters to the patient.[63]

Deep Brain Stimulation

Case reports provide limited evidence for DBS effects on posttraumatic DOC, pain, movement disorders, and behavioral disturbances, but no randomized controlled trials of DBS in TBI have been completed. A total of seven TBI cases have been reported with DBS for MCS (n = 3[64]; n = 3[65]; n = 1[66,67]), most of whom had the implant in the thalamus and emerged to a conscious state. A total of 40 TBI cases have been reported with thalamic or reticular formation DBS for VS (n = 8[68]; n = 23[69]; n = 9[65,70]). Although less than half of the VS cohort emerged to a conscious state, one group[68,69] reported a better recovery rate among nine patients with TBI in VS with DBS than 18 patients with TBI in VS and no DBS. Conversely, Cohadon[70] proposed that failure to respond clinically to thalamic DBS signified loss of cortical connectivity predictive of irreversible VS. DBS parameters for posttraumatic movement disorders are based on Food and Drug Administration (FDA)-approved protocols for essential tremor and Parkinson disease, with similar complications and rates of success. Six cases of TBI with thalamic or internal globus pallidus (GPi) DBS for dystonia have been reported (n = 1[71]; n = 1[72]; n = 4[73]), all of whom improved, but many had postsurgical complications or unwanted stimulation side effects. Twelve cases of TBI with GPi or ventralis intermedius nucleus DBS for tremor have been reported (n = 3[74]; n = 1[75]; n = 5[76]; n = 1[77]; n = 1[78]), most of whom improved with DBS. Two cases of TBI with DBS for pain (n = 1 GPi[79]; n = 1 precentral gyrus[80]) and five cases of TBI for behavioral modification (n = 1 posterior hypothalamus[81]; n = 4 bilateral nucleus accumbens and anterior limb of internal capsule[82]) have been reported, all with improvement in symptoms.

Transcranial Focused Ultrasound Stimulation

TFUS is an emerging technology with the potential to modulate activity in deep brain structures without the morbidity associated with neurosurgery. One case report of low-intensity, thalamic TFUS for MCS after acute, severe TBI has been reported (n = 1).[83] The patient emerged to consciousness 3 days posttreatment, although it is unclear whether recovery was spontaneous or a treatment effect. No randomized controlled trials of TFUS in TBI have been completed, and long-term outcomes of TFUS are unknown.

Vagal Nerve Stimulation

Vagal nerve stimulation (VNS) is approved in humans for treatment-refractory depression and epilepsy.[84]

Preclinical trials have demonstrated the potential to facilitate motor and cognitive recovery after TBI with VNS, but no TBI-specific clinical trials have been completed.[85,86] Potential adverse events associated with VNS are related to postoperative complications (e.g., infection, device failure) or stimulation side effects (e.g., vocal cord paralysis, cough, dyspnea, facial weakness). The left vagus nerve is preferentially used for stimulation to minimize the effects on cardiac function.

Summary

Brain stimulation methods, including TMS, tDCS, DBS, epidural or subdural cortical stimulation, TFUS, and VNS have not been cleared by the FDA for clinical use and remain investigational. As a result, expert consensus is to provide these treatments to patients with TBI only in the context of clinical trials or for palliation of medically intractable syndromes when all other options are exhausted.

BRAIN-COMPUTER INTERFACES

BCI systems are composed of electrodes that stimulate or record neural activity, a signal processing and decoding module, and an environmental interface to capture or produce changes in physical states that are also experienced by others, facilitating communication of thoughts, social interaction, and reaction to and control over the physical world. Electrodes may range from large and noninvasive, e.g., scalp electroencephalography (EEG) montages or transcutaneous EMG arrays, to subdural or epidural electrocorticography (eCoG) grids and small, implanted, intracortical or deep brain microelectrode arrays (MEA). MEAs stimulate and record from very focal areas, with the potential for single-neuron resolution. Noninvasive electrodes stimulate and record from distributed networks, with the potential for detecting and modulating population responses in neural circuits. EEG-based BCI systems have been used to enable communication by patients who are "locked in" and unable to speak or move using event-related potentials (e.g., P300[87]), steady-state evoked potentials,[88] event-related desynchronization,[89] or hybrid combinations of these.[90] EEG-based BCI has been successfully used in clinical trials to spell letters on a computer screen, play VR games,[91] control power chairs, and for other tasks. eCoG and intracortical MEA-based BCI systems have been used by paralyzed individuals to control computer cursors,[92] robotic arms,[93] exoskeletons,[94] as well as evoked movements of their own paralyzed limbs (Table 17.3).[98]

Brain-Computer Interfaces in Traumatic Brain Injury

Although visual dysfunction, auditory dysfunction, and neuromotor deficits are common after TBI, there have been no reported studies trialing cochlear or brainstem auditory implants, visual neuroprosthetics, or BCI for motor control after TBI.[99] TBI has been seen as a relative contraindication for implanted sensorimotor BCI systems, although this attitude may be changing. Defense Advanced Research Projects Agency (DARPA) has recognized the need for BCI neuroprosthetics to address memory impairments after TBI[100] and has funded the development of a hippocampal neuroprosthetic that is currently being tested in animals.[101] Other groups have demonstrated that a cortico-cortico BCI can functionally relink premotor and somatosensory activity after TBI, restoring upper limb reaching and grasping ability in rats.[102] These innovative technologies are not yet ready for human trials but have the potential to augment neurorecovery after TBI beyond the brain's intrinsic ability to heal. BCI systems are being used in pilot trials to help identify patients with DOC with residual cognitive function who appear behaviorally unresponsive on the Coma Recovery Scale- Revised. EEG-based systems that were originally developed for tetraplegic or "locked-in" patients have been adapted for the DOC TBI

TABLE 17.3 Definitions	
BCI	Neuroprosthetic device that replaces biological motor output pathways from the brain, sensory input pathways to the brain, or cognitive processes mediated by connections within the central nervous system, allowing the user to interact freely with his or her environment. Different BCI systems may bypass, replace, or compensate for lost sensorimotor, visual, auditory, cognitive, affective, or volitional functions of an individual[95]
Cochlear implant	Type of BCI that transduces pressure changes associated with sound waves into electrical auditory nerve stimulation, which evokes auditory cortex activity and the subjective perception of sound. Cochlear implants are used to restore hearing to patients with damaged sensory hair cells[96]
Visual neuro-prosthetic	Type of BCI that captures visual images with a camera, encodes visual information in electrical stimulation patterns of visual pathway neurons, and evokes neural activity in the visual cortex associated with the subjective perception of shape, motion, depth, and other visual information[97] Visual neuroprosthetic devices are used to restore vision to blind patients

BCI, brain-computer interface.

population.[103] Due to intrinsic cognitive, attentional, and arousal deficits in TBI, these BCI implementations have prioritized simplicity and real-time audiovisual feedback to motivate and engage users.[104,105] In addition, lessons from clinical trials of BCI systems with "locked-in" patients emphasize the need for user-centered design to minimize cognitive workload and optimize the interface to the strengths of the user.[106] In the first case series, one patient with TBI in MCS used an EEG-based BCI to accurately distinguish left from right using imagined hand versus foot movements.[104] In the second experiment, of two patients, one with TBI-MCS was accurately able to use a hybrid Steady State Visual Evoked Potentials (SSVEP) and P300 BCI to selectively attend to one of two cued photographs, whereas the patient with TBI-VS was unable to perform better than chance.[107] A hybrid BCI was also used to evaluate the ability to recognize, compare, and compute numbers by selectively attending to one of two numbers on a screen. Two of six patients in VS, two of three patients in MCS, and two of two patients who had emerged from DOC performed the task significantly better than chance with the BCI.[108] Last, an EEG-based BCI was used to evaluate yes or no accuracy to CRS-R-style questions in two patients with TBI-MCS and two patients with TBI-VS. Both patients with MCS and none of the patients with VS accurately distinguished yes from no using BCI responses to audiovisual cues and feedback.[109] These small studies suggest that many patients with TBI in MCS have sufficient capacity for sustained attention, two alternative forced choice response selection, working memory, language comprehension, and visual or auditory acuity to use the BCI for functional communication.

Summary

Closed-loop BCI systems that restore intracortical connections and facilitate memory encoding are an emerging technology that may provide cybernetic hope for enhanced recovery after TBI. Audiovisually engaging, EEG-based BCI systems offer a means to communicate with behaviorally unresponsive patients in MCS. Neuroprosthetics for sensory dysfunction or paralysis have not been evaluated in TBI.

ETHICAL ISSUES

Ethical considerations in neuroprosthetics surround risk versus benefit, selection criteria, and access. Risk versus benefit considerations include potential benefits of altering neural circuits versus risk of neurophysiologic and psychologic sequelae.[95] For example, cochlear implants and visual prosthetics are beneficial because they improve deafness[96] and blindness,[97] respectively, and can allow a person to have improved independence. However, sudden change in hearing or seeing for an individual can create difficulty with adjustment to different sensory and experiential worlds. This adjustment in behavior can be beneficial or detrimental to people who have regained hearing or sight depending on the extent to which they have to reconstruct their conception of the world and their image of self.

Risk versus benefit for implantable devices such as DBS are even more complicated. DBS can be beneficial when used to enhance motor control, arousal, cognition, mood, and motivation.[66,67,82] However, neurosurgical implantation involves serious risks, including intra- or postoperative complications, e.g., infection, seizures, intracranial hemorrhage, cerebral edema, and device malfunction; unwanted side effects of stimulation, i.e., hypomania, compulsive behaviors, suicidality, sensorimotor changes, and cognitive deficits; as well as the risk of the intervention having no benefit. Furthermore, when used for psychiatric sequelae of TBI, concerns involving capacity for informed consent must be addressed—including uncertainties over whether a given patient has the capacity to give consent for the procedure and whether the capacity level depends on device utilization. In addition, both DBS and BCI-mediated cognition and behaviors raise philosophical (and potentially legal) questions about whether the person is thinking and acting through his or her own free will or the device is controlling the thoughts and behaviors outside of a person's conscious awareness.[95]

Finally, there are ethical concerns about access to care and subject selection for neuroprosthetics or neuromodulation with devices such as tDCS, TMS, BCI systems, FES, and Myopro. Appropriate selection criteria to optimize treatment effects for tDCS, and indeed most of the interventions, remain to be elucidated. Furthermore, many of these treatments, although promising, remain investigational and can offer false hope to patients who do not benefit. Some devices are expensive and available only at large clinical centers during clinical trials or to economically advantaged individuals (e.g., TMS, BCI, Myopro) because treatments with them are often not covered by insurance companies. Social justice issues are therefore a concern because economically disadvantaged, underinsured, or regionally remote individuals who might otherwise benefit may not have access to facilities that have these devices. Alternatively, clinicians may be faced with decisions about whether it is ethical to trial someone on these devices in therapy knowing that home use would be economically prohibitive. Finally, some inexpensive and portable devices, such as tDCS, may be amenable to supervised home use or teletherapy.[110,111] However, proper supervision, training safeguards, education (including for stimulation techniques and locations for stimulation), caregiver support, and follow-up are essential, and as a result, not all patients with brain injury will be good candidates.

In summary, neuroprosthetics are an emerging technology that holds promise for neurorehabilitation, although ethical considerations should be weighed and discussed carefully with patients and families before trialing these devices for persons with TBI.

REFERENCES

1. Naik G. Emerging Theory and Practice in Neuroprosthetics. In: Naik G, Guo Y, eds. Hershey, PA: IGI Global; 2014: 1–8.
2. Brunner M, Hemsley B, Togher L, Palmer S. Technology and its role in rehabilitation for people with cognitive-communication disability following a traumatic brain injury. *Brain Inj.* 2017;31(8):1–16.
3. Dowd MM, Lee PH, Sheer JB, et al. Electronic reminding technology following traumatic brain injury: effects on timely task completion. *J Head Trauma Rehabil.* 2011; 26(5):339–347.
3a. Lannin N, Carr B, Allaous J, et al. A randomized controlled trial of effectiveness of handheld computers for improving everyday memory functioning in patients with memory impairments after acquired brain injury. *Clin Rehabil.* 2014;28(5):470–481.
4. Evald L. Prospective memory rehabilitation using smartphones in patients with TBI: what do participants report? *Neuropsychol Rehabil.* 2015;25(2):283–297.
5. Blumenfeld L, Hahn Y, Lepage A, et al. Transcutaneous electrical stimulation versus traditional dysphagia: a nonconcurrent cohort study. *Otolaryngol Head Neck Surg.* 2006;135(5):754–757.
6. Park JW, Kim Y, Oh JC, et al. Effortful swallowing training combined with electrical stimulation in post-stroke dysphagia: a randomized controlled study. *Dysphagia.* 2012;27(4):521–527.
7. Permsirivanich W, Tipchatyotin S, Wongchai M, et al. Comparing the effects of rehabilitation swallowing therapy vs neuromuscular electrical stimulation therapy among stroke patients with persistent pharyngeal dysphagia: a randomized controlled study. *J Med Assoc Thai.* 2009;92(2):259–265.
8. Bethoux F, Rogers HL, Nolan KJ, et al. The effects of peroneal nerve functional electrical stimulation versus ankle-foot orthosis in patients with chronic stroke: a randomized controlled study. *Neurorehabil Neural Repair.* 2014;28(7):668–697.
9. Gervasoni E, Parelli R, Uszynski M, et al. Effects of functional electrical stimulation on reducing falls and improving gait parameters in multiple sclerosis and stroke. *PM R.* 2017;9(4):339–347.
10. Sabut SK, Sikdar C, Kumar R, et al. Functional electrical stimulation of dorsiflexor muscle: effects on dorsiflexor strength, plantarflexor spasticity, and motor recovery in stroke patients. *Neurorehabilitation.* 2011;29(4): 393–400.
11. Everaert DG, Thompson AK, Chong SL, et al. Does functional electrical stimulation for foot drop strengthen corticospinal connections? *Neurorehabil Neural Repair.* 2010;24(2):168–177.
12. Cecatto RB, Maximino JR, Chadi G. Motor recovery and cortical plasticity after functional electrical stimulation in a rat model of focal stroke. *Am J Phys Med Rehabil.* 2014;93(9):791–800.

13. Taylor P, Humphreys L, Swain I. The long-term cost-effectiveness of the use of functional electrical stimulation for the correction of dropped foot due to upper motor neuron lesion. *J Rehabil Med*. 2013;45(2):154–160.

14. Ring H, Rosenthal N. Controlled study of neuroprosthetic functional electrical stimulation in sub-acute post-stroke rehabilitation. *J Rehabil Med*. 2005;37(1):32–36.

15. Alon G, Levitt AF, McCarthy PA. Functional electrical stimulation enhancement of upper extremity functional recovery during stroke rehabilitation: a pilot study. *Neurorehabil Neural Repair*. 2007;21(3):207–215.

16. Shin HK, Cho SH, Jeon HS, et al. Cortical effect and functional recovery by the electromyography-triggered neuromuscular stimulation in chronic stroke patients. *Neurosci Lett*. 2008;442(3):174–179.

17. Peters HT, Page SJ, Persch A. Giving them a hand: wearing a myoelectric elbow-wrist-hand orthosis reduces upper extremity impairment in chronic stroke. *Arch Phys Med Rehabil*. 2017. [epub ahead of print].

18. Page SJ, Hill V, White S. Portable upper extremity robotics is as efficacious as upper extremity rehabilitative therapy: a randomized controlled pilot trial. *Clin Rehabil*. 2013;27(6):494–503.

19. Kwakkel G, Kollen BJ, Krebs HI. Effects of robot-assisted therapy on upper limb recovery after stroke: a systemic review. *Neurorehabil Neural Repair*. 2008;22(2):111–121.

20. Bonnechère B, Jansen B, Omelina L, Van Sint Jan S. The use of commercial video games in rehabilitation: a systematic review. *Int J Rehabil Res*. 2016;39(4):277–290.

21. Straudi S, Severini G, Charabati AS, et al. The effects of video game therapy on balance and attention in chronic ambulatory traumatic brain injury: an exploratory study. *BMC Neurol*. 2017;17:86.

22. Besnard J, Richard P, Banville F, et al. Virtual reality and neuropsychological assessment: the reliability of a virtual kitchen to assess daily-life activities in victims of traumatic brain injury. *Appl Neuropsychol Adult*. 2016;23(3):223–235.

23. Kim BR, Chun MH, Kim LS, Park JY. Effect of virtual reality on cognition in stroke patients. *Ann Rehabil Med*. 2011;35(4):450–459.

24. Biffi E, Beretta E, Cesareo A, et al. An immersive virtual reality platform to enhance walking ability of children with acquired brain injuries. *Methods Inf Med*. 2017;56(2):119–126.

25. Salisbury DB, Dahdah M, Driver S, Parsons TD, Richter KM. Virtual reality and brain computer interface in neurorehabilitation. *Proc (Bayl Univ Med Cent)*. 2016;29(2):124–127.

26. Glegg SMN, Holsti L, Stanton S, et al. Evaluating change in virtual reality adoption for brain injury rehabilitation following knowledge translation. *Disabil Rehabil Assist Technol*. 2017;12(3):217–226.

27. Robitaille N, Jackson PL, Hébert LJ, et al. A Virtual Reality avatar interaction (VRai) platform to assess residual executive dysfunction in active military personnel with previous mild traumatic brain injury: proof of concept. *Disabil Rehabil Assist Technol*. 2017;12(7):758–764.

28. Bolognini N, Pascual-Leone A, Fregni F. Using non-invasive brain stimulation to augment motor training-induced plasticity. *J Neuroeng Rehabil*. 2009;6:8.

29. Li S, Zaninotto AL, Neville I, et al. Clinical utility of brain stimulation modalities following traumatic brain injury: current evidence. *Neuropsychiatr Dis Treat*. 2015;11:1573–1586.

30. Adkins DL. Cortical stimulation-induced structural plasticity and functional recovery after brain damage. In: Kobeissy FH, ed. *Brain Neurotrauma: Molecular, Neuropsychological, and Rehabilitation Aspects*. Boca Raton (FL): CRC Press/Taylor & Francis; 2015 [chapter 43].

31. Villamar MF, Santos Portilla A, Fregni F, Zafonte R. Noninvasive brain stimulation to modulate neuroplasticity in traumatic brain injury. *Neuromodulation*. 2012;15(4):326–338.

32. Takai H, Tsubaki A, Sugawara K, et al. Effect of transcranial direct current stimulation over the primary motor cortex on cerebral blood flow: a time course study using near-infrared spectroscopy. In: Elwell CE, Leung TS, Harrison DK, eds. *Oxygen Transport to Tissue XXXVII (Advances in Experimental Medicine and Biology*. vol. 876. New York (NY): Springer; 2016:335–341.

33. Koski L, Kolivakis T, Yu C, et al. Noninvasive brain stimulation for persistent postconcussion symptoms in mild traumatic brain injury. *J Neurotrauma*. 2015;32(1):38–44.

34. Leung A, Fallah A, Shukla S, et al. rTMS in alleviating mild TBI related headaches–a case series. *Pain Physician*. 2016;19(2):E347–E354.

35. Manganotti P, Formaggio E, Storti SF, et al. Effect of high-frequency repetitive transcranial magnetic stimulation on brain excitability in severely brain-injured patients in minimally conscious or vegetative state. *Brain Stimul*. 2013;6(6):913–921.

36. Pistoia F, Sacco S, Carolei A, Sarà M. Corticomotor facilitation in vegetative state: results of a pilot study. *Arch Phys Med Rehabil*. 2013;94(8):1599–1606.

37. Pape TLB, Rosenow J, Lewis G, et al. Repetitive transcranial magnetic stimulation-associated neurobehavioral gains during coma recovery. *Brain Stimul*. 2009;2(1):22–35.

38. Pape TLB, Rosenow JM, Patil V, et al. RTMS safety for two subjects with disordered consciousness after traumatic brain injury. *Brain Stimul*. 2014;7(4):620–622.

39. Giovannelli F, Chiaramonti R, Bianco G, et al. P699: lack of behavioural effects of high-frequency rTMS in vegetative state: a randomised, double blind, sham-controlled, cross-over study. *Clin Neurophysiol*. 2014;125:S243.

40. Fitzgerald PB, Hoy KE, Maller JJ, et al. Transcranial magnetic stimulation for depression after a traumatic brain injury: a case study. *J ECT*. 2011;27(1):38–40.

41. Nielson DM, McKnight CA, Patel RN, et al. Preliminary guidelines for safe and effective use of repetitive transcranial magnetic stimulation in moderate to severe traumatic brain injury. *Arch Phys Med Rehabil*. 2015;96(4):S138–S144.

42. George MS, Raman R, Benedek DM, et al. A two-site pilot randomized 3 day trial of high dose left prefrontal repetitive transcranial magnetic stimulation (rTMS) for suicidal inpatients. *Brain Stimul.* 2014;7(3):421–431.

43. Bonnì S, Mastropasqua C, Bozzali M, et al. Theta burst stimulation improves visuo-spatial attention in a patient with traumatic brain injury. *Neurol Sci.* 2013;34(11): 2053.

44. Pachalska M, Łukowicz M, Kropotov JD, et al. Evaluation of differentiated neurotherapy programs for a patient after severe TBI and long term coma using event-related potentials. *Med Sci Monit.* 2011;17(10):CS120.

45. Cosentino G, Giglia G, Palermo A, et al. A case of post-traumatic complex auditory hallucinosis treated with rTMS. *Neurocase.* 2010;16(3):267–272.

46. Kreuzer PM, Landgrebe M, Frank E, Langguth B. Repetitive transcranial magnetic stimulation for the treatment of chronic tinnitus after traumatic brain injury: a case study. *J Head Trauma Rehabil.* 2013;28:386–389.

47. Neville IS, Hayashi CY, Hajj SA, et al. Repetitive transcranial magnetic stimulation (rTMS) for the cognitive rehabilitation of traumatic brain injury (TBI) victims: study protocol for a randomized controlled trial. *Trials.* 2015;16(1):440.

48. Cavinato M, Iaia V, Piccione F. Repeated sessions of sub-threshold 20-Hz rTMS. Potential cumulative effects in a brain-injured patient. *Clin Neurophysiol.* 2012;123(9):1893–1895.

49. Fregni F, Nitsche MA, Loo CK, et al. Regulatory considerations for the clinical and research use of transcranial direct current stimulation (tDCS): review and recommendations from an expert panel. *Clin Res Regul Affairs.* 2015;32(1):22–35.

50. Bikson M, Grossman P, Thomas C, et al. Safety of transcranial direct current stimulation: evidence based update 2016. *Brain Stimul.* 2016;9(5):641–661.

51. Woods AJ, Antal A, Bikson M, et al. A technical guide to tDCS, and related non-invasive brain stimulation tools. *Clin Neurophysiol.* 2016;127(2):1031–1048.

52. Pinchuk D, Pinchuk O, Sirbiladze K, Shugar O. Clinical effectiveness of primary and secondary headache treatment by transcranial direct current stimulation. *Front Neurol.* 2013;4:25.

53. de Amorim RLO, Brunoni AR, de Oliveira MAF, et al. Transcranial direct current stimulation for post-concussion syndrome: study protocol for a randomized crossover trial. *Front Neurol.* 2017;8:164.

54. Middleton A, Fritz SL, Liuzzo DM, et al. Using clinical and robotic assessment tools to examine the feasibility of pairing tDCS with upper extremity physical therapy in patients with stroke and TBI: a consideration-of-concept pilot study. *Neurorehabilitation.* 2014;35(4): 741–754.

55. Ulam F, Shelton C, Richards L, et al. Cumulative effects of transcranial direct current stimulation on EEG oscillations and attention/working memory during subacute neurorehabilitation of traumatic brain injury. *Clin Neurophysiol.* 2015;126(3):486–496.

56. Sacco K, Galetto V, Dimitri D, et al. Concomitant use of transcranial direct current stimulation and computer-assisted training for the rehabilitation of attention in traumatic brain injured patients: behavioral and neuroimaging results. *Front Behav Neurosci.* 2016;10:57.

57. O'Neil-Pirozzi TM, Doruk D, Thomson JM, Fregni F. Immediate memory and electrophysiologic effects of prefrontal cortex transcranial direct current stimulation on neurotypical individuals and individuals with chronic traumatic brain injury: a pilot study. *Int J Neurosci.* 2017;127(7):592–600.

58. Kang EK, Kim DY, Paik NJ. Transcranial direct current stimulation of the left prefrontal cortex improves attention in patients with traumatic brain injury: a pilot study. *J Rehabil Med.* 2012;44(4):346–350.

59. Leśniak M, Polanowska K, Seniów J, Czlonkowska A. Effects of repeated anodal tDCS coupled with cognitive training for patients with severe traumatic brain injury: a pilot randomized controlled trial. *J Head Trauma Rehabil.* 2014;29(3):E20–E29.

60. Angelakis E, Liouta E, Andreadis N, et al. Transcranial direct current stimulation effects in disorders of consciousness. *Arch Phys Med Rehabil.* 2014;95(2):283–289.

61. Thibaut A, Bruno MA, Ledoux D, et al. tDCS in patients with disorders of consciousness Sham-controlled randomized double-blind study. *Neurology.* 2014;82(13): 1112–1118.

62. Naro A, Calabrò RS, Russo M, et al. Can transcranial direct current stimulation be useful in differentiating unresponsive wakefulness syndrome from minimally conscious state patients? *Restor Neurol Neurosci.* 2015;33(2): 159–176.

63. Datta A, Bikson M, Fregni F. Transcranial direct current stimulation in patients with skull defects and skull plates: high-resolution computational FEM study of factors altering cortical current flow. *Neuroimage.* 2010;52(4):1268–1278.

64. Hassler R, Ore GD, Bricolo A, et al. EEG and clinical arousal induced by bilateral long-term stimulation of pallidal systems in traumatic vigil coma. *Electroencephalogr Clin Neurophysiol.* 1969;27(7):689.

65. Yamamoto T, Katayama Y. Deep brain stimulation therapy for the vegetative state. *Neuropsychol Rehabil.* 2005;15(3–4):406–413.

66. Schiff ND, Giacino JT, Kalmar K, et al. Behavioural improvements with thalamic stimulation after severe traumatic brain injury. *Nature.* 2007;448(7153):600–603.

67. Giacino J, Fins JJ, Machado A, Schiff ND. Central thalamic deep brain stimulation to promote recovery from chronic posttraumatic minimally conscious state: challenges and opportunities. *Neuromodulation.* 2012;15(4):339–349.

68. Tsubokawa T, Yamamoto T, Katayama Y, et al. Deep-brain stimulation in a persistent vegetative state: follow-up results and criteria for selection of candidates. *Brain Inj.* 1990;4(4):315–327.

69. Yamamoto T, Katayama Y, Kobayashi K, et al. Deep brain stimulation for the treatment of vegetative state. *Eur J Neurosci.* 2010;32(7):1145–1151.

70. Cohadon F, Richer E. Deep brain stimulation in patients with post-traumatic persistent vegetative state: 25 cases. *Neurochirurgie.* 1993;39(5):281–292.

71. Sellal F, Hirsch E, Barth P, et al. A case of symptomatic hemidystonia improved by ventroposterolateral thalamic electrostimulation. *Mov Disord.* 1993;8(4):515–518.

72. Capelle HH, Grips E, Weigel R, et al. Posttraumatic peripherally-induced dystonia and multifocal deep brain stimulation: case report. *Neurosurgery.* 2006;59(3):E702.

73. Kim JP, Chang WS, Chang JW. The long-term surgical outcomes of secondary hemidystonia associated with post-traumatic brain injury. *Acta Neurochir.* 2012;154(5):823–830.

74. Foote KD, Seignourel P, Fernandez HH, et al. Dual electrode thalamic deep brain stimulation for the treatment of posttraumatic and multiple sclerosis tremor. *Oper Neurosurg.* 2006;58(suppl 4):ONS-280.

75. Reese R, Herzog J, Falk D, et al. Successful deep brain stimulation in a case of posttraumatic tremor and hemiparkinsonism. *Mov Disord.* 2011;26(10):1954–1955.

76. Issar NM, Hedera P, Phibbs FT, et al. Treating posttraumatic tremor with deep brain stimulation: report of five cases. *Parkinsonism Relat Disord.* 2013;19(12):1100–1105.

77. Carvalho KS, Sukul VV, Bookland MJ, et al. Deep brain stimulation of the globus pallidus suppresses posttraumatic dystonic tremor. *J Clin Neurosci.* 2014;21(1):153–155.

78. Follett MA, Torres-Russotto D, Follett KA. Bilateral deep brain stimulation of the ventral intermediate nucleus of the thalamus for posttraumatic midbrain tremor. *Neuromodulation.* 2014;17(3):289–291.

79. Loher TJ, Hasdemir MG, Burgunder JM, Krauss JK. Long-term follow-up study of chronic globus pallidus internus stimulation for posttraumatic hemidystonia: case report. *J Neurosurg.* 2000;92(3):457–460.

80. Son BC, Lee SW, Choi ES, et al. Motor cortex stimulation for central pain following a traumatic brain injury. *Pain.* 2006;123(1):210–216.

81. Kuhn J, Lenartz D, Mai JK, et al. Disappearance of self-aggressive behavior in a brain-injured patient after deep brain stimulation of the hypothalamus: technical case report. *Neurosurgery.* 2008;62(5):E1182.

82. Rezai AR, Sederberg PB, Bogner J, et al. Improved function after deep brain stimulation for chronic, severe traumatic brain injury. *Neurosurgery.* 2016;79(2):204–211.

83. Monti MM, Schnackers C, Korb A, et al. Non-invasive ultrasonic thalamic stimulation in disorders of consciousness after severe brain injury: a first-in-man report. *Brain Stimul.* 2016;9:940–941.

84. Larkin M, Meyer RM, Szuflita NS, et al. Post-traumatic, drug-resistant epilepsy and review of seizure control outcomes from blinded, randomized controlled trials of brain stimulation treatments for drug-resistant epilepsy. *Cureus.* 2016;8(8):744.

85. Neren D, Johnson MD, Legon W, et al. Vagus nerve stimulation and other neuromodulation methods for treatment of traumatic brain injury. *Neurocrit Care.* 2016;24(2):308–319.

86. Shi C, Flanagan SR, Samadani U. Vagus nerve stimulation to augment recovery from severe traumatic brain injury impeding consciousness: a prospective pilot clinical trial. *Neurol Res.* 2013;35(3):263–276.

87. Farwell L, Donchin E. Talking off the top of your head: toward a mental prosthesis utilizing event-related brain potentials. *Electroencephalogr Clin Neurophysiol.* 1988;70:510–523.

88. Herrmann CS. Human EEG responses to 1–100 Hz flicker: resonance phenomena in visual cortex and their potential correlation to cognitive phenomena. *Exp Brain Res.* 2001;137:346–353.

89. Pfurtscheller G, Neuper C. Motor imagery and direct brain-computer communication. *Proc IEEE.* 2001;89:1123–1134.

90. Pfurtscheller G, Allison BZ, Brunner C, et al. The hybrid BCI. *Front Neurosci.* 2010;4:42.

91. Holz EM, Höhne J, Staiger-Sälzer P, et al. Brain-computer interface controlled gaming: evaluation of usability by severely motor restricted end-users. *Artif Intell Med.* 2013;59(2):111–120.

92. Wang W, Collinger JL, Degenhart AD, et al. An electrocorticographic brain interface in an individual with tetraplegia. *PLoS One.* 2013;8(2):e55344.

93. Collinger JL, Wodlinger B, Downey JE, et al. High-performance neuroprosthetic control by an individual with tetraplegia. *Lancet.* 2013;381(9866):557–564.

94. Ajiboye AB, Willett FR, Young DR, et al. Restoration of reaching and grasping movements through brain-controlled muscle stimulation in a person with tetraplegia: a proof-of-concept demonstration. *Lancet.* 2017;389(10081):1821–1830.

95. Glannon W. Ethical issues in neuroprosthetics. *J Neural Eng.* 2016;13(2):021002.

96. Wilson BS, Dorman MF. Cochlear implants: a remarkable past and a brilliant future. *Hear Res.* 2008;242(1):3–21.

97. Schiller PH, Tehovnik EJ. Visual prosthesis. *Perception.* 2008;37(10):1529–1559.

98. Bouton CE, Shaikhouni A, Annetta NV, et al. Restoring cortical control of functional movement in a human with quadriplegia. *Nature.* 2016;533(7602):247–250.

99. Eapen BC, Murphy DP, Cifu DX. Neuroprosthetics in amputee and brain injury rehabilitation. *Exp Neurol.* 2017;287:479–485.

100. Miranda RA, Casebeer WD, Hein A, et al. DARPA-funded efforts in the development of novel brain-computer interface technologies. *J Neurosci Methods.* 2014;244:52–67.

101. Berger TW, Song D, Chan RHM, et al. A hippocampal cognitive prosthesis: multi-input, Multi-output nonlinear modeling and VLSI implementation. *IEE Trans Neural Syst Rehabil Eng.* 2012;20(2):198–211.

102. Guggenmos DJ, Azin M, Barbay S, et al. Restoration of function after brain damage using a neural prosthesis. *Proc Natl Acad Sci USA*. 2013;110(52):21177–21182.

103. Chatelle C, Chennu S, Noirhomme Q, et al. Brain–computer interfacing in disorders of consciousness. *Brain Inj*. 2012;26(12):1510–1522.

104. Coyle D, Stow J, McCreadie K, et al. Motor imagery BCI with auditory feedback as a mechanism for assessment and communication in disorders of consciousness. In: Guger C, Allison B, Ushiba J, eds. *Brain-Computer Interface Research a State-of-the-Art Summary 5*. New York (NY): Springer International Publishing; 2017:51–69.

105. Coyle D, Stow J, McCreadie K, et al. Sensorimotor modulation assessment and brain-computer interface training in disorders of consciousness. *Arch Phys Med Rehabil*. 2015;96(3):S62–S70.

106. Schreuder M, Riccio A, Risetti M, et al. User-centered design in brain–computer interfaces—a case study. *Artif Intell Med*. 2013;59(2):71–80.

107. Pan J, Xie Q, He Y, et al. Detecting awareness in patients with disorders of consciousness using a hybrid brain–computer interface. *J Neural Eng*. 2014;11(5):056007.

108. Li Y, Pan J, He Y, et al. Detecting number processing and mental calculation in patients with disorders of consciousness using a hybrid brain-computer interface system. *BMC Neurol*. 2015;15(1):259.

109. Wang F, He Y, Qu J, et al. Enhancing clinical communication assessments using an audiovisual BCI for patients with disorders of consciousness. *J Neural Eng*. 2017;14:046024.

110. March 29, 2017: 12th World Congress on Brain Injury – International Brain Injury Association, New Orleans, LA. In: Zasler N, Bockbrader M, Park MJ, Rosenthal J, eds. *Preconference Workshop Session PreA2, Emerging Neuromodulation Techniques for the Treatment of Post-traumatic Cephalalgias*.

111. Bockbrader MA. Physician-monitored home tDCS for post-brain injury fatigue, depression and headache: a case report. *Brain Stimul J*. 2017;10(4):e33–e34.

CHAPTER 18

Community Reintegration

TRACY KRETZMER, PHD • KATHRYN KIEFFER, MS, CCC-SLP • JAMES M. KAPLAN, MED, CTRS, ATP, CBIS • BARBARA J. DARKANGELO, PT, DPT, NCS • BRYAN GARRISON, RKT, CDRS • FAIZA HUMAYUN, MD • HEATHER G. BELANGER, PHD

Community reintegration (CR), defined here as the process of integrating back into society following a traumatic brain injury (TBI), is arguably the primary goal of acute brain injury rehabilitation. Implicit in this definition is the belief that CR is a desirable outcome, such that patients are able to pursue previously (or newly learned) meaningful activities, either as they used to perform them or via adaptive means. Sander et al.[1] contend that most clinicians would include these key elements in their conceptualization of CR: independent living, social and leisure activity, and work or other productive activity. As might be apparent, however, the most salient aspects of CR (and what it means) may vary from patient to patient, based on subjective and cultural factors. As such, an individualized approach to CR is frequently needed.

Successful CR requires rehabilitation specialists to assess and address each patient's priorities, which may in part be determined by their age, personal experiences, values, and culture. For example, in a sample of 167 patients, Sander et al.[2] found that at an average of 8 months post-TBI blacks and Hispanics placed more importance than whites on domestic activities (like cooking and housekeeping).

Measures of CR and participation are increasingly becoming the most common and important outcome measures in rehabilitation research. As medicine moves toward more personalized care, this trend will likely continue. Current measures of CR reflect the many aspects of CR. Three common measures of CR include the Community Integration Measure,[3] which assesses how comfortable people feel in their community, their perceptions of belonging, whether they feel useful, etc.; the Participation Objective, Participation Subjective questionnaire (POPS),[4] which assesses both objective and subjective aspects of community participation; and the Mayo-Portland Adaptability Inventory-4, which measures abilities, adjustment, and participation.[5] A measure of CR for use specifically with veteran and military populations is the Measure of Community Reintegration of Injured Service Members.[6] For more details on outcome measures, please see Chapter 16.

Despite rehabilitation efforts to enhance CR, evidence suggests that most patients who have sustained a moderate to severe TBI have continued CR challenges well after discharge. For example, despite intensive TBI rehabilitation, Ponsford et al.[7] found in their sample of 175 patients that over half were not working 2 years later, a third still needed assistance with community skills and transport, and most reported ongoing cognitive, behavioral, and emotional challenges. At 5 years postinjury, these researchers found that although there were improvements (from 2 to 5 years postinjury) in terms of increased independence in activities of daily living and use of transport, the reported cognitive, behavioral, and emotional difficulties became even more common.[8] At 5 years, 32% were not employed. At 10 years postinjury,[8] problems that were evident at 2 years postinjury persisted.

The goal of this chapter is to highlight the challenges related to CR in patients with a history of moderate to severe TBI. Although details surrounding these numerous challenges are many, the focus will be on providing rehabilitation specialists with important considerations in working with this population to maximize CR.

GENERAL HEALTH AND WELL-BEING

In recent years, the view of TBI as a singular, time-limited, "event" such that once the individual was medically stable and rehabilitative goals had plateaued they returned to a general care milieu has been challenged. Today, the view of TBI as a chronic or "lifelong" condition that requires continued specialty care, or at least closer coordination with primary care providers, is recommended.[9] This is particularly salient given that a large proportion of individuals with TBI experience their injuries as young adults.[10] This, in conjunction with increased survival rates,[11] indicates that a percentage of individuals with TBI have decades of life ahead of them, thereby pointing to the increased importance of CR-focused rehabilitation and treatment. As we have come to better understand both the long-term symptoms and the changing nature of post-TBI sequelae over the life course, the role of providers and treatments focused on improving CR have become paramount. Previous chapters have focused on the role of medical, behavioral and cognitive care over the TBI course, whereas the following section will discuss some of the most common "well-being" issues that can negatively affect the CR for individuals who had a moderate to severe TBI.

Mental Health

Change in mood, including depression and anxiety, is a common presentation for many individuals following moderate to severe TBI. Although the factors underlying its occurrence remain unclear, it is likely that physiologic changes,[12,13] reaction to changes in functioning,[14,15] and premorbid factors play multifactorial roles.[16–18] Regardless of the cause, the literature is clear—individuals experiencing moderate to severe TBI are at an increased risk of developing disorders, such as depression, anxiety, posttraumatic stress disorder (PTSD), obsessive compulsive disorder (OCD), substance abuse, and/or psychosis. As with other rehabilitation and medical populations, the presence of psychologic comorbidities often serves as a limiting factor to better functional outcomes and can play a particularly negative role in socialization, relationships, employment, and independence.

Mood and anxiety disorders

The most common mood disorder experienced by individuals who sustained a moderate to severe TBI is depression.[19] Numerous studies have demonstrated that throughout the post-TBI course, 30%–50% of individuals with moderate to severe TBI will at some point meet the criteria for depression.[19] Although prevalence rates vary across studies likely due to the methodological differences in how and when depression is assessed, depression rates in TBI are considerably higher than the general population rate (7%).[20]

Premorbid factors, including younger age at injury, premorbid psychiatric history, lower levels of education, premorbid history of substance abuse, and poor vocational and social functioning before injury, are associated with increased risk of developing depression postinjury.[17–19] Depression within the first year following injury also increases the risk of continued depression at 2 years postinjury.[21] Notably, this is often a period during which many individuals are engaging in CR activities and therapies.

Symptoms of depression post-TBI may be difficult to parse out as many symptoms overlap with TBI symptoms, such as poor sleep, fatigue, irritability, and poor concentration. However, Cook and colleagues[22] demonstrated that symptoms of depression reported by individuals with TBI are generally consistent with depressive symptoms reported in the general population. By examining the validity of response patterns across primary care and TBI populations, they found that the Patient Health Questionnaire 9 was a valid tool for measuring depressive symptoms post-TBI. Although this tool is commonly used in TBI populations, further psychologic evaluation is needed, as depressive symptoms may present differently, such as increased irritability or acting out. Furthermore, in cases in which aphasia, poor awareness (anosognosia), or pseudobulbar affect are present, determining the presence of true psychologic distress can be difficult. Therefore the inclusion of mental health providers with TBI expertise is often required to help accurately assess and diagnose post-TBI depression or other psychologic disorders.

As with the general population, individuals experiencing post-TBI depression are at increased risk of suicide. Individuals with TBI are at three to four times greater risk for committing suicide than individuals in the general population.[23] They also demonstrate higher rates of suicide attempt and suicidal ideation.[24] Therefore all individuals with a history of TBI should be screened for suicidal ideation. Individuals with a history of TBI and comorbid psychiatric disorders, substance abuse, premorbid history of suicide, attempt or TBI-related neurobehavioral disturbances (i.e., aggression, impulsivity) are at further increased risk of suicide.[25] According to Simpson and Tate,[26,27] warning signs and preceding events that increased suicide attempt in a study of 43 persons with TBI included feelings of depression and hopelessness, relationship conflicts and breakdowns, daily functioning, social isolation, and intolerable levels of stress, and hopelessness about symptom resolution. Forty-eight percent of these individuals also had at least one other suicide attempt in the recent past. Based on these findings, they recommend that all persons with TBI who have attempted suicide be closely monitored for 1 year following their first attempt.

Generalized anxiety disorder and PTSD are the most common anxiety-related disorders diagnosed post-TBI.[28] Prevalence rates vary across studies because of methodological and population differences but consistently remain higher than the general population.[20] Potential mechanisms underlying the development of post-TBI anxiety are unclear but likely include a combination of premorbid, physiologic, and psychologic factors. To date, the literature has demonstrated that individuals experiencing moderate to severe TBI are at increased risk of developing post-TBI anxiety when they have a history of premorbid anxiety, are females, are older and, are unemployed at the time of injury.[29-31] Post-TBI depression also increases the risk of developing an anxiety disorder because anxiety is more commonly diagnosed in depressed individuals with a history of TBI, followed by those with a history TBI without depression.[17]

Both post-TBI depression and anxiety have been associated with poorer CR outcomes. For example, individuals with post-TBI depression experience more vocational difficulties, including adjusting to work, completing work responsibilities, and/or returning to work.[32-34] Post-TBI depression and anxiety are also related to poorer relationships with family and less socialization,[35] increased substance abuse,[36] decreased quality of life, and poorer life satisfaction.[17,37] Hart and colleagues[38] demonstrated a relationship between depression severity and outcome, with worse symptoms associated with the poorest outcomes in community participation, disability, functional outcomes, and satisfaction with life.

Treatment

With accurate diagnosis, treatment is often needed. Psychopharmacologic and psychologic interventions are available, and often both are utilized to provide the most efficacious treatment available. To date, there is limited consistent empirical evidence to provide specific recommendations about the most efficacious interventions for individuals with TBI experiencing depression and/or anxiety. For some, psychotherapy utilizing cognitive behavioral therapy (CBT) paradigms to address specific psychologic disorders has been demonstrated in the literature to be helpful.[39,40] Although the specific steps of various CBT protocols too extensive to review in detail in this chapter, most protocols include modifications to traditional framework, such as (1) utilizing adaptations of treatment material to address specific cognitive deficits present (e.g., use of less abstract thoughts, limiting information on work sheets, providing homework assignments in writing) and (2) modifying treatment sessions (e.g., shorter sessions, smaller groups, taking breaks). Additional therapies modified for a TBI population have begun to be examined in the literature, including substance abuse,[41-43] suicidal prevention,[44,45] and PTSD.[46,47] Methodological differences and the need to modify psychotherapy interventions on an individualized basis make generalizations or the use of standardized protocols difficult.

Substance Abuse

For a percentage of individuals, following moderate to severe TBI, there is an increased risk of substance abuse. Most research has examined the impact of alcohol abuse in TBI, and although more studies are beginning to examine the impact of other substances, much of what we understand about substance abuse following TBI is based on alcohol abuse. In a study surveying 1606 adults 1 year post-TBI, approximately 30% reported moderate to heavy levels of drinking in the previous month.[36] Those reporting high levels of alcohol consumption were more likely to have a premorbid history of substance abuse, be a single male, have a diagnosis of depression, be younger, and have better physical functioning. With estimated rates of individuals in inpatient TBI rehabilitation centers having a premorbid history of substance abuse ranging from 30% to 58%, the risk of continued substance abuse following TBI is concerning.[48] Although premorbid abuse is a significant risk factor for postinjury abuse, individuals with no premorbid history of substance abuse also remain at increased risk for abusing substances postinjury.[49]

Research has demonstrated that patterns of abuse following TBI can vary over time. Initially, there may be a period of abstinence and sobriety, but over time the percentage of those who engage in substance abuse appears to increase.[50] This increase in proportion of abuse is particularly noted 1–3 years postinjury. Although the literature is limited in explaining the timing of this pattern, hypothesized potential contributing factors include difficulties with CR, such as poor psychosocial adjustment, poor coping abilities, poor adjustment to disabilities/loss of independence, loss of leisure and social engagement, or unemployment and feelings of nonproductivity. The potential impact of cognitive and behavioral TBI-related sequelae potentially affecting substance abuse following TBI is less well understood.

One of the most consistent CR outcomes associated with TBI and substance abuse is that it is often associated with postinjury unemployment.[51,52] Unemployment following TBI, in and of itself, leads to its own myriad of negative outcomes on finances, family distress, mood, and social engagement. Additional negative outcomes associated with TBI and comorbid substance abuse include increased engagement in aggressive behaviors,[53] increased risk for seizure,[54] comorbid depression,[55] poorer cognitive abilities,[56] lower perceived sense of well-being,[57] and increased risk of suicide.[58] In addition, several studies have demonstrated the negative impact of substance abuse on brain functioning and structure in an already neurologically compromised brain.[59,60]

The severity of such implications on health, mortality, and successful CR necessitate that TBI providers attempt to identify which individuals with a history of TBI are at the highest risk of developing a substance abuse problem, engage in best prevention practices, and intervene when substance abuse is present. Unfortunately, the empirical literature is limited on how best to treat individuals with TBI and substance abuse,[61] and at present there are no standardized protocols available. Programs specific to TBI and substance abuse are rare; however, The TBI Network[41] is a unique treatment paradigm that integrates substance abuse treatment and vocational rehabilitation following brain injury.[41,62] The program model is guided by coordinated and integrated care with multiple community providers. Several studies have revealed positive effects of this model, yet many CR programs have yet to incorporate it. Therefore many rehabilitation and substance abuse therapists treat this population with traditional individual or group therapy substance abuse paradigms, such as behavioral distraction/activation, motivational interviewing, Alcoholics Anonymous, and/or behavioral management with token reinforcements. Protocols may be modified to address cognitive, physical, and/or behavioral limitations, but they are often provided without the benefit of a coordinated community TBI care program. Outcomes following such protocols in a TBI population are not well understood.

For other providers working with this population, best practice guidelines at this time include patient and family education independent of prior substance use, routine substance screening, and referral to treatment resources for those at most risk. According to Corrigan,[61] education should include a frank discussion about the risk factors for abuse (premorbid use, younger age, single male), potential consequences of abuse (seizure, slowed neurorecovery, exacerbation of TBI sequelae, interaction with medications, and varying impact on an already compromised brain), and the fact that for individuals with TBI, there is no true "safe" amount to drink. With regard to community referral for more intensive substance abuse interventions, providers are strongly recommended to utilize a coordinated community care milieu and provide education to community providers about the patient's unique TBI-related needs to ensure the most effective treatment and outcome.

Exercise and Nutrition

At the most fundamental level, proper diet and adequate physical activity are necessary for lifelong health. In a brain injured population, weight management and routine exercise can be challenging for a variety of reasons, including apathy, impulsivity, physical limitations, and/or cognitive impairments. Weight gain during the chronic phase of TBI is a common outcome[63] that has additional health implications given that obesity and limited exercise increase the risk of developing diabetes, hypertension, and hypocholesterolemia. Such vascular risk factors increase the risk for stroke and myocardial infarction, which may result in further neuroinsult. A longitudinal study of 107 patients by Crenn et al.[64] found that hyperphagia and behavioral dysexecutive function were predictive factors for weight gain in patients with TBI, with 42% gaining an average of 19.8 lbs during the chronic phase of TBI. Additional factors associated with weight gain following moderate to severe TBI include memory deficits, larger calorie intake per meal, poor response to social eating cues, and poor satiety awareness.[63]

Physical, cognitive, and behavioral limitations can negatively affect one's ability to plan and organize daily meals, complete cooking tasks, manage/navigate grocery stores, and/or engage in routine exercise. Occupational, physical, and cognitive rehabilitation therapists can provide treatment, assistive technology, and/or compensatory strategies to improve functional independence on return to the community. For example, memory boards, meal/exercise alarms, limiting availability of high-calorie foods, and/or utilization of premade meals can increase healthy eating and routine exercise. Referral to a nutritionist may also be helpful, especially in cases in which weight loss is needed. In cases of very severe injury, however, caregivers may need to provide assistance in the form of establishing a daily eating and exercise routine, and healthy meal planning on the patient's behalf.[65]

In addition to the aforementioned benefits of healthy eating and exercise on overall health and weight, TBI research has also demonstrated that consistent and routine exercise can lower depressive symptoms, improve the quality of life,[66] improve learning ability, and improve reaction times,[67] as well as improve balance, self-esteem, and social participation.[68] Given the data supporting the cognitive, emotional, and physical benefits of regular exercise in the TBI population, scheduled physical activity is an essential tool in promoting successful reentry into the community. Because individuals with TBI may struggle to convey or even recognize healthcare needs as a result of their cognitive and/or behavioral sequelae, TBI providers should address weight, nutrition, wellness, and exercise needs directly and consistently given the increased risk of additional health comorbidities post-TBI. Education, encouragement, and helping the patients and their caregiver develop specific wellness plans and healthier lifestyle habits should be a routine focus of care.[69]

Leisure Activities

Leisure activities provide an important outlet to stimulate interpersonal interactions, enhance socialization, improve peer relationship development, and increase life satisfaction.[70] Leisure activities that enhance CR include reengagement with family, friends, and activities that promote self-esteem, self-efficacy, health, and well-being. Studies have shown that people with TBI are less active in social and recreational activities than people with no disability.[71] A study examining 130 moderate to severe TBI participants 1 year postinjury demonstrated that the majority of individuals reported a significant reduction in leisure engagements and that they were moderately to severely bothered by this change.[72] Many of these individuals tended to engage in more "at-home" and sedentary leisure activities such as watching television or using the computer, thereby increasing their isolation. Reduction in leisure engagement has been consistently linked to decreased satisfaction with life. In a population already at risk for depression, isolation, and weight gain, the impact of reduced leisure engagement and a more sedentary lifestyle may be a more important focus of CR treatment than many providers realize.

There is no single defining characteristic that causes decreased leisure participation but rather a broad spectrum of TBI sequelae. Studies have shown that factors such as cognitive deficits, depression, emotional/behavioral outbursts, fatigue, inability to manage environmental factors (heat, light sensitivity, noise, etc.), and lack of initiation/motivation can negatively affect an individual's ability to participate in recreational and social activities.[73] In addition, there are also secondary factors that may limit leisure activity engagement, such as limited finances, lack of transportation, and few TBI-focused community programs that provide consistent structured and goal-oriented leisure activity interventions.

Wise and colleagues[72] provide helpful recommendations for rehabilitation providers, including the need to rethink the way leisure activities are utilized in a chronic TBI population. For those who are not in the workforce, goal-oriented leisure activities may build a bridge to vocational engagement, as individuals are able to work on skills to improve social interactions, self-esteem, and communication abilities. They further suggest that leisure activity goals postinjury may not be as simple as modifying and adapting preinjury leisure interests, particularly when there have been significant physical and cognitive changes. Rather, assisting the individual to choose alternative leisure activities that may result in the same types of satisfaction that they

received from previous (i.e., body motion, being outside, compete, socializing) leisure activities may be more successful.

MOBILITY

Deficits in mobility are a major barrier to CR for many individuals with TBI. Deficits in gait following TBI may include slower walking speed, increased double support times, and biomechanical errors (most commonly excessive knee flexion at initial foot contact) that increase risk for falls.[74] Despite mobility being an area showing the greatest functional improvement during acute inpatient rehabilitation,[75] up to 83% of patients continue to have deficits after returning home.[76] Interestingly, although spasticity is associated with mobility impairments, the severity and distribution of lower limb spasticity does not ultimately affect mobility outcome.[77,78] Importantly, individuals can make significant functional gains (which are maintained at 3 months) in gait, mobility, and balance with intensive, multifaceted therapy.[79]

In terms of maximizing CR, planning for discharge is a continual process. A person's independence in the community is affected by his or her abilities and barriers, which are addressed through rehabilitation or environmental modifications. While the participants are in inpatient rehabilitation setting, the therapeutic recreation, physical, and occupational therapists will assess their ability to function inside and outside of the hospital environment. One component of this evaluation is mobility in the community including locomotion (walking or wheelchair), transfers in and out of private or public vehicles, getting around a store or restaurant (managing purchases), accessing their home environment, and physically managing household maintenance tasks. When assessing mobility in the community, many factors need to be assessed including safety awareness, physical ability, equipment needs, problem solving, and memory. During a community evaluation, the patient is allowed to make safe mistakes to assess his or her abilities. Throughout the rehabilitation process, patients need to be challenged across a variety of environments to ensure that their new skills are transferred into the home and community.[80]

The need for speed and distance requirements in the community should be considered when prescribing assistive devices. The specific requirements for community mobility are well documented in the research literature.[81] Successful community locomotor speeds range from 0.9 to 1.2 m/s to safely cross streets and function in society.[81,82] In addition to speed of mobility, there are distance requirements to access the community. The distance from disabled parking areas and the size of stores make it necessary to propel a wheelchair or ambulate closer to 600 m compared to previous benchmarks of 62 m referenced on the Functional Independence Measure (FIM).[81] Hoenig and colleagues[83] compared the speed of mobility with varied devices in community and household settings. They found that, in general, participants performed more quickly with a wheeled walker than with a manual or power wheelchair in community and household settings. Gait speed is a critical outcome measure to use when assessing readiness to return to the community. A few scales used to assess readiness for community mobility include Community Balance and Mobility Scale, FIM, High-Level Mobility Assessment Tool, Dynamic Gait Index, Tinetti Balance Assessment, Berg Balance, and Mini-Balance Evaluation Test (Mini-Bestest). More information on outcome measures can be found in Chapter 16.

As patients are transitioned from inpatient facilities to communities, these increased physical requirements for success need to be addressed and trained. It is very important that mobility training be performed in more challenging real-world settings as soon as safety can be ensured. Practice should include ramps, curbs, curb cuts, deep grass, sand, uneven pavement, gravel, and loose stones. If these opportunities are not available in the practice setting, patients can be challenged in a different manner by using floor mats with objects under them to simulate uneven outdoor surfaces, with steps of different heights, with increasing required locomotor distances, and with dual tasking to prepare them for community mobility. Many clinics are now equipped with overhead harness systems that allow patients to be challenged in a safe setting.

Another important consideration as patients get ready to transition to the community is the physical environment. Fleming and colleagues[84] found, after controlling for injury and disability factors, that community-dwelling individuals with brain injury at 6 months postdischarge were most affected and limited in CR by physical barriers such as the design and layout of buildings, the natural environment, and other aspects such as crowds or noise. These findings stress the importance of adequate follow-up in the community either pre- or postdischarge to identify and modify environmental factors that may potentially limit engagement in home or community. Therapists need to know what specific physical and environmental obstacles the patient will be facing upon return to daily life. Home and community mobility assessments allow therapists to assist in problem-solving approaches to

teach safe strategies to overcome identified barriers, decrease fall risks, and enhance independence with daily activities. There are many forms for the completion of home assessments that can be found online. If families want to assess their home, a Home Safety Self-Assessment Tool v.4 is available for download at www.agingresearch.buffalo.edu.[85]

Once the environmental barriers are identified, they will need to be removed, modified structurally, or addressed with equipment provisions. Alternatively, the patient may learn new techniques to limit the impact of obstacles on functional independence. An example would be a partially ambulatory client who has two steps to enter the home with no railing and is either trained to negotiate the stairs with a cane or has a railing installed. Bathrooms are also a significant barrier in many homes. For example, many bathrooms are not wheelchair accessible, so potential interventions include making the door wider (changing door type, changing hinges, or widening the frame), making the wheelchair smaller (by removing push rims from the wheels to gain 2 inches of clearance), or training the patient to use a commode chair in the bedroom. These decisions are dictated by financial resources available to the patient and family and other factors.

RETURN TO WORK/SCHOOL
Employment
One of the major rehabilitative goals following TBI is return to work (RTW). With higher survival rates and younger survivors, the need to RTW is paramount not only for financial reasons but also for psychosocial health. TBI-related changes, including physical, sensory, cognitive, and/or behavioral deficits, may prevent a successful return to previous employment levels. RTW following injury may require minimal cognitive and/or environmental modifications to ensure vocational success. For others, however, considerable changes may be needed, including working in a new position that requires less cognitive or physical demands, working in a sheltered program, or working without compensation. RTW is often considered a separate and specialized therapy focus in CR treatment programs because of the complexity and individualized interventions needed to assist individuals with the RTW goals.

Dikmen and colleagues[86] reported in their study of 366 adults with TBI admitted to a level 1 trauma center that 38% with severe TBI and 66% with moderate TBI RTW within 2 years of injury. However, rates of RTW following moderate to severe TBI vary widely across the literature depending on how and when the RTW was measured, how the severity of TBI was determined, and inconsistent ways of defining employment status. Factors that influence RTW include TBI severity, age at injury, marital status, preinjury employment status, education level, diagnosis of depression, current substance abuse, level of social support, violent behavior, financial disincentives, physical disability, and cognitive issues.[87]

Among the myriad of deleterious consequences following TBI, persistent cognitive deficits are likely one of the most significant factors that will predict RTW and CR outcomes more generally.[88] Research has consistently demonstrated the impact that cognitive deficits can have on the ability of an individual with TBI to achieve successful CR. Cognitive and behavioral barriers may include decreased communication-related skills such as spoken language processing, reading and writing abilities,[89] attentional and executive impairments,[90] anosognosia,[91] challenging or disinhibited behavior,[92] lack of compensatory cognitive strategies, and poor social and problem-solving skills.[93]

Muelenbroek and colleagues[89] found seven skills necessary for individuals with TBI to succeed in mid-level jobs, including spoken language processing, verbal memory, reading and writing, verbal reasoning, expressive pragmatics, multitasking, and social cognition. They further suggested that disordered communication behaviors after TBI, including the use of irrelevant comments and insensitivity to the conversational needs of others, reflect underlying impairments in executive functions, processing speed, attention, working memory, and social cognition, which make employment and social functions much more challenging for individuals with TBI. Kelley et al.[91] suggested that awareness of cognitive, behavioral, and/or physical deficits is one of the strongest predictors of ability to RTW, with individuals who are most aware of their deficits and abilities having the most successful outcomes in the workplace. Given the consistent findings in the literature, CR rehabilitation programs should provide extensive focus and treatment in these areas.

The role of vocational rehabilitation specialists is a vital one in CR programs given the importance that RTW or, actually return to productivity, has on mood, functioning, and quality of life factors. Vocational Rehabilitation interventions are labor intensive because they often require providers to go to a work site to provide education and make environmental modifications. They may also require job shadowing or work trials with problem-solving-specific issues at multiple steps of the process. Although structured CR programs with intensive RTW therapy are limited, the impact that vocational therapies

provide has been demonstrated. A review of RTW studies suggests that without specialized vocational rehabilitation, less than 30%–40% of individuals with moderate to severe TBI RTW, whereas RTW is much higher among those receiving vocational rehabilitation (60%–70%).[94,95] Vocational rehabilitation services include assistance to people with disabilities in attaining skills for education, job placement, and job retention. The Americans with -Disabilities Act (ADA) provides protection to qualified individuals with disabilities. According to the Equal Employment Opportunity Commission:

> to be protected under the ADA an individual must have, have a record of, or be regarded as having a substantial impairment. A substantial impairment is one that significantly limits or restricts a major life activity such as hearing, seeing, speaking, breathing, performing manual tasks, walking, caring for oneself, learning or working.[96]

Under the ADA, employers are responsible for providing reasonable accommodations to employees with special needs. A reasonable accommodation, as seen in Box 18.1, is a change to the working conditions, environment, job tasks, or responsibilities that allows persons with disabilities to perform the required duties of their job.

Academic

Relative to RTW, much less is known about return to school following TBI. Most studies are limited to surveys, pediatric populations, small sample sizes, or poor clarification of TBI severity. Given that the largest proportion of individuals who sustain a moderate to

---

BOX 18.1
Examples of Reasonable Return to Work Accommodations

1. Acquiring or modifying equipment or devices
2. Job restructuring
3. Part-time or modified work schedules
4. Reassignment to a vacant position
5. Adjusting or modifying training materials or policies
6. Modifying the office layout, desks, or computer stations

It is important to note that there are limitations to the responsibility of employers. If an accommodation would provide an undue hardship on the business or employer, they are not required to provide it. An undue hardship as defined under ADA would alter the nature of the business or be unduly costly, extensive, substantial, or disruptive to the business.

ADA, Americans with Disabilities Act.

severe TBI tend to be young adults,[10] it is surprising that not more is understood about return to school following TBI.

A survey of college students with a history of moderate to severe TBI indicated that although cognitive difficulties were the most significant academic challenge they faced, other factors such as such as depression, anger, fatigue, headaches, and relationship difficulties also adversely affected their academic performance.[97] In terms of cognitive difficulties, memory and organizational difficulties are particularly salient barriers in successful academic and vocational reintegration.[98] Unfortunately, a survey by Kennedy and colleagues[97] revealed that only 50% of the responders were aware of campus disability services.

Under the Individuals with Disabilities Education Act,[99] qualifying students are entitled to educational assistance such as Individualized Education Plans, which include educational goals, objectives, and interventions based on the student's needs, abilities, and expectations. Accommodations may include physical (modification of classroom setup and environment, modification of classroom equipment, etc.), cognitive (use of assistive technology devices, modified classroom assignments, modified testing procedures, etc.) and/or psychosocial (behavior plans, behavior modeling) modifications. Assistive technologies available to assist individuals with TBI-related cognitive or mobility sequelae returning to college are discussed in Chapter 17.

DRIVING

Driving and/or transportation is one of the most important aspects of independent living and therefore a crucial element of successful CR.[100,101] Driving is a complex task that requires the integration of cognitive, physical, cognitive, and behavioral repertoires. Individuals often continue to experience physical, sensory, and cognitive limitations following moderate to severe TBI that can negatively affect the reaction time, visual scanning, route planning, and mental flexibility.[102–105] In addition, behavioral sequelae that are common following TBI can also negatively affect driving, including disinhibition, aggression, impulsivity, and apathy.[106] Despite the presence of deficits that can negatively impact the ability to drive safely, prevalence studies suggest that between 38% and 78% of patients return to driving post-TBI, with many not receiving a formal driver evaluation (DE).[107]

Clinicians have often relied on neuropsychologic evaluation as a way to make determinations about a patient's ability to drive safely, and although such information can be informative in some cases, research has demonstrated varying degrees of validity in predicting who is safe to drive based on cognitive test results.[108,109] Therefore a formal DE is a critical step in determining if an individual is ready to safely return to driving after TBI.[110] Although there is a significant need for professionals who can address this area, often most healthcare providers do not know where to find them.[110] A certified driver rehabilitation specialist (CDRS) is a healthcare professional (usually occupational therapist, kinesiotherapist, physical therapist, or driver educator) who has completed additional training and education in the field of driver rehabilitation. To locate a driver rehabilitation specialist near you, simply go to the link provided (http://www.aded.net/).

Initial DE referrals typically require medical clearance (i.e., seizure free, visual abilities), a valid driver's license or learner's permit, and often a recent neuropsychologic evaluation report. It should be noted that specific driver requirements differ across states, particularly with regard to seizure-free period durations and visual abilities. During a formal DE, individuals will complete a battery of tests designed to assess driving knowledge, reaction time, visual abilities, and cognitive skills as they specifically relate to driving. Some tools used include Trails Making Tests A & B,[111] traffic sign identification exam, Saint Louis University Mental Status Exam,[112] state rules of the road exam, and the Snellgrove Maze Test.[113] When available, driving simulators can be helpful in assessing decision making, information processing, sensation, proprioception, strength, range of motion, and coordination in a closed and safe environment. However, there has not been enough research to evaluate the extent to which driving simulation predicts actual driving behavior and safety.[114] When deemed reasonably safe after screening measures, a full behind-the-wheel assessment is recommended in those with histories of moderate to severe TBI who wish to drive. Behind-the-wheel DE includes conditional assessment of (1) basic vehicle maneuvers (i.e., turns, use of signals, emergency stops, reverse driving, parking), often completed in a parking lot or low-traffic area; (2) residential driving where speeds are increased up to 25 mph and skills such as visual scanning and sign recognition are assessed; (3) commercial driving with multilane turns, unprotected turns, turns into the flow of traffic, merging, lane changes, and lane reduction situations; and (4) highway/interstate driving, including highway entry and exit, active lane selection, and speed maintenance. In all areas of driving, appropriate anticipatory skills, spatial awareness, proper integration with traffic, proper response to changes in traffic situations, and use of any identified compensatory skills must be demonstrated.

Following completion of the DE, the CDRS will make specific recommendations to the individual and their family, which may include cessation of driving, engagement in formal driving rehabilitation therapy, or education regarding alternative forms of transportation, including community and private services. On-road training lessons for drivers with TBI histories have demonstrated utility in improving back-to-driving outcomes in those with initial failed DEs,[115] requiring an average of seven driving lessons. For some, assistive devices may be recommended, which will allow the individual to return to safe driving and increase the likelihood of successful CR. Some specific assistive devices that may be recommended include mechanical hand controls designed for those no longer safe to operate a motor vehicle with their feet or assistive devices designed to operate the ignition, signal lights, horn, wipers, dimmers, air-conditioner, windows, and/or gear selection. More advanced devices that are particularly helpful for individuals with severe mobility limitations include digital accelerator rings and electronic mobility controls that require more training and typically have a higher cost of installation.

SUMMARY

Over the past several decades, there has been increased recognition that more structured and empirically supported interventions aimed specifically at CR are both needed and beneficial for individuals following TBI. Although arguably the primary goal of acute brain injury rehabilitation is assisting individuals to returning to the community with as much independence as possible, for many, acute rehabilitation stays are brief and therefore unable to cover the range of CR needs. Over time, patient's abilities change with continued recovery, and updated evaluations and interventions are needed. Primary issues such as cognitive, physical, and behavioral sequelae are typically addressed throughout the lifetime following TBI. However, the literature discussed earlier demonstrates the importance of TBI providers to also address mood, substance abuse, diet/exercise, engagement in leisure activities, productivity through vocational or academic means, and ability to drive given the long-term implications that they can have on an individual's functioning, relationships, well-being, and quality of life. As summarized in Table 18.1, various recommendations for these areas may assist providers and caregivers in identifying the needs based on the patient's current physical and cognitive functional abilities.

Successful CR requires a range of rehabilitation professionals to address the multiple facets of long-term TBI needs. Physiatrists, neuropsychologists, as well as occupational, physical, and speech therapists are commonly employed to assist individuals with TBI, but additional expertise in psychology, vocational rehabilitation, driving, and recreational interventions are also essential. Holistic approaches that include a coordinated community care approach to address the multiple and changing needs of individuals with TBI and their families throughout the lifetime are most effective and should be the gold standard of care in chronic TBI. Such coordination often falls to the physician or (when possible) social worker working with the individual. Interdisciplinary (or multidisciplinary, transdisciplinary) teams help to maximize CR, by addressing both the specific individual's CR goals and ensuring that interventions provided consider the unique cognitive, physical, behavioral, and psychosocial abilities and disabilities present.

TABLE 18.1
Darkangelo Community Reintegration Checklist

	ADL and IADL	Mobility	Driver Training	Vocational Rehabilitation	Assistive Technology	Leisure Activities
PHYSICAL LEVEL						
Low level: FIM scores 1–3 for the majority of physical tasks (ADLs and mobility) indicating being dependent to moderate assistance needed	Family training for assisting the participant; family education on use of assistive devices to maximize patient independence and caregiver body mechanics	Family and patient training for transfers (manual and mechanical); equipment including wheelchairs, hospital beds, and home therapy equipment	Assessing family and participant for vehicle ingress/egress and mobility aid carrier; wheelchair accessible van when appropriate	Examining family and patient financial benefits	Explore technology that would assist patient in moving around safely and efficiently (i.e., power assist wheels or power wheelchair)	Explore options for caregiver-assisted leisure and recreation activities
Mid level: FIM scores 4–5 indicating need for assistance or supervision for the majority of physical tasks (ADLs and mobility)	Family and patient are trained in performance of skills; assistive devices may be prescribed to aid in independence	Family and patient training, equipment for assistance including wheelchairs, assistive devices for walking, transfer aids, bracing	Assessing family and participant for vehicle ingress/egress and mobility aid carrier DE with adaptive equipment to participate if cognitive and visual evaluations passed	Evaluation to determine school or work possibilities May need physical accommodations or modifications	Explore technology that would assist the patient in completing tasks due to physical deficits	Caregiver-supervised leisure activities such as biking, adaptive sports, yoga, gardening, fishing
High level: FIM scores 6–7 indicating independently able to perform ADLs and mobility items with or without extra time	Patient evaluated and trained in all tasks Assistive devices recommended if needed for safety or efficiency	Individual training in all environments with emphasis on client's independence and safe performance of activities with the goal of independent living	DE if participant passed cognitive and visual evaluations	Vocational evaluation to determine school and employment possibilities	Explore technology that would remind them of safety issues	Educate patient on leisure and recreational activities in the community

TABLE 18.1
Darkangelo Community Reintegration Checklist—cont'd

	ADL and IADL	Mobility	Driver Training	Vocational Rehabilitation	Assistive Technology	Leisure Activities
COGNITIVE LEVEL						
Low level: FIM scores 1–3 for the majority of cognitive components indicating being dependent to moderate assistance needed for problem solving, comprehension, expression, and memory	Family training is paramount for performance and assisting in organizing, cueing, and creating an environment conducive to maximizing the function of participant	Family and patient training to assist in safety in most situations	Education for family on transportation needs	Explore family and patient benefits for transition to home environment	Explore technology to assist with memory or communication	Educate caregiver in options for directly supervised and structured activities
Mid level: FIM scores 4–5 for the majority of cognitive components indicating being dependent to moderate assistance needed for problem solving, comprehension, expression, and memory	Family and patient training to use compensatory mechanisms to cue themselves to perform ADL and IADL activities	Family and individual training for use of compensatory tools to aid mobility such as checklists and reminders	Driver training to evaluate participant's fitness to operate a motor vehicle	Vocational assessment to determine if home, school, or work is a goal and begin to work with participant to coordinate assistance and accommodations as needed Explore sheltered work setting or job coaching	Explore technology to assist with memory, follow-through, sequencing	Explore supervised activities of interest, set alerts and reminders to attend
High level: FIM scores 6–7 for the majority of cognitive components indicating independence or extra time for problem solving, comprehension, expression, and memory	Patient trained to cue self or use assistive technology independently to perform all functions in the ADL and IADL categories	Patient challenged and should experience independence with some assistive technology	Driving evaluation completed to ensure fitness to operate a motor vehicle postinjury	Vocational assessment to assist in transitioning client back to community with full involvement in work, school, or home management	Explore technology that will maximize independence with reminders for memory	Encourage involvement in community activities

ADL, activities of daily living; *IADL*, instrumental activities of daily living; *DE*, driver evaluation; *FIM*, functional independence measure.

REFERENCES

1. Sander AM, Clark A, Pappadis MR. What is community integration anyway? defining meaning following traumatic brain injury. *J Head Trauma Rehabil.* 2010;25:121–127.
2. Sander AM, Pappadis MR, Clark AN, Struchen MA. Perceptions of community integration in an ethnically diverse sample. *J Head Trauma Rehabil.* 2011;26:158–169.
3. McColl MA, Davies D, Carlson P, Johnston J, Minnes G. The community integration measure: development and preliminary validation. *Arch Phys Med Rehabil.* 2001;82:429–434.
4. Brown M, Dijkers M, Gordon W, Ashman T, Charatz H, Cheng Z. Participation objective, participation subjective: a measure of participation combining outsider and insider perspectives. *J Head Trauma Rehabil.* 2004;19:459–481.
5. Malec J. *The Mayo Portland Adaptability Inventory.* The Center for Outcome Measurement in Brain Injury Web site. http://www.tbims.org/combi/mpai.
6. Resnik L, Plow M, Jette A. Development of CRIS: measure of community reintegration of injured service members. *J Rehabil Res Dev.* 2009;46:469–480.
7. Ponsford JL, Olver JH, Curran C. A profile of outcome: 2 years after traumatic brain injury. *Brain Inj.* 1995;9:1–10.
8. Ponsford JL, Downing MG, Olver J, et al. Longitudinal follow-up of patients with traumatic brain injury: outcome at two, five, and ten years post-injury. *J Neurotrauma.* 2014;31:64–77.
9. Masel BE, DeWitt DS. Traumatic brain injury: a disease process, not an event. *J Neurotrauma.* 2010;27(8):1529–1540.
10. *Traumatic Brain Injury and Concussion: How Big Is the Problem?* Centers for Disease Control and Prevention Website. https://www.cdc.gov/traumaticbraininjury/get_the_facts.html.
11. Harrison-Felix C, Whiteneck G, DeVivo M, Hammond FM, Jha A. Mortality following rehabilitation in the traumatic brain injury model systems of care. *Neurorehabilitation.* 2004;19:45–54.
12. Jorge RE, Starkstein SE. Pathophysiologic aspects of major depression following traumatic brain injury. *J Head Trauma Rehabil.* 2005;20(6):475–487.
13. Jorge RE, Acion L, Starkstein SE, Magnotta V. Hippocampal volume and mood disorders after traumatic brain injury. *Biol Psychiatr.* 2007;62(4):332–338.
14. Pagulayan KF, Hoffman JM, Temkin NR, Machamer JE, Dikmen SS. Functional limitations and depression after traumatic brain injury: examination of the temporal relationship. *Arch Phys Med Rehabil.* 2008;89(10):1887–1892.
15. Schonberger M, Ponsford J, Gould KR, Johnston L. The temporal relationship between depression, anxiety and functional status after traumatic brain injury: a cross-lagged analysis. *J Int Neuropsychol Soc.* 2011;17(5):781–787.
16. Jorge RE, Robinson RG, Arndt SV, Starkstein SE, Forrester AW, Geisler F. Depression following traumatic brain injury: a 1 year longitudinal study. *J Affect Disord.* 1993;27(4):233–243.
17. Bombardier CH, Fann JR, Temkin NR, Esselman PC, Barber J, Dikmen SS. Rate of major depressive disorder and clinical outcomes following traumatic brain injury. *JAMA.* 2010;303(19):1938–1945.
18. Dikmen SS, Bombardier CH, Machamer JE, Fann JR, Temkin NR. Natural history of depression in traumatic brain injury. *Arch Phys Med Rehabil.* 2004;85(9):1457–1464.
19. Clark AN. Emotional distress following traumatic brain injury. In: Sherer M, Sander AM, eds. *Handbook on the Neuropsychology of Traumatic Brain Injury.* New York, NY: Springer; 2014:257–269.
20. Kessler RC, Chiu WT, Demler O, Merokangas KR, Walters EE. Prevalence, severity, and comorbidity of 12-month DSM-IV disorders in the national comorbidity survey replication. *Arch Gen Psychiatr.* 2005;62(6):617–627.
21. Hart T, Hoffman JM, Pretz C, Kennedy R, Clark AN, Brenner LA. A longitudinal study of major and minor depression following traumatic brain injury. *Arch Phys Med Rehabil.* 2012;93(8):1343–1349.
22. Cook KF, Bombardier CH, Bamer AM, Choi SW, Kroenke K, Fann JR. Do somatic and cognitive symptoms of traumatic brain injury confound depression screening? *Arch Phys Med Rehabil.* 2011;92(5):818–823.
23. Simpson G, Tate R. Suicidality after traumatic brain injury: demographic, injury and clinical correlates. *Psychol Med.* 2002;32(4):687–697.
24. Tsaousides T, Cantor JB, Gordon WA. Suicidal ideation following traumatic brain injury: prevalence rates and correlates in adults living in the community. *J Head Trauma Rehabil.* 2011;26(4):265–275.
25. Brenner LA, Carlson NE, Harrison-Feliz C, Ashman T, Hammond FM, Hirschberg RE. Self-inflicted traumatic brain injury: characteristics and outcomes. *Brain Inj.* 2009;23(13–15):991–998.
26. Simpson G, Tate R. Clinical features of suicide attempts after traumatic brain injury. *J Nerv Ment Dis.* 2005;193(10):680–685.
27. Simpson G, Tate R. Preventing suicide after traumatic brain injury: implication for general practice. *Med J Aust.* 2007;187(4):229–232.
28. Gould KR, Ponsford JL, Johnston L, Schonberger M. The nature, frequency and course of psychiatric disorders in the first year after traumatic brain injury: a prospective study. *Psychol Med.* 2011;41:2099–2109.
29. Ashman TA, Spielman LA, Hibbard MR, Silver JM, Chandna T, Gordon WA. Psychiatric challenges in the first 6 years after traumatic brain injury: cross-sequential analyses of axis I disorders. *Arch Phys Med Rehabil.* 2004;85(4 suppl 2):S36–S42.
30. Whelan-Goodinson R, Ponsford J, Schonberger M. Association between psychiatric state and outcome following traumatic brain injury. *J Rehabil Med.* 2008;40(10):850–857.
31. Whelan-Goodinson R, Ponsford J, Schonberger M, Johnston L. Predictors of psychiatric disorders following traumatic brain injury. *J Head Trauma Rehabil.* 2010;25(5):320–329.

32. Seel RT, Kreutzer JS, Rosenthal J, Hammond FM, Corrigan JD, Black K. Depression after traumatic brain injury: a National Institute on Disability and Rehabilitation Research Model Systems multicenter investigation. *Arch Phys Med Rehabil.* 2003;84(2):177–184.

33. Franulic A, Carbonell CG, Pinto P, Sepulveda I. Psychosocial adjustment and employment outcomes 2, 5 and 10 years after TBI. *Brain Inj.* 2004;18(2):119–129.

34. McGarity S, Barnett SD, Lamberty G, et al. Community reintegration problems among veterans and active duty service members with traumatic brain injury. *J Head Trauma Rehabil.* 2017;32(1):34–45.

35. Groom KN, Shaw TG, O'Connor ME, Howard NI, Pickens A. Neurobehavioral symptoms and family functioning in traumatically brain-injured adults. *Arch Clin Neuropsychol.* 1998;13(8):695–711.

36. Horner MD, Ferguson PL, Selassie AW, Labbate LA, Kniele K, Corrigan JD. Patterns of alcohol use one year after traumatic brain injury: a population-based, epidemiological study. *J Int Neuropsychol Soc.* 2005;11:322–330.

37. Hibbard MR, Ashman TA, Spielman LA, Chun D, Charatz HJ, Melvin S. Relationship between depression and psychosocial functioning after traumatic brain injury. *Arch Phys Med Rehabil.* 2004;85(4 suppl 2):S43–S53.

38. Hart T, Brenner L, Clark AN, et al. Major and minor depression after traumatic brain injury. *Arch Phys Med Rehabil.* 2011;92(8):1211–1219.

39. Khan-Bourne N, Brown RG. Cognitive behavioral therapy for the treatment of depression in individuals with brain injury. *Neuropsychol Rehabil.* 2003;13(1–2): 89–107.

40. Hsieh MY, Ponsford J, Wong D, Schonberger M, McKay A, Haines K. A cognitive behaviour therapy (CBT) programme for anxiety following moderate-severe traumatic brain injury (TBI): two case studies. *Brain Inj.* 2012;26(2):126–138.

41. Corrigan JD, Lamb-Hart GL, Rust E. A program of intervention for substance abuse following traumatic brain injury. *Brain Inj.* 1995;9:221–236.

42. Corrigan JD, Bogner JA, Lamb-Hart GL. Substance abuse and brain injury. In: Rosenthal M, Griffith ER, Miller JD, Kreutzer J, eds. *Rehabilitation of the Adult and Child with Traumatic Brain Injury.* 3rd ed. Philadelphia, PA: FA Davis Co; 1999.

43. Heinemann AW, Corrigan JD, Moore D. Case management for traumatic brain injury survivors with alcohol problems. *Rehabil Psychol.* 2004;49(2):156–166.

44. Dennis JP, Ghahramanlou-Holloway M, Cox DW, Brown GK. A guide for the assessment and treatment of suicidal patients with traumatic brain injury. *J Head Trauma Rehabil.* 2011;26(4):244–256.

45. Simpson GK, Tate RL, Whiting DL, Cotter RE. Suicide prevention after traumatic brain injury: a randomized controlled trial of a program for the psychological treatment of hopelessness. *J Head Trauma Rehabil.* 2011;26(4):290–300.

46. Wolf GK, Strom TQ, Kehle SM, Eftekhari A. A preliminary examination of prolonged exposure therapy with Iraq and Afghanistan veterans with a diagnosis of posttraumatic stress disorder and mild to moderate traumatic brain injury. *J Head Trauma Rehabil.* 2012;27(1):26–32.

47. Wolf GK, Kretzmer T, Crawford E, et al. Prolonged exposure therapy with veterans and active duty personnel diagnosed with PTSD and traumatic brain injury. *J Trauma Stress.* 2015;28(4):339–347.

48. Corrigan JD, Bogner JA, Lamb-Hart GL, Sivak-Sears N. *Problematic Substance Use Identified in the TBI Model Systems National Dataset.* Center for Outcome Measurement in Brain Injury (COMBI); 2003. Available at: https://www.tbims.org/subst/index.html.

49. Corrigan JD, Rust E, Lamb-Hart GL. The nature and extent of substance abuse problems among persons with traumatic brain injuries. *J Head Trauma Rehabil.* 1995;10(3):29–45.

50. Bombardier CH, Temkin NR, Machamer J, Dikmen SS. The natural history of drinking and alcohol-related problems after traumatic brain injury. *Arch Phys Med Rehabil.* 2003;84:185–191.

51. Sherer M, Bergloff P, High W, Nick TG. Contribution of functional ratings to prediction of longterm employment outcome after traumatic brain injury. *Brain Inj.* 1999;13(12):973–987.

52. MacMillan PJ, Hart RP, Martelli MM, Zasler ND. Preinjury status and adaptation following traumatic brain injury. *Brain Inj.* 2002;16(1):41–49.

53. Bogner JA, Corrigan JD, Mysiw WJ, Clinchot D, Fugate L. Comparison of substance abuse and violence in the prediction of long-term rehabilitation outcomes after traumatic brain injury. *Arch Phys Med Rehabil.* 2001;82:571–577.

54. Verma NP, Policherla H, Buber B. Prior head injury accounts for the heterogeneity of the alcohol-epilepsy relationship. *Clin Electroencephalogr.* 1992;23(3):147–151.

55. Silver JM, Kramer R, Greenwald S, Weissman M. The association between head injuries and psychiatric disorders: findings from the New Haven Epidemiologic Catchment Area Study. *Brain Inj.* 2001;15(11):935–945.

56. Dikmen SS, Machamer JE, Donovan DM, Winn HR, Temkin NR. Alcohol use before and after traumatic head injury. *Ann Emerg Med.* 1995;26:167–176.

57. Corrigan JD, Bogner JA, Mysiw WJ, Clinchot D, Fugate L. Life satisfaction following traumatic brain injury. *J Head Trauma Rehabil.* 2001;16(6):543–555.

58. Teasdale TW, Engberg AW. Suicide after traumatic brain injury: a population study. *J Neurol Neurosurg Psychiatr.* 2001;71:436–440.

59. Bigler ED, Blatter DD, Johnson SC, et al. Traumatic brain injury, alcohol and quantitative neuroimaging: preliminary findings. *Brain Inj.* 1996;10(3):197–206.

60. Baguley IJ, Felmingham KL, Lahz S, Gordon E, Lazzoro I, Schotte DE. Alcohol abuse and traumatic brain injury: effect on event-related potentials. *Arch Phys Med Rehabil.* 1997;78(11):1246–1253.

61. Corrigan JD. The treatment of substance abuse in persons with TBI. In: Zasler ND, Katz DI, Zafonte R, eds. *Brain Injury Medicine Principles and Practice.* New York, NY: Demos Medical Publishing; 2007:1105–1115.

62. Bogner JA, Corrigan JD, Spafford DE, Lamb-Hart GL. Integrating substance abuse treatment and vocational rehabilitation after traumatic brain injury. *J Head Trauma Rehabil.* 1997;12(5):57–71.

63. Henson MB, De Castro JM, Stringer AY, Johnson C. Food intake by brain-injured 342 humans who are in the chronic phase of recovery. *Brain Inj.* 1993;7:169–178.

64. Crenn P, Hamchaoui S, Bourget-Massari A, Hanachi M, Melchior JC, Azouvi P. Changes in weight after traumatic brain injury in adult patients: a longitudinal study. *Clin Nutr.* 2014;33:348–353.

65. Keatley MA, Whittemore LL. *Feed Your Body, Feed Your Brain: Nutritional Tips to Speed Recovery*; 2010. BrainLine.org Website. http://www.brainline.org/content/2010/12/feed-your-body-feed-your-brain-nutritional-tips-to-speed-recovery.html.

66. Wise E, Hoffman J, Powell J, Bombardier CH, Bell KR. Benefits of exercise maintenance after traumatic brain injury. *Arch Phys Med Rehabil.* 2012;93:1319–1323.

67. Grealy M, Johnson D, Rushton S. Improving cognitive function after brain injury: the use of exercise and virtual reality. *Arch Phys Med Rehabil.* 1999;80:661–667.

68. Thornton M, Marshall S, McComas J, Finestone H, McCormick A, Sveistrup H. Benefits of activity and virtual reality based balance exercise programmes for adults with traumatic brain injury: perceptions of participants and their caregivers. *Brain Inj.* 2005;19:989–1000.

69. Malec JF. Comprehensive brain injury rehabilitation in post-hospital treatment settings. In: Sherer M, Sander AM, eds. *Handbook on the Neuropsychology of Traumatic Brain Injury.* New York, NY: Springer; 2014: 283–307.

70. Specht J, King G, Brown E, Foris C. The importance of leisure in the lives of persons with congenital physical disabilities. *Am J Occup Ther.* 2002;56:436–445.

71. Brown W, Gordon W, Speilman L. Participation in social and recreational activity in the community by individuals with traumatic brain injury. *Rehabil Psychol.* 2003;48(4): 266–274.

72. Wise EK, Mathews-Dalton C, Dikmen S, et al. Impact of traumatic brain injury on participation in leisure activities. *Arch Phys Med Rehabil.* 2010;91(9):1357–1362.

73. Burleigh SA, Farber RS, Gillard M. Community integration and life satisfaction after traumatic brain injury: long term findings. *Am J Occup Ther.* 1998;52: 45–52.

74. Williams G, Morris ME, Schache A, McCrory PR. Incidence of gait abnormalities after traumatic brain injury. *Arch Phys Med Rehabil.* 2009;90(4):587–593.

75. McLafferty FS, Barmparas G, Ortega A, et al. Predictors of improved functional outcome following inpatient rehabilitation for patients with traumatic brain injury. *Neurorehabilitation.* 2016;39(3):423–430.

76. Langlois JA, Rutland-Brown W, Wald MM. The epidemiology and impact of traumatic brain injury: a brief overview. *J Head Trauma Rehabil.* 2006;21(5): 375–378.

77. Williams G, Banky M, Olver J. Distribution of lower limb spasticity does not influence mobility outcome following traumatic brain injury: an observational study. *J Head Trauma Rehabil.* 2015;30(5):E49–E57.

78. Williams G, Banky M, Olver J. Severity and distribution of spasticity does not limit mobility or influence compensatory strategies following traumatic brain injury. *Brain Inj.* 2015;29(10):1232–1238.

79. Peters DM, Jain S, Liuzzo DM, et al. Individuals with chronic traumatic brain injury improve walking speed and mobility with intensive mobility training. *Arch Phys Med Rehabil.* 2014;95(8):1454–1460.

80. Darragh AR, Sample P, Fisher AG. Environment effect on functional task performance in adults with acquired brain injuries: use of the assessment of motor and process skills. *Arch Phys Med Rehabil.* 1998;79:418–423.

81. Andrews AW, Chinsworth SA, Boursassa M, et al. Update on distance and velocity requirements for community ambulation. *J Geriatr Phys Ther.* 2010;33(3):128–134.

82. Gates TJ, Noyce DA, Bill AR, Van Ee A. Recommended walking speeds for pedestrian clearance timing based on pedestrian characteristics. In: *Paper Presented at: 85th Annual Meeting of the Transportation Research Board; January 22-26, 2006; Washington DC.* 2006.

83. Hoenig H, Cone C, Morgan M, Landerman LR, Caves K. Effects of wheelchair type on mobility performance in community and home environments. In: *Paper Presented at: Annual Conference of the Rehabilitation Engineering and Assistive Technology Society of North America; June 28-July 3, 2012; Baltimore, MD.* 2012.

84. Fleming J, Nalder E, Alves-Stein S, Cornwell P. Environmental barriers on community integration for individuals with moderate to severe traumatic brain injury. *J Head Trauma Rehabil.* 2014;29(2):125–135.

85. Tomita MR, Saharan S, Rajendran S, Nochajski SM, Schweitzer JA. Psychometrics of the home safety self-assessment tool (HSSAT) to prevent falls in community-dwelling older adults. *Am J Occup Ther.* 2014;68(6):711–718.

86. Dikmen SS, Temkin NR, Machamer JE, Holubkov K, Fraser RT, Winn HR. Employment following traumatic head injuries. *Arch Neurol.* 1994;51:177–186.

87. West M, Targett P, Yasuda S, Wehman P. Return to work following TBI. In: Zasler ND, Katz DI, Zafonte DR, eds. *Brain Injury Medicine Principles and Practice.* New York, NY: Demos Medical Publishing; 2007:1131–1147.

88. Fleming J, Tooth L, Hassell M, Chan W. Prediction of community integration and vocational outcome 2-5 years after traumatic brain injury rehabilitation in Australia. *Brain Inj.* 1999;13(6):417–431.

89. Meulenbroek P, Bowers B, Turkstra L. Characterizing common workplace communication skills for disorders associated with traumatic brain injury: a qualitative study. *J Voc Rehabil.* 2016;44:15–31.

90. Libin AV, Scholten J, Maitland-Schladen M, et al. Executive functioning in TBI from rehabilitation to social reintegration: COMPASS goal, a randomized controlled trial. *Mil Med Res.* 2015;152:32.

91. Kelley E, Sullivan C, Loughlin J, et al. Self-awareness and neurobehavioral outcomes, 5 years or more after moderate to severe brain injury. *J Head Trauma Rehabil.* 2014;29(2):147–152.

92. Winkler D, Unsworth C, Sloan S. Factors that lead to successful community integration following severe traumatic brain injury. *J Head Trauma Rehabil.* 2006;21(1):8–21.

93. Hawkins BL, McGuire FA, Linder SM, et al. Understanding contextual influences of community reintegration among injured service members. *J Rehabil Res Dev.* 2015;52(5):527–542.

94. Malec JF. Vocational rehabilitation. In: High WM, Sander AM, Struchen MS, Hart KA, eds. *Rehabilitation for Traumatic Brain Injury.* New York, NY: Oxford University Press; 2005.

95. Malec JF, Moessner AM. Replicated positive results for the VCC model of vocational intervention after ABI within the social model of disability. *Brain Inj.* 2006;20(3): 227–236.

96. US Equal Employment Opportunity Commission. *Equal Employment Opportunity Act*; 2017. https://www.eeoc.gov/.

97. Kennedy MR, Krause MO, Turkstra LS. An electronic survey about college experiences after traumatic brain injury. *Neurorehabilitation.* 2008;23:511–520.

98. Stewart-Scott AM, Douglas JM. Education outcome for secondary and postsecondary students following traumatic brain injury. *Brain Inj.* 1998;12:317–331.

99. US Department of Education. *Individuals with Disabilities Education Act (IDEA)*; 1997. http://idea.ed.gov/.

100. Fox GK, Bashford GM, Caust SL. Identifying safe versus unsafe drivers following brain impairment: the Coorabel Programme. *Disabil Rehabil.* 1992;14:140–145.

101. Pietrapiana P, Tamietto M, Torrini G, et al. Role of premorbid factors in predicting safe return to driving after severe TBI. *Brain Inj.* 2005;19:197–211.

102. McDonald BC, Flashman LA, Saykin AJ. Executive dysfunction following traumatic brain injury: neural substrates and treatment strategies. *Neurorehabilitation.* 2002;17:333–344.

103. Mathias JL, Wheaton P. Changes in attention and information processing speed following severe traumatic brain injury: a meta-analytic review. *Neuropsychology.* 2007;21:212–223.

104. Fortin S, Godbout L, Braun CM. Cognitive structure of executive deficits in frontally lesioned head trauma patients performing activities of daily living. *Cortex.* 2003;39:273–291.

105. Eby DW, Molnar LJ. Driving fitness and cognitive impairment. *JAMA.* 2010;303(16):1642–1643.

106. Tateno A, Jorge RE, Robinson RG. Clinical correlates of aggressive behavior after traumatic brain injury. *J Neuropsychiatr Clin Neurosci.* 2003;15:155–160.

107. Fisk G, Schneider JJ, Novack TA. Driving following traumatic brain injury: prevalence, exposure, advice and evaluations. *Brain Inj.* 1998;12:683–695.

108. McKay A, Liew C, Schonberger M, Ross P, Ponsford J. Predictors of the on-road driving assessment after traumatic brain injury: comparing cognitive tests, injury factors, and demographics. *J Head Trauma Rehabil.* 2016;31(6):E44–E52.

109. Ortoleva C, Brugger C, Van der Linden M, Walder B. Prediction of driving capacity after traumatic brain injury: a systematic review. *J Head Trauma Rehabil.* 2012;27(4):302–313.

110. Hopewell CA. Driving assessment issues for practicing clinicians. *J Head Trauma Rehabil.* 2002;17:48–61.

111. Arbuthnott K, Frank J. Trail making test, part B as a measure of executive control: validation using a set-switching paradigm. *J Clin Exp Neuropsychol.* 2000;22:518–528.

112. Tariq SH, Tumosa N, Chibnall JT, Perry III MH, Morley JE. Comparison of the Saint Louis University mental status examination and the mini-mental state examination for detecting dementia and mild neurocognitive disorder-a pilot study. *Am J Geriatr Psychiatr.* 2006;14(11):900–910.

113. Snellgrove C. *Cognitive Screening for the Safe Driving Competence of Older People with Mild Cognitive Impairment or Early Dementia*; 2005. https://infrastructure.gov.au/roads/safety/publications/2005/pdf/cog_screen_old.pdf.

114. Imhoff S, Lavalliere M, Teasdale N, Fait P. Driving assessment and rehabilitation using a driving simulator in individuals with traumatic brain injury: a scoring review. *Neurorehabilitation.* 2016;39(2):239–251.

115. Ross PE, DiStefano M, Charlton J, Spitz G, Ponsford JL. Interventions for resuming driving after traumatic brain injury. *Disabil Rehabil.* 2017:1–11. https://doi.org/10.1080/09638288.2016.1274341.

Index

Note: Page numbers followed by "f" indicate figures, "t" indicate tables and "b" indicate boxes.

Printed in the United States
By Bookmasters